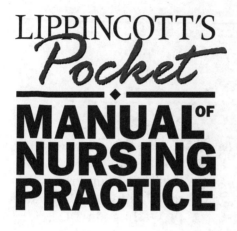

LIPPINCOTT'S
Pocket

MANUAL OF
NURSING
PRACTICE

Sandra M. Nettina, RN,C, MSN, ANP

Adjunct Assistant Professor
George Washington University
Washington, DC

and

George Mason University
Fairfax, Virginia
Primary Care Nurse Practitioner
Greenbelt, Maryland

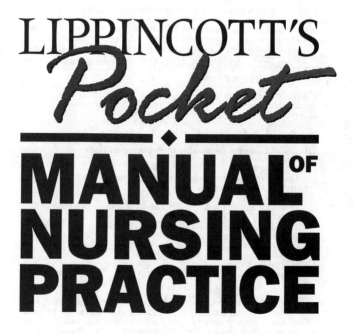

LIPPINCOTT'S
Pocket
MANUAL OF
NURSING
PRACTICE

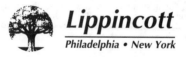

Lippincott
Philadelphia • New York

Acquisitions Editor: Lisa Stead
Editorial Assistant: Brian MacDonald
Project Editor: Barbara Ryalls
Production Manager: Helen Ewan
Production Coordinator: Kathryn Rule
Design Coordinator: Doug Smock
Indexer: Anne Cope

9   8   7   6   5   4   3   2   1

Library of Congress Cataloging in Publications Data

Nettina, Sandra M.
    Lippincott's pocket manual of nursing practice / Sandra M. Nettina.
        p.   cm.
    Companion v. to The Lippincott manual of nursing practice.
    ISBN 0-397-55355-2
    1. Nursing—Handbooks, manuals, etc.   I. Title.
    [DNLM: 1. Nursing Care—handbooks.   WY 49 N474L 1997]
RT51.N377   1997
610.73—dc20
DNLM/DLC
for Library of Congress   96-15107
                                                                          CIP

Care has been taken to confirm the accuracy of the information presented and to describe generally accepted practices. However, the authors, editors, and publishers are not responsible for errors or omissions or for any consequences from application of the information in this book and make no warranty, express or implied, with respect to the contents of the publication.

The authors, editors and publishers have exerted every effort to ensure that drug selection and dosage set forth in this text are in accordance with current recommendations and practice at the time of publication. However, in view of ongoing research, changes in government regulations, and the constant flow of information relating to drug therapy and drug reactions, the reader is urged to check the package insert for each drug for any change in indications and dosage and for added warnings and precautions. This is particularly important when the recommended agent is a new or infrequently employed drug.

Some drugs and medical devices presented in this publication have Food and Drug Administration (FDA) clearance for limited use in restricted research settings. It is the responsibility of the health care provider to ascertain the FDA status of each drug or device planned for use in their clinical practice.

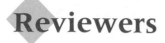Reviewers

Cynthia Bumgarner, RN, MSN
Clinical Consultant
Hill-Rom, a Hillenbrand Industry
Alexandria, Virginia

Lynne Hutnik Conrad, RN, C, MSN, BSN
Program Director, ObGyn
Elkins Park Hospital
Elkins Park, Pennsylvania

Betsy A. Finklemeier, RN, MS
Manager of Clinical Services
Division of Cardiothoracic Surgery
Northwestern University Medical School

Clinical Appointment
Department of Nursing
Northwestern Memorial Hospital
Chicago, Illinois

Gina Haas, RN, BSN
Department of Obstetrics and Childbirth Education
George Washington University Medical Center
Washington, DC

Ruth Lebet, MSN, RN, CCRN
Nurse Manager, Pediatric Emergency Department
The Johns Hopkins Childrens Center
Baltimore, Maryland

Mary Anne McKenna, BSN, MSN
Assistant Professor of Nursing
Delaware County Community College
Media, Pennsylvania

Edna Michel-Moyer, RN, MS, CS, CRNP
Associate Professor of Nursing
Catonsville Community College
Baltimore, Maryland

Barbara Resnick, MSN, CRNP
Geriatric Nurse Practitioner
School of Nursing and Department of Family Practice
University of Maryland
Baltimore, Maryland

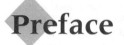

Preface

*L*ippincott's Pocket Manual of Nursing Practice has been prepared as a companion handbook to *The Lippincott Manual of Nursing Practice*, 6/E. It is designed for use by practicing and student nurses in the clinical area. *Lippincott's Pocket Manual of Nursing Practice* is compact enough to carry in one's pocket, concise enough to review quickly while providing patient care, and thorough enough to consult with confidence even as complex situations arise. Like its parent book, *The Lippincott Manual of Nursing Practice*, the *Pocket Manual* contains comprehensive assessment, treatment, and nursing intervention information on the most common medical–surgical, pediatric, psychiatric, and maternity conditions. The *Pocket Manual* is the only comprehensive handbook covering all major areas of nursing practice.

Medical–surgical, pediatric, and psychiatric conditions are presented in alphabetical order with extensive cross-referencing. Where warranted, adult medical–surgical and pediatric care topics are integrated, with clearly highlighted differences between adult and pediatric presentations, treatments, and nursing interventions for those conditions. Common surgical procedures are covered as distinct entries with their own format, focusing on potential complications, preoperative care, postoperative care, and patient education. Because maternity conditions do not fit into the alphabetical organization of diseases and disorders, they are grouped together following the alphabetical entries. The Maternity Nursing section focuses on prenatal physiology of the mother and fetus, labor and delivery, and postpartum physiology of the mother and neonate, as well as obstetric and nursing care for both. Complications of childbearing are listed alphabetically within the Maternity section and follow the same consistent format.

Nursing Alerts, Gerontologic Alerts, Pediatric Alerts, and **Community Care Considerations** appear within entries to quickly highlight important patient care information across the lifespan. Subheads in the condition entries include Assessment, Diagnostic Evaluation, Collaborative Management, and Nursing Interventions. Collaborative Management is categorized by Therapeutic Interventions, Pharmacologic Interventions, and Surgical Interventions. Nursing Interventions are categorized by Monitoring, Supportive Care, and Patient (or Family) Education and Health Maintenance. Through these subheads, *Lippincott's Pocket Manual of Nursing Practice* maintains a broad focus of information for nursing care in the acute care setting, the outpatient center, the home, or the long-term care facility.

Lippincott's Pocket Manual of Nursing Practice is designed to accompany the nurse wherever patient care is provided. Its parent book, *The Lippincott Manual of Nursing Practice*, 6/E remains the comprehensive reference at the nurses' station, on your desk, or in the trunk of your car if you are a home care nurse. Together, these companion books will increase your wealth of knowledge and your love of nursing.

Sandra M. Nettina, RN,C, MSN, ANP

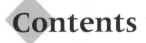

Contents

H

I

K

L

M

N

O

P

R

S

T

U

V

W

Part Two
MATERNITY NURSING **887**

◆ The Usual Childbearing Experience **889**

◆ Complications of the Childbearing Experience **950**

Index **980**

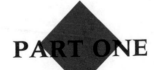

PART ONE

Diseases and Disorders

Abdominal Surgery
See Gastrointestinal or Abdominal Surgery

Acquired Immunodeficiency Syndrome
See HIV Disease and AIDS

ADD
See Attention Deficit Disorder and Learning Disabilities

Addison's Disease
See Adrenocortical Insufficiency

Adrenocortical Insufficiency

Adrenocortical insufficiency occurs when the adrenal cortex secretes inadequate amounts of adrenocortical hormones, primarily glucocorticoids and mineralocorticoids. The disorder occurs in two forms in adults and children. Primary adrenocortical insufficiency (Addison's disease) results from destruction and subsequent hypofunction of the adrenal cortex, usually caused by an autoimmune process. Presentation may be insidious or acute. Secondary adrenocortical insufficiency occurs because of adrenocorticotropic hormone (ACTH) deficiency from pituitary disease, or from suppression of the hypothalamic–pituitary axis by corticosteroids administered to treat nonendocrine disorders, which causes the adrenal cortex to atrophy.

Inadequate aldosterone produces disturbances of sodium, potassium, and water metabolism. Cortisol deficiency produces abnormal fat, protein, and carbohydrate

A

metabolism. Absence of cortisol during a period of stress can precipitate Addisonian (adrenal) crisis, an exaggerated state of adrenal cortical insufficiency, which is fatal if not quickly treated.

◆ Assessment

1. Hyponatremia and hyperkalemia
2. Hypotension, low basal metabolic rate (BMR), increased insulin sensitivity
3. Muscular weakness, fatigue, weight loss
4. Anorexia, nausea, vomiting, diarrhea, constipation, abdominal pain; craving salty foods
5. Mental changes, such as depression, irritability, anxiety, and apprehension; behavioral problems in children
6. Hyperpigmentation (''bronzing'') of skin caused by melanocyte-stimulating hormone (MSH) secretion from the pituitary

PEDIATRIC ALERT
Newborns with the condition are gravely ill after birth, with tachycardia, tachypnea, fever, cyanosis, cold and clammy skin, and hypotension.

◆ Diagnostic Evaluation

1. Decreased glucose, decreased sodium, increased potassium
2. Increased lymphocytes on complete blood count (CBC)
3. Low fasting plasma cortisol levels; low aldosterone levels
4. 24-hour urine studies show decreased levels of 17-ketosteroids, 17-hydroxycorticoids, and 17-ketogenic steroids.
5. ACTH stimulation test may show no increase in plasma cortisol and urinary 17-ketosteroids.
6. Possibly increased adrenal antibody titers in children

◆ Collaborative Management

Therapeutic Interventions

1. High-sodium, low-potassium diet and fluids to restore normal fluid and electrolyte balance
2. Cardiovascular support may be indicated, with cardiac and hemodynamic monitoring, oxygen therapy.
3. Recognition and treatment of underlying cause of Addisonian crisis (eg, treatment of infection)

Pharmacologic Interventions

1. Hydrocortisone or prednisone to treat glucocorticoid deficiency.

GERONTOLOGIC ALERT
The elderly and patients with chronic obstructive pulmonary disease (COPD) and heart failure may require preparations with low mineralocorticoid activity, such as methylprednisolone, to prevent fluid retention.

2. Fludrocortisone to treat mineralocorticoid deficiency.

NURSING ALERT
Overtreatment may be manifested by hypertension, edema from sodium and water retention, and weakness caused by potassium loss.

3. If Addisonian crisis or circulatory collapse is imminent, provide immediate treatment:
   a. Intravenous sodium chloride solution to replace sodium ions
   b. IV hydrocortisone
   c. Injection of circulatory stimulants such as atropine, calcium chloride, and epinephrine

◆ Nursing Interventions

Monitoring

1. Monitor vital signs frequently; a decrease in blood pressure and increase in temperature may suggest an impending crisis.

A

2. Monitor serum sodium and potassium levels.
3. Monitor intake and output, daily weight, and edema during corticosteroid therapy.

Supportive Care

1. Encourage high-calorie, high-protein diet rich in sodium and fluid content, if tolerated.
2. Administer or teach self-administration of prescribed glucocorticoids and mineralocorticoids; document response.
3. Administer IV infusions of sodium, water, and glucose as indicated.
4. Assess comfort and emotional status of the patient. Minimize stressful situations to avoid risk of adrenal crisis.
5. Protect the patient from infection by using good handwashing technique and avoiding contact with staff and visitors who may be carriers.
6. Assist the patient with activities of daily living if weak and fatigued.
7. Provide periods of rest and activity to avoid overexertion.
8. Maintain constant room temperature and avoid drafts, dampness, or extremes in temperature to prevent Addisonian crisis.
9. Observe and report early signs of Addisonian crisis (sudden decrease in blood pressure, nausea and vomiting, high temperature).

Family Education and Health Maintenance

1. Instruct about the need for lifelong therapy and follow-up.
   a. Emphasize the importance of not missing a dose and of taking more hormones when under stress. Dose may be doubled for minor illness, tripled for illness keeping patient home from school or work. An injection of hydrocortisone may be needed for trauma, surgery, severe fatigue, and other highly stressful situations.
   b. Suggest that the patient carry an identification card indicating medication being taken and health care provider's telephone number.
2. Teach intramuscular injection technique as indicated.

3. Advise the patient that excessive long-term use of corticosteroids may cause dangerous side effects such as fluid overload, osteoporosis, hyperglycemia, masking of signs of infection, etc.

PEDIATRIC ALERT:
In children, weight gain and poor growth may occur.

---

4. Identify actions to take to avoid factors that may precipitate Addisonian crisis (infection, extremes of temperature, trauma).

Aldosteronism, Primary

Primary aldosteronism refers to excessive secretion of aldosterone by the adrenal cortex, which is usually caused by a cortical adenoma or bilateral adrenal hyperplasia. Hyperaldosteronism in turn causes excessive sodium and water retention and excessive potassium excretion by the kidneys and gastrointestinal (GI) tract. A secondary form of the disease occurs in conjunction with heart failure, renal dysfunction, or cirrhosis of the liver. One to two percent of cases of hypertension are caused by primary aldosteronism; this usually can be treated successfully by adrenalectomy.

Seventy percent of patients with aldosterone-secreting adenomas are women, and the incidence of primary aldosteronism is four times higher among African Americans than among the general population. Complications include the long-term effects of untreated hypertension—stroke, renal failure, and heart failure.

◆ Assessment

1. Hypertension
2. Muscle weakness caused by hypokalemia
3. Possible paresthesias, tetany, and polyuria caused by alkalosis
4. Excessive thirst (polydipsia) caused by hypernatremia

A

◆ Diagnostic Evaluation

1. Suspect primary aldosteronism in all hypertensive patients with spontaneous hypokalemia; also suspect it if hypokalemia develops concurrently with start of diuretics and remains after diuretics are discontinued.
2. Salt-loading screening test—ingestion of at least 200 mEq/day (approximately 12 g salt) for 4 days will depress serum potassium to less than 3.5 mEq/L in a patient with aldosteronism. No effect is seen if aldosteronism is absent.
3. Computed tomography (CT) scanning to determine and localize cortical adenoma.

◆ Collaborative Management

Pharmacologic Interventions

1. Spironolactone, a potassium-sparing diuretic to treat both hypertension and potassium depletion
   a. Therapy is needed 4 to 6 weeks before the full effect on blood pressure is seen.
   b. Side effects include reduced testosterone in men or boys (decreased libido, impotence, gynecomastia) and gastrointestinal discomfort. Amiloride may be given instead in sexually active men or in cases of gastrointestinal intolerance.
   c. Restrict sodium: Avoid saline infusions, give low-sodium diet.
   d. Give potassium supplement if indicated by severity of hypokalemia.
2. Antihypertensive agent such as thiazide diuretic may be needed.
3. Management of underlying cause of secondary aldosteronism (heart, kidney, or liver disease)

Surgical Interventions

1. Unilateral adrenalectomy may be done to remove adrenal tumor.

◆ Nursing Interventions

Monitoring

1. Monitor fluid intake and output and daily weights.
2. Monitor serum potassium and observe for electrocardiogram (ECG) changes caused by hypokalemia.

3. Monitor blood pressure.
4. Monitor for complications of adrenalectomy (hemorrhage, adrenal crisis).
5. After adrenalectomy, monitor serum sodium, potassium, and glucose; report abnormalities.
   a. Sodium and potassium may normalize, or potassium may become elevated (because of transient adrenal insufficiency after surgery).
   b. Electrolyte imbalances may persist for 4 to 18 months after surgery.
   c. Hypertension may persist for 3 to 6 months after surgery.
   d. Temporary corticosteroid treatment causes glucose level to increase and worsens control in diabetics; may require additional treatment.

Supportive Care

1. Provide low-sodium diet and potassium supplements as ordered and teach patient to carry out these measures.
2. Administer or teach self-administration of antihypertensives as ordered.
3. Assess for dependent edema; encourage activity, frequent repositioning, and elevation of feet periodically to reduce edema.
4. Prepare the adrenal surgery patient by reinforcing explanation of procedure given by health care provider; describe nursing care.
5. Advise about the need for frequent blood pressure checks and glucocorticoid infusions before and after surgery to cover period of stress (surgery), because one adrenal gland is removed and it will take time for the remaining gland to compensate.
6. Perform usual postoperative care for abdominal surgery, including frequent check of vital signs, assessing for hemorrhage, turning, coughing and deep breathing, early ambulation, slow progression of diet when bowel sounds return, and control of pain with scheduled narcotic administration or patient-controlled analgesia.
7. Administer hydrocortisone IV as ordered.
8. Maintain nonstressful environment, promote rest, and provide meticulous care to protect the patient against

A

infection and other complications that could cause adrenal crisis.

Patient Education and Health Maintenance

1. Instruct the patient regarding the nature of illness, the necessary treatment, and the need for continued medical care.
2. Instruct the patient on the importance of following prescribed medical treatments.
   a. The patient must remain on spironolactone (Aldactone) for life. Advise on reporting significant side effects and if drug interferes with sexual performance and quality of life.
   b. Advise the patient that glucocorticoid administration may be temporary after subtotal or unilateral adrenalectomy, long-term for bilateral adrenalectomy; dose may need to be increased during times of illness or stress.
3. Teach the patient and family members how to take blood pressure readings, if indicated.

AIDS
See HIV Disease and AIDS

ALS
See Amyotrophic Lateral Sclerosis

Alzheimer's Disease

Alzheimer's disease is a degenerative disorder of the cerebral cortex characterized by dementia with progressive impairment of memory, cognitive function, language, and self-care ability. There is no known cause, but neurochemical, viral, and environmental factors are being studied. In addition, a genetic abnormality linked to the disorder has recently been located on chromosome 21. Profound structural changes in brain tissue are known to occur (amyloid deposition, granulovascular degeneration, and neurofibrillary tangles). Complications include infection, injury, and malnutrition.

◆ Assessment

1. Stage I—poor recent memory, mildly impaired remote recall, impaired visual–spatial skills, mild language impairment, indifference, and occasional irritabiltiy
2. Stage II—severe memory impairment, spatial disorientation, fluent aphasia, inability to make calculations, indifference, irritability, apraxia, delusions, and restlessness with pacing
3. Stage III—very poor cognitive function, rigidity of the extremities, flexion posture, urinary and fecal incontinence

◆ Diagnostic Evaluation

1. Imaging studies such as magnetic resonance imaging (MRI) and computed tomography (CT) scan of the brain to rule out treatable forms of dementia
2. Neuropsychological evaluation to establish clinical criteria for diagnosis
3. Laboratory testing such as blood chemistry, thyroid function tests, and urinalysis to rule out metabolic disorders

◆ Collaborative Management

Therapeutic Interventions

1. Environmental control to provide structure and routine that the patient can cope with
2. Frequent reorientation and cuing to facilitate activities of daily living

Pharmacologic Interventions

1. Antipsychotic agents such as haloperidol to help control agitation and hallucinations
2. Tacrine, a cholinesterase inhibitor, improves cognitive functioning and quality of life for some patients

A

   a. May cause elevation of liver enzymes; monitor liver function tests frequently

   b. May interact with many other drugs, including theophylline, cimetidine, anticholinergics, and nonsteroidal antiinflammatory drugs

3. Antidepressants may be helpful.

NURSING ALERT

Acute catastrophic reactions, characterized by agitation or insomnia, occur in the patient with Alzheimer's disease when coping mechanisms fail. Reactions may be precipitated by the strange environment of the hospital. They may be managed by haloperidol 2 to 5 mg PO or IM; lorazepam 5 mg PO or 1 mg IM; nortriptylline or trazodone if accompanied by depression; antihistamines; chloral hydrate; and maintenance of a simple, quiet, softly lit environment.

◆ Nursing Interventions

Monitoring

1. Watch for signs and symptoms of respiratory and urinary tract infections.
2. Monitor fluid and food intake to check for malnutrition or imbalances caused by inattention to mealtime and hunger or lack of ability to prepare meals. Monitor intake and output, and weigh patient weekly.
3. Inspect the skin for evidence of injury attributable to lack of insight, hallucinations, and confusion.
4. Monitor neurologic function, including emotional and mental states and motor capabilities, for changes indicating further deterioration.
5. Monitor response to antipsychotic medications.

Supportive Care

1. Simplify the patient's environment.
   a. Reduce noise levels.
   b. Provide a structured routine to reduce the number of choices available to the patient. Use lists and written instructions as reminders to daily activities.

A

    c. Provide cues in the environment: post large calendar and clock in patient's view; use pictures to identify activities; orient frequently to time, person, and place.

    d. Maintain consistency in interactions, and introduce new people slowly.

2. Protect the patient from accidents.

    a. Try to avoid using restraints, but keep the patient under observation as needed.

    b. Provide adequate lighting to help the patient interpret environment.

    c. Remove unneeded furniture and other obstacles from the room to reduce risk of falling.

    d. Make sure patient's shoes or slippers are easy to put on and to remove.

◆

COMMUNITY CARE CONSIDERATIONS

Remind family members of possible dangers around the house as patient becomes less responsible for behavior. Encourage them to reduce the temperature of hot water heater, remove dials from the stove and other electrical appliances, remove matches and lighters, and store tools and other potentially dangerous items safely.

3. Provide the patient with an identification tag or medical alert bracelet.

4. If possible, help the patient maintain a level of social interaction.

    a. Instruct the family that their presence is helpful even though actual interaction with the patient may be limited.

    b. Encourage the family to interact at a level meaningful to the patient. Have them bring objects from home that are meaningful.

5. Ensure adequate rest, alternating with periods of exercise to expend energy.

6. Maintain usual sleep habits and a bedtime ritual, including changing into pajamas, bedtime snack or warm noncaffeinated beverage, listening to music, or prayer.

7. Provide familiar foods that are high in calories and fiber in small, frequent meals. Include finger foods and adequate liquids.
8. Ensure that dentures fit well and that dental care is maintained.
9. Provide support to the caregiver.

Family Education and Health Maintenance

1. Advise caregiver to encourage activities that provide physical exercise and repetitive movement but take little thought, such as dancing, painting, doing laundry, or vacuuming.
2. Teach about catastrophic reactions and their cause and treatment.

COMMUNITY CARE CONSIDERATIONS
Episodes of catastrophic reactions and insomnia can be managed at home by using soft background music or white noise, having the patient wear a wander alarm, and providing repetitive stimulation such as music or rocking.

3. Teach the elimination of stimulants such as caffeine from diet.
4. Discuss the need to organize finances, and make advance directive decisions and guardianship arrangements before they are needed, to allow patient to participate in the process.
5. Tell family members that avoidance of aluminum-containing antacids, aluminum cooking utensils, and aluminum-containing deodorants reduces aluminum intake, which is thought to be one of the environmental factors that may cause this disorder.
6. For additional information, refer to agencies such as:

Alzheimer's Association
919 North Michigan Ave.
Suite 1000
Chicago, IL 60611
800-272-3900

Amnesic Disorder
See Delirium, Dementia, and Amnesic Disorder

Amputation

Amputation is the total or partial surgical removal of an extremity or digit. It is done in cases of inadequate tissue perfusion not responsive to other treatments, such as diabetes mellitus or other peripheral vascular diseases; severe trauma; malignant tumor; or in congenital deformity. The extent of amputation is based on the level of maximal viable tissue available for wound healing.

In a closed amputation, the stump is covered by a flap of skin sutured posteriorly; this is the most common procedure. Open (guillotine) amputation is used in emergencies, such as in severe infection and in patients who are poor surgical risks; the wound heals by granulation or secondary closure in approximately a week. Dressings may be either soft or rigid. Soft dressings permit wound inspection and are used primarily in patients who should avoid early weight-bearing (eg, those with peripheral vascular disease). Rigid dressings shape the residual limb, reduce edema, and allow early ambulation and attachment of a prosthesis.

◆ Potential Complications

1. Infection, sepsis
2. Hematoma, necrosis
3. Unrelieved phantom pain
4. Delayed healing of residual limb

◆ Collaborative Management

Preoperative Care
1. Hemodynamic evaluation is performed through testing such as angiography or arterial blood flow xenon 133 scan—to determine optimal amputation level.
2. Culture and sensitivity tests of draining wounds are done to assist in control of infection preoperatively.

A

3. Evaluation of contralateral extremity is performed to determine functional postoperative potential.
4. Evaluation of cardiovascular, respiratory, renal, and other body systems is needed to determine preoperative condition of the patient and reduce the risks of surgery by optimizing function.

GERONTOLOGIC ALERT
Amputation of the lower extremity can be a life-threatening procedure, especially in patients older than 60 years of age with peripheral vascular disease. In such patients, significant morbidity accompanies above-knee amputations because of associated poor health and disease as well as the complications of sepsis and malnutrition and the physiologic insult of amputation.

5. Nutritional status is evaluated, and supplemental protein may be added to enhance wound healing.
6. Exercises are taught to patients with a lower-limb amputations to strengthen upper-extremity muscles for use of ambulatory aids.
7. The patient is familiarized with ambulatory aids to instill self-confidence and prepare for postoperative mobility.

Postoperative Care

1. Monitor for signs of excessive blood loss: hypotension, tachycardia, diaphoresis, decreased alertness.
2. Watch for excessive wound drainage.
   a. Keep tourniquet ready to apply to residual limb if excessive bleeding occurs.
   b. Reinforce dressing as required, using aseptic technique.
   c. Maintain accurate record of bloody drainage on dressing and in drainage system.
3. Monitor intake and output for fluid balance.
4. Elevate residual limb to promote venous return.
5. Maintain pressure dressing; reapply if necessary, using sterile dressing secured with elastic bandage.
6. Notify surgeon if rigid cast dressing comes off.
7. Control surgical pain with narcotics as prescribed, and

use other techniques such as progressive muscle re-laxation and imagery.

8. Recognize that increasing discomfort may indicate presence of hematoma, infection, or necrosis.

9. Use physical modalities (eg, wrapping, temperature changes) and transcutaneous electrical nerve stimulation (TENS), if prescribed, to relieve phantom limb pain, and encourage patient activity to decrease awareness of pain.

10. Reassure patient that phantom limb pain will diminish over time.

11. Support patient through psychological acceptance of body image change.

12. Encourage participation in rehabilitation planning and self-care.

13. Teach the patient to avoid long periods in bed in one position, to prevent dependent edema, flexion deformity, and skin pressure areas.
    a. Lower-extremity amputations—hip flexion contracture (avoid placing residual limb on pillow; encourage prone position twice a day) and abduction deformity (use trochanter roll; avoid pillow between legs)
    b. Upper-extremity amputations—postural abnormalities (encourage good posture)

14. Encourage active range-of-motion and muscle-strengthening exercises when prescribed, to minimize atrophy, increase muscle strength, and prepare residual limb for prosthesis.

15. Promote reestablishment of balance (amputation alters distribution of body weight).
    a. Transfer the patient to a chair within 48 hours of surgery.
    b. Instruct and guard lower-limb amputee during balance exercises.

GERONTOLOGIC ALERT
Diabetes mellitus, heart disease, infection, stroke, chronic obstructive pulmonary disease (COPD), peripheral vascular disease, and increasing age are factors limiting rehabilitation.

A

◆ Patient Education and Health Maintenance

1. Teach the patient and family how to wrap residual limb with elastic bandage to control edema and to form a firm conical shape for prosthesis fitting.
2. Teach the patient residual limb conditioning:
   a. Push the residual limb against a soft pillow.
   b. Gradually push residual limb against harder surfaces.
   c. Massage healed residual limb to soften scar, decrease tenderness, and improve vascularity.
3. Instruct the patient to wash and dry limb thoroughly at least twice a day, removing all soap residue, to prevent skin irritation and infection. Avoid soaking residual limb, because this results in edema.
4. Inspect residual limb and skin under prosthesis harness daily for pressure, irritation, and actual skin breakdown.
5. Have patient wear residual limb sock or cotton underwear, to absorb perspiration and to avoid direct contact between prosthetic socket or harness and skin. Avoid wrinkles in residual limb sock to prevent potential pressure areas.
6. Wipe the socket of prosthesis with a damp cloth when prosthesis is removed for evening.
7. Have prosthesis checked periodically.
8. Teach the patient to protect the remaining extremity from injury and to secure prompt treatment of problems.

Amyotrophic Lateral Sclerosis

Amyotrophic lateral sclerosis (ALS), also known as Lou Gehrig's disease, is an incapacitating disease of unknown cause that results from degeneration of upper and lower motor neurons. This causes progressive loss of voluntary muscle contraction and functional capacity, accompanied by other lower motor neuron signs such as atrophy or fasciculations. ALS usually affects men in their 50s and 60s. It is invariably fatal; death usually results from a complication such as respiratory failure, aspiration pneumonia, or cardiopulmonary arrest.

◆ Assessment

1. Progressive weakness and wasting of muscles of arms, trunk, and legs
2. Muscle fasciculations and spasticity
3. Cranial nerve dysfunction, particularly gag reflex and swallowing difficulty, as well as nasal and unintelligible speech
4. Tachypnea, hypopnea, restlessness, poor sleep, and excessive fatigue caused by hypoxia from respiratory weakness

◆ Diagnostic Evaluation

1. Electromyography to evaluate denervation and muscle atrophy; nerve conduction testing to evaluate nerve pathways
2. Pulmonary function testing to evaluate respiratory status
3. Barium swallow to evaluate ability to control swallowing
4. Brain imaging such as magnetic resonance imaging (MRI) and computed tomography (CT) scanning to rule out other disorders
5. Laboratory testing such as creatine kinase, heavy metal screen, thyroid function tests, and cerebrospinal fluid evaluation to rule out other disorders

◆ Collaborative Management

Therapeutic Interventions
1. Enteral nutrition through gastrostomy or jejunostomy tube when high risk for aspiration develops
2. Intubation, tracheostomy, and mechanical ventilation when indicated for respiratory failure

Pharmacologic Interventions
1. Antispasticity drugs such as baclofen and diazepam
2. Antidepressants and sleep aids as needed

◆ Nursing Interventions

Monitoring

1. Monitor respiratory rate, depth, and tidal volume frequently. Document pattern and report any decrease below patient's baseline.
2. Monitor for drooling or regurgitation of liquids through nose, indicating deteriorating swallowing ability.
3. Monitor for fever and tachycardia and obtain sputum, urine, and other cultures as indicated to evaluate for infection.
4. Because standard call lights cannot be activated by the severely disabled ALS patient, arrange constant monitoring and surveillance to meet patient needs.

Supportive Care

1. Position the patient upright, suction the upper airway, and perform chest physical therapy as tolerated to enhance respiratory function.
2. Encourage use of an incentive spirometer to exercise respiratory muscles.
3. Establish the patient's wishes regarding life support measures; obtain a copy of living will for chart, if applicable.
4. Provide meticulous care to patient with artificial airway to prevent infection.
5. Encourage the patient to continue usual activities as long as possible, but alternate with naps to avoid fatigue.
6. Encourage physical therapy exercises to strengthen unaffected muscles and carry out range-of-motion exercises to prevent contractures.
7. Obtain assistive devices as needed to help patient maintain independence, such as special feeding devices, remote controls, and a motorized wheelchair.
8. Provide high-calorie, small frequent feedings to patient who can still swallow.
   a. Semisolids are usually easiest to swallow.
   b. Position patient upright for meals with neck flexed to protect the airway.
   c. Instruct the patient to take a breath before swal-

lowing, hold breath to swallow, exhale or cough after swallowing, and swallow again.
9. Examine the oral cavity before and after swallowing and provide frequent mouth care.
10. Encourage rest periods before meals to alleviate muscle fatigue.
11. Remember that the patient with ALS maintains full alertness, sensory function, and intelligence. Use mechanical speech aids or communication board when needed. Eye movements/blinking may be the last voluntary movement; develop a code system to serve as a communication method.

Patient Education and Health Maintenance
1. Stress the importance of maintaining physical exercise; discourage bed rest to prevent pulmonary stasis.
2. Review with the patient and family proper eating mechanics to avoid fatigue and aspiration of food.
3. Inform the patient of right to make decisions regarding a living will if he or she decides against artificial ventilation.
4. Encourage the family to seek support and respite care.
5. Remind the family that the patient with ALS maintains full alertness, sensory function, and intelligence. Encourage them to maintain interaction, socialization, and stimulation.
6. Refer the family for counseling as needed and to supportive agencies such as:

> **The Amyotrophic Lateral Sclerosis Association**
> 21021 Ventura Blvd.
> Suite 321
> Woodland Hills, CA 91364
> 800-782-4747

Anaphylaxis

Anaphylaxis is an immediate, life-threatening systemic reaction that occurs on exposure to a particular substance. It results from a type I hypersensitivity reaction in which release of chemical mediators from mast cells results in

A

massive vasodilation, increased capillary permeability, bronchoconstriction, and decreased peristalsis. Anaphylaxis may be caused by immunotherapy, skin testing, medications, contrast media infusion, insect stings, foods, or exercise. Prompt identification of signs and symptoms and immediate intervention is essential; the more quickly a reaction occurs, the more severe it tends to be. Complications include cardiovascular collapse and respiratory failure.

> **NURSING ALERT**
> With immunotherapy (allergy shots), the risk of systemic reaction is always present. Skin testing can also cause systemic reactions. Have epinephrine 1:1,000 (with syringe and tourniquet) available during these procedures and observe the patient for at least 30 minutes after administration.

◆ Assessment

1. Immediately assess airway, breathing, and circulation (ABCs) if severe presentation and intervene with cardiopulmonary resuscitation (CPR) as appropriate.
2. If less severe presentation, assess vital signs, degree of respiratory distress, and presence of angioedema.
3. Signs and symptoms include:
   a. Laryngeal edema, bronchospasm, cough, wheezing, feeling of lump in throat
   b. Hypotension, tachycardia, palpitations, syncope
   c. Urticaria (hives), angioedema, pruritus, flushing
   d. Nausea, vomiting, diarrhea, abdominal pain, bloating

> **NURSING ALERT**
> Before administering any medication, ask patients if they have ever had a reaction to it. Do not rely on the chart alone.

◆ Diagnostic Evaluation

None necessary; diagnosis is made by clinical presentation.

◆ Collaborative Management

Therapeutic and Pharmacologic Interventions

1. Immediate treatment should include application of a tourniquet above site of antigen injection (allergy injection, insect sting, etc.) or skin test site, to slow the absorption of antigen into the system.
2. Epinephrine (Adrenalin) 0.1 to 0.5 mg (0.01 mg/kg) is injected into opposite arm SQ or IM. May repeat every 15 to 20 minutes if necessary, to cause vasoconstriction, decrease capillary permeability, relax airway smooth muscle, and inhibit mast cell mediator release.
3. Subsequently, an adequate airway is established and hypotension and shock are treated with fluids and vasopressors.
4. Bronchodilators are given to relax bronchial smooth muscle.
5. Antihistamines such as diphenhydramine and possibly H_2 histamine blockers such as ranitidine may be given to block the effects of histamine.
6. Corticosteroids are given to decrease vascular permeability and diminish the migration of inflammatory cells; may be helpful in preventing late-phase responses.

◆ Nursing Interventions

Monitoring

1. Continually monitor respiratory rate and depth and breath sounds for respiratory effort and effectiveness of ventilation.
2. Monitor blood pressure by continuous automatic cuff, if available.
3. Monitor central venous pressure (CVP) to ensure adequate fluid volume and to prevent fluid overload.
4. Insert indwelling catheter and monitor urine output hourly to ensure kidney perfusion.

Supportive Care

1. Establish and maintain an adequate airway. If epinephrine has not stabilized bronchospasm, assist with endotracheal intubation, emergency tracheostomy, or cricothyroidotomy as indicated.

2. Administer nebulized epinephrine and or other bronchodilators, as ordered. Monitor heart rate (increased with bronchodilators).

3. Provide oxygen by nasal cannula at 2 to 5 L/min or by alternate means, as ordered.

4. Rapidly infuse IV fluids to fill vasodilated circulatory system and raise blood pressure. Titrate vasopressors based on blood pressure response.

5. Remain responsive to the patient, who may remain alert but not completely coherent because of hypotension, hypoxemia, and effects of medication.

6. When the patient is stable and alert, give simple, honest explanation of anaphylaxis and the treatment that was given.

7. Keep family and significant others informed of the patient's condition and the treatment being given.

Family Education and Health Maintenance

1. Instruct the patient to read labels and be familiar with the scientific name of the drug thought to cause a reaction.

2. Advise patient to discard all unused drugs. Make sure any drug kept in the medicine cabinet is clearly labeled.

3. Help the patient become familiar with drugs that may cross-react with the allergen.

4. Advise extreme care about diet if patient has known sensitivity to a food product—allergic compounds (such as monosodium glutamate) are often hidden in a preparation.

5. Teach the patient at risk for anaphylaxis about the potential seriousness of these reactions.

6. Educate patients to recognize the early signs and symptoms of anaphylaxis.

7. Instruct a patient allergic to bee stings to avoid wearing brightly colored or black clothes, perfumes, and hair spray. Shoes should be worn at all times.

8. For exercise-induced anaphylaxis, patients should exercise in moderation, preferably with another person, and in a controlled setting where assistance is readily available.

9. If food is associated with exercise-induced anaphy-

laxis, instruct patient to wait at least 2 hours after eating to exercise.

10. Instruct the patient to wear a medical alert bracelet or tag at all times.

COMMUNITY CARE CONSIDERATIONS
Instruct the patient in self-injection of epinephrine (Epi-Pen; Ana-Kit) and to carry it at all times. Explain about drug action, possible side effects, and the importance of prompt administration at the first sign of a systemic reaction. Check medication periodically to make sure it has not expired.

Anemia, Iron Deficiency and Other Types

Iron deficiency anemia is a condition in which total body iron content is inadequate for optimal development of red blood cells (RBC). The defective RBCs are fewer in number and have lower hemoglobin content. This reduces the blood's ability to deliver sufficient oxygen to the tissues.

Iron deficiency anemia is the most common type of anemia in all age-groups and results from one or more of several causes: 1) chronic blood loss; 2) iron malabsorption, as in small bowel disease or gastroenterostomy; 3) increased iron requirement, as in pregnancy or periods of rapid growth; or 4) insufficient intake caused by inadequate diet or weight loss. The disease primarily occurs in premenopausal women, children in rapid growth spurts, and pregnant women. Without treatment, advanced disease may cause growth retardation in children, heart failure, and ischemic organ damage such as myocardial infarction or cerebrovascular accident.

Other major types of anemia include pernicious anemia, folic acid deficiency anemia, aplastic anemia, and thalassemia major (Table 1).

GERONTOLOGIC ALERT
The elderly person who may be eating a soft diet because of dental problems is also at risk for iron deficiency anemia.

A

TABLE 1 Other Important Anemias

Type and Causes	Features	Treatment
Pernicious Anemia		
A megaloblastic anemia associated with vitamin B_{12} deficiency from small-bowel disease, gastric resection, or genetic malabsorption	In addition to anemia, causes GI symptoms and neuropathy. RBC indices reveal increased MCV. Schilling test is positive (decreased absorption of B_{12}).	Parenteral replacement with cyanocobalamin (B_{12}). Administered monthly for rest of patient's life. Therapy is monitored every 6 months.
Folic Acid Deficiency		
A megaloblastic anemia caused by dietary deficiency, alcoholism, jejunal malabsorption, pregnancy, and some medications (methotrexate, phenytoin, sulfamethoxazole, etc.)	Implicated in congenitally acquired neural tube defects. Folate level is decreased, and MCV is increased.	Oral folic acid replacement and adjustment of diet. Counseling and additional medical care for alcoholic patient, as needed.
Aplastic Anemia		
Bone marrow hypoplasia resulting in pancytopenia (insufficient numbers of RBCs, WBCs, and platelets). May be idiopathic or caused by exposure to chemical toxins, radiation, viral infections, certain drugs (chloramphenicol), or may be congenital.	In addition to anemia, causes increased risk of overwhelming infection due to neutropenia, and gross and occult bleeding due to thrombocytopenia. Course is variable; if severe, is often fatal.	Removal of causative agent or toxin. Allogeneic bone marrow transplantation (BMT) is treatment of choice in severe cases. Immunosuppressants and bone marrow stimulators are given. Supportive treatment, including platelet and red blood cell transfusions, antibiotics, and antifungals.
Thalassemia Major (Cooley's anemia)		
A genetic microcytic, hemolytic anemia most commonly seen in people of Mediterranean descent. The heterozygous form, beta-thalassemia minor, does not cause the severe manifestations.	In addition to anemia, causes skeletal deformities, growth failure, heart failure, hepatosplenomegaly, and hemosiderosis (deposition of iron in skin and internal organs). RBC indices indicate low MCV and MCHC.	Frequent transfusions of packed RBCs for hemoglobin less than 10. Iron chelation therapy with deferoxamine to decrease iron effects on body. Splenectomy may be done. BMT has been tried.

◆ Assessment

1. Headache, dizziness, tinnitus, fatigue
2. Tachycardia, palpitations, chest pain
3. Dyspnea on exertion
4. Pallor of conjunctivae, nail beds, skin, lips, and oral mucosa
5. Smooth, sore tongue
6. Lesions at corners of mouth (cheilosis)
7. Spoon-shaped fingernails (koilonychia)
8. Irritability, inability to concentrate, possible pica (craving to eat unusual substances, eg, mud, ice)

◆ Diagnostic Evaluation

1. Complete blood count shows decreased hemoglobin and hematocrit and elevated red cell distribution width (RDW).
2. Iron profile shows decreased serum iron and ferritin, and normal or elevated total iron-binding capacity.
3. Determination of source of chronic blood loss may include sigmoidoscopy, colonoscopy, upper and lower gastrointestinal (GI) studies, stool and urine for occult blood examination.

◆ Collaborative Management

Pharmacologic Interventions

1. Iron therapy—oral ferrous sulfate is the therapy of choice and continues until hemoglobin level is normalized and iron stores are replaced (up to 6 months); parenteral therapy is rarely used because of risk of anaphylaxis.
2. Source of blood loss is treated (treatment of ulcers, menorrhagia, etc.).

◆ Nursing Interventions

Supportive Care

1. Assess diet for inclusion of foods rich in iron. Arrange nutritionist referral as appropriate.
2. Use Z-track method of deep IM injection for parenteral iron.

A

NURSING ALERT

Anaphylactic reactions may occur after parenteral iron administration. Monitor patient closely for hypotension, angioedema, and stridor after injection. Do not administer in conjunction with oral iron.

---

3. Determine activities that cause fatigue; assist in developing a schedule of activity, rest periods, and sleep.
4. Encourage conditioning exercises to increase strength and endurance.
5. Assess patient for palpitations, chest pain, dizziness, and shortness of breath; minimize any activities that cause these symptoms.
6. Elevate head of bed and provide supplemental oxygen as ordered.

Family Education and Health Maintenance

1. Educate patient on proper nutrition and good sources of iron: select a well-balanced diet including animal proteins, iron-fortified cereals and bread, green leafy vegetables, dried fruits, legumes, nuts.
2. Teach patient about iron supplementation:
   a. Take iron on empty stomach with full glass of water or fruit juice. (Iron is absorbed best in acidic environment).
   b. Liquid forms may stain teeth; mix well and use straw. Dental stains can be removed by brushing teeth with sodium bicarbonate.
   c. Limit amount of milk to 16 to 24 ounces per day and do not give with iron because it impairs iron absorption.
   d. Anticipate some epigastric discomfort, change in color of stool to green or black, and in some cases nausea, constipation, or diarrhea.

COMMUNITY CARE CONSIDERATIONS

Ensure that iron medications are kept secure and away from children: overdose may be fatal.

---

3. Encourage follow-up laboratory studies and visits to health care provider, especially for children for evaluation of growth and development.

Aneurysm, Aortic

An *aneurysm* is distention of an artery caused by structural weakening of the arterial wall. Under hemodynamic pressure, the weakened area enlarges, causing serious complications by compressing surrounding structures. Aneurysms result from degeneration of the medial wall, which occurs as a normal part of the aging process, in hypertension, and as a complication of Marfan syndrome. Two major classes of aneurysms are described:

Thoracoabdominal aortic aneurysms may originate in the ascending aorta and aortic arch (frequent site of dissection) or in the lower descending thoracic aorta and upper abdominal aorta.

Abdominal aneurysms originate in the abdominal aorta, typically between the renal arteries and iliac branches. Many of these patients are asymptomatic; most are male (9:1). Aneurysms also may occur in peripheral arteries (femoral, popliteal, renal, subclavian) or any major artery. Aneurysms may be saccular (distention of vessel projecting from one side), fusiform (distention of entire circumference), or dissecting (tear of the intima and separation of the medial layers causing hemorrhage or intramural hematoma). Complications include fatal hemorrhage, paraplegia caused by interruption of anterior spinal artery, abdominal ischemia, stroke, and cardiac tamponade.

◆ Assessment

1. Thoracoabdominal aortic aneurysm.
   a. Pain is constant, boring pressure in chest
   b. May also be intermittent neuralgic pain caused by nerve compression
   c. Pain of sudden onset, or that is sharp, ripping or tearing, or located in the anterior chest, epigastric area, shoulders or back, indicates acute dissection or rupture.

A

    d. Dyspnea, cough, and hoarseness may result from pressure against trachea and recurrent laryngeal nerve.

    e. Dysphagia may occur because of pressure on esophagus.

    f. Dilated superficial veins of chest and cyanosis caused by compression of chest vessels

    g. Ipsilateral dilatation of pupils caused by pressure against cervical sympathetic chain

    h. Pulse or blood pressure variations between arms caused by interference with circulation in left subclavian artery.

2. Abdominal aneurysm

    a. Persistent or intermittent abdominal pain, often localized to middle or lower left side of abdomen

    b. Pain is intense in low back with rapid expansion, followed by syncope, tachycardia, and hypotension

    c. Pulsating mass with bruit

    d. Blood pressure elevated in arm more than in thigh

3. Predisposing factors include:

    a. Local infection, pyogenic or fungal (mycotic aneurysm)

    b. Congenital weakness of vessels

    c. Arteriosclerosis

    d. Trauma

    e. Syphilis

GERONTOLOGIC ALERT
Most abdominal aneurysms occur between the ages of 60 and 90 years. Rupture is likely if there is coexistent hypertension or if the aneurysm is larger than 6 cm (2.4 in).

◆ Diagnostic Evaluation

1. Abdominal or chest radiographs may show calcification that outlines the aneurysm.

2. Computed tomography (CT) and ultrasonography are used to detect and monitor size of aneurysm.

3. Aortography allows visualization of aneurysm and vessel.

A

◆ Collaborative Management

Therapeutic Interventions

1. Reassure the patient that small aneurysms (4 cm [1.5 in] or less) may be monitored with CT scans or ultrasound every 6 months, concurrent with aggressive blood pressure control.

Surgical Interventions

1. Surgery may be required to remove the aneurysm and restore vascular continuity with a bypass graft. Complications of surgery include arterial occlusion, graft hemorrhage, infection, ischemic colon, and impotence.

◆ Nursing Interventions

Monitoring

1. Monitor for signs and symptoms of spinal cord ischemia—pain, numbness, paresthesias, weakness—caused by dissection
2. Monitor for signs of stroke or cardiac tamponade caused by dissection.
3. Postoperatively, monitor vital signs continuously.
4. Monitor for arterial occlusion: Check extremities for sensation, temperature, pulses, color, capillary refill, and petechiae.
5. Monitor for bleeding from the wound and for signs of hemorrhage: hypotension, tachycardia, pallor, diaphoresis.
6. Monitor temperature and incision for signs of infection.
7. Measure abdominal girth or limb girth (of graft site) daily.
8. Monitor for watery, bloody diarrhea, which indicates ischemic bowel caused by reduced perfusion during surgery.
9. Monitor urinary output hourly.

Supportive Care

1. Maintain IV infusion to administer blood pressure medications and provide fluids postoperatively.
2. Administer antibiotics, if ordered, to prevent infection.
3. Administer pain medication as ordered or monitor patient-controlled analgesia.

A

4. Position the patient to enhance circulation.
   a. Elevate the head of the bed no more than 45 degrees for first 3 days postoperatively to prevent pressure on the repair and graft site.
   b. Warn the patient not to cross legs or sit for long periods to prevent thrombus formation.

Patient Education and Health Maintenance

1. Teach the patient about blood pressure medications and the importance of taking them as prescribed.
2. Teach the patient to recognize and report signs and symptoms of an expanding aneurysm or rupture.
3. For postsurgical patients, discuss warning signs of postoperative complications (fever, inflammation of operative site, bleeding, and swelling).
4. Encourage adequate nutritional intake to enhance wound healing.
5. Teach the patient to maintain a postoperative exercise schedule.

Aneurysm, Intracranial, or Ruptured Arteriovenous Malformation

An *intracranial aneurysm* is a saccular dilation of a cerebral artery whose walls are congenitally weakened. Consistent blood flow against the weakened area causes the aneurysm to grow; the enlarging aneurysm may compress nearby cranial nerves or brain tissue to cause symptoms, or it may rupture. The resulting hemorrhage within the subarachnoid space causes increased intracranial pressure, vasospasm, and ischemia, producing symptoms of a hemorrhagic stroke. Intracranial aneurysm may result from unknown causes or may be related to atherosclerosis, intracranial arteriovenous malformation (AVM; see below), hypertensive vascular disease, or head trauma.

An *arteriovenous malformation (AVM)* is a tangle of abnormally formed cerebral arteries and veins that lack a normal interconnecting capillary bed. Because of backflow pressure, a fistula develops, resulting in vascular dilatation and chronic hypoperfusion. Approximately 50% of patients with AVMs present with hemorrhage.

Intracranial aneurysm and AVM are graded from 0 (unruptured, asymptomatic) to IV (deep coma, decerebrate rigidity). Complications include rebleeding, cerebral vasospasm, hydrocephalus, and seizures.

◆ Assessment

1. Sudden onset of severe headache, nausea, and photophobia but no neurologic deficits may result from a "warning bleed" caused by leaking of aneurysm or rupture of the AVM.
2. Decreasing level of consciousness and focal neurologic deficits caused by vasospasm. The patient may present with loss of consciousness and severe deficits if bleed is massive.
3. Visual disturbances, dizziness, nuchal rigidity, hemiparesis, and papilledema may also be present.

◆ Diagnostic Evaluation

1. Computed tomography (CT) and magnetic resonance imaging (MRI) scans of the head to determine presence of blood in subarachnoid space and rule out other lesions
2. Cerebral angiography may be done to detect presence and location of cerebral aneurysm and provide information about vasospasm.
3. Lumbar puncture to check for blood in cerebrospinal fluid (CSF); observe for elevated opening pressure

◆ Collaborative Management

Pharmacologic Interventions

1. Osmotic diuretics to control increased intracranial pressure (IICP)
2. Antifibrinolytic therapy to inhibit clot lysis and prevent additional bleeding
3. Nitroprusside to manage systemic hypertension. Monitor closely to prevent sharp decrease in blood pressure, aggravating ischemia.
4. Calcium-channel blockers and plasma expanders, to prevent vasospasm
5. Seizure prophylaxis

A

Surgical Interventions

1. Craniotomy and clipping or ligation of the affected vessel
2. Strengthening the vessel wall by wrapping if it is inaccessible to clipping or ligation
3. Embolization with particles (AVM) or balloon angioplasty (aneurysm)
4. Procedures done to prevent rebleeding. Studies show surgery is more effective if done before vasospasm occurs.
5. See p. 226 for care of craniotomy patient.

◆ Nursing Interventions

Monitoring

1. Monitor for signs of IICP—increasing temperature, decreasing pulse, increasing blood pressure, widening pulse pressure, tachypnea, decreased level of consciousness, pupillary changes, and vomiting.
2. Document findings and report changes; subtle change in level of consciousness such as drowsiness and slurred speech may be first sign of deterioration.
3. Be alert for increasing headache, which may indicate rebleeding (highest incidence in first 3 weeks).

Supportive Care

1. Keep the patient free from agitation, and institute seizure precautions.
2. Institute subarachnoid precautions:
   a. Maintain absolute bed rest with head elevated 15 to 30 degrees to reduce cerebral edema.
   b. Maintain quiet, tranquil environment with low lighting and no noise or unnecessary activity to prevent photophobia, agitation, and pain.
   c. Provide physical care such as bathing and feeding.
   d. Restrict visitors to the immediate family or significant other who have been counseled to ensure tranquility.
   e. Encourage the conscious patient to avoid activities that increase blood pressure or intracranial pressure (ICP) (Valsalva maneuver for position changing, straining, sneezing, acute flexion or rotation of the neck, cigarette smoking).

f. Teach the conscious patient to exhale through the mouth during defecation to reduce strain; administer stool softeners as ordered.

g. Advise the patient to avoid caffeinated beverages.

3. Assess level of pain and pain relief; report any increase in headache.

4. If narcotic is being given with a sedative, monitor for central nervous system (CNS) depression, decreased respirations, decreased blood pressure.

5. Use reassurance and therapeutic conversation to relieve the patient's fear and anxiety.

6. Encourage distraction with soft music and other measures that will promote calm.

7. Prepare patient and family for surgery (see p. 226).

8. Encourage discussion of risks and benefits with the surgeon.

Patient Education and Health Maintenance

1. Educate the patient to the risk of rebleed, which is highest within first 3 weeks of rupture, but may remain for rest of their life.

2. Advise the patient to avoid strenuous activities to prevent sudden increased intracranial pressure—heavy lifting, straining, etc.

3. Encourage lifelong medical follow-up and immediate attention if severe headache develops.

4. Teach the patient and family how to deal with permanent neurologic deficits, and ensure that they obtain rehabilitation referral.

Anorexia Nervosa
See Eating Disorders

Anxiety, Somatoform, and Dissociative Disorders

Anxiety is a subjective feeling of apprehension and tension that is manifested by psychophysiologic arousal and a variety of behavioral patterns. The common theme among

A

all anxiety-related disorders is that affected persons experience a level of anxiety that interferes with functioning in personal, occupational, or social spheres, as well as with psychophysiologic well-being.

Anxiety-related disorders are divided into three broad groups by the *Diagnostic and Statistical Manual, 4th edition (DSM-IV)*:

1. *Anxiety disorders,* including panic disorder, phobias, obsessive-compulsive disorder, posttraumatic stress disorder, acute stress disorder, generalized anxiety disorder, and substance-induced anxiety disorder
2. *Somatoform disorders,* including somatization disorder, undifferentiated somatoform disorder, conversion disorder, pain disorder, hypochondriasis, and body dysmorphic disorder
3. *Dissociative disorders,* including dissociative amnesia, dissociative fugue, dissociative identity disorder, and depersonalization disorder

Anxiety-related disorders result from combinations of many psychological and physiologic factors. Psychological factors may include unconscious childhood conflicts; emotional distress from unmet (early) needs; or dissociation of certain mental processes, which may protect the person from specific painful and anxiety-producing memories. Physiologic factors may include abnormal neurotransmission or other biochemical imbalances in the locus coeruleus in the pons, limbic system, prefrontal cortex, frontal lobes, basal ganglia, or other brain centers. Genetic factors are also important.

♦ **Assessment**

Diagnostic criteria for common anxiety, somatoform, and dissociative disorders are as follows:

1. Panic disorder
   a. Recurrent unexpected anxiety attacks; onset is sudden, and patient experiences intense apprehension and dread
   b. Four or more of the following symptoms: dyspnea, chest discomfort, dizziness, hot or cold flashes, tingling of hands or feet, feelings of unreality, palpitations, syncope, diaphoresis, trembling, or fear of losing control, going crazy, or dying

2. Posttraumatic stress disorder
   a. After experiencing a psychologically traumatic event outside the range of usual experience (eg, rape, combat, bombings, kidnapping), the person re-experiences the event through recurrent and intrusive dreams and flashbacks.
   b. Emotional numbness, detachment, and estrangement may be used to defend against anxiety
   c. May experience sleep disturbance, hypervigilance, guilt about surviving, poor concentration, and avoidance of activities that trigger memory of the event
3. Phobias—irrational fear of an object or situation that persists, although the person may recognize it as unreasonable. Anxiety is severe if the object, situation, or activity cannot be avoided. Types include:
   a. Agoraphobia: fear of being alone or in public places where escape might be difficult; may not leave home
   b. Social phobia: fear of situations in which one might be seen and embarrassed or criticized; fear of eating in public, public speaking, or performing
   c. Specific phobia: fear of a single object, activity, or situation (eg, snakes, closed spaces, and flying)
4. Obsessive-compulsive disorder
   a. Preoccupation with persistent intrusive thoughts (obsessions), repeated performance of rituals designed to prevent some event (compulsions), or both
   b. Anxiety occurs if obsessions or compulsions are resisted and from feeling powerless to resist the thoughts or rituals
5. Substance-induced anxiety disorder
   a. Prominent anxiety, panic attacks, or obsessions or compulsions predominate
   b. Symptoms developed within 1 month of substance intoxication or withdrawal
   c. Medication use is related to disturbance
   d. The disturbance does not occur exclusively during the course of delirium.
   e. Significant distress or impaired social and occupational functioning results

A

6. Generalized anxiety disorder—persists for at least 6 months. Symptoms present from three of the four following categories:
   a. Motor tension
   b. Autonomic hyperactivity
   c. Apprehensiveness
   d. Hypervigilance

7. Acute stress disorder—person has witnessed or experienced a traumatic event; duration of 2 days to 4 weeks. Develops three or more of the following dissociative symptoms:
   a. Subjective sense of numbing
   b. Absence of emotional responsiveness
   c. Feeling dazed
   d. Derealization
   e. Depersonalization
   f. Dissociative amnesia

8. Somatization disorder—history of many physical complaints beginning before age 30 years, occurring over a period of years, and resulting in a change of lifestyle. Complaints must include all of the following:
   a. History of pain in at least four different sites or functions
   b. History of at least two gastrointestinal symptoms other than pain
   c. History of at least one sexual or reproductive symptom
   d. History of at least one symptom defined as, or suggesting, a neurologic disorder

9. Hypochondriasis
   a. Preoccupation with fears of having, or the idea that one has, a serious disease
   b. Preoccupation persists despite appropriate medical tests and assurances to the contrary
   c. Other disorders are ruled out, for example, somatic delusional disorders
   d. Preoccupation causes significantly impaired social or occupational functioning or causes marked distress

10. Body dysmorphic disorder
    a. Preoccupation with some imagined defect in appearance in a normal-appearing person (if the defect is present, concern is excessive)

      b. Preoccupation causes significantly impaired social or occupational functioning or causes marked distress

11. Conversion disorder
    a. Development of a symptom or deficit suggesting a neurologic disorder or involuntary motor function
    b. Not caused by malingering or factitious disorder and not culturally sanctioned
    c. Causes impairment in social or occupational functioning, causes marked distress, or requires medical attention

12. Pain disorder
    a. Pain in one or more anatomic sites is a major part of the clinical picture
    b. Causes significantly impaired occupational or social functioning or causes marked distress
    c. Psychological factors are thought to cause onset, severity, or exacerbation.
    d. If a medical condition is present, it plays a minor role in accounting for pain.

13. Undifferentiated somatoform disorder—one or more physical complaints: fatigue, loss of appetite, GI or urinary symptoms

14. Dissociative amnesia
    a. One or more episodes of inability to recall important information—usually of a traumatic or stressful nature
    b. Other psychological (eg, multiple personality disorder) and physical (eg, substance-induced) disorders are ruled out.

15. Dissociative identity disorder
    a. Presence of two or more distinct identities, each with its own patterns of relating, perceiving, and thinking
    b. At least two of these identities take control of the person's behavior
    c. Inability to recall important personal information too extensive to be explained by ordinary forgetfulness
    d. Other causes ruled out

16. Dissociative fugue
    a. Sudden, unexpected travel away from home or

A

one's place of work, with inability to remember past

b. Confusion about personal identity or assumption of new identity

17. Depersonalization disorder
  a. Persistent or recurrent experience of feeling detached from and outside of one's mental processes or body
  b. Reality testing remains intact
  c. The experience causes significantly impaired occupational or social functioning or causes marked distress.
  d. Does not occur exclusively during course of another mental disorder

◆ Diagnostic Evaluation

1. Measurement tools for anxiety:
  a. Manifest Anxiety Scale
  b. Institute for Personality and Ability Testing Anxiety Scale Questionnaire
  c. Sheehan Anxiety Scale
  d. Total Anxiety Scale
  e. Yale-Brown Obsessive-Compulsive Scale
2. Dissociation Experiences Scale—measurement tool for dissociation
3. Sodium lactate infusion or carbon dioxide inhalation will likely produce a panic attack in a person with panic disorder.
4. Increased arousal may be measured through studies of autonomic functioning (eg, heart rate, electromyography, sweat gland activity) in a person with posttraumatic stress disorder.

◆ Collaborative Management

Therapeutic Interventions

1. Determine the level and place of care to be provided: psychiatric inpatient, outpatient, psychiatric home care.
2. Psychoeducational strategies:
  a. Relaxation techniques
  b. Progressive muscle relaxation
  c. Guided imagery

3. Psychotherapy
   a. Psychodynamic: Assist persons in understanding their experiences by identifying unconscious conflicts and developing effective coping behaviors.
   b. Behavioral: Focus on the person's problematic behavior and work to modify or extinguish the behavior. Systematic desensitization is often successful.
   c. Hypnotherapy can be used as part of therapy for those suffering dissociative disorders.
4. Biofeedback: Relaxation through biofeedback is achieved when a person learns to control physiological mechanisms that are not ordinarily within his or her awareness. Awareness and control are accomplished by monitoring body processes, including muscle tone, heart rate, and brain waves.

Pharmacologic Interventions

1. Psychopharmacologic intervention directed at targeted symptoms with specific desired outcomes to prevent polypharmacy. Anxiolytics most often used.
2. Narcotherapy: Sodium amytal or IV sodium pentothal may assist the therapist in gaining access to a patient's repressed memories and buried conflicts.
   a. In a person experiencing dissociative amnesia or dissociative fugue, the therapist may explore dissociated events.
   b. If the person is diagnosed with dissociative identity disorder, this type of interview may facilitate the access of other personalities.

◆ Nursing Interventions

Monitoring

1. Monitor for objective and subjective manifestations of anxiety.
   a. Tachycardia, tachypnea
   b. Verbalization of feelings of anxiety
   c. Signs and symptoms associated with autonomic stimulation: perspiration, difficulty concentrating, insomnia
2. Monitor effects of medication and functional ability.

Supportive Care

1. Help patient identify anxiety-producing situations and plan for such events.

A

2. Assist patient to develop assertiveness and communication skills.

3. Practice stress reduction techniques with patient.

4. Use short, simple sentences when communicating with patient.

5. Maintain a calm, serene manner.

6. Use adjuncts to verbal communication, such as visual aids and role playing, to stimulate memory and retention of information.

7. Teach relaxation techniques to diminish distress that interferes with concentration ability.

8. Encourage patient to discuss reasons for and feelings about social isolation.

9. Help patient identify specific causes or situations that produce anxiety that inhibits social interaction.

10. Recommend participation in programs directed at specific conflict areas or skill deficiencies. Such programs may focus on assertiveness skills, body awareness, managing multiple role responsibilities, and stress management.

11. Identify secondary benefits, such as decreased responsibility and increased dependency, that inhibit patient's move to independence.

12. Provide experiences in which patient can be successful.

13. Explore alternative methods of meeting dependency needs.

14. Explore beliefs that support a helpless or dependent mode of behavior.

15. Teach and role-play assertive behaviors in specific situations.

16. Assist patient to improve skills based on performance.

17. Develop an honest, nonjudgmental relationship with the patient.

18. Try to establish communication between patient's subpersonalities.

19. Do not overwhelm patient with information or memories.

20. Assist patient to incorporate dissociated material into conscious memories by encouraging the sharing of painful, repressed memories.

Patient Education and Health Maintenance

1. Teach patient and family members about anxiety.
2. Describe the medication regimen.
3. Identify, describe, and practice deep-muscle relaxation techniques, relaxation breathing, imagery, and other relaxation therapies.
4. Teach family to give positive reinforcement for use of healthy behaviors.
5. Teach family not to assume responsibilities or roles normally assigned to the patient.
6. Teach family to give attention to the patient, not to the patient's symptoms.
7. Teach alternative ways to perform activities of daily living if physical disability inhibits function and performance.
8. For additional information and support, refer to agencies such as:

> **Anxiety Disorders Association of America**
> 6000 Executive Blvd.
> Suite 200
> Rockville, MD 20852
> 301-231-9350

Aortic Aneurysm
See Aneurysm, Aortic

Appendicitis

Appendicitis is inflammation of the vermiform appendix caused by an obstruction attributable to infection, stricture, fecal mass, foreign body, or tumor. Appendicitis can affect any age group, but is most common in males 10 to 30 years of age. Appendicitis is the most common major surgical disease. If left untreated, appendicitis may progress to abscess, perforation, subsequent peritonitis, and death.

◆ Assessment

1. Generalized or localized abdominal pain occurs in the epigastric or periumbilical areas, and the upper right abdomen.
2. Within 2 to 12 hours, the pain localizes in the right lower quadrant and intensity increases.
3. Anorexia, fever, nausea, and vomiting also may occur.

GERONTOLOGIC ALERT
Be aware of vague symptoms in elderly patients: milder pain, low-grade fever, and leukocytosis with shift to the left on white blood cell (WBC) differential.

4. Bowel sounds may be diminished.
5. Tenderness anywhere in the right lower quadrant
   a. Often localized over McBurney's point, just below midpoint of line between umbilicus and iliac crest on the right side
   b. Guarding and rebound tenderness in right lower quadrant and referred rebound when palpating the left lower quadrant
6. Positive psoas sign
   a. Have the patient attempt to raise the right thigh against the pressure of your hand placed over the right knee.
   b. Increased abdominal pain indicates inflammation of the psoas muscle in acute appendicitis.
7. Positive obturator sign
   a. Flex the patient's right hip and knee and rotate the leg internally.
   b. Hypogastric pain indicates inflammation of the obturator muscle.

◆ Diagnostic Evaluation

1. WBC count shows moderate leukocytosis (10,000 to 16,000/mm) with shift to the left (increased immature neutrophils) in WBC differential.
2. Urinalysis to rule out urinary disorders
3. Abdominal x-ray to visualize shadow consistent with fecalith in appendix

4. Tests to rule out other conditions, such as pelvic sonogram to rule out ovarian cyst or ectopic pregnancy

◆ **Collaborative Management**

Surgical Interventions

1. Surgical removal is the only effective treatment (simple appendectomy or laparoscopic appendectomy).
2. Preoperatively, maintain patient on bed rest, nothing by mouth (NPO) status, IV hydration, possible antibiotic prophylaxis, and analgesia, as directed.

NURSING ALERT

When appendicitis is suggested, analgesics with antipyretic property may be avoided to prevent masking of fever, and cathartics are contraindicated because they may cause rupture.

◆ **Nursing Interventions**

Monitoring

1. Monitor frequently for signs and symptoms of worsening condition, indicating perforation, abscess, or peritonitis: increasing severity of pain, tenderness, rigidity, distention, ileus, fever, malaise, tachycardia.
2. Notify health care provider immediately if pain suddenly ceases; indicates perforation, a medical emergency.

Supportive Care

1. Assist patient to position of comfort, such as semi-Fowler's with knees flexed.
2. Restrict activity that may aggravate pain, such as coughing and ambulation.
3. Apply ice bag to abdomen for comfort.
4. Avoid indiscriminate palpation of the abdomen to avoid increasing the patient's discomfort.
5. Promptly prepare patient for surgery once diagnosis is established (see p. 350).

Family Education and Health Maintenance

1. Explain signs and symptoms of postoperative complications to report—elevated temperature, nausea or

A

vomiting, abdominal distention; may indicate infection.
2. Instruct patient on turning, coughing, deep breathing, use of incentive spirometer, ambulation. Discuss purpose and continued importance of these maneuvers during the recovery period.
3. Teach incisional care and avoidance of heavy lifting or driving until cleared by surgeon.
4. Advise avoidance of enemas or harsh laxatives; increased fluids and stool softeners may be used for postoperative constipation.

Arterial Occlusive Disease

Arterial occlusive disease is a common complication of arteriosclerosis in which the vascular system of the legs become blocked. Chronic occlusive arterial disease occurs much more frequently than acute disease (which usually results from sudden and complete blocking of a vessel by a thrombus or embolus).

There are two main types of occlusive arterial disease: *arteriosclerosis obliterans* occurs at bifurcations of a vessel, most commonly at aorto-iliac, femoro-popliteal, and popliteal-tibial sites. *Thromboangiitis obliterans,* or Buerger's disease, occurs because of thrombi originating in the left side of the heart caused by atrial fibrillation or mitral stenosis, and from sites of atherosclerotic plaque. Untreated, chronic occlusive arterial disease may progress to ulceration of feet and toes; severe occlusion causes gangrene and may necessitate partial or complete limb amputation.

Acute occlusive disease results from an arterial embolus that causes complete arterial obstruction; such emboli tend to lodge at bifurcations and atherosclerotic narrowings.

◆ Assessment

1. Intermittent claudication or pain in extremity.
   a. The chronic disorder begins with tingling and numbness of toes; later, pain occurs in the leg, even

when at rest. Patients may report excruciating cramplike pain in calf muscles.

b. Pain occurs at night, requiring patients to get out of bed to walk to relieve the pain.

c. Acute onset of severe pain may signal an acute arterial embolism. Pain may be aggravated by movement of and pressure on the extremity.

2. Changes in color (pallor to mottling in acute arterial embolism), sensation, and temperature (coldness) from one side to the other

3. Loss of pulses distal to occlusion (Fig. 1); bruits on auscultation

4. Thickened and opaque nails; shiny, atrophic, hairless skin with dry appearance reflect long-term changes

5. Possible ulcers of toes and feet

6. Collapse of superficial veins because of decreased blood flow to the extremity in acute arterial embolism

7. Sharp line of color and temperature demarcation distal to the site of occlusion as a result of ischemia in acute arterial embolism

◆ Diagnostic Evaluation

1. Vascular examination, including brachial and ankle systolic pressures, before and after exercise

2. Doppler ultrasound may show increased flow velocity through a stenotic vessel, or total occlusion; segmental plethysmography, which may indicate decreased flow.

3. Imaging studies (angiography, radionuclide scan) confirm arterial occlusion.

◆ Collaborative Management

Therapeutic Interventions

1. Conservative treatment to manage intermittent claudication includes walking, weight reduction, smoking cessation, and control of other conditions such as hypertension and diabetes mellitus

Pharmacologic Interventions

1. Pentoxifylline may be given to improve blood flow; drug increases erythrocyte flexibility and reduces blood viscosity.

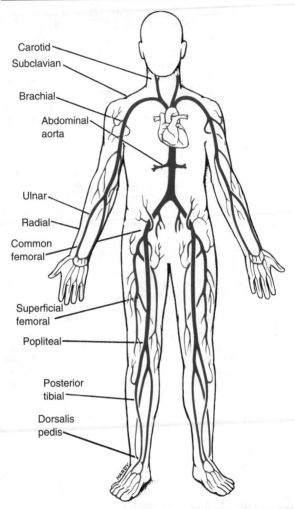

FIGURE 1 Salient points in evaluating peripheral arterial insufficiency. Reduced or absent femoral pulses indicate aortoiliac disease. Absent popliteal pulses indicate superficial femoral occlusion. Pulse deficits in one extremity, with normal pulses in contralateral extremity, suggest acute arterial embolus. Absent pedal pulses indicate tiboperoneal artery involvement.

2. Anticoagulants and thrombolytics to treat acute arterial embolism
   a. Heparin IV reduces tendency of emboli to form or expand (useful in smaller arteries).
   b. Thrombolytics IV dissolve clot.
3. Treatment of shock in the event of acute arterial embolism of large artery

---

NURSING ALERT

Arterial embolization of a large artery, such as the iliac, that has major systemic effects is life-threatening and requires emergency surgical intervention.

Surgical Interventions

1. Reconstructive arterial surgery (endarterectomy, arterial bypass grafting, or a combination) may be required.
2. Percutaneous transluminal angioplasty (PTA) may be used alone or with reconstructive surgery to dilate localized noncalcified segments of narrowed arteries.
3. Microvascular surgery may be required for small-artery occlusive disease.
4. Embolectomy, which must be performed within 6 to 10 hours of acute arterial occlusion, to prevent muscle necrosis and loss of extremity

◆ Nursing Interventions

Monitoring

1. Monitor the condition of extremities for injury, ulceration, and signs of infection.
2. In anticoagulant therapy for acute arterial embolism, monitor patient for signs of bleeding (gums, urine, stool). Also monitor prothrombin and partial thromboplastin times.
3. Monitor the postoperative embolectomy patient for tachycardia, fever, pain, erythema, warmth, swelling, and drainage at the incision site, indicating infection.

A

Supportive Care

1. In acute arterial embolism, protect the extremity by keeping it at or below the body's horizontal plane.
2. Provide and encourage a well-balanced diet to enhance sound healing.
3. Encourage walking or performance of range-of-motion exercises to increase blood flow.
4. Teach Buerger-Allen exercises, by which gravity alternately fills and empties the blood vessels:
   a. Begin with the patient lying flat in bed. Elevate legs to above the level of the heart for 2 minutes or until blanching takes place.
   b. Allow legs to dangle; exercise feet for 3 minutes or until legs are pink.
   c. Instruct the patient to lie flat for 5 minutes.
   d. Have the patient repeat each step 5 times and do the entire set of exercises 3 times a day.
5. Postoperatively, check the surgical wound for bleeding, swelling, erythema, and discharge.
6. Provide and teach proper foot care:
   a. Encourage the patient to wear protective footwear such as rubber-soled slippers or shoes with closed, wide toebox when out of bed.
   b. Avoid using adhesive tape on affected skin.
   c. Wash and carefully dry feet, trim toenails, and inspect feet daily.
   d. Apply lanolin or petrolatum to lower extremities to prevent drying and cracking of skin.
   e. Encourage the patient to wear clean hose daily; woolen socks for winter, cotton for summer.

Patient Education and Health Maintenance

1. Teach patient the importance of maintaining/improving circulation:
   a. Walking.
   b. Not sitting or standing in one position for long periods; not crossing legs when sitting or lying.
   c. Not using tight-fitting elastic-topped socks.
2. Teach patient methods to promote vasodilation by keeping extremity warm, not smoking, and stopping use of other vasoconstricting substances such as caffeine.
3. Reinforce dietary teaching to promote healing.

4. Tell patient to have a podiatrist cut corns and calluses; do not use corn pads or strong medications.
5. Teach the patient to recognize and report important signs:
   a. Redness, swelling, irritation, blistering
   b. Itching, burning—athlete's foot
   c. Bruises, cuts, and other skin lesion

Arteriovenous Malformation, Ruptured
See Aneurysm, Intracranial

Arthritis
See Osteoarthritis, Rheumatoid Arthritis, and Rheumatoid Arthritis, Juvenile

Arthroplasty and Total Joint Replacement

Arthroplasty is reconstructive surgery to restore joint motion and function and to relieve pain. It generally involves replacement of bony joint structure by a prosthesis. In total joint replacement, both articulating surfaces are replaced with metal or plastic components. The most common types of joint replacement (Fig. 2) are total hip replacement, usually with a metal femoral component topped by a spherical ball fitted into a plastic acetabular socket; and total knee replacement, an implant procedure in which tibial, femoral, and patellar joint surfaces are replaced.

Indications for total joint replacement include unremitting pain and irreversible joint damage, as in primary degenerative arthritis (osteoarthritis) and rheumatoid arthritis; selected fractures (eg, femoral neck fracture); failure of previous reconstructive surgery; congenital hip disease; pathologic fractures from metastatic cancer; and joint instability.

A

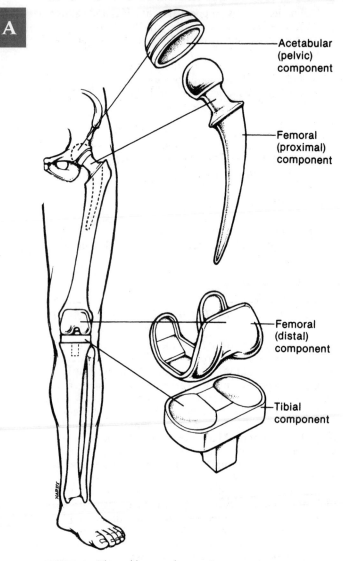

- Acetabular
  (pelvic)
  component

- Femoral
  (proximal)
  component

- Femoral
  (distal)
  component

- Tibial
  component

FIGURE 2 Hip and knee replacement.

◆ Potential Complications

1. Deep infection, sepsis, thromboembolism
2. Increased pain or decreased function associated with loosening of prosthetic components
3. Implant wear
4. Dislocation or fracture of components
5. Avascular necrosis or dead bone caused by loss of blood supply
6. Heterotrophic ossification (formation of bone in peri-prosthetic space)

◆ Collaborative Management

Preoperative Care

1. Assess the patient for bladder, dental, or skin infections that may be a source for prosthesis infections.
2. Provide preoperative patient teaching.
   a. Educate the patient concerning postoperative regimen (eg, extended exercise program).
   b. Teach isometric exercises (muscle setting) of quadriceps and gluteal muscles; teach active ankle motion.
   c. Teach bed-to-wheelchair transfer without going beyond the hip flexion limits (usually 90 degrees).
   d. Practice non–weight- and partial weight-bearing ambulation with ambulatory aid (walker, crutches) to facilitate postoperative ambulation.
   e. Demonstrate abduction splint, knee immobilizer, or continuous passive motion if equipment will be used postoperatively.
3. Use antiembolism stockings to minimize development of thrombophlebitis.
4. Give meticulous skin preparation with antimicrobial solution to minimize potential infection.
5. Administer antibiotics as prescribed to assure therapeutic blood levels during and immediately after surgery.
6. Thoroughly assess cardiovascular, respiratory, renal, hepatic, hydration, and nutritional status and institute measures to maximize general health condition.

Postoperative Care

1. Employ appropriate positioning to prevent dislocation of prosthesis.

A

2. After *hip arthroplasty,* position the patient supine in bed. Keep the affected extremity in slight abduction using an abduction splint or pillow or Buck's extension traction to prevent dislocation of the prosthesis.

> **NURSING ALERT**
> The patient must not adduct or flex operated hip—may produce dislocation. Signs of joint dislocation include shortened extremity, increasing discomfort, inability to move joints.

  a. With the aid of a coworker, turn the patient on unoperated side while supporting operated hip securely in an abducted position; support the entire leg on pillows.
  b. Use overhead trapeze to assist with position changes.
  c. The bed is usually not elevated more than 45 degrees; placing the patient in an upright sitting position puts a strain on the hip joint and may cause dislocation.
  d. Use a fracture bedpan when needed. Instruct the patient to flex the unoperated hip and knee and pull up on the overhead trapeze to lift buttocks onto pan. Instruct the patient *not* to bear down on the operated hip in flexion when getting off the pan.
3. After *knee arthroplasty,* immobilize the knee in extension with a firm compression dressing and an adjustable soft extension splint or long-leg plaster cast.
  a. Elevate the leg on pillows to control swelling.
  b. Alternatively, initiate continuous passive motion to facilitate joint healing and restore range of motion.
4. Promote early mobility. When the patient is ready to ambulate, teach to advance the walker and then advance the operated extremity to the walker to permit weight bearing as prescribed.
  a. Use an abduction splint or pillows while assisting the hip replacement patient to get out of bed.
  b. Keep the hip at maximum extension.
  c. Instruct the patient to pivot on unoperated extremity.
  d. Assess the patient for orthostatic hypotension.

   e. With increased joint stability, assist the patient to use crutches or cane as prescribed.

   f. Encourage practicing physical therapy exercises to strengthen muscles and prevent contractures.

5. Assist the knee replacement patient with transfer out of bed into wheelchair with extension splint in place.

   a. Ensure that no weight bearing is permitted until prescribed by the orthopedic surgeon.

   b. Apply continuous passive motion equipment or carry out passive range-of-motion exercises as prescribed.

◆ Patient Education and Health Maintenance

1. Advise wearing elastic stockings until full activities are resumed.

2. Warn against excessive hip adduction, flexion, and rotation after hip arthroplasty:

   a. Avoid sitting in low chair/toilet seat.

   b. Keep knees apart; do *not* cross legs.

   c. Limit sitting to 30 minutes at a time—to minimize hip flexion and risk of prosthetic dislocation, and to prevent hip stiffness and flexion contracture.

3. Encourage quadriceps setting and range-of-motion exercises as directed.

   a. Have a *daily* program of stretching, exercise, and rest throughout lifetime.

   b. Do not participate in activities that place undue or sudden stress on joint (eg, jogging, jumping, lifting heavy loads, becoming obese, excessive bending and twisting).

   c. Use a cane when taking fairly long walks.

4. Teach patient to use self-help and energy-saving devices:

   a. Handrails by toilet

   b. Raised toilet seat if there is some residual hip flexion problem

   c. Bar-type stool for shower and kitchen work

5. Tell the patient to lie prone twice daily for 30 minutes.

6. Encourage follow-up evaluation.

7. Teach proper use of supportive equipment (crutches, canes, raised toilet seat) as prescribed.

A

8. Advise patient to notify dentist and other doctors of need to take prophylactic antibiotic if undergoing any procedure (tooth extraction, manipulation of genitourinary tract) known to cause bacteremia.
9. Advise of need to avoid magnetic resonance imaging (MRI) studies because of implanted metal component.

Asthma

Asthma is a disease characterized by variable, recurrent, reversible airway obstruction with intermittent episodes of wheezing and dyspnea. It is associated with bronchial hypersensitivity and inflammation caused by various stimuli. Asthma is the most common chronic disease of childhood, with 5% to 10% of school-aged children having symptoms of asthma. Asthma may develop in infants, but it usually develops after the third birthday. It is more common in African Americans from urban settings.

Asthma is classified into six main types: *extrinsic asthma,* caused by inhaled allergens (eg, dust, dust mites, mold, pollens, feathers, and animal dander) and mediated by immunoglobulin E (IgE); *intrinsic asthma,* caused by infection (often viral) and environmental stimuli (such as air pollution), with no inciting allergen; *mixed asthma,* in which type I (immediate) reactivity appears to be combined with intrinsic factors; *aspirin-induced asthma,* caused by ingestion of aspirin and related compounds; *exercise-induced asthma,* in which respiratory symptoms occur within 5 to 20 minutes after exercise; and *occupational asthma,* caused by industrial fumes, dust, and gases.

Severe, acute asthma that fails to respond to bronchodilators is called *status asthmaticus* and is a medical emergency (Box 1). Other complications include pneumonia, atelectasis, dehydration, dysrrhythmias, cor pulmonale, respiratory failure, and death.

◆ Assessment

1. Feeling of chest tightness
2. Episodes of coughing
3. Wheezing, dyspnea

A

■ BOX 1 STATUS ASTHMATICUS

Status asthmaticus is a severe form of acute asthma in which airway obstruction resists conventional drug therapy and lasts longer than 24 hours. Unless treated promptly, status asthmaticus progresses to respiratory failure. Status asthmaticus is characterized by:

1. Labored respirations, with increased effort on expiration.
2. Distended neck and face veins.
3. Fatigue, headache, irritability, dizziness, impaired mental functioning caused by hypoxia.
4. Muscle twitching, somnolence, diaphoresis caused by CO_2 retention.
5. Tachycardia, elevated blood pressure.
6. Heart failure and death from suffocation.

■ Management and Nursing Interventions

1. Continuously or frequently monitor arterial blood gases (ABGs), blood pressure, ECG, and respiratory rate.

NURSING ALERT
In status asthmaticus, the return to a normal or increasing Pco_2 does not necessarily mean that the patient is improving. It may indicate a fatigue state that develops just before the patient slips into respiratory failure. Correlate ABGs with respiratory effort and level of consciousness.

2. Administer repeated aerosol treatments with bronchodilators such as albuterol. However, administer cautiously until metabolic and respiratory acidosis and hypoxemia have been corrected.

continued

A

■ **BOX 1** *(Continued)*

3. Administer aminophylline as prescribed through IV infusion. Be alert for signs of theophylline toxicity (tachycardia, nausea, vomiting, restlessness, dizziness).

4. Give prescribed IV corticosteroids to treat inflammation of airways. Because these act slowly, their beneficial effects may not be apparent for several hours.

5. Give fluids to treat dehydration and loosen secretions.

6. Provide continuous humidified oxygen via nasal cannula as prescribed. Use oxygen cautiously in patients with chronic obstructive pulmonary disease, because hypoxemia stimulates their respiratory drive.

7. Initiate mechanical ventilation for severe acidosis, hypoxemia, or respiratory fatigue.

8. Perform chest physiotherapy (chest wall percussion and vibration), administer expectorant and mucolytic drugs as prescribed, and suction as needed to prevent obstruction by secretions. Bronchoscopy may be needed.

9. Alleviate the patient's anxiety and fear by acting calmly and reassuring the patient during an attack. Stay with the patient until the attack subsides.

---

4. Anxiety, apprehension
5. Nasal flaring, use of accessory muscles

❖

NURSING ALERT
Do not be misled by lack of wheezing on auscultation when the patient complains of severe shortness of breath. Airflow may be so restricted that wheezing ceases.

A

◆ Diagnostic Evaluation

1. Increased levels of IgE in allergic asthma
2. Pulmonary function testing shows obstruction, especially decreased forced expiratory volume
3. Bronchial methacholine challenge test (inhalation of a cholinergic agent in serial concentrations delivered by nebulizer)—demonstrates airway hyperreactivity; positive response is indicated by a 20% decrease in the forced expiratory volume in 1 second (FEV_1) from the control value
4. Skin tests to identify causative allergens
5. Sputum and nasal cytology may detect eosinophilia.
6. Chest X-ray to rule out other lung diseases

◆ Collaborative Management

Therapeutic Interventions

1. Environmental control
   a. Minimize contact with offending allergens, regardless of other treatment.
   b. Dust mites can be removed from carpeting through treatment with 3% tannic acid or benzyl benzoate (Ascarosan).
2. Foods that contain tartrazine (yellow dye #5) may cause asthma in aspirin-sensitive patients and should be avoided.
3. Regular aerobic exercise. Use of an inhaled beta-agonist or cromolyn taken 15 to 20 minutes before exercise will decrease postexercise bronchospasm.
4. Prompt recognition and treatment of respiratory infections and exacerbation of asthma symptoms.
5. During acute attacks:
   a. Supplemental oxygen is given to maintain oxygen saturation above 95%.
   b. Cardiorespiratory monitoring and possible placement of arterial line for frequent blood gas measurements
   c. Respiratory support may be necessary with mechanical ventilation.
   d. Dehydration and thickened secretions caused by fever and increased insensible loss (through expired air) may require IV fluids.

A

Pharmacologic Interventions

1. Medications are used in a stepwise fashion, with additional therapies added as needed.
   a. Inhaled beta-agonist bronchodilators—first-line therapy; used for maintenance and increased with acute attacks
   b. Inhaled corticosteroids—added for exacerbations and may be needed for maintenance therapy in moderate asthma
   c. Inhaled cromolyn sodium—used prophylactically in extrinsic asthma
   d. Oral corticosteroids and oral beta-agonist or methylxanthine bronchodilators are added as second-line therapy for moderate to severe asthma.
   e. Inhaled anticholinergics may be tried if condition is unresponsive to beta-agonists.
2. Immunotherapy—desensitization of immune system to a known allergen(s) that causes type I (immediate) hypersensitivity

> **NURSING ALERT**
> Beta-adrenergic blocking agents such as propranolol should not be given to patients with asthma because of the potential to cause bronchoconstriction. They also should not be given to patients receiving immunotherapy, because they would make it difficult to reverse a systemic reaction, should one occur.

◆ Nursing Interventions

Monitoring

1. Monitor vital signs, skin color, and degree of restlessness, which may indicate hypoxia.
2. Monitor airway functioning through peak flow meter or spirometry to assess effectiveness of treatment.
3. Monitor oxygen saturation through finger oximetry and correlate to arterial blood gas measurement as indicated.

NURSING ALERT

Be aware of the following demographic and history factors that increase risk of asthma-related death: adolescence, African American ethnicity, exacerbation requiring hospitalization within the last year, exacerbation requiring intubation, and history of depression.

Supportive Care

1. Provide nebulization and oxygen therapy as prescribed.
2. Encourage fluid intake to liquefy secretions.
   a. Avoid iced fluids, which may cause bronchospasm.
   b. Avoid carbonated beverages, which may contribute to acidosis.
3. Instruct patient on positioning to facilitate breathing, for example, sitting upright (leaning forward on a table).
4. Employ chest physical therapy and postural drainage to mobilize secretions as needed.
5. Encourage patient to use pursed-lip breathing to decrease the work of breathing.

Family Education and Health Maintenance

1. Provide information on the nature of asthma and methods of treatment, including proper use of inhaler devices; warn against overuse of inhalers and nebulizers.

COMMUNITY CARE CONSIDERATIONS

Review technique for use of metered dose inhaler at every follow-up visit. If patient has difficulty with device, suggest that the health care provider prescribe a spacer to enhance inhalation technique.

2. Demonstrate the use of peak flow meter and recording of peak flow measurements.
3. Help patient to identify what triggers asthma, warning

A

signs of an impending attack, and strategies for preventing an attack. Advise of association of attacks with emotional stress.

4. Warn the patient to avoid taking sleeping pills after an asthma attack, because these medications slow respirations and make breathing more difficult.

5. Teach deep-breathing exercises to prevent atelectasis. Suggest breathing exercises for children at home, such as blowing a cotton ball across a table top or blowing large soap bubbles.

6. Discuss methods of environmental control.
   a. Avoid persons with respiratory infections.
   b. Avoid substances and situations known to precipitate bronchospasm, such as irritants, gases, fumes, and smoke.
   c. Wear a scarf across nose and mouth if cold weather precipitates bronchospasm.
   d. Stay inside when air pollution is high.

7. Promote optimal health practices, including nutrition, rest, and exercise.
   a. Encourage regular exercise to improve cardiorespiratory and musculoskeletal conditioning.
   b. Drink liberal amounts of fluids to keep secretions thin.
   c. Try to avoid upsetting situations.
   d. Use relaxation techniques, biofeedback management.
   e. Use community resources for smoking cessation classes, stress management, exercises for relaxation, etc.

8. Assist families to maintain sense of normalcy in everyday activities despite chronic disease. Suggest counseling as needed.

9. For additional information and support, refer to:

Asthma & Allergy Foundation of America
1125 15th St. NW, Suite 502
Washington, DC 20005
202-466-7643

Atopic Dermatitis
See Dermatitis, Atopic

Attention Deficit Disorder and Learning Disabilities

A

Attention deficit disorder (ADD), also known as attention deficit hyperactivity disorder, is characterized by a cluster of symptoms, including developmentally inappropriate short attention span, impulsivity, and distractibility. Hyperactivity is not always present. Learning disabilities (LD) and ADD often occur together. Learning disabilities are defined as a group of disorders manifested by significant difficulties in the acquisition of listening, speaking, reading, writing, reasoning, or mathematical abilities, or of social skills.

The exact causes of ADD and LD are not known; chromosomal abnormalities, inborn errors of metabolism, various prenatal and postnatal factors, neurotransmitter disturbances in the brain, and affinity with other handicapping conditions (eg, spina bifida, cerebral palsy, and seizure disorders) are being investigated. There is no evidence that ADD or LD are associated with a history of birth trauma or brain damage.

Estimates of the incidence of ADD among children range from 5% to 30%; LD is reportedly present in approximately 13% of children at the end of second grade. Boys are diagnosed twice as frequently as girls, and girls are less likely to exhibit disruptive behaviors.

◆ Assessment

1. ADD—according to the American Psychiatric Association, a child must have at least 8 of the 14 listed symptoms for more than 6 months:
   a. Fidgeting with hands or feet or squirming in seat
   b. Difficulty remaining seated when required to do so
   c. Easily distracted by extraneous stimuli
   d. Difficulty awaiting his or her turn
   e. Blurts out answers to questions before they have been completed
   f. Difficulty following instructions from others
   g. Difficulty sustaining attention in tasks or play activities

A

h. Shifts from one uncompleted activity to another
i. Difficulty playing quietly
j. Talks excessively
k. Interrupt or intrudes on others
l. Does not seem to listen to what is being said to him or her
m. Often loses things necessary for tasks or activities at school or at home
n. Often engages in physically dangerous activities without considering possible consequences

2. LD:
   a. School achievement is significantly below potential.
   b. Perceptual-motor impairments
   c. Emotional lability
   d. Speech and language disorders
   e. Coordination deficits
   f. Intelligence is usually normal or above normal.

◆ Diagnostic Evaluation

1. Complete medical review, family history, and physical examination, including vision and hearing assessment and neurologic evaluation, are done to rule out other disorders.
2. Psychological testing is done to determine the exact nature of cognitive and perceptual dysfunctions.
3. Behavioral and social assessment
4. Assessment of academic performance
5. Magnetic resonance imaging, electroencephalogram, or positron-emission tomography may be done to determine underlying neurologic abnormality.

NURSING ALERT

Historically, preschool and kindergarten screening tools have not been accurate in predicting LD; newer tests of language and memory appear to be better predictors.

◆ Collaborative Management

A

Therapeutic Interventions

1. Behavioral therapy and individual or family counseling may be necessary to deal with the emotional and social problems that arise from these disorders.
2. For children with LD, special teaching strategies:
   a. For visual perceptual deficit: present material verbally; use hands-on experience; tape-record teaching sessions.
   b. For auditory perceptual deficit: provide materials in written form; use pictures; provide tactile learning.
   c. For integrative deficit: use multisensory approaches; print directions while you verbalize them; use calendars and lists to organize tasks and activities.
   d. For motor/expressive deficits: break down skills and projects into their multiple component parts; verbally describe the component parts; provide extra time to perform; allow child to type work rather than using cursive writing.
   e. For highly distractible child—provide a structured environment; have child sit in front of class; place child away from doors or windows; decrease clutter on desk.

Pharmacologic Interventions

1. Central nervous system (CNS) stimulants such as methylphenidate or dextroamphetamine are effective in 70% to 75% of ADD children (usually reserved for children older than 7 years of age).
2. Side effects of central nervous system (CNS) stimulants:
   a. Insomnia may result from decreased dosage or if administered too late in the day.
   b. Anorexia and temporary growth retardation: height will catch up after medication is discontinued
   c. Increased pulse and respiratory rates, nervousness, nausea, and stomach ache
   d. Liver dysfunction with pemoline; periodic liver function tests are required

e. Altered effects of many antiseizure drugs and tri-cyclic antidepressants
3. Do not cause euphoric effect or addiction in children

B

◆ Nursing Interventions

Supportive Care and Family Education

1. Teach parents to administer medications before break-fast and lunch (sustained-release forms do not require a lunchtime dose).
2. Work with school system to insure lunch dose is given.
3. Recommend "drug holidays" during vacations and weekends to monitor effectiveness and the need for change; this is especially recommended at the start of each academic school year.
4. Advise parents that the child is usually started on a small dose, which is gradually increased until the de-sired response is achieved.
5. Evaluate the child's response to medication by direct observation and consultation with others, such as par-ent and teachers.
6. Refer to resource groups such as:

> **Council for Learning Disabilities**
> P.O. Box 40303
> Overland Park, KS 66204
> 913-492-8755

Back Pain, Low

Low back pain is characterized by an uncomfortable or acute pain in the lumbosacral area associated with severe spasm of the paraspinal muscles, often with radiating pain. Low back pain may result from many causes, including joint, muscular, or ligamentous sprains; disk infection, degeneration or herniation; lack of physical activity and exercise; arthritis; bone diseases; metastatic carcinoma; spinal cord tumors; congenital or systemic disorders; or vertebral infections. It may also result from referred pain from other areas. Complications include spinal instability, sensory and motor deficits, and chronic pain. In some cases low back pain may lead to malingering and other psychosocial reactions.

B

◆ Assessment

1. Pain localized to low back or radiating to buttocks or one or both legs
2. Paresthesias, numbness, weakness of lower extremities
3. Reflex loss
4. Bowel or bladder dysfunction (with cauda equina compression)

◆ Diagnostic Evaluation

1. X-rays of lumbar spine are usually negative.
2. Computed tomography of spine to detect arthritic changes, degenerative disk disease, tumor, and other abnormalities
3. Myelography to confirm and localize disk herniation
4. Magnetic resonance imaging to detect any pathology: disc herniation, soft tissue injury, etc.
5. Electromyography of lower extremities to detect nerve changes related to back pathology
6. Diskogram to detect herniated disk

◆ Collaborative Management

For management of herniated disk, see p. 428.
For management of spinal cord tumors, see p. 428.

Therapeutic Interventions

1. Bed rest in a supine to semi-Fowler's position with hips and knees flexed. Relieves painful muscle and ligament sprain, heals soft tissue injury, removes stress from lumbar sacral area and sciatic nerves, and opens the posterior part of the intervertebral spaces.

B

    a. Acute spasm and pain should subside in 3 to 7 days if there is no nerve involvement or other serious underlying disease.

    b. Isometric exercises should be done hourly while on bed rest if possible.

2. Heat or ice used to relax muscle spasm and relieve discomfort. Follow heat by massage.

3. Lumbosacral support may be used to provide abdominal compression and decreases load on lumbar intervertebral disks.

4. Transcutaneous electrical nerve stimulation (TENS) may be helpful in relieving pain.

5. Psychiatric intervention may be needed for the patient with chronic depression, anxiety, and low back syndrome.

6. Focus on getting back to functional state after long disability.

Pharmacologic Interventions

1. Oral pain medication and muscle relaxants: nonsteroidal antiinflammatory drugs (NSAIDs) are frequently used.

2. Painful trigger points may be injected with hydrocortisone or xylocaine for pain relief.

3. Parenteral and narcotic pain medication may be used in acute severe pain syndromes.

4. Psychotropic medication may be used for chronic pain and treatment of depression and anxiety, which potentiate pain.

◆ Nursing Interventions

Monitoring

1. Monitor pain level and compliance with activity restrictions.

2. Monitor for neurologic deficits indicating spinal nerve involvement, including reflex, sensory, and strength changes.

Supportive Care

1. Advise the patient to rest in bed on firm mattress or with bedboards beneath mattress for support. Bed rest may eliminate the need for pain medications.

2. Keep pillow between flexed knees while in side-lying position to minimize strain on back muscles.

3. Apply heat or ice as prescribed.
4. Administer or teach self-administration of pain medications and muscle relaxants as prescribed.
   a. Give NSAIDs with meals to prevent GI upset and bleeding.
   b. Muscle relaxants may cause drowsiness.
5. Encourage range-of-motion exercises of all uninvolved muscle groups.
6. Suggest gradual increase of activities and alternating activities with rest in semi-Fowler's position.
7. Avoid prolonged periods of sitting.
8. Encourage the patient to discuss problems that may be contributing to backache.
9. Encourage the patient to do prescribed back exercises to keep postural muscles strong, help recondition the back and abdominal musculature, and allow an outlet for emotional tension.

Patient Education and Health Maintenance

1. Instruct the patient to avoid recurrences as follows:
   a. Avoid prolonged sitting (intradiskal pressure in lumbar spine is higher during sitting), standing, and driving.
   b. Change positions and rest at frequent intervals.
   c. Avoid assuming tense, cramped positions.
   d. Sit in a straight-back, fairly high-seated chair. Sit with the knees higher than the hips. Use a footstool.
   e. Flatten the hollow of the back by sitting with the buttocks "tucked under." Pelvic tilt (small of back is pressed against a flat surface) decreases lordosis.
   f. Avoid knee and hip extension. When driving a car, have the seat pushed forward as necessary for comfort. Place a cushion in the small of the back for support.
2. Tell the patient to rest one foot on a small stool to relieve lumbar lordosis when sitting or standing for period of time.
3. Tell the patient to avoid fatigue, which contributes to spasm of back muscles.
4. Teach how to pick up objects or loads correctly:
   a. Maintain a straight spine.
   b. Flex knees and hips while stooping.
   c. Keep load close to body.
   d. Lift with the legs.

B

    e. Avoid twisting trunk while lifting.
    f. Avoid lifting above waist level and reaching up for any length of time.
5. Reinforce that daily exercise and maintenance of ideal weight is important to prevent back problems.
    a. Do prescribed back exercises twice daily to strengthen back, leg, and abdominal muscles.
    b. Walking outdoors (progressively increasing distance and pace) is recommended.

Bacterial Endocarditis

See Endocarditis, Infective

Bartholin Cyst or Abscess

Bartholin cyst or abscess, also called bartholinitis, results from obstruction and infection of the greater vestibular (Bartholin's) glands, which lie on both sides of the vagina at the base of the labia minora and serve to lubricate the vagina (Fig. 3). The abscess or cyst may spontaneously rupture or enlarge and become painful. Infection is often caused by sexually transmitted disease (STD).

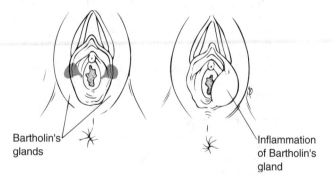

Bartholin's glands

Inflammation of Bartholin's gland

FIGURE 3   *Site and infection of vestibular gland.*

◆ Assessment

1. May be asymptomatic
2. Warmth, erythema, pain, swelling in labia minora
3. If abscess is present—pain, edema, cellulitis

◆ Diagnostic Evaluation

1. Culture of drainage or aspirated fluid to identify infectious organisms

◆ Collaborative Management

Therapeutic and Pharmacologic Interventions

1. Provide warm soaks or sitz baths.
2. If cellulitis or STD is present, administer antibiotics.

Surgical Interventions

1. Abscess or cyst may require incision and drainage. This provides immediate relief, but problem may recur.
2. Marsupialization, for recurrent abscesses:
   a. Contents are opened and drained, then edges of abscess are sutured to edges of external incision to keep cavity open.
   b. Healing occurs from within the area of the abscess.

◆ Nursing Interventions

Supportive Care

1. Administer pain medications as indicated.
2. Instruct the patient to apply warm soaks or take sitz bath three to four times a day for 15 to 20 minutes to promote comfort and drainage.
3. Encourage the patient to remain in bed as much as possible, because pain is exacerbated by activity.
4. Prepare the patient for incision and drainage if indicated.
5. For marsupialization: apply ice packs intermittently for 24 hours to reduce edema and provide comfort; thereafter warm sitz baths or a perineal heat pack or lamp can be used to provide comfort.
6. Explain to the patient that infection may have been caused by STD:

   a. Tell the patient to instruct her partner to be tested for sexually transmitted diseases.

   b. Advise the patient to abstain from intercourse until cyst or abscess has completely resolved and she has completed all her antibiotics.

Patient Education and Health Maintenance

1. Review principles of perineal hygiene with the patient.
2. Discuss sexually transmitted diseases and methods of prevention.
3. Encourage patient to follow-up for recurrent abscess, because surgical treatment is often necessary.

Bipolar Disorders

Bipolar disorders are characterized by depressive episodes and one or more elated mood episodes. Cause is unknown, but genetic, physiologic, and psychological factors are involved. In the most intense presentation, the bipolar individual experiences altered thought processes that can produce bizarre delusions. Untreated bipolar disorder can lead to physical exhaustion.

◆ Assessment

Characteristics according to the American Psychological Association *Diagnostic and Statistical Manual IV (1994):*

1. Bipolar I disorder
   a. Presence of only one manic episode
   b. No past major depressive episodes
   c. Manic episode is not accounted for by schizoaffective disorder.
   d. Manic episode is not superimposed on schizophrenia, schizophreniform disorder, delusional disorder, or psychotic disorder.
   e. May be further specified as: with mixed symptoms, psychotic, in remission, with catatonic features, or postpartum onset
2. Bipolar II disorder
   a. Presence/history of one or more major depressive episodes

  b. Presence/history of at least one hypomanic episode
  c. No manic or mixed episodes have occurred.
  d. The symptoms cause clinically significant distress or impaired social or occupational functioning.
  e. May be further specified as hypomanic or depressed

B

3. Cyclothymic disorder
  a. Over a period of 2 years, there are numerous periods without hypomanic symptoms and numerous periods with depressive symptoms that do not meet criteria for a major depressive episode.
  b. During the 2-year period, the patient has not been without these symptoms for more than 2 months at a time.
  c. During the 2-year period, no major depressive episode, manic episode, or mixed episode has occurred.
  d. Symptoms are not caused by physiologic aspects.
  e. Symptoms cause clinically significant distress or impairment in all aspects of functioning.

◆ Diagnostic Evaluation

1. Rating scale assessment tools:
  a. Mania Rating Scale
  b. Mini Mental Status Examination
2. Complete psychophysiological examination

◆ Collaborative Management

Therapeutic Interventions

1. Psychotherapy includes individual therapy and family therapy.
2. Psychiatric home care nursing may be required to facilitate compliance with medications and therapeutic interventions.
3. Community-based support group participation may be recommended.

Pharmacologic Interventions

1. For acute mania; usually treated in the hospital to ensure a safe environment to initiate and stabilize medication:
  a. Lithium carbonate is the drug of choice.

B

   b. Adjunctive treatment includes neuroleptic agents such as haloperidol, benzodiazepines such as clonazepam, and anticonvulsants such as carbamazepine for mood-stabilizing properties.
   c. Combination therapy consisting of lithium and an anticonvulsant may be used.
2. For acute depression:
   a. Lithium carbonate
   b. Combination therapy consisting of antidepressant and lithium
   c. Monoamine oxidase (MAO) inhibitors
3. Maintenance therapy is instituted once stabilized.

◆ Nursing Interventions

Monitoring

1. Monitor mood for range of affect.
2. Monitor behavior for hyperactivity, increased appetite, indiscriminate sexual activity, poor concentration, little or no sleep, spending large sums of money, and other inappropriate acts.
3. Monitor thought processes for flight of ideas, sexually explicit speech, delusions, hallucinations, and clang associations (sound of word, rather than meanings, directs subsequent associations).
4. Monitor vital signs, weight, and urine output for patient in acute mania.
5. Monitor serum thyroid function test and electrolyte results for patient on lithium.

Supportive Care

1. Assess patient's degree of distorted thinking; redirect the patient if difficult to follow patient's thought processes.
2. Use brief explanations; remain consistent in approach and expectations.
3. Frequently reality-orient the patient; speak in a clear, simple manner.
4. Provide the patient with a relaxing area with decreased environmental stimulation.
5. Assist the patient with a gradual and progressive integration into the social environment while observing

for behavioral changes that indicate readiness for participation in further activities.

6. To facilitate adequate sleep, establish a distraction-free environment at bedtime, and help the patient avoid caffeine and nicotine intake.

7. Administer prescribed medications as ordered and monitor the patient's response.

8. Maintain accurate documentation of food and fluid intake.

9. Offer small, frequent meals of high-calorie food. Include food that the patient likes and can be eaten "on the move."

10. Serve the patient meals in a low-stimulus environment.

11. Observe and assess interaction patterns within the family and discuss their influence on the patient and his or her family functioning.

Patient Education and Health Maintenance

1. Reinforce instructions to patient and family about bipolar illness; teach about symptoms of relapse.

2. Instruct patient and family members about psychopharmacologic treatment, including its purpose, effects, side effects, and management.

3. Advise patient and family members about community-based support groups or health care agencies that are relevant to their care.

Bladder Cancer
See Cancer, Bladder

Bone Cancer
See Cancer, Bone

Brain Tumors in Adults

A *brain tumor* is a localized intracranial neoplasm. Tumors may originate in any tissue in the central nervous system

B

(CNS) or metastasize from tumors elsewhere in the body. There are many types of benign or malignant brain tumors, and all produce effects of a space-occupying lesion (cerebral edema, increased intracranial pressure [IICP]). Malignancy may be related not to cell type or invasiveness, but, rather, to location and inoperability.

Tumor types include astrocytoma (arising from connective tissue of the brain, highly invasive); glioblastoma (grade 3 and 4 astrocytomas); oligodendroglioma (arising from frontal and temporal lobes of the cerebrum); colloid cyst (develop with lateral or third ventricles); meningioma (arising from linings of the brain); acoustic neuroma (develops in or on eighth cranial nerve); metastatic lesions (usually multiple and unresectable); pituitary or pineal tumors; hemangioma (from blood vessels of the brain); and congenital tumors. Complications include IICP and brain herniation and neurologic deficits from the expanding tumor or treatment.

◆ Assessment

1. Signs and symptoms of tumor caused by IICP, including morning headaches, vomiting, papilledema, altered mental status, and malaise
2. Cranial nerve, motor, sensory, behavioral, affect, and cognitive dysfunction are possible.
3. Focal neurologic deficits related to region of tumor:
   a. Parietal area—motor or sensory alterations, speech and memory disturbances, visuospatial deficits
   b. Frontal lobe—personality changes, contralateral motor weakness, Broca's aphasia
   c. Temporal area—memory disturbances, auditory hallucinations, Wernicke's aphasia, complex partial seizures, visual field deficits
   d. Occipital area—visual agnosia and visual field deficits
   e. Cerebellar area—coordination, gait and balance disturbances
   f. Brain stem—dysphagia, incontinence, cardiovascular instability, cranial nerve dysfunction
   g. Hypothalamus—loss of temperature control, diabetes insipidus
   h. Pituitary/sella turcica—visual field deficits, amen-

orrhea, galactorrhea, impotence, Cushingoid symptoms

◆ Diagnostic Evaluation

1. Computed tomography or magnetic resonance imaging to visualize a tumor, associated edema, and shift of structures caused by mass effect
2. EEG detects locus of irritability.
3. Stereotactic biopsy/surgery may be done to confirm the diagnosis and identify tumor type.

◆ Collaborative Management

Therapeutic and Pharmacologic Interventions

1. Effectiveness of treatment depends on tumor type and location, capsulation or infiltrative status. Tumors in vital areas such as the brain stem or those that are nonencapsulated and infiltrating may not be surgically accessible, and treatment may produce severe neurologic deficits (blindness, paralysis, mental impairment).
2. Whole-brain radiation may begin after scalp incision heals (may cause brain edema and delayed necrosis) or brachytherapy (radioisotopes implanted directly into tumor to permit high doses) may be performed.
3. Single or combination chemotherapy may be used. Autologous bone marrow transplantation may be desirable, in which bone marrow is aspirated before chemotherapy and reinfused afterward to treat bone marrow depression.

Surgical Interventions

1. Procedures include stereotaxic resection, with preceding corticosteroid and anticonvulsant therapy, laser resection, or ultrasonic aspiration

◆ Nursing Interventions

Monitoring

1. Monitor the patient's responses to therapy. Be alert for change in level of consciousness, neurologic deficits, IICP, abnormal respirations.

2. Report any signs of IICP (decreased level of consciousness, elevated temperature, widening pulse pressure, bradycardia, irregular respirations, pupillary changes, headache, vomiting) or worsening condition immediately.
3. Monitor for seizure activity and have medications available for management of status epilepticus.
4. Monitor fluid and electrolyte balance to prevent dehydration.

Supportive Care

1. Provide analgesics and comfort measures according to patient's level of pain, as ordered.
   a. Maintain a quiet environment to increase the patient's pain tolerance.
   b. Provide scheduled rest periods to help the patient recuperate from stress of pain.
   c. Darken the room or provide sunglasses if the patient is photophobic.
2. Instruct the patient to lie with the operative side up.
3. Maintain the head of the bed at 15 to 30 degrees to reduce cerebral venous congestion; if the patient is dysphagic or unconscious, position the head to the side to prevent aspiration.
4. Position dysphagic patient upright and instruct in sequenced swallowing to facilitate feeding.
   a. Keep oxygen and suction equipment at bedside in case of aspiration.
   b. Alter diet as tolerated if the patient has pain when chewing.
5. If the patient has visual field deficits, place materials in visual field; teach the patient to scan to the "other side" and place weak extremities in safe position when moving in bed or chair.
6. Pad the side rails of the bed to prevent injury if seizures occur.
7. Provide appropriate care and teaching for the patient receiving chemotherapy, radiation, or craniotomy.

Patient Education and Health Maintenance

1. Explain the side effects of treatment, such as nausea, vomiting, alopecia, bone marrow depression.
2. Encourage close follow-up after diagnosis and treatment.

3. Explain the importance of continuing corticosteroids and how to manage side effects such as weight gain and hyperglycemia.
4. Encourage the use of community resources for physical and psychological support, such as transportation to medical appointments, financial assistance, respite care.
5. Refer the patient and family to:

> **American Brain Tumor Association**
> 2720 River Rd.
> Desplains, IL 60018
> 708-827-9910

Brain Tumors in Children

Brain tumors in children, as in adults, are localized intracranial neoplasms that produce effects of a space-occupying lesion. Approximately 20% of malignant tumors that occur in children are brain tumors. In children, they most commonly occur between ages 2 and 12 years, and they are one of the most common causes of death from cancer. Tumors commonly occurring in children fall into four main types:

Cerebellar astrocytoma is a slow-growing, often cystic type of tumor of the cerebellum, and accounts for about 10% to 20% of all pediatric brain tumors.

Medulloblastoma is a highly malignant, rapidly growing tumor, usually found in the cerebellum. As the tumor grows, it seeds along cerebrospinal fluid pathways. It is the single most common CNS tumor in children.

Brain stem glioma interferes early with the function of cranial nerve nuclei, pyramidal tracts, and cerebellar pathways. This type accounts for approximately 15% of brain tumors in children.

Ependymoma is a tumor derived from the ependyma, the lining of the central canal of the spinal cord and cerebral ventricles. It commonly arises on the floor of the fourth ventricle, obstructing the flow of cerebrospinal fluid. These tumors may invade the cardiorespiratory center, cerebellum, and spinal cord. Ependymomas represent about 5% to 10% of all primary childhood CNS tumors.

Prognosis is improved with early diagnosis and adequate therapy. The 5-year survival rate is increasing, especially in children with low-grade astrocytomas or ependymomas. Without treatment, however, brain stem herniation and hydrocephalus may occur.

B

◆ Assessment

1. Cerebellar astrocytoma—insidious onset and slow course
   a. Increased intracranial pressure (IICP)—headache, visual disturbances, papilledema, and personality changes
   b. Cerebellar signs—ataxia, dysmetria (inability to control the range of muscular movement), and nystagmus
   c. Behavioral changes
2. Medulloblastoma
   a. Similar to manifestations of cerebellar astrocytoma, but condition develops more rapidly
   b. The child may present with unsteady gait, anorexia, vomiting, and early-morning headache, and later develop ataxia, nystagmus, papilledema, drowsiness, and increased head circumference.
3. Brain stem glioma
   a. Cranial nerve palsies, such as strabismus, fasciculations of the tongue, and swallowing difficulties
   b. Hemiparesis, cerebellar ataxia
   c. Signs of increased intracranial pressure (rare)
4. Ependymoma of the fourth ventricle
   a. Signs of IICP
   b. Unsteady gait/ataxia, dysmetria
   c. Focal motor weakness, visual disturbances, seizures
5. Observe for the appearance or disappearance of any of the clinical manifestations described above. Report these to the health care provider and record each in detail.

◆ Diagnostic Evaluation

1. Several or all of the following procedures may be used to localize and determine tumor extent:
   a. Computed tomography

b. Angiography
c. Magnetic resonance imaging
d. Myelogram
e. Positron emission tomography
f. Lumbar puncture
g. Electroencephalogram—of limited value, but possibly useful when seizures are manifested

◆ Collaborative Management

Surgical Interventions

1. Surgery is performed to determine the type of the tumor and the extent of invasiveness, and to excise as much of the lesion as possible.
2. A ventriculoperitoneal shunt is often necessary for children who develop hydrocephalus.

Therapeutic and Pharmacologic Interventions

1. Radiation therapy is usually initiated as soon as the diagnosis is established and the surgical wound healed.
2. Chemotherapy is used in children younger than age 4 years with medulloblastoma to avoid early radiation, and in children with ependymomas.

◆ Nursing Interventions

Monitoring

1. Monitor vital signs, level of consciousness, and pupillary reaction frequently.
2. Observe for signs of brain stem herniation—should be considered a neurosurgical emergency.
   a. Attacks of opisthotonos (excessive arching of back)
   b. Tilting of the head; neck stiffness
   c. Poorly reactive pupils
   d. Increased blood pressure; widened pulse pressure
   e. Change in respiratory rate and nature of respirations
   f. Irregularity of pulse or lowered pulse rate
   g. Alterations of body temperature

B

❖

NURSING ALERT

Signs of brain stem herniation, especially opisthotonos, are ominous. The health care provider should be called immediately and the child prepared for ventricular tap to relieve pressure. Have resuscitation equipment on hand.

3. Monitor temperature closely after surgery.
   a. A marked rise in temperature may be attributable to trauma, disturbance of the heat-regulating center, or to intracranial edema.
   b. If hyperthermia occurs, administer antipyretics and sponge baths as ordered. Temperature should not be reduced too rapidly.
4. Observe for signs of shock, increased intracranial pressure, and altered level of consciousness.

Supportive Care

1. Prepare the parents for the postoperative appearance of their child; advise that the child might be comatose immediately after surgery.
2. Prepare the child for surgery; explain procedures at the appropriate developmental level.
3. Prepare the child for postoperative expectations (ie, child may feel sleepy or have a headache and will need to remain supine).
4. Administer narcotics as ordered in the immediate postoperative period; assess the child's level of consciousness before administration.
5. Position the child according to surgeon's request; usually on unaffected side with head level. Raising the foot of the bed may increase intracranial pressure and bleeding.
6. Change the child's position frequently and provide meticulous skin care to prevent hypostatic pneumonia and pressure sores.
7. Move the child carefully and slowly, being certain to move the head in line with the body.
8. Support paralyzed or spastic extremities with pillows, towel rolls, or other means.
9. Initiate feeding of the child when the child is fully

alert. Refeed the child after he or she vomits. (Vomiting is not usually associated with nausea.)

10. If the child is unable to eat, provide tube feedings. A gastrostomy tube may be inserted.

11. Maintain IV hydration or hyperalimentation and intralipids if indicated.

12. Check the surgical dressing for bleeding and for drainage of cerebrospinal fluid.

13. Assess the child for edema of the head, face, and neck.

14. Carefully regulate fluid administration to prevent increased cerebral edema.

15. Have equipment readily available for cardiopulmonary resuscitation, respiratory assistance, oxygen inhalation, blood transfusion, ventricular tap, and other potential emergency situations.

16. If the child is receiving chemotherapy or radiation, instruct the parents to report a fever of over 101°F (38.4°C) or nausea and vomiting unrelated to chemotherapy.

17. Encourage the child to express feelings regarding the threat to body image.

18. Reassure the child that he or she will be able to wear a wig or a hat after recovery; hair will grow back.

19. Help the parents to see the child's increasing capabilities and encourage them to foster independence.

Family Education and Health Maintenance

1. Provide parents with written information regarding the child's needs—medications, activity, care of the incision, and follow-up appointments.

2. Teach the parents about radiation or chemotherapy treatments and their side effects.

3. If a child has a ventriculoperitoneal shunt, teach parents to recognize and report fever, nausea, vomiting, irritability, or a bulging anterior fontanelle.

4. Initiate a referral to a community health nurse to reinforce teaching and to maintain therapeutic support for the family.

5. For additional resources, refer family to agencies such as:

American Brain Tumor Association
2720 River Rd.
Des Plaines, IL 60018
708-827-9910

Breast Cancer
See Cancer, Breast

B

Bronchiectasis

Bronchiectasis is a chronic dilatation of the bronchi and bronchioles caused by inflammation and destruction of bronchiolar walls. Sputum accumulates and obstructs the bronchioles; poor airway clearance results in severe coughing, which permanently dilates the bronchi. This disorder usually involves the lower lung lobes, and may progress to atelectasis, fibrosis, and respiratory insufficiency. Bronchiectasis is commonly caused by pulmonary infections; bronchial obstruction; aspiration of foreign bodies, vomitus or material from the upper respiratory tract; and immunologic disorders.

Complications include progressive suppuration, major pulmonary hemorrhage, emphysema, and chronic respiratory insufficiency.

◆ Assessment

1. Persistent cough, with copious amounts of purulent sputum; intermittent hemoptysis; breathlessness
2. Diffuse rhonchi and coarse crackles heard over involved lobes during inspiration
3. Recurrent fever and pulmonary infections
4. Finger clubbing commonly occurs late in the disorder.

◆ Diagnostic Evaluation

1. Chest x-rays detect areas of atelectasis with possibly widespread dilatation of bronchi.
2. Sputum specimens for smears and cultures to identify causative organisms

◆ Collaborative Management

Therapeutic Interventions
1. Smoking cessation program

2. Chest physiotherapy and postural drainage to mobilize bronchial secretions

Pharmacologic Interventions

1. Antimicrobials to treat exacerbations of infection
2. Bronchodilators are effective for selected patients with increased airway hyperreactivity.
3. Influenza immunization yearly and pneumococcal pneumonia vaccine to protect the patient against potential pulmonary pathogens

Surgical Interventions

1. Segmental resection of the lung is done when conservative management fails (see p. 827).

◆ Nursing Interventions

Supportive Care

1. Use percussion, vibration, postural drainage, and encourage productive coughing to help mobilize secretions.
2. Encourage increased fluid intake and use a vaporizer to reduce viscosity of sputum and facilitate expectoration.
3. Be alert to exacerbations characterized by change in sputum production.

Patient Education and Health Maintenance

1. Instruct the patient to avoid noxious fumes, dusts, smoke, and other pulmonary irritants.
2. Teach the patient to watch for and report changes in sputum quantity or character.
3. Encourage regular dental care because copious sputum production may affect dentition.
4. Instruct the patient and family to implement drainage exercises and chest physical therapy. Encourage the patient to use postural drainage before rising in the morning, to remove nocturnal sputum accumulation.
5. Advise engaging in physical activity throughout day to help mobilize secretions.
6. Emphasize the importance of influenza and pneumonia immunizations and prompt treatment of all respiratory infections.
7. Monitor response to therapy. Be alert to exacerbations characterized by change in sputum production.

Bronchitis, Acute

B

Acute bronchitis is an infection of the lower respiratory tract that generally follows an upper respiratory tract infection. As a result of this viral (most common) or bacterial infection, the airways become inflamed and irritated, and mucus production increases.

◆ Assessment

1. Cough with clear to purulent sputum production
2. Diffuse rhonchi and crackles (contrast with localized crackles usually heard with pneumonia)
3. Fever, tachypnea, pleuritic chest pain may be present.

◆ Diagnostic Evaluation

1. Chest x-ray may be taken to rule out pneumonia. In bronchitis, films show no evidence of lung infiltrates or consolidation.

◆ Collaborative Management

Therapeutic Interventions
1. Chest physiotherapy if indicated to mobilize secretions
2. Hydration to liquefy secretions

Pharmacologic Interventions
1. Antibiotics for 7 to 10 days to treat the causative infection
2. Inhaled bronchodilators to reduce bronchospasm and promote sputum expectoration

◆ Nursing Interventions

Supportive Care
1. Encourage mobilization of secretions through ambulation, coughing, and deep breathing.
2. Ensure adequate fluid intake to liquefy secretions and prevent dehydration caused by fever and tachypnea.
3. Encourage rest, avoidance of bronchial irritants, and good diet to facilitate recovery.

Patient Education and Health Maintenance

1. Instruct the patient to complete the full course of prescribed antibiotics and explain the effect of meals on drug absorption.

2. Caution the patient on using over-the-counter cough suppressants, antihistamines, and decongestants that may cause drying and retention of secretions. However, cough preparations containing the mucolytic guaifenesin may be appropriate.

3. Advise the patient that a dry cough may persist after bronchitis because of irritation of airways. Suggest avoiding dry environments and using a humidifier at bedside.

4. Teach the patient to recognize and immediately report early signs and symptoms of acute bronchitis.

Bronchogenic Cancer
See Cancer, Lung

Bulimia Nervosa
See Eating Disorders

Burns

Burns are a form of traumatic injury caused by thermal, electrical, chemical, or radioactive agents. Most burn-related accidents occur at home, and most others occur at work. Flame injury is the leading cause of accidents for adults, and scalding is the leading cause of accidents for children.

Burns may be partial or full thickness (Fig. 4). *Partial-thickness* burn injuries involve the epidermis and upper portions of the dermis. Some of the dermal appendages remain, from which the wound can spontaneously reepithelialize. In *full-thickness* injuries, all layers of the skin and sometimes underlying tissues are destroyed. Grafting usually is required to close the wound.

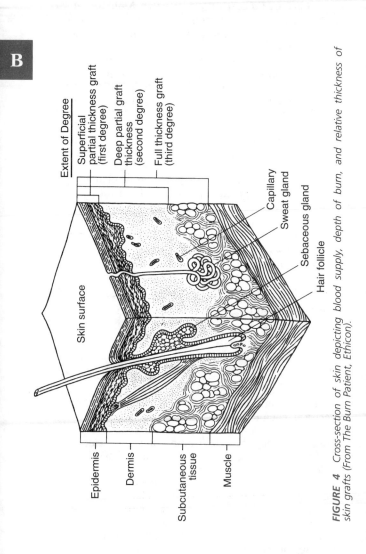

FIGURE 4 *Cross-section of skin depicting blood supply, depth of burn, and relative thickness of skin grafts (From The Burn Patient, Ethicon).*

Extent of Degree

Superficial partial thickness graft (first degree)

Deep partial graft thickness (second degree)

Full thickness graft (third degree)

Skin surface

Capillary

Sweat gland

Sebaceous gland

Hair follicle

Epidermis

Dermis

Subcutaneous tissue

Muscle

Inhalation injury (from smoke particles, toxic gases such as carbon monoxide, sulfur dioxide, nitrous oxide, and fumes from burning plastics) causes 50% to 60% of fire deaths.

Infection and pulmonary complications also significantly increase morbidity and mortality.

B

◆ Assessment

1. Assess airway, breathing, and circulation as indicated and intervene as necessary.
2. Assess burn severity.
   a. Depth: 1st-, 2nd-, 3rd-degree (Table 2)
   b. Extent: percent total body surface area (TBSA). Use "rule of nines" chart (Fig. 5) or Lund and Browder chart for children.

NURSING ALERT:
Burns affecting hands, feet, face, and perineum require specialized care. Circumferential burns also require special attention and may require escharotomy.

3. Assess for signs of smoke inhalation: upper body burns; erythema or blistering of lips, buccal mucosa or pharynx; singed nares hair; soot in oropharynx; dark gray or black sputum; hoarseness; crackles on auscultation.

NURSING ALERT:
Increasing hoarseness, stuttering, or drooling indicate need for intubation.

4. Evaluate all patients in closed-space fires for symptoms of carbon monoxide poisoning: headache, visual changes, confusion, irritability, decreased judgment, nausea, ataxia, collapse.

TABLE 2 Assessment of Burn Injuries

Degree and Assessment	Treatment Considerations
First-Degree Burn	
1. Pink to red; slight edema, subsides quickly	1. Epidermis peels in about 5 days
2. Pain may last up to 48 hours, relieved by cooling	2. Itching and pink skin persist for about 1 week
	3. No scarring occurs
	4. Heals spontaneously in 10 days to 2 weeks in absence of infection
Second-Degree Burn	
1. Superficial	1. Takes several weeks to heal
a. Pink or red; vesicles form—weeping, edematous	2. Scarring may occur
b. Superficial skin layers destroyed; leaves moist, painful wound	
2. Deep dermal	
a. Mottled white and red; edematous reddened areas blanch on pressure	
b. May be yellowish, soft and elastic; may or may not be sensitive to touch; sensitive to cold air	
Third-Degree Burn	
1. Destruction of epidermis, dermis, fat, muscle, and bone	1. Eschar must be removed by debridement. Granulation tissue forms to nearest epithelium from wound margins or support graft
2. Reddened areas do not blanch with pressure	2. Grafting is required for areas larger than 3 to 5 cm (1.2–1.9 in)
3. Wound not painful; inelastic; coloration varies from waxy white to brown (leathery devitalized tissue—eschar)	3. Expect scarring and loss of skin function

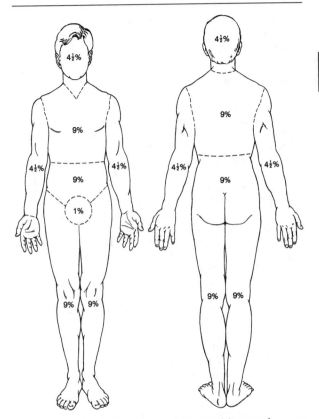

FIGURE 5 *Rule of nines for calculating total burn surface area (TBSA).*

◆ Diagnostic Evaluation

1. Arterial blood gases (ABGs), carboxyhemoglobin levels and spirometry may be measured to assess for inhalation injury.
2. Bronchoscopy may be needed to visualize vocal chord damage.
3. A chest x-ray should be done to obtain baseline information.

4. CBC, BUN, and creatinine, electrolytes, and other laboratory tests will be performed at baseline and monitored periodically.

B

◆ Collaborative Management

Therapeutic Interventions

1. Immediate intravenous fluid resuscitation is indicated for:
   a. Adults with burns over more than 15% to 20% of body surface area
   b. Children with burns involving more than 10% of body surface area
   c. Patients with electrical injury, the elderly, or anyone with cardiac or pulmonary disease and compromised response to burn injury
2. Generally a crystalloid (Ringer's lactate) solution is used initially. Colloid is used during the second day (5% albumin or plasma).
3. The Parkland formula is most commonly used to determine fluid requirements in the first 48 hours. The Brooks & Evans formulas may also be used. Parkland formula is as follows.
   a. First 24 hours: 4 mL Ringer's lactate × weight in kg × %TBSA burned.
   b. Half the fluid is given in the first 8 hours, calculated from the time of injury. If the starting of fluids is delayed, then the same amount of fluid is given over the remaining time.
   c. The remaining half of the fluid is given over the next 16 hours.
   d. Second 24 hours: 0.5 mL colloid × weight in kg × %TBSA + 2000 mL 5% D/W run concurrently over the 24-hour period
   e. Boluses of crystalloid or colloid may be necessary to maintain urinary output of 0.5 to 1 mL/kg/hr.
4. Initially, the patient is kept NPO until bowel sounds return (1–2 days). However, small amounts (5–10 mL/hr) of isotonic enteral tube feedings are often started within 24 hours to help maintain a functioning gastrointestinal tract. Small amounts of erythromycin may be used to encourage gastrointestinal motility.

5. When caloric requirements cannot be met by enteral feedings, total parenteral nutrition is initiated.
6. Treatment of the burn wound includes daily or twice-daily wound cleansing with debridement, or hydrotherapy (tubbing) and dressing changes. Enzymatic agents may be applied to speed debridement.
7. Burn wound coverings are applied to close the wound temporarily, protect granulation tissue, reduce pain, and help determine when granulating wounds will accept an autograft successfully.
   a. *Biologic dressings* are used to cover large surfaces of the body. Usually they are split-thickness grafts harvested either from human cadavers or other mammalian donors such as pigs. Human amnion also may be used.
   b. *Biosynthetic dressings* are used when permanent autografts are unavailable or not necessary (as when partial-thickness wounds will heal spontaneously over time).
   c. *Artificial dermis* material is being studied in selected burn centers to improve survival of patients with massive burns and little available donor skin.
8. Physical therapy, occupational therapy, and psychiatric support are provided.

Pharmacologic Interventions

1. Narcotics to control pain
2. Topical antimicrobials are applied directly to the burn area or incorporated in single-layer dressings that do not stick to the wound but permit drainage.
3. Intravenous antibiotics may be given prophylactically to prevent gram-positive infection.
4. Wounds, urine, sputum, and so forth are cultured and specific antibiotics given as indicated.

Surgical Interventions

1. Early excision of nonviable skin and grafting reduces wound infection and speeds recovery; however, this incurs significant blood loss and increases metabolic demands.
   a. Tangential excision (excision of thin layers of damaged skin until live tissue is evidenced by capillary bleeding) is used with deep partial-thickness burns.

B

b. Fascial (primary) excision (skin, lymphatics, and subcutaneous tissue removed down to fascia) is done for full-thickness burns.

2. Skin grafting is usually required or preferred with full-thickness burns greater than 2 cm in diameter or in deep partial-thickness wounds.

3. Grafts of the patient's own skin (autografts) are applied after gradual eschar removal and development of a base of granulating tissue, or in the presence of viable tissue following excision. Sheet grafts or meshed grafts, which provide wider expansion from donor sites, may be used.

4. Three to 4 days after grafting, blood flow is established, and after 7 to 10 days, vascular continuity and wound closure are established.

5. Cultured epithelial autografts (CEAs) may be used for patients with large burns and little available donor skin.

◆ Nursing Interventions

Monitoring

1. Check vital signs every 15 minutes until stabilized, then as often as needed.

2. Monitor respiratory rate, depth, rhythm, cough; observe for signs of respiratory distress.

3. Monitor tidal volume in the patient with chest burns; report decreasing volume to health care provider.

4. Monitor central venous pressure and pulmonary artery pressure as indicated to help guide fluid resuscitation.

5. Monitor peripheral pulses hourly. Use Doppler as necessary.

6. Monitor hydration status, intake and output, daily weight, and urine specific gravity.

7. Monitor serum levels of potassium and other electrolytes.

8. Monitor temperature, white blood cell count, and differential.

9. In inhalation injury, monitor ABGs and oxygen saturation.

10. Monitor wounds for signs of infection.

11. Monitor the patient's response to pain control.

B

Supportive Care

1. Provide humidified 100% oxygen until blood level of carbon monoxide is known. (**Caution**: Adjust oxygen flow rate for the patient with chronic obstructive pulmonary disease [COPD] as prescribed.) If the patient is stable, try to get the initial ABG on room air.
2. Assess for signs of hypoxemia (anxiousness, tachypnea, tachycardia) and differentiate this from pain.
3. In mild inhalation injury, provide humidification of inspired air and encourage coughing and deep breathing.
4. In moderate to severe inhalation injury, initiate frequent suctioning, administer bronchodilator treatments, and monitor closely.
5. Be prepared to intubate patient and provide mechanical ventilation, continuous positive airway pressure, or positive end-expiratory pressure if requested.
6. Place the patient in semi-Fowler's position to permit maximal chest excursions if there are no contraindications, such as hypotension or spinal cord injury.
7. Ensure that chest dressings are not constricting.
8. Elevate extremities to prevent edema.
9. Monitor tissue pressure surrounding burns and prepare the patient for escharotomy if circulation is impaired.
10. Be alert to signs of fluid overload and congestive heart failure, especially during initial fluid resuscitation and immediately after, when fluid mobilization is occurring.

GERIATRIC ALERT
The elderly and those with impaired renal function, cardiovascular disease, and pulmonary disease are more likely to develop fluid overload from fluid replacement therapy. Proceed with caution.

11. Administer diuretics as ordered.
12. Cleanse wounds and change dressings twice daily. Use an antimicrobial solution and saline solution, or mild soap and water. Dry gently. This may be done in the hydrotherapy tank, bathtub, shower, or at the bedside.

B

13. Perform debridement of dead tissue at this time. May use gauze, scissors, or pickups or forceps as appropriate. Try to limit time to 20 to 30 minutes, depending on the patient's tolerance. Additional analgesia may be necessary.

14. Apply topical antimicrobial agents as directed. Cream or ointment is applied ⅛″ to ¼″ thick unless otherwise indicated.

15. Dress wounds as appropriate, using burn pads, gauze rolls, or any combination. Dressings may be held in place as necessary with gauze rolls or netting.

16. Describe hydrotherapy to the patient who is experiencing it for the first time, coordinate timing of pain medication, and assure the patient that you will stay.
    a. If the patient has an indwelling catheter, drain and plug it, or maintain a closed system to avoid contamination.
    b. Use aseptic technique in preparing the patient for hydrotherapy, during hydrotherapy, and in redressing wounds after therapy.
    c. After cleansing of the wounds, debride wound, shave adjacent areas at health care provider's direction, shampoo hair, and gently wash normal skin.
    d. Limit hydrotherapy to as brief a time as possible to minimize loss of body heat and subsequent chilling.

17. For grafted areas, use extreme caution in removing dressings; observe for and report serous or sanguineous blebs or purulent drainage. Redress grafted areas according to protocol.

18. Observe all wounds daily, and document wound status on the patient's record.

19. Use radiant warmers, warming blankets, or adjust the room temperature to keep the patient warm because thermoregulatory ability is impaired.

20. Use meticulous handwashing and barrier garments (isolation gown or plastic apron) for all care requiring contact with the patient or the patient's bed; cover hair and wear mask when wounds are exposed or when performing a sterile procedure.

21. Check history of tetanus immunization and provide passive or active tetanus prophylaxis as indicated.

22. Ensure consultation with physical and occupational therapists who will exercise the patient at least once

or twice daily, and order splints to prevent contractures.

23. Consult with dietitian for calculation of nutritional needs based on age, weight, height, and burn size.

24. Administer potassium, vitamins and mineral supplements as prescribed.

25. Check amount and pH of gastric drainage after down time of tube feedings and administer H_2 blockers and antacids as prescribed to prevent stress ulcers.

26. Explore with the patient alternative mechanisms for coping with the burn injury and its consequences.

27. Facilitate psychological counseling as indicated.

28. Arrange for the patient to see face (if burned) with appropriate supportive personnel before being transferred to a room with a mirror.

29. Encourage participation in a burn survivors' group, such as the Phoenix Society.

30. Use and emphasize the concept of being a burn survivor, rather than a "burn victim," which enhances the sick role.

Family Education and Health Maintenance

1. Demonstrate and explain wound care procedures to be continued after discharge:
   a. Wash hands.
   b. Cleanse small open wounds with mild soap in tub or shower.
   c. Rinse well with tap water.
   d. Pat dry with clean towel.
   e. Apply prescribed topical agent or dressing.

2. Teach the patient to recognize and report local signs of wound infection.

3. Instruct the patient in measures to lubricate and enhance comfort of healing skin:
   a. After cleansing, use moisturizers such as cocoa butter or other nonperfumed hand lotion at least twice a day.
   b. Wear clean, white underwear and clothing free of irritating dyes.
   c. Apply antipruritics as prescribed.
   d. Stay in a cool environment if itching occurs.
   e. Protect skin from further trauma, use a sunscreen with SPF of 24 or higher.

    f. Discuss summer precautions to include a hat with a full wide brim if there were facial or neck burns. Also limit exposure to sun because the affected areas will sunburn more easily and tan more deeply.

4. Advise the patient that, if wearing a pressure vest with or without sleeves or tights, the OSHA (Occupational Safety & Health Administration) standards for work in a hot environment as well as the need for oral fluid replacement should be used.

5. Advise the patient to develop a schedule to incorporate exercise regimen as prescribed by physical therapist.

6. Instruct the patient in use and care of splints and pressure garments.

7. Review with the patient and family common emotional responses during convalescence (depression, withdrawal, grieving, dreaming, anxiety, guilt, excessive sensitivity, emotional lability, insomnia, fear of future) and discuss usual temporary nature of these and effective coping mechanisms. Make sure that the patient has a phone number or referral to the counselor for follow-up appointments if desired.

Cancer, Bladder

Cancer of the bladder is the second most common urologic malignancy. Approximately 90% of all bladder cancers arise from the epithelial lining of the urinary tract. The remaining 10% are adenocarcinoma, squamous cell carcinoma, or sarcoma. Most are superficial papillary tumors that are easily resected, but metastasis may occur to the bladder wall and pelvis, para-aortic or supraclavicular nodes, and the liver, lungs, and bone.

Although the specific cause is unknown, bladder cancers have been linked to cigarette smoking (2–3 times higher risk), prolonged exposure to aromatic amines (industrial dyes), to the drug cyclophosphamide, to pelvic radiation therapy, and to chronic bladder irritation (as in long-term indwelling catheterization). Bladder cancer occurs 3 times more frequently in men, with peak incidence between ages 60 and 80 years.

C

◆ Assessment

1. Painless hematuria, either gross or microscopic, is the most characteristic sign.
2. Dysuria, frequency, urgency
3. Pelvic or back pain may indicate distant metastases; leg edema may result from invasion of pelvic lymph nodes.

◆ Diagnostic Evaluation

1. Cystoscopy to visualize the number, location, and appearance of tumors, and to obtain biopsy specimens
2. Urine and bladder washing for cytology to detect cancer cells.
3. Urine flow cytometry uses fluorescence microscopy to scan for abnormal cells
4. Intravenous pyelography (IVP); may show a filling defect indicative of bladder cancer; also helps determine status of upper urinary tract.
5. Additional tests to evaluate metastatic disease, such as endoscopy, pelvic examination, computed tomography (CT) or magnetic resonance imaging (MRI), bone scan

◆ Collaborative Management

Therapeutic and Pharmacologic Interventions

1. Intravesical (within the bladder) chemotherapy allows a high concentration of drug to come in contact with the tumor and urothelium with minimal systemic toxicity.
2. Instillation of immunotherapeutic agent, Bacillus

Calmette-Guérin (BCG) to stimulate immune response to prevent recurrence of transitional cell tumors

   a. Adverse reaction is a systemic BCG reaction—fever greater than 100°F for more than 24 hours
   b. Treated with antituberculosis agents
   c. Weekly instillations may be performed for 6 to 8 weeks.
3. Systemic chemotherapy to treat metastatic bladder cancer; combination therapy
4. Radiation therapy may be internal or external.

Surgical Interventions

1. Transurethral resection and fulguration may be used for superficial tumors; usually with intravesical chemotherapy to prevent tumor recurrence. (Some tumors may be treated with lasers, but this does not allow biopsies.)
2. Partial cystectomy may be used when tumors are located only in the dome of the bladder, away from the ureteral orifices.
3. Radical cystectomy (bladder removal) may be used for invasive or poorly differentiated tumors.
   a. Requires urinary diversion
   b. *In the male,* includes removal of bladder, prostate and seminal vesicles, proximal vas deferens, and part of proximal urethra
   c. *In the female,* includes anterior exenteration with removal of bladder, urethra, uterus, fallopian tubes, ovaries, and segment of anterior wall of the vagina
   d. Cystectomy may be combined with chemotherapy and radiation

◆ **Nursing Interventions**

Monitoring

1. Monitor for postoperative complications:
   a. Hemorrhage, infection, bladder perforation, and temporary irritative voiding in transurethral resection
   b. Urinary tract infection, irritative voiding symptoms, allergic reaction, bone marrow suppression or systemic BCG reaction in intravesical chemotherapy

2. After transurethral surgery, monitor intake and output, including irrigation solution.
3. Monitor urine output for clearing of hematuria.

Supportive Care
1. After transurethral surgery, maintain patency of indwelling urinary drainage catheter. Manual irrigation is not recommended because of the risk of bladder perforation. Continuous bladder irrigation may be used if necessary. Do not irrigate unless specifically ordered.
2. Ensure adequate hydration, either orally or IV.
3. Administer analgesic medication for pelvic discomfort.
4. Administer anticholinergic medications or belladonna and opium (B & O) suppositories to relieve bladder spasms.
5. Remove indwelling catheter as soon as possible after procedure, to reduce risk of infection.
6. To relieve anxiety, allow the patient to verbalize fears and concerns, and provide information about diagnostic studies, surgery, and treatments.
7. For intravesical chemotherapy:
    a. Minimize fluids and avoid diuretics for several hours before instillation to maximize concentration of drug during treatment.
    b. Help patient change position as directed during instillation to allow drug to contact as much of urothelial surface as possible.
    c. Tell the patient not to void for 1 to 2 hours after instillation; then have the patient increase fluid intake and void frequently.
    d. Tell the patient to wash hands and perineal area after voiding, to prevent contact dermatitis, caused by medication.

Patient Education and Health Maintenance
1. Advise the patient that irritative voiding symptoms and intermittent hematuria are possible for several weeks after transurethral resection.
2. Teach the patient importance of adhering to follow-up schedule; cystoscopy every 3 months for 1 year, then every 6 months to 1 year thereafter for the rest of the patient's life (70% of superficial tumors will recur).
3. Encourage cessation of smoking.

Cancer, Bone

Bone cancer refers to primary malignant tumors, such as chondrosarcoma and osteogenic sarcoma, which arise from the cartilage or bone structure and eventually may spread to the lung; and metastatic bone tumors (seeded from another site), which may accompany cancers of the breast, the prostate, and, most commonly, the lung. Metastatic tumors most frequently occur in the vertebrae and cause pathologic fractures. Benign bone tumors include osteoid osteoma, chondroma, and benign giant cell tumors; some may metastasize.

◆ Assessment

1. Generally mild to constant pain, which may be worse at night or with activity. Pain will be acute with pathologic fracture.
2. Neurological symptoms may present with nerve root compression.
3. Swelling and limitation of motion and joint effusion
4. Palpable, tender, fixed bony mass
   a. Increase in skin temperature over mass
   b. Superficial veins dilated and prominent

◆ Diagnostic Evaluation

1. X-ray studies show increased or decreased bone density, indicating tumor activity.
2. Bone scan to detect extent of malignancy, and help follow therapy
3. CT and MRI demonstrate soft tissue involvement and location of tumor(s).
4. Serum alkaline phosphatase usually elevated
5. Bone biopsy may be necessary to confirm diagnosis.
6. Additional tests include arteriography to further assess soft tissue involvement, and chest x-ray and lung scan to detect metastasis.

◆ Collaborative Management

Therapeutic Interventions
1. Radiation therapy may be used to irradiate tumors, often in combination with other therapies.

2. Prophylactic radiation to lungs may suppress metastases.
3. If pathologic fracture occurs, the fracture is managed conservatively or with open reduction and internal fixation as appropriate.

Pharmacologic Interventions

1. Chemotherapy may be administered before surgery to shrink the tumor and afterward to prevent metastases.
   a. May be used in combination with other therapies to achieve greater patient response at lower toxicity, and to minimize potential drug resistance problems.
   b. May be given in varying courses separated by rest periods.
2. Immunotherapy may be used.
3. Hormone therapy may be used to treat metastatic tumors of the breast and prostate.

Surgical Interventions

1. Tumor curettage or resection with bone grafting may be used.
2. Limb-salvaging procedures involve resection of affected bone and surrounding normal muscle tissue, with reconstruction using metallic prostheses or allografts and skin grafts as needed.
3. Amputation is necessary in some cases.

◆ Nursing Interventions

Monitoring

1. Monitor the patient's response to pain control measures.
2. Monitor for side effects of chemotherapy.
3. Monitor for side effects of radiation therapy.

Supportive Care

1. Prepare the patient for amputation (p. 15) or other orthopedic surgery (p. 622) as indicated.
2. Administer pain medications $\frac{1}{2}$-hour before ambulation or other uncomfortable movement; use relaxation and diversion techniques, as well.
3. Support painful extremities on pillows; support joints when repositioning the patient.

4. Assist the patient in movement with gentleness and patience.
5. Avoid jarring the patient or the bed.
6. To avoid pathologic fractures, create a hazard-free environment.
7. Create a supportive environment to help family deal with diagnosis of cancer and possible amputation.
8. Answer questions and clear up misconceptions about treatment options. Refer for counseling as indicated.

Patient Education and Health Maintenance

1. Teach the patient about the particular treatment selected.
2. Encourage appropriate follow-up and diagnostic testing for recurrence.
3. Refer for additional information and support to:

American Cancer Society
1599 Clifton Rd., NE
Atlanta, GA 30329
800-ACS-2345

Cancer, Breast

Breast cancer or carcinoma is the leading type of cancer in American women. Approximately 182,000 new cases (1,000 male) are reported yearly. It is second only to lung cancer as the highest cause of cancer deaths in American women; estimated deaths in 1994 were 46,000 (approximately 300 men also died of it). Most breast cancer begins in the lining of the milk ducts, sometimes in the lobule. Eventually the cancer grows through the wall of the duct and into the fatty tissue. Breast cancer metastasizes most commonly to axillary nodes, lung, bone, liver, and the brain.

Age, staging, histological differentiation, and treatment are important prognostic factors for survival. If the cancer is localized to the breast, the 5-year survival rate is 94% in white women, 84% in black women. If the cancer spreads to the nodes, these rates decrease to 74% and 57%, respectively.

Women at high risk for breast cancer include those with prior breast cancer, and a family history (especially mother, sisters), and who are older. Other probable risk factors include nulliparity, first child after age 30, late menopause, early menarche, and benign breast disease. Possible (controversial) risk factors may include oral contraceptive use, estrogen replacement therapy, alcohol use, obesity, and increased dietary fat intake.

C

GERONTOLOGIC ALERT
Age is the greatest single risk factor for the development of cancer. Cancer warning signals may be unheeded in older women.

◆ Assessment

1. A firm lump or thickening in breast, usually painless; 50% are located in the upper outer quadrant of the breast
2. Enlargement of axillary or supraclavicular lymph nodes may indicate metastasis
3. Spontaneous nipple discharge; may be bloody, clear, or serous
4. Nipple retraction or scaliness—especially in Paget's disease
5. Asymmetry of the breasts—may be noted as the woman changes positions; compare one breast with the other

GERONTOLOGIC ALERT
Normal breast changes in the elderly include drooping, flaccid breasts caused by decreased subcutaneous tissue from decreased estrogen levels. Nipple size and erection are also reduced.

6. Late signs of breast cancer include pain, ulceration, edema, orange peel skin (*peau d'orange*) from impaired lymphatic drainage.

C

◆ Diagnostic Evaluation

1. Mammography (most accurate method of detecting nonpalpable lesions); shows lesions and cancerous changes, such as microcalcification. Ultrasonography may be used to distinguish cysts from solid masses.
2. Biopsy or aspiration, to confirm a diagnosis and determine the type of breast cancer.
3. Estrogen/progesterone receptor assays, proliferation/S phase study (tumor aggressiveness), and other tests of tumor cells are performed to determine appropriate treatment and prognosis.
4. Blood testing to detect metastasis includes liver function tests to detect liver metastasis; calcium and alkaline phosphatase levels to detect bony metastasis
5. Chest x-rays, bone scans, or possible brain and chest CT scans to detect metastasis

◆ Collaborative Management

Measures are based on the type and stage of breast cancer, receptor studies, and menopausal status. For women with localized breast cancer, clinical trials indicate that treatment with a breast-preserving surgery yields similar survival rates to modified radical mastectomy.

Therapeutic Interventions

1. Radiation is an adjuvant therapy to breast-preserving surgery to decrease incidence of local tumor recurrence.
   a. Radiation is directed to breast, chest wall, and remaining lymph nodes.
   b. A course usually involves five treatments a week for 6 or 7 weeks. A "booster" or second phase of treatment may be given.
   c. May include implants of radioactive material after external treatments are completed

2. Also used as primary therapy to shrink a large tumor to operable size, and to alleviate pain caused by metastasis

Pharmacologic Interventions

1. Chemotherapy is primarily used as adjuvant treatment postoperatively; usually begins 4 weeks after surgery (very stressful for a patient who just finished major surgery).
   a. Treatments are given every 3 to 4 weeks for 6 to 9 months. Because the drugs differ in their mechanisms of action, various combinations are used to treat cancer.
   b. Principal breast cancer drugs include cyclophosphamide, methotrexate, fluorouracil, and doxorubicin.
   c. Paclitaxel, an antimitotic cytotoxic agent, is being used now for advanced cancer.
2. Indications for chemotherapy include:
   a. Premenopausal women with positive lymph nodes, regardless of hormone-receptor status.
   b. Premenopausal women with negative lymph nodes and poor prognostic factors.
   c. Postmenopausal women with positive lymph nodes and negative hormone-receptor status.
3. Chemotherapy is also used as primary treatment in inflammatory breast cancer and as palliative treatment in metastatic disease or recurrence.
4. Anti-estrogens, such as tamoxifen, are used as adjuvant systemic therapy after surgery.
   a. Given orally for at least 2 years
   b. Greatest benefit is seen in estrogen- or progesterone-receptor–positive patients; it also may be used for metastases or recurrence.
   c. For postmenopausal women with positive nodes and positive hormone-receptor status, tamoxifen is the treatment of choice.
5. Hormonal agents may be used in advanced disease to induce remissions that last for months to several years. Agents commonly used include:
   a. Estrogens, such as diethylstilbestrol or ethinyl estradiol, given in high doses to suppress follicle-stimulating hormone (FSH) and luteinizing hormone (LH); may also reduce endogenous estrogen production

C

    b. Progestins may decrease estrogen receptors.
    c. Androgens may suppress FSH and estrogen production.
    d. Aminoglutethimide suppresses estrogen production by blocking adrenal steroids; this "medical adrenalectomy" is especially useful for women with bone and soft tissue metastases.
    e. Corticosteroids suppress estrogen-progesterone secretion from the adrenals.

Surgical Interventions

1. Surgeries include lumpectomy (breast-preserving procedure), mastectomy (breast removal), and mammoplasty (reconstructive surgery). See p. 561.
2. Endocrine-related surgeries to reduce endogenous estrogen as a palliative measure:
    a. Oophorectomy (removal of ovaries) is used to treat recurrent or metastatic disease in estrogen receptor–positive premenopausal women. This deprives the breast tumor of its primary estrogen source and obtains remissions of 3 months to several years.
    b. Adrenalectomy (removal of adrenal glands) eliminates androgens, which convert to estrogen. Although this procedure yields remissions of 6 months to several years, it is rarely done because of need for long-term steroid replacement therapy.
3. Bone marrow transplantation may be combined with chemotherapy.
    a. Autologous method after high-dose chemotherapy; may be curative because it allows for high doses of drugs
    b. Especially indicated for stage 3 disease

◆ Nursing Interventions

Monitoring

1. Monitor for side effects of radiation therapy:
    a. Mild fatigue, sore throat, dry cough, nausea, anorexia; later, skin will look and feel sunburned, and eventually the breast becomes more firm.
    b. Complications include increased arm edema, decreased arm mobility, pneumonitis, and brachial nerve damage.

2. Monitor for side effects of chemotherapy: bone marrow suppression, nausea and vomiting, alopecia, weight gain/loss, fatigue, stomatitis, anxiety, and depression.
3. Monitor for side effects of endocrine therapy: hot flashes, irregular periods, vaginal irritation, nausea and vomiting, headaches.

Supportive Care

1. Realize that a diagnosis of breast cancer is a devastating emotional shock to the woman. Provide psychological support to the patient throughout the diagnostic and treatment process.
2. Interpret the results of each diagnostic test in language the patient can readily understand.
3. Involve the patient in planning treatment.
4. Describe surgical procedures.
5. Prepare the patient for the effects of chemotherapy and plan ahead for alopecia, fatigue, etc.
6. Administer antiemetics prophylactically, as directed, for patients receiving chemotherapy.
7. Encourage frequent light meals and fluids as tolerated.
8. Administer IV fluids and hyperalimentation as indicated.
9. Help patient identify and use support persons in family or community.

Patient Education and Health Maintenance

1. Encourage the patient to continue in close postoperative follow-up. Most women are scheduled for examinations every 3 months for the first 2 years, every 6 months for the next 3 years, and once a year after 5 years.
2. Stress importance of continued yearly mammogram.

COMMUNITY CARE CONSIDERATIONS

Fewer than half of women obtain regular screening mammograms based on the established guidelines. Because health teaching is an important nursing role, nurses should be educating women about the importance of routine screening.

3. Suggest to the patient that psychological intervention may be necessary for anxiety, depression, or sexual problems.

4. Teach all women the recommended cancer screening procedures:
   a. Breast self-examination: once a month, age 20 and older
   b. Clinical examination by a doctor or nurse every 3 years (ages 20–40), or every year (older than age 40).
   c. Mammography: have first mammogram by age 40; have a mammogram every 1 to 2 years (ages 40–49); every year (age 50 and older).
5. Refer for additional information to:
   a. National Cancer Institute, 800-4-CANCER
   b. American Cancer Society, 800-ACS-2345

Cancer, Cervical

Cervical cancer is a common gynecologic malignancy. Preinvasive types include dysplasia (atypical cells with some degree of surface maturation) and carcinoma in situ (CIS), which is confined to the cervical epithelium. In invasive carcinomas, the stroma is involved; 90% are of the squamous cell type. Invasive cancer spreads by local invasion and lymphatics to the vagina and beyond.

Cervical cancer most commonly occurs in women aged 35 to 55. Incidence is higher in blacks and in lower socioeconomic levels.

Major risk factors include early sexual activity, multiple sexual partners, and history of sexually transmitted diseases, especially human papilloma virus (HPV) and herpes simplex virus. Cervical cancer may involve the bladder and rectum and metastasize to the lungs, mediastinum, bones, and liver.

◆ Assessment

1. Early disease is usually asymptomatic.
2. Initial symptoms are postcoital bleeding, irregular vaginal bleeding or spotting between periods or after menopause, and malodorous discharge.
3. As disease progresses, bleeding becomes more constant

and is accompanied by pain that radiates to buttocks and legs.
4. Weight loss, anemia, and fever signal advanced disease.

◆ Diagnostic Evaluation

1. Papanicolaou (Pap) smear for cervical cytology is usual screening test. A computerized screening program may increase the accuracy of manual laboratory Pap screening by as much as 30%.
2. If Pap is abnormal, colposcopy and biopsy or conization may be done.
3. In advanced disease, staging laparotomy is done to evaluate metastasis outside the pelvis.
4. Additional testing includes metastatic workup (intravenous pyelogram, cystoscopy, sigmoidoscopy).

◆ Collaborative Management

Therapeutic and Pharmacologic Interventions

1. Radiation therapy is the usual treatment for all stages. Therapy is individualized according to the stage of disease and the patient's response to and tolerance of radiation.
2. Intracavitary—radium via applicator in endocervical canal
   a. Applicator remains in place 24 to 72 hours.
   b. Complications include cystitis, proctitis, vaginal stenosis, uterine perforation.
3. External—via linear accelerator or cobalt
   a. External radiation over pelvis may supplement intracavitary to eliminate cancer spread via lymphatic system.
   b. Complications include bone marrow depression, bowel obstruction, fistula.
4. Laser therapy may be used to treat dysplasia.
5. Chemotherapy may be used as adjuvant to surgery or radiation treatments.

Surgical Interventions

1. Conization is performed if childbearing is desired, depends on stage of cancer.

2. Cryosurgery may be employed to destroy cancer cells by freezing.
3. Loop electrosurgical excision procedure (LEEP) may be used to remove abnormal tissue with thin wire loop.
4. Hysterectomy
   a. Performed if childbearing no longer desired
   b. Usually combined with radiation therapy for CIS and invasive carcinoma
   c. May cause impaired bladder function
5. Pelvic exenteration
   a. Removal of the vagina, uterus, uterine tubes, ovaries, bladder, rectum, and supporting structures
   b. Creation of an ileal conduit and fecal stoma
   c. Performed for very advanced disease if radiation therapy cannot be used; also for recurrent cancer
   d. Vaginal reconstruction may be done.

◆ Nursing Interventions

Monitoring

1. During intracavitary radiation, check radioisotope applicator position every 8 hours, and monitor amount of bleeding and drainage (a small amount is normal).
2. Observe for signs and symptoms of radiation sickness—nausea, vomiting, fever, diarrhea, abdominal cramping.
3. Monitor for complications of surgery—bleeding, infection.

Supportive Care

1. Assist the patient to seek information on stage of cancer, treatment options.
2. Prepare the patient for hysterectomy or other surgery (see p. 495).
3. Prepare the patient for radiation therapy to the uterus (see p. 159).
4. Provide emotional support during treatment.

Patient Education and Health Maintenance

1. Advise patient on expected discharge after surgical procedure and need to report excessive, foul-smelling discharge or bleeding.
2. Explain the importance of life-long follow-up regard-

less of treatments, to determine the response to treatment and detect spread of cancer.
3. Refer the patient to a local cancer support group.

Cancer, Colorectal

Colorectal cancer refers to malignancies of the colon and rectum. Colorectal tumors are nearly always adenocarcinomas, and they represent the second most common visceral cancer in the United States.

Colorectal tumors occur most frequently in the rectum and sigmoid areas. A tumor starts in the mucosal layers of the colonic wall and eventually penetrates the wall and invades surrounding structures and organs (bladder, prostate, ureters, vagina). Cancer spreads by direct invasion, and through the lymph system and bloodstream. The liver and lungs are the most common metastatic sites. Other complications are hemorrhage, obstruction, and anemia.

Risk factors include age (older than 50), chronic ulcerative colitis (increasing risk after 10-year history), Crohn's disease, previous history of resected colorectal cancer, high-fat and low-fiber diet, genetic predisposition, polyposis syndromes, and immunodeficiency diseases.

◆ Assessment

1. May be asymptomatic or symptoms vary according to the location of the tumor and the extent of involvement
2. Right-sided tumors—change in bowel habits, usually diarrhea; vague abdominal discomfort; black tarry stools, anemia, weakness, weight loss, palpable mass in right lower quadrant
3. Left-sided tumors—change in bowel habits, often increasing constipation with bouts of diarrhea caused by partial obstruction; bright red blood in stool; cramping pain; weight loss, anemia; palpable mass
4. Rectal tumors—change in bowel habits with possibly urgent need to defecate, alternating constipation and diarrhea, and narrowed caliber of stool; bright red

blood in stool; feeling of incomplete evacuation; rectal fullness progressing to dull constant ache

◆ Diagnostic Evaluation

1. Digital rectal examination detects 15% of tumors.
2. Fiberoptic sigmoidoscopy or colonoscopy to detect tumor
3. Stools for occult blood—often reveals evidence of carcinoma when the patient is otherwise asymptomatic
4. Intravenous pyelography and possible cystoscopy, which may be indicated to assess whether malignancy has spread locally to involve ureter or bladder
5. CT scan of liver, lung, and brain may show metastatic disease.
6. Carcinoembryonic antigen (CEA)— elevated with metastasis or tumor recurrence

◆ Collaborative Management

Therapeutic Interventions

1. Blood replacement or other treatment if severe anemia exists
2. Radiation therapy may be used preoperatively to improve resectability of the tumor or postoperatively as adjuvant therapy to treat residual disease.

Pharmacologic Interventions

1. Chemotherapy may be used as adjuvant therapy to improve survival time
2. May be used for residual disease, recurrence of disease, unresectable tumors, and metastatic disease

Surgical Interventions

1. Wide segmental bowel resection of tumor, including regional lymph nodes and blood vessels
2. Low anterior resection (LAR) for upper rectal tumors; possible temporary diversion loop colostomy while rectal anastomosis heals; second procedure for takedown of colostomy
3. Abdominoperineal resection (APR) with permanent end colostomy—for lower rectal tumors when adequate margins cannot be obtained or anal sphincters are involved

4. Temporary loop colostomy to decompress bowel and divert fecal stream, followed by later bowel resection, anastomosis, and takedown of colostomy
5. Diverting colostomy or ileostomy as palliation for obstructing, unresectable tumor
6. Total protocolectomy and possible ileal reservoir—anal anastomosis for patients with familial adenomatous polyposis and chronic ulcerative colitis (CUC) before cancer is confirmed
7. More extensive surgery involving removal of other organs if cancer has spread (bladder, uterus, small intestine)

◆ Nursing Interventions

Monitoring

1. Monitor amount, consistency, frequency, occult blood, and color of stools.
2. Monitor the patient's dietary intake and weight.
3. Monitor for excess fluid loss through vomiting and diarrhea and watch for dehydration.
4. Monitor the patient's response to radiation or chemotherapy and watch for adverse reactions.

Supportive Care

1. Meet the patient's nutritional needs by serving a high-calorie, low-residue diet for several days before surgery, if condition permits.
2. Serve smaller meals spaced throughout the day to maintain adequate calorie and protein intake if not NPO.
3. Adjust diet before and after treatments such as chemotherapy or radiation. Serve clear liquids, bland diet, or NPO as prescribed.
4. Maintain hydration through IV therapy and record urinary output. Metabolic tissue needs are increased, and more fluids are needed to eliminate waste products.
5. Instruct the patient to take prescribed antiemetic as needed, especially if receiving chemotherapy.
6. For constipation, encourage exercise and adequate fluid/fiber intake to promote bowel motility.
7. For diarrhea related to radiation or chemotherapy

(not caused by obstruction), administer antidiarrheal medications and discuss foods that may slow transit time of bowel, such as bananas, rice, peanut butter, and pasta.

8. Evaluate effectiveness of analgesic regimen. Investigate different approaches, such as relaxation techniques, repositioning, imaging, laughter, music, reading, and touch for control or relief of pain.

9. Institute an individualized activity plan after assessing the patient's activity level and tolerance, noting shortness of breath or tachycardia. Allow for frequent rest periods to regain energy.

10. To minimize fear, provide information and answer questions regarding disease process, treatment modalities, and complications. Offer additional educational materials and refer to American Cancer Society for information and support.

Patient Education/Health Maintenance

1. Teach and demonstrate colostomy management skills. Enlist the help of an enterostomal therapist.

2. Initiate a home care nursing referral to assist with wound care and management of treatment side effects, and to continue teaching colostomy care.

Cancer, Esophageal

Esophageal cancer occurs in four types worldwide: squamous cell, adenocarcinoma, carcinosarcoma, and sarcoma. Its cause is unknown, but predisposing factors include Barrett's esophagus (epithelial changes in esophagus), other head and neck cancers, achalasia, long-term alcohol and tobacco use, genetic predisposition (more common in nonwhite men), and chemical esophagitis, which causes esophageal strictures. Squamous cell and adenocarcinoma are the most common types.

Complications include malnutrition, aspiration pneumonitis, hemorrhage, sepsis, and tracheoesophageal fistula. Postoperatively, dumping syndrome, nutritional deficiencies, reflux esophagitis, and leakage of anastamosis may occur.

◆ Assessment

1. Dysphagia is late, but is usual presenting sign.
   a. Mild, atypical chest pain associated with eating usually precedes dysphagia, but is overlooked.
   b. Pain on swallowing (odynophagia) may occur.
2. Progressive weight loss and dietary changes
3. Cough and hoarseness are evident with laryngeal involvement. Later, hiccups, respiratory difficulty, foul breath, and regurgitation of food and saliva may occur.
4. Supraclavicular or cervical lymphadenopathy and hepatomegaly occur with metastatic involvement.

◆ Diagnostic Evaluation

1. Chest x-ray may show adenopathy, mediastinal widening, metastasis, or a tracheoesophageal fistula.
2. Barium swallow shows polypoid, infiltrative, or ulcerative lesions.
3. Endoscopy is done to obtain biopsy specimen.
4. Computed tomography (CT) may be helpful in delineating the extent of the tumor, as well as in identifying adjacent tissue invasion and metastases.

◆ Collaborative Management

Therapeutic and Pharmacologic Interventions

1. The goal of treatment may be cure or palliation, depending on the tumor stage and the patient's overall condition. Palliative treatment aims to reduce tumor-related complications and improve quality of life. One or more therapies can be used for palliative treatment. The wide variety of treatments reflects overall poor results from a single approach.
2. Radiation and chemotherapy appear to be more effective when used in combination.
3. Endoscopy or laser dilation provide palliative treatment of dysphagia.

Surgical Intervention

1. Lesions of the middle and lower esophagus are excised via thoracotomy with esophagogastrectomy or colon

interposition (section of colon is used to replace the excised portion of the esophagus).
2. Lesions of the cervical esophagus are excised via bilateral neck dissection and esophagogastrectomy; laryngectomy and thyroidectomy may be necessary.
3. A two-step approach may be selected, in which resection with cervical esophagostomy and feeding gastrostomy are performed initially, followed by reconstructive surgery.

◆ Nursing Interventions

Monitoring

1. Monitor nutritional status.
2. Monitor vital signs to note early onset of hemorrhage, infection, dysrhythmias, aspiration, or anastomosis leakage.
3. Observe drainage from incision or chest tube for bleeding or purulence.
4. Be alert for pain caused by dumping syndrome or reflux esophagitis.

Supportive Care

1. Administer oxygen as prescribed to facilitate tissue oxygenation.
2. Provide nutritional supplements as indicated. Expect to provide IV hyperalimentation if the patient is unable to take adequate calories.
3. Postoperatively, administer IV fluids as prescribed. Initially the patient may require large volumes if many lymph nodes were removed.
4. Assess for return of bowel sounds postoperatively, and administer fluids by nasogastric tube as prescribed.
5. Encourage the patient to advance diet from liquids to soft foods.
6. Remind the patient to remain in upright position for approximately 2 hours after eating to promote digestion and discourage reflux.
7. Provide mouth care for comfort and hygiene.

Patient Education and Health Maintenance

1. Encourage the patient to avoid overeating, take small bites, chew food well; avoid chunks of meat and stringy raw vegetables and fruit.

2. Depending on type of surgery, frequent small meals may be better tolerated.
3. Encourage rest postoperatively, advancing activities as tolerated.
4. Instruct patient regarding signs and symptoms of complications to report: nausea, vomiting, elevated temperature, cough, difficulty in swallowing.

Cancer, Gastric

Gastric cancer, or malignant tumor of the stomach, is usually an adenocarcinoma. It spreads rapidly to the lungs, lymph nodes, and liver. Risk factors include chronic atrophic gastritis with intestinal metaplasia; pernicious anemia or having had gastric resections (greater than 15 years); high alcohol consumption; and smoking. This cancer is most common in men older than 40 years. The incidence of gastric cancer in the United States has been declining in recent years.

◆ Assessment

1. Most often the patient presents with the same symptoms as gastric ulcer. Later evaluation shows the lesion to be malignant.
2. Gastric fullness (early satiety), dyspepsia lasting more than 4 weeks, progressive loss of appetite, vomiting (may be coffee-ground appearance) are initial symptoms.
3. Stool specimens are positive for occult blood.
4. Later manifestations include pain in back or epigastric area (often induced by eating, relieved by antacids or vomiting); weight loss; hemorrhage; gastric obstruction.

◆ Diagnostic Evaluation

1. Upper GI x-ray with contrast media may initially show suspicious ulceration that requires further evaluation.
2. Endoscopy with biopsy and cytology to confirm malignant disease

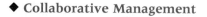

3. Imaging studies (bone scan, liver scan, CT scan) to help determine metastasis

◆ Collaborative Management

Surgical Interventions

1. The only successful treatment of gastric cancer is gastric *resection,* surgical removal of part of the stomach.
2. If tumor is localized to stomach and can be removed, 5-year survival rates are still poor.
3. Palliative surgery such as subtotal gastrectomy with or without gastroenterostomy may be performed to maintain continuity of the GI tract.
4. Surgery may be combined with chemotherapy to provide palliation and prolong life.

◆ Nursing Interventions

Monitoring

1. Monitor nutritional intake and weigh patient regularly.
2. Monitor CBC and serum vitamin B_{12} levels.
3. Monitor for signs of dumping syndrome after gastric resection—nausea, weakness, perspiration, palpitations, syncope, and diarrhea.

Supportive Care

Also see Gastrointestinal surgeries, p. 350.

1. Provide comfort measures and administer analgesics as ordered.
2. Frequently turn the patient and encourage deep breathing to prevent vascular and pulmonary complications and to promote comfort.
3. Maintain nasogastric suction to remove fluids and gas in the stomach and prevent painful distention.
4. Provide oral care to prevent dryness and ulceration.
5. Keep the patient NPO as prescribed to promote gastric wound healing. Administer parenteral nutrition, if ordered.
6. When nasogastric drainage has decreased and bowel sounds have returned, begin oral fluids and progress slowly.
7. Avoid high-carbohydrate foods, such as milk, that may

trigger dumping syndrome because of excessively rapid emptying of gastric contents.
8. Administer protein and vitamin supplements to foster wound repair and tissue building.

Patient Education and Health Maintenance

1. Instruct the patient to avoid dumping syndrome:
   a. Eat small, frequent meals rather than three large meals.
   b. Suggest a diet high in protein and fat and low in carbohydrates, and avoid meals high in sugars, milk, chocolate, salt.
   c. Reduce fluids with meals, but take them between meals.
   d. Take anticholinergic medication before meals (if prescribed) to lessen gastrointestinal activity.
   e. Relax when eating; eat slowly and regularly and rest after meals.
2. Teach the patient how to avoid phytobezoar formation (mass of compact vegetable matter that does not pass into intestine):
   a. Avoid fibrous foods such as citrus fruits, skins and seeds because they tend to form phytobezoars.
   b. Chew food adequately before swallowing.
3. Provide information on support groups for patients with cancer.
4. Stress the importance of vitamin B_{12} injections after gastrectomy to prevent surgically induced pernicious anemia.
5. Encourage follow-up visits with the health care provider and routine blood studies and other testing to detect complications or recurrence.

Cancer, Laryngeal

Laryngeal cancer refers to carcinoma of the vocal cords or other portions of the larynx, which occurs predominantly in men older than age 60. In North America, approximately two thirds of carcinomas of the larynx arise in the vocal cords (glottis), almost one third arise in the supraglottic region, and approximately 3% arise in the subglottic region. Carcinoma of the vocal cords spreads slowly because of minimal blood supply. Other laryngeal cancers spread more rapidly because of abundant supply of blood and lymph and soon involve the lymph nodes of the neck. However, if treated early, these cancers may be cured.

Risk factors include a history of smoking, high alcohol intake, vocal straining, chronic laryngitis, industrial exposure, nutritional deficiency, and family predisposition.

C

◆ Assessment

1. Supraglottic cancer
   a. Tickling sensation in throat
   b. Dryness and fullness (lump) in throat
   c. Painful swallowing (odynophagia)—associated with invasion of extralaryngeal musculature
   d. Coughing on swallowing
   e. Pain radiating to ear (late symptom)
2. Glottic (vocal cord) cancer
   a. Hoarseness or voice change
   b. Aphonia (loss of voice)
   c. Dyspnea
   d. Pain (in later stages)
3. Subglottic cancer
   a. Coughing
   b. Short periods of difficulty in breathing
   c. Hemoptysis; fetid odor—results from ulceration and disintegration of tumor

◆ Diagnostic Evaluation

1. Indirect mirror examination of larynx or direct laryngoscopy and biopsy to identify lesion
2. CT scan and other special radiologic tests to detect tumor
3. Laryngography—contrast study of larynx to define blood vessels and lymph nodes

◆ Collaborative Management

Therapeutic Interventions
1. Endoscopic removal of early malignancy
2. Radiation

a. Administered alone or in combination with surgery
b. Complications of radiation: edema of larynx; soft tissue and cartilage necrosis; chondritis (inflammation of cartilage)

Surgical Interventions

1. Carbon dioxide laser: to treat early-stage lesions
2. Partial laryngectomy: removal of small lesion on true cord, along with adjacent healthy tissue
3. Supraglottic laryngectomy: removal of hyoid bone, epiglottis, and false vocal cords; tracheostomy may be done to maintain adequate airway; radical neck dissection may be done
4. Hemilaryngectomy: removal of one true vocal cord, false cord, one half of thyroid cartilage, arytenoid cartilage
5. Total laryngectomy: removal of entire larynx. A radical neck dissection also may be done because of metastasis to cervical lymph nodes
6. Total laryngectomy with laryngoplasty: voice rehabilitation may be attempted through the Asai operation to construct a tube from the upper end of the trachea, which may be blocked by finger to produce speech
7. Postoperative complications include salivary fistula, carotid artery rupture, stomal stenosis, aspiration, and recurrence of cancer in stoma.

◆ Nursing Interventions

Monitoring

1. Postoperatively, monitor for signs of difficult breathing; suprasternal and intercostal retractions, tachypnea, dyspnea, tachycardia, decreased alertness.
2. Monitor intravenous fluids during first few postoperative days; assess hydration and measure intake and output.
3. Monitor for saliva collecting beneath the skin flaps or leaking through suture line or drain site; indicates salivary fistula. Management includes nasogastric tube feeding, meticulous local wound care with frequent dressing changes, and promotion of drainage.

C

4. Monitor nutritional status through frequent weighing.

Supportive Care

1. Prepare the patient before surgery for alternate means of communication until speech can be relearned.
2. Arrange for the patient to be visited by laryngectomee for hope and encouragement.
3. Provide information about alternate modes of restoring communication, eg, artificial larynx, Electrolarynx, tracheoesophageal puncture (TEP) with voice prosthesis, esophageal speech (accomplished by training the patient to force air down the esophagus and release it in a controlled manner), and surgical reconstructive procedures to restore voice.
4. Postoperatively, suction secretions frequently to prevent obstruction or aspiration. Employ chest physical therapy and humidification through tracheal collar to help remove secretions.

5. Be aware that the postoperative patient is unable to cough. Teach to bend forward until stoma is below lung level and to exhale rapidly, then wipe resultant secretions away from tracheostoma with a handkerchief.
6. Encourage breathing exercises, because most patients have been heavy smokers.

7. To provide adequate nutrition, administer tube feedings until sufficient healing of pharynx has occurred (10–12 days) and the patient can consume sufficient oral feedings to meet body needs.
8. Encourage the patient to relearn swallowing. Have standby suction available.
   a. Place the patient in sitting position, leaning slightly forward, which allows larynx to move forward and hypopharynx to partially open. (Explain that the epiglottis normally prevents fluid and food from entering larynx during swallowing.)
   b. Teach patient to inhale before swallowing, swallow, cough gently while exhaling, and reswallow. This leaves enough air in the lungs to cough out any obstruction, thus preventing aspiration.
9. Encourage communication by writing and agreed-on signals until voice work can begin with speech therapist. Discourage forced whispering, which increases pharyngeal tension.
10. Perform and teach tracheostoma care and changing gauze dressing and tracheostomy ties when they become soiled. A laryngectomy or tracheostomy tube is worn until stoma heals (1–2 months); the patient then starts gradual process of leaving tube out 1 hour at a time.

COMMUNITY CARE CONSIDERATIONS
Teach patient to wash hands before touching stoma and clean tracheostoma with warm water and clean wash cloth. Avoid using soap, tissues, and cotton balls, which may enter airway.

Patient Education and Health Maintenance

1. Advise the patient to provide humidification at home; use pans of water in the rooms, a humidifier, or a cool mist vaporizer, especially in the bedroom.
2. Advise use of stoma cover made of cotton or crocheted yarn; or wearing ascot, turtle neck, or scarf over stoma to filter air and manage secretions. Use a protective shield for bathing, showering, shampooing or cutting hair.

3. Encourage intake of fluids liberally (2–3 liters daily) to help liquefy secretions.
4. Tell patient to counteract any loss of smell and impairment of taste sensation with additional seasoning of food.
5. Advise high-fiber diet and use of stool softeners, because patient may not be able to hold breath and bear down for bowel movement.
6. Advise avoidance of antihistamines and medications that tend to dry mucous membranes.
7. Advise reporting the following: pain, difficulty in breathing or swallowing, the appearance of pus or blood-streaked sputum.
8. Advise that swimming is not recommended.
9. Encourage the patient to join local laryngectomy support group (Lost Chord Club; New Voice Club).

Cancer, Liver

Liver cancer occurs in three major forms: hepatocellular carcinoma, a primary cancer of the liver, arises in normal tissue as a discrete tumor or in end-stage cirrhosis in a multinodular pattern. Cholangiocarcinoma is a primary malignant tumor of the bile ducts, which can be intrahepatic or extrahepatic. The third type of liver cancer results from metastasis from an extrahepatic site, and invades the liver through the portal system, lymphatic channels, or by direct extension from an abdominal tumor.

The incidence of hepatocellular carcinoma is increasing in the United States in the younger population and in women. Cirrhosis, hepatitis B virus, and hepatitis C virus have been implicated in its cause. Rarer associated causes include hemochromatosis; alpha 1-antitrypsin deficiency; aflatoxins; chemical toxins, such as vinyl chloride and Thorotrast; carcinogens in herbal medicines; nitrosamines; and ingestion of hormones, as in oral contraceptives.

Without cirrhosis and with good liver function, a liver tumor may grow to huge proportions before becoming symptomatic, but in a cirrhotic patient, the lack of hepatic reserve usually leads to a more rapid course. Major complications include malnutrition, biliary obstruction with jaundice, fulminant liver failure, and metastasis.

◆ Assessment

1. Most common presenting symptom is right upper quadrant abdominal pain, usually dull or aching and may radiate to the right shoulder
2. Right upper quadrant mass, abdominal distention, fever, malaise, and anorexia become evident.
3. Jaundice is present in few patients at diagnosis in primary liver cancer. In cholangiocarcinoma, the presenting symptom is usually obstructive jaundice.
4. If there is portal vein obstruction, ascites and esophageal varices occur.

◆ Diagnostic Evaluation

1. Serum bilirubin, alkaline phosphatase, and serum transaminases are all increased.
2. Alpha-fetoprotein: principal tumor marker for hepatocellular carcinoma—elevated in 70% to 95% of patients with the disease.
3. Ultrasonography, CT, and MRI are used to detect cancer and assess if the tumor can be surgically removed.
4. Arteriography helps determine resectability of liver tumor.
5. Percutaneous needle biopsy or biopsy through ultrasonography may be done.
6. Laparoscopy with liver biopsy may be performed.

◆ Collaborative Management

Therapeutic Interventions

1. Radiation therapy can help reduce pain and discomfort.
2. Liver cancer is radiosensitive, but treatment is restricted by the limited radiation tolerance of normal liver.
3. Hyperthermia has been used to treat hepatic metastases.
4. Management of ascites and edema through fluid restriction, albumin, and diuretics

C

Pharmacologic Interventions

1. Chemotherapy is used as an adjuvant therapy after surgical resection of liver cancer.
   a. Systemic chemotherapy is the only treatment applicable once the cancer has spread outside the liver.
   b. Regional infusion chemotherapy by implantable pump has been used to deliver a high concentration of chemotherapy directly to the liver through the hepatic artery.
2. Hepatic artery occlusion and embolization with chemotherapeutic agents is another possible method.
3. Immunotherapy is currently under investigation.

Surgical Intervention

1. Surgery is the best treatment but is only feasible in 25% of cases, after the extent of tumor and hepatic reserve have been considered.
2. Surgical resection may be along anatomic divisions of the liver or nonanatomic resections. Care of the patient after liver surgery is similar to that for general abdominal surgery (see p. 350).
3. Freezing hepatic tumors by cryosurgery is a new modality that preserves normal liver.
4. Liver transplantation has been performed to treat liver tumors, but results have been poor because of the high rate of recurrent primary liver malignancy. It is now recommended that the patient be treated before and after transplantation with chemotherapy and radiation therapy.
5. Percutaneous transhepatic biliary drainage (PTBD) is used to drain obstructed biliary ducts in patients with inoperable tumors or in patients considered poor surgical risks. A percutaneous catheter drains the biliary tree to relieve jaundice, decrease pruritus, and decrease anorexia.
6. Percutaneous or endoscopic placement of internal stents may also be used as palliative treatment for a patient with obstructed bile ducts with a terminal diagnosis.

◆ Nursing Interventions

Monitoring

1. Assess the patient's response to pain control measures.

2. Monitor vital signs, intake and output, and daily weights to detect fluid balance.
3. Measure and record abdominal girth daily.
4. Monitor laboratory values for liver function.
5. Note subtle changes in mental status indicating hepatic encephalopathy.
6. Monitor for signs of malnutrition, including weight loss, loss of strength, anemia.

C

Supportive Care

1. Administer pain control agents as ordered, keeping in mind decreased liver metabolism. Monitor for signs of drug toxicity.
2. Provide nonpharmacologic methods of pain relief, such as massage and guided imagery.
3. Position the patient for comfort—usually in semi-Fowler's position.
4. Encourage the patient to eat small meals and supplementary liquid feedings.
5. Assess and report factors that may increase nutritional needs: increased body temperature, pain, signs of infection, stress level. Encourage additional calories as tolerated.
6. Restrict sodium and fluid intake as prescribed.
7. If the patient has PTBD, monitor catheter exit site for bleeding or bile drainage and assess drainage in bag for color, amount, and consistency. The drainage initially may have some blood mixed with bile but should clear within a few hours.
   a. Flush catheter if ordered.
   b. Check for and report signs of peritonitis from bile leaking into abdomen: fever, chills, abdominal pain and tenderness, distention.

Patient Education and Health Maintenance

1. Instruct the patient and family on preparation for surgery; reinforce and clarify proposed surgical procedure; and review postoperative instructions.
2. Instruct the patient to recognize and report signs and symptoms of complications.
3. Instruct the patient in continued surveillance for recurrence.
4. Instruct the patient and family in care of any tubes or drains.

Cancer, Lung

Lung cancer or *bronchogenic cancer* is a malignant tumor of the lung arising within the bronchial wall or epithelium. Bronchogenic cancer is classified according to cell type: epidermoid (squamous cell—most common), adenocarcinoma, small cell (oat cell) carcinoma, and large cell (undifferentiated) carcinoma. The lung is also a common site of metastasis from cancer elsewhere in the body through venous circulation or lymphatic spread.

The primary predisposing factor in lung cancer is cigarette smoking. Lung cancer risk is also high in persons occupationally exposed to asbestos, arsenic, chromium, nickel, iron, radioactive substances, isopropyl oil, coal tar products, and petroleum oil mists. Complications include superior vena cava syndrome, hypercalcemia (from bone metastasis), syndrome of inappropriate antidiuretic hormone (SIADH) secretion, pleural effusion, pneumonia, brain metastasis, and spinal cord compression.

◆ Assessment

1. New or changing cough, dyspnea, wheezing, excessive sputum production, hemoptysis, chest pain (aching, poorly localized), malaise, fever, weight loss, fatigue, or anorexia.
2. Decreased breath sounds, wheezing, and possible pleural friction rub (with pleural effusion) on exam.

NURSING ALERT
Suspect lung cancer in susceptible patients who have repeated unresolved respiratory infections.

◆ Diagnostic Evaluation

1. Chest x-ray may be suspicious for mass; computed tomography (CT) will better visualize tumor.
2. Sputum and pleural fluid samples for cytologic examination may show malignant cells.
3. Fiberoptic bronchoscopy to determine the location and

extent of the tumor and obtain biopsy. Lymph node biopsy and mediastinoscopy may also be ordered to establish lymphatic spread and help plan treatment.
4. Pulmonary function tests, which may be combined with a split-function perfusion scan to determine if the patient will have adequate pulmonary reserve to withstand surgical procedure

◆ Collaborative Management

Therapeutic Interventions
1. Oxygen through nasal cannula based on level of dyspnea
2. Enteral or total parenteral nutrition for malnourished patient who is unable or unwilling to eat
3. Removal of pleural fluid (by thoracentesis or tube thoracostomy) and instillation of sclerosing agent to obliterate pleural space and prevent fluid recurrence

Pharmacologic Interventions
1. Expectorants and antimicrobial agents to relieve dyspnea and infection
2. Analgesics given regularly to maintain pain at tolerable level. Titrate dosages to achieve pain control.
3. Chemotherapy, immunotherapy, and radiation treatments may be indicated.

Surgical Interventions
1. Resection of tumor, lobe, or lung (see p. 827)

◆ Nursing Interventions

Monitoring
1. Monitor for signs of metastasis: bone pain; abdominal discomfort, nausea, and vomiting from liver involvement; pancytopenia from bone marrow involvement; headache from brain metastasis; lymphadenopathy.
2. Monitor for metabolic or neurologic disturbances due to paraneoplastic syndrome (secretion of substances by the tumor).
3. Monitor nutritional status through serial weights, anthropometric measurements, dietary log, and biochemical laboratory tests.

C

Supportive Care

1. Elevate the head of the bed to ease the work of breathing and to prevent fluid collection in upper body (from superior vena cava syndrome).
2. Teach breathing retraining exercises to increase diaphragmatic excursion and reduce work of breathing.
3. Augment the patient's ability to cough effectively.
   a. Splint the patient's chest manually with hands.
   b. Instruct the patient to inspire fully and cough 2 to 3 times in one breath.
   c. Provide humidifier or vaporizer to provide moisture to loosen secretions.
4. Teach relaxation techniques to reduce anxiety associated with dyspnea. Allow the severely dyspneic patient to sleep in a reclining chair.
5. Encourage the patient to conserve energy by decreasing activities.
6. Ensure adequate protein intake—milk, eggs, oral nutritional supplements; and chicken, fowl, and fish if other meats are not tolerated, to promote healing and prevent edema.
   a. Advise the patient to eat small amounts of high-calorie and high-protein foods frequently, rather than three daily meals.
   b. Suggest eating the major meal in the morning if rapid satiety is a problem.
   c. Change diet consistency to soft or liquid if patient has esophagitis from radiation therapy.
7. Consider alternative pain control methods, such as cognitive and behavioral training, biofeedback, or relaxation, to increase the patient's sense of control.
   a. Evaluate problems of insomnia, depression, anxiety, etc., that may be contributing to the patient's pain.
   b. Suggest referral to pain clinic/specialist if pain does not respond to usual control methods.

Patient Education and Health Maintenance

1. Teach the patient to use prescribed medications as needed for pain without being overly concerned about addiction.
2. Advise the patient to report any new or persistent pain;

it may be attributable to some other cause, such as arthritis.

3. Encourage the patient to keep busy and to continue with usual activities (work, recreation, sexual) as much as possible.

4. Suggest talking to a social worker about financial assistance or other services that may be needed.

5. For additional information and support, refer to:
   American Cancer Society—call local chapter or 1-800-ACS-2345

C

Cancer, Oral

Cancers of the oral cavity may arise from the lips, buccal mucosa, gums, hard palate, floor of the mouth, salivary glands, and the anterior two thirds of the tongue. The disorder is often asymptomatic in early stages. Predisposing factors include use of tobacco and alcohol (particularly in combination); use of smokeless tobacco (snuff); pipe smoking; and chronic sun exposure. Approximately 90% of lesions are squamous cell carcinomas. This type of cancer is most prevalent in men aged 50 to 70 years. Oral cancers may spread to the larynx, hypopharynx, esophagus, and lungs. Depending on the stage of cancer at diagnosis, the overall 5-year survival rate is 30% to 40%.

◆ Assessment

1. Changes in swallowing, smell, taste, or voice; salivation; discomfort when eating; sore throat; foul breath odor.

2. Mucosal erythroplasia—red inflammatory or erythroplastic mucosal changes; appears smooth, granular, and minimally elevated, with or without a white component (leukoplakia), persisting longer than 10 to 14 days.

3. Although often asymptomatic in early stages, specific presentations include:
   a. Cancer of the lip—presence of a lesion that fails to heal
   b. Cancer of the tongue—swelling, ulceration, areas

C

      of tenderness or bleeding, abnormal texture, or limited tongue movement

    c. Cancer of the floor of the mouth—red, slightly elevated, mucosal lesions with ill-defined borders, leukoplakia, induration, ulceration, or wartlike growths

4. Advanced stages characterized by ulceration, bleeding, pain, induration, and cervical lymphadenopathy

◆ Diagnostic Evaluation

1. Inspection of the oral cavity and pharynx with indirect mirror to locate abnormal tissue
2. Staining of oral lesions with toluidine blue to distinguish abnormal from normal tissue (lesions stain dark blue after rinsing with acetic acid; normal tissues retain their pink color)
3. Chest x-ray to detect local invasiveness and metastasis
4. Excisional biopsy of suspected mass to identify or rule out malignancy

◆ Collaborative Management

Surgical Interventions

1. Selection of treatment depends on size and site of lesion and involvement of surrounding tissues. Surgery, radiation, and chemotherapy may be considered.
2. Small lesions can be excised widely or treated with radiation therapy or interstitial irradiation.
3. Large lesions may be excised widely or treated by radical neck dissection for extensive lymphatic involvement, followed by external irradiation to decrease recurrence rate while preserving external appearance.
4. Complications of surgery may include transient salivary outflow obstruction, infection, voice changes, fistula formation, loss of swallowing ability, and cosmetic defects.

Other Interventions

1. Radiation therapy may be palliative, if not tried earlier.
2. Complications of radiation therapy may include temporary loss of taste, xerostomia (decreased salvation), radiation caries, and osteoradionecrosis.

3. Chemotherapy of previously untreated patients with locally advanced tumors has shown high response rates in clinical trials. Side effects include nausea and vomiting, alopecia, and bone marrow suppression.

◆ Nursing Interventions

(Also see p. 601 if radical neck dissection has been performed).

Monitoring

1. Evaluate the patient's emotional status as well as adjustment to cancer and altered appearance with therapy.
2. Monitor nutritional status through intake and output, weight, and laboratory studies.

Supportive Care

1. Provide analgesics and comfort measures.
2. If the patient can tolerate it, provide mouth care with soft toothbrush and flossing between teeth.
   a. If patient cannot tolerate brushing and flossing, provide gentle oral lavage with nonirritant mouthwashes.
   b. Use power water spray to clean inaccessible areas.
3. Manage excessive salivation and mouth odors by insertion of a gauze wick in corner of mouth to absorb excess saliva, suctioning of secretions, and instruction to the patient on suctioning methods.
4. Manage decreased salivation, if necessary, by intake of adequate fluids; avoidance of dry, bulky, and irritating foods; and lozenges or chewing gum to stimulate salivation.
5. Encourage oral feedings and supplements high in protein and vitamin content and low in acidity and salt or provide alternate enteral or parenteral nutrition as indicated.
6. Maintain clean and odor-free environment for meals.
7. If swallowing difficulties persist, suggest occupational or speech therapist consultation.
8. Assist the patient in caring for personal appearance and provide emotional support.
9. Observe for reaction to cancer such as acting out or

withdrawn behavior and suggest psychological consultation, if necessary.

Patient Education and Health Maintenance

1. Reinforce teaching about good oral hygiene.
2. Emphasize adequate nutrition and food preparation with blender, if necessary.
3. Provide detailed instructions on postoperative wound care.
4. Advise reporting of any bleeding, infection, problems with salivation, or depression.
5. Encourage cessation of high-risk behaviors: smoking, alcohol consumption, use of smokeless tobacco, pipe smoking.
6. Emphasize the need for routine follow-up examinations.

Cancer, Ovarian

Ovarian cancer is a common gynecologic malignancy that carries a high mortality because it is not usually diagnosed until well advanced. Although its exact cause is not known, ovarian cancer has been linked to high-fat diet, smoking, alcohol, use of talcum powder perineally, patient history of breast, colon, or endometrial cancer, and family history of breast or ovarian cancer. Ninety percent of ovarian tumors arise in epithelial tissue, with germ cell and stromal tissue making up the rest. Incidence peaks in women aged 50 years or older. Ovarian tumors spread intraabdominally and through the lymph system.

◆ Assessment

1. First manifestations include vague abdominal discomfort, indigestion, flatulence, anorexia, pelvic pressure, weight loss or gain, and palpable ovarian enlargement.
2. Late manifestations include abdominal pain, ascites, pleural effusion, and intestinal obstruction.

> **NURSING ALERT**
> A combination of a long history of ovarian dysfunction and persistent undiagnosed GI complaints raises the suspicion of ovarian cancer. A palpable ovary in a postmenopausal woman is abnormal and should be evaluated as soon as possible.

◆ Diagnostic Evaluation

1. Pelvic sonography and CT scan—unfortunately are not sensitive to early detection of ovarian cancer.
2. Laparoscopy is more sensitive to visualize mass.
3. Laparotomy is necessary to stage the disease and determine effectiveness of treatment.
4. Paracentesis or thoracentesis are done if ascites or pleural effusion are present.
5. CA 125 is a serum tumor marker that is not reliable for screening, but an increase signifies progression of disease.

◆ Collaborative Management

Therapeutic and Pharmacologic Interventions

1. Chemotherapy—more effective if tumor is optimally debulked; usually follows surgery because of frequency of advanced disease; may be given IV or intraperitoneally
2. Immunotherapy with interferon or hormonal therapy with tamoxifen, an antiestrogen agent, may be used.
3. Radiation therapy (intraperitoneal or external) is usually adjuvant to chemotherapy, and is individualized according to the stage of disease and the patient's response to and tolerance of radiation.

Surgical Interventions

1. Total abdominal hysterectomy with bilateral salpingo-oophorectomy and omentectomy is usual treatment because of delayed diagnosis.
2. Second-look laparotomy may be done after adjunct therapies to take multiple biopsy specimens and determine effectiveness of therapy.

C

◆ Nursing Interventions

Supportive Care

1. Administer anxiolytic and analgesic medications as prescribed and provide support through the diagnostic process.
2. Administer or teach the patient or caregiver to administer antiemetics as needed for nausea and vomiting.
3. Encourage small, frequent, bland meals or liquid nutritional supplements as able. Assess the need for IV fluids if the patient is vomiting.
4. Prepare the patient for body image changes resulting from chemotherapy, for example, hair loss. Encourage the patient to prepare ahead of time with turbans, wig, hats, etc.
5. Encourage the patient to enhance appearance with makeup, clothing, jewelry, and so forth, as appropriate.
6. Stress the positive effects of the patient's treatment plan.
7. Prepare the patient for surgery as indicated; explain the extent of incision, presence of IVs, catheter, packing and drain tubes expected (see p. 350).
8. Postoperatively, reposition frequently and encourage early ambulation to promote comfort and prevent side effects.
9. Refer the patient to cancer support group.

Patient Education and Health Maintenance

1. Explain to the patient that ovary removal will cause menopausal symptoms.
2. Tell the patient that disease progression will be monitored closely by laboratory tests, and second-look laparoscopy may be necessary.
3. Explain that female relatives of the patient should notify their doctors; biannual pelvic examinations may be necessary.
4. Advise that, for women who have not had breast or ovarian cancer, oral contraceptives may decrease the risk of ovarian and endometrial cancer.

Cancer, Pancreatic

Pancreatic cancer is the fourth leading cause of cancer deaths, and its incidence is increasing, especially among persons aged 60 to 80 years. Most pancreatic cancers (70%) occur in the head of the pancreas. The tumor may block bile flow as it compresses the common bile duct, causing pain and digestive enzyme dysfunction as well. Symptoms are often vague and nonspecific, preventing early detection. Risk factors include smoking, prolonged exposure to industrial chemicals, high-fat diet, excessive alcohol intake, diabetes mellitus, and chronic pancreatitis. In rare cases, hyperinsulinism may result from islet cell tumors.

◆ Assessment

1. Gnawing or boring pain usually occurs in the upper abdomen and may radiate to the back.
   a. Pain is often worse at night. Patients tend to lie with legs drawn up. Patient bends over while walking.
   b. Pain becomes more localized, severe, and unremitting as the disease progresses.
2. Pancreatic enzyme dysfunction causes early satiety and a feeling of bloating after.
3. Biliary obstruction produces jaundice, tea-colored urine, clay-colored stools, and pruritus.
4. Anorexia, weight loss, weakness, nausea and vomiting, steatorrhea, and dehydration eventually occur.

◆ Diagnostic Evaluation

1. Elevated liver function tests and prolonged coagulation studies; possibly elevated levels of carcinoembryonic antigen and CA 19-9.
2. Ultrasound and CT studies detect tumors larger than 2 cm.
3. Endoscopic retrograde cholangiopancreatography is performed to visualize structures and obtain biopsy specimen.
4. Percutaneous needle aspiration or biopsy through ultrasonography may be performed.

C

5. Angiography may be performed to assess for any vascular involvement.

◆ Collaborative Management

Pharmacologic Interventions

1. Chemotherapy may be used in combination with radiation therapy for resectable and unresectable tumors with and without surgery.
2. Radiation therapy may be used alone for palliation or as adjuvant to surgery.
   a. External beam irradiation for local control, reduction of pain, and to palliate obstruction.
   b. Intraoperative radiation therapy has been successful in some centers for palliation.
3. Chemical splanchnicectomy may be performed to denervate the pancreas for pain relief; may be performed intraoperatively or percutaneously under CT guidance.

Surgical Interventions

1. Whipple procedure (pancreatoduodenectomy) for carcinoma of the head of the pancreas, periampullary area, chronic pancreatitis of the head of the pancreas, and trauma
2. Total pancreatectomy including a splenectomy may be performed for diffuse tumor throughout the pancreas.
3. Distal pancreatectomy, removal of the distal pancreas and spleen for tumors localized in the body and tail
4. Palliative bypass of the bile duct (choledochojejunostomy or cholecystojejunostomy) or stomach (gastrojejunostomy) for unresectable pancreatic tumors
5. Care as for abdominal surgery (see p. 350).
6. Endoscopic or percutaneous stent may be placed to relieve biliary obstruction.

◆ Nursing Interventions

Monitoring

1. Monitor fluid status through vital signs, intake and output, and daily weights.
2. Monitor for changes in vital signs or increased pain, which may indicate hemorrhage or leak from anastomosis.

3. Monitor serum glucose level for hyperglycemia or hypoglycemia.

Supportive Care

1. Administer narcotics as ordered or monitor patient-controlled analgesia. Assess the patient's response to pain control measures and consider consultation with hospice service for pain control if tumor is nonresectable.
2. Teach relaxation techniques such as relaxation breathing, progressive muscle relaxation, and imagery as adjuncts for pain relief.
3. Assist with frequent turning and comfortable positioning.
4. Administer parenteral nutrition as prescribed preoperatively and postoperatively.
5. Maintain nasogastric decompression and measure and record gastric output.
6. Progress diet slowly when oral intake is tolerated; observe for nausea, vomiting, and gastric distention.
7. Administer high-protein, high-carbohydrate diet with vitamin supplements and pancreatic enzymes as prescribed.
8. Evaluate laboratory values for hypoalbuminemia, hyponatremia, hypochloremia, and metabolic alkalosis; give replacement as prescribed.
9. Observe skin for jaundice, breakdown, irritation, or excoriation. Administer antipruritics, provide frequent skin care without soap and thorough rinsing, apply emollient lotions, and keep fingernails short to prevent scratching.
10. Inspect skin around drains and tubes for irritation and protect from fluid leakage.
11. Inspect surgical dressings and incision for bleeding, drainage, or signs of infection.
12. Prevent tension on suture lines of anastamoses by monitoring for abdominal distention and maintaining patency of tubes and drains.

Patient Education and Health Maintenance

1. Instruct the patient and family on self-care measures for pancreatic insufficiency.
   a. Glucose monitoring, insulin administration, signs and symptoms of hypoglycemia and hyperglycemia

b. Pancreatic enzyme replacement, high-protein, high-carbohydrate diet
2. Teach wound and drain care.

COMMUNITY CARE CONSIDERATIONS
Advise that skin around drainage tubes can be washed with soap and water, dried well, and then protected by generous application of petroleum jelly or zinc oxide before dressing applied.

3. Explore options for pain management.
4. Coordinate referral for home care for IV therapy, postoperative management, or hospice care.

Cancer, Prostate

Cancer of the prostate is the second leading cause of cancer death among American men and is the most common carcinoma in men older than age 65 years. Incidence of prostate cancer is 40% higher in African American men. The cause of prostate cancer is unknown; there is an increased risk for persons with a family history of the disease. Most prostate cancers are palpable on rectal examination because they arise from the peripheral zone of the gland. Prostate cancer can spread by local extension, by lymphatics, or through the bloodstream. Complications include bone metastasis leading to vertebral collapse, spinal cord compression, and pathologic fractures, or spread to urinary tract or pelvic lymph nodes.

◆ Assessment

1. First symptoms are caused by obstructed urinary flow, including hesitancy and straining on voiding, frequency, nocturia, reduced size and force of urinary stream.
2. Symptoms due to metastasis include:
   a. Pain in lumbosacral area radiating to hips and down legs (from bone metastases)

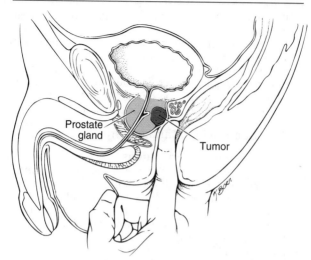

FIGURE 6 *The prostate gland can be felt through the wall of the rectum. The size of the gland, overall consistency, and the presence of any firm areas and nodules are noted.*

    b. Perineal and rectal discomfort
    c. Anemia, weight loss, weakness, nausea, oliguria (from uremia)
    d. Hematuria (from urethral or bladder invasion, or both)
    e. Lower-extremity edema—occurs when pelvic node metastases compromise venous return
2. Rectal examination to detect nodules on prostate (Fig. 6).

◆ Diagnostic Evaluation

1. Needle biopsy (through anterior rectal wall or through perineum) for histologic study of biopsy tissue or aspiration for cytologic study
2. Transrectal ultrasonography delineates tumor.
3. Prostate-specific antigen (PSA)—usually greater than 10 ng/mL

4. Prostatic acid phosphatase—elevated in advanced prostatic cancer
5. Excretory urography may be ordered to demonstrate changes due to ureteral obstruction.
6. Metastatic workup may include chest x-ray, intravenous pyelography, bone scan, and CT or MRI (recently developed method of performing prostatic MRI with endorectal coil provides detailed images)

C

◆ Collaborative Management

Therapeutic Interventions

1. In many patients older than age 70, no treatment may be indicated, because the cancer may be slow-growing and will not be the cause of death. Instead, these patients should be followed closely with periodic serum PSA testing and examined for evidence of metastases.
2. In advanced prostatic cancer not responsive to treatment, palliative measures include:
   a. Analgesics and narcotics to relieve pain
   b. Short course of radiation therapy for specific sites of bone pain
   c. Intravenous administration of a beta-emitter agent (strontium chloride 89) to directly irradiate metastatic sites
   d. Transurethral resection to remove obstructing tissue if bladder outlet obstruction occurs
   e. Suprapubic catheter placement
3. External beam radiation (using linear accelerator) focused on the prostate: Focuses maximum radiation on tumor while sparing uninvolved tissues.
4. Interstitial radiation (brachytherapy): interstitial implantation of isotopes into prostate delivers radiation directly to tumor while sparing uninvolved tissue.
   a. Complications include radiation cystitis (urinary frequency, urgency, nocturia), urethral injury (stricture), radiation enteritis (diarrhea, anorexia, nausea), radiation proctitis (diarrhea, rectal bleeding), impotence.

Pharmacologic Interventions

1. Hormone manipulation deprives tumor cells of androgens or their by-products and thereby alleviates symptoms and retards progress of disease.

2. Estrogen therapy suppresses release of luteinizing hormone, thereby indirectly decreasing testosterone levels.
   a. Therapy with estrogens leads to water retention, cardiovascular side effects, and gynecomastia (soreness and enlargement of breasts).
3. Analogs of luteinizing hormone–releasing hormone (LHRH) such as leuprolide reduce testosterone levels as effectively as orchiectomy or estrogen.
4. Antiandrogen drugs (megestrol and flutamide) block androgen action directly at the target tissues (testes and adrenals) and block androgen synthesis within the prostate gland.
5. Combination therapy with LHRH analogs and flutamide blocks the action of all circulating androgen.
6. Complications of hormonal manipulation include hot flashes, nausea and vomiting, gynecomastia, and sexual dysfunction.

Surgical Interventions

1. Radical prostatectomy—removal of entire prostate gland, prostatic capsule, and seminal vesicles; may include pelvic lymphadenectomy (see p. 689)
   a. Complications include urinary incontinence, impotence, and rectal injury.
   b. Sexual potency may be preserved with better surgical dissection techniques.
2. Laparoscopic pelvic lymph node dissection may be performed before prostatectomy to accurately stage disease; positive lymph nodes would preclude radical prostatectomy.
3. Cryosurgery freezes prostate tissue, killing tumor cells without prostatectomy.
4. Bilateral orchiectomy (removal of testes) results in reduction of the major circulating androgen, testosterone, as a palliative measure to reduce symptoms and progression.

◆ **Nursing Interventions**

Supportive Care

1. Assess pain control. Be sure that the patient is not undermedicated; help the family and patient understand that addiction is not a concern.

2. Teach relaxation techniques such as imagery, music therapy, progressive muscle relaxation as adjunct to pain control.
3. Employ safety measures to prevent pathologic fractures, such as prevention of falls if bone metastasis is present.
4. To reduce anxiety, give repeated explanations of diagnostic tests and treatment options, and help the patient gain some feeling of control over disease and decisions.
5. To help achieve optimal sexual function, give the patient the opportunity to communicate his concerns and sexual needs.
6. Inform the patient that decreased libido is expected after hormonal manipulation therapy, and impotence may result from some surgical procedures and radiation.
7. Suggest options such as sexual counseling, learning other options of sexual expression, and consideration of penile implant.

Patient Education and Health Maintenance

1. Teach patient importance of follow-up for check of PSA levels and evaluation for disease progression.
2. Teach IM or subcutaneous administration of hormonal agents as indicated.
3. If bone metastasis has occurred, encourage safety measures around the home to prevent pathologic fractures, such as removal of throw rugs, using hand rail on stairs, using nightlights.
4. Advise reporting of symptoms of worsening urethral obstruction such as increased frequency, urgency, hesitancy, and urinary retention.
5. Encourage all men to seek medical screening for prostate cancer.

❖

NURSING ALERT
The American Cancer Society recommends an annual rectal examination for all men older than age 40. Annual rectal examination and PSA blood testing is recommended for all men older than age 50.

5. For additional information and support, refer to agencies such as

> **US TOO International Inc.**
> 930 North York Rd., Suite 50
> Hensdale, IL 60521
> 800-808-7866

Cancer, Renal Cell

Renal cell carcinoma is the most common malignant renal tumor, occurring twice as frequently in men as in women. Most renal cell tumors arise in the renal parenchyma and develop with few if any symptoms. There is no known cause, although they may be associated with cigarette smoking.

Renal tumors are aggressive and metastasize rapidly, often before diagnosis. They most frequently occur in persons aged 50 to 60 years.

◆ Assessment

1. Often asymptomatic and may be found late on routine examination as palpable abdominal mass
2. Fatigue, anemia, weight loss, fever may be first manifestations.
3. Classic triad (late symptoms)
   a. Hematuria: intermittent or continuous, microscopic or gross
   b. Flank pain: from distention of renal capsule, invasion of surrounding structures
   c. Palpable mass in flank

◆ Diagnostic Evaluation

1. Intravenous pyelography (IVP) is usual initial screening procedure.
2. Renal ultrasonography is used to differentiate renal cysts from renal tumors; used as a complement to IVP.
3. CT or MRI scans for patients with urographic findings suggesting tumor; useful to detect, categorize, and stage a renal mass

◆ Collaborative Management

Pharmacologic Interventions

1. Renal cell carcinomas are generally refractory to chemotherapeutic agents, radiation, and hormonal therapy.
2. Interleukin-2 (a lymphokine that stimulates growth of T lymphocytes) may offer some benefit in metastatic disease, but toxicity is severe.
3. Interferon is also being investigated for treating metastatic cancer.

Surgical Interventions

1. Radical nephrectomy:
   a. Removal of kidney and associated tumor, adrenal gland, surrounding perirenal fat, Gerota's fascia, and possibly regional lymph nodes to provide maximum opportunity for disease control
   b. Performed through a vertical midline, subcostal, thoracoabdominal, or flank incision
2. Renal artery embolization:
   a. Preoperative occlusion of renal artery followed by nephrectomy, performed if the patient has large vascular tumor
   b. Embolizing material (Gelfoam, steel coils, blood clot) is injected through catheter into the renal artery and carried with arterial blood flow to occlude the tumor vessels.
   c. Procedure decreases tumor vascularity, minimizes blood loss, relieves pain, and devitalizes the tumor, thereby decreasing the chance for tumor cell implantation at time of surgery.
   d. Complications include postinfarction syndrome, arterial obstruction, bleeding, and reduced renal function.

◆ Nursing Interventions

Monitoring

1. Monitor patient comfort level and need for additional analgesia.
2. If renal artery embolization is performed, monitor for postinfarction syndrome (lasts 2–3 days): severe abdominal pain, nausea, vomiting, diarrhea, fever.

Supportive Care

1. Assess the patient's understanding about diagnosis and treatment options. Answer questions and encourage more thorough discussion with health care provider as needed.
2. Encourage the patient to discuss fears and feelings; involve family and significant others in teaching.
3. To control symptoms of postinfarction syndrome:
   a. Administer analgesics as prescribed to control flank and abdominal pain.
   b. Encourage rest and assist with positioning for 2 to 3 days until syndrome subsides.
   c. Obtain temperature every 4 hours and administer antipyretics as indicated.
   d. Restrict oral intake and provide IV fluids and antiemetics to control nausea.
4. Provide postoperative nephrectomy care (see p. 514).

Patient Education and Health Maintenance

1. Ensure that the patient understands where and when to go for follow-up (nephrologist; surgeon; primary care provider; oncologist and radiologist for metastatic workup and treatment).
2. Explain the importance of follow-up for hypertension and evaluation of renal function, even if the patient feels well.
3. Advise the patient with one kidney to wear a medical alert bracelet and notify all health care providers, because all potentially nephrotoxic medications and procedures must be avoided.

Cancer, Skin

Skin cancer is the most common malignancy. Three major types of skin cancer are recognized. The most common type, *basal cell carcinoma,* arises from basal layers of the epidermis or hair follicles and rarely metastasizes. *Squamous cell carcinoma* arises from the epidermis; metastasis occurs more often than with basal cell carcinoma. *Malignant melanoma,* the rarest type, arises from nevocytic cells in the upper dermis and metastasizes widely. Most basal and squamous cell carcinomas are located on sun-exposed areas and are directly related to ultraviolet radiation. These carcinomas are easily curable, however, because of early diagnosis and slow progression. Untreated skin cancer may progress to regional or systemic metastasis (frequently to the central nervous system).

Risk factors for skin cancer include: fair complexion, blue eyes, blond or red hair; working outdoors; elderly with sun-damaged skin; history of x-ray treatment of skin conditions; exposure to certain chemical agents (arsenicals, nitrates, tar and pitch, oils and paraffins); burn scars, damaged skin in areas of chronic osteomyelitis, fistulae openings; long-term immunosuppressive therapy; genetic susceptibility; and family history of dysplastic or congenital nevi.

C

◆ **Assessment**

NURSING ALERT
Any skin lesion that changes in size or color, bleeds, ulcerates, or becomes infected may be skin cancer.

1. Basal cell carcinoma
   a. Lesions often begin as small nodules with a rolled, pearly, translucent border with telangiectasia, crusting, and occasionally ulceration.
   b. Appear most frequently on sun-exposed skin, frequently on face between hair line and upper lip
   c. If neglected, may cause local destruction, hemorrhage, and infection of adjacent tissues, producing severe functional and cosmetic disabilities
2. Squamous cell carcinoma
   a. Appears as reddish rough, thickened, scaly lesion with bleeding and soreness, or may be asymptomatic; border may be wider, more infiltrated, and more inflammatory than basal cell carcinoma
   b. May be preceded by leukoplakia (premalignant lesion of mucous membrane) of the mouth or tongue, actinic keratoses, scarred or ulcerated lesions

c. Seen most commonly on lower lip, rims of ears, head, neck, and backs of the hands
3. Malignant melanoma
   a. Melanoma in situ: earliest phase, difficult to recognize because clinical changes are minimal
   b. Superficial spreading melanoma (most common)—circular, with irregular outer portions; the margins may be flat or elevated and palpable; has combination of colors—hues of tan, brown, and black mixed with gray, bluish-black, or white; may be dull pink-rose color in a small area within the lesion; occurs anywhere on body; usually affects middle-aged persons
   c. Nodular melanoma—spherical blueberry-like nodule with relatively smooth surface and relatively uniform blue-black, blue-gray, or reddish-blue color; may be polypoidal and elevated, with smooth surface of rose-gray or black color; occurs commonly on torso and extremities; invades directly into the subjacent dermis (vertical growth) and hence has a poorer prognosis
   d. Lentigo—malignant melanoma—first appears as tan, flat macule; malignant degeneration is manifested by changes in color, size, and topography; slowly evolving; occurs on exposed skin surfaces of persons in the fifth or sixth decade
   e. Acrolentiginous melanoma (uncommon, except in black-skinned individuals)—irregular pigmented macules, which develop nodules; may become invasive early; occurs commonly on palms, soles, nail beds, and rarely on mucous membranes

◆ Diagnostic Evaluation

1. Excisional biopsy for histopathologic diagnosis and microstaging, to determine thickness and level of invasion and guide treatment and prognosis

◆ Collaborative Management

Therapeutic Interventions

1. Prepare the patient for prescribed radiation therapy: can be done for cancer of eyelid, tip of nose, in or near

vital structures (eg, facial nerve), where tissue sparing is difficult, with other forms of treatment; also used for extensive malignancies where goal is palliation or when other medical conditions contraindicate other forms of therapy.
2. Photoradiation may be used.

Pharmacologic Interventions

1. Regional perfusion chemotherapy—agent may be perfused directly into area containing melanoma by mechanically controlling arterial and venous blood flow; allows higher concentration of cytotoxic drug to be delivered to site, with less systemic toxicity
2. Systemic chemotherapy: generally used for recurrence of metastasis or palliation; may be combined with autologous bone marrow transplantation or several agents used in combination
3. Other regimens include topical fluorouracil, interferon, retinoids.

Surgical Interventions

1. Curettage followed by electrodessication—usually done on small tumors of basal or squamous cell type (smaller than 1–2 cm)
2. Surgical excision; may be followed by simple closure, flap or graft
3. Microscopically controlled surgery—immediate microscopic examination is made of frozen or chemically fixed sections for evidence of cancer cells. Layers are removed until no more cancer cells are seen.

◆ Nursing Interventions

Supportive Care and Patient Education

1. Teach the patient and all individuals to use a sunscreen with a sun protection factor of at least 15 routinely for the rest of life and *never become sunburned.* Teach methods of minimizing sun exposure with appropriate clothing and hats.
2. Encourage lifelong follow-up with dermatologist or primary care provider, with skin examinations every 6 months.
3. Encourage all individuals to have moles removed that

are accessible to repeated friction and irritation, congenital, or suspicious in any way.

4. Demonstrate skin self-examination to all individuals, using mirrors and magnifying glass to examine all skin surfaces, including scalp, genital area, buttocks, feet, etc., for suspicious lesions.

5. Encourage reporting any skin lesion that changes in size or color, bleeds, ulcerates, or becomes infected.

C

Cancer, Testicular

Testicular cancer is a disease that occurs in younger men between the ages of 25 and 35 years. Most testicular cancers originate in the germ cells, and most are potentially curable. The most common germinal tumors in adults are seminoma, embryonal carcinoma, teratoma, and choriocarcinoma. The direct cause of testicular cancer is unknown; it has been linked to cryptorchidism (failure of the testes to descend into the scrotum). Complications include metastasis to the retroperitoneal lymph nodes with subsequent involvement of the mediastinal lymph nodes, lungs, and liver, resulting in death.

◆ Assessment

1. Painless swelling or enlargement of the testis; accompanied by sensation of heaviness in scrotum
2. Pain in the testis (if patient has epididymitis or bleeding into tumor)
3. Signs and symptoms of metastatic disease: cough, lymphadenopathy, back pain, abdominal mass

◆ Diagnostic Evaluation

1. Elevated serum markers of human chorionic gonadotropin (hCG) and alpha-fetoprotein (AFP); tumor marker assays also used for diagnosis, detection of early recurrence, staging of tumors, and monitoring response to therapy
2. Scrotal ultrasonography to locate tumor and differentiate between solid and cystic lesions

3. Chest x-rays to locate pulmonary or mediastinal metastases
4. CT scanning of chest, abdomen, and pelvis, to evaluate retroperitoneal lymph nodes and to follow progress of therapy

◆ Collaborative Management

Therapeutic and Pharmacologic Interventions

1. Radiation therapy to lymphatic drainage pathways is used after orchiectomy in seminomas.
   a. Achieves close to 99% cure rate
   b. During this therapy, the uninvolved testicle is shielded, usually preserving fertility.
2. Chemotherapy with cisplatin combination therapy is used to treat nonseminomatous primary tumor and regional lymphatic metastases and in managing distant metastatic disease.

Surgical Interventions

1. Inguinal orchiectomy: removal of testis and its tunica and spermatic cord
2. Retroperitoneal lymph node dissection (RPLND): usually performed after orchiectomy in nonseminomas for staging and therapeutic purposes
3. Modified nerve-sparing unilateral lymphadenectomy can be done on selected patients, thus preserving ejaculation.
4. Complications of surgery
   a. RPLND causes infertility because of retrograde ejaculation.
   b. Unilateral orchiectomy eliminates half of germinal cells, thus reducing sperm count.
   c. Libido and ability to attain an erection are preserved in both procedures.

◆ Nursing Interventions

Supportive Care

1. Provide routine postoperative care, including early ambulation, respiratory care, and administration of pain medication.

2. After RPLND, monitor for paralytic ileus, which is common after extensive resection.
   a. Auscultate bowel sounds frequently and observe for abdominal distention.
   b. Withhold oral fluids until bowel sounds have returned.
   c. Report complaints of nausea and any vomiting.
   d. Begin nasogastric decompression, if indicated.
3. For patients receiving chemotherapy, intervene for common side effects, including nausea and vomiting, alopecia, myalgias, abdominal cramping, and mucositis.
4. Encourage the younger patient to investigate depositing sperm in sperm bank before surgery if fertility may be desired in the future.
5. Provide realistic information about impending surgery or treatment; dispel myths associated with testicular disease, and emphasize high positive cure rates.
6. Reassure the patient that orchiectomy will not diminish virility, and retroperitoneal lymph node dissection may cause retrograde ejaculation (into the urinary bladder) but not affect libido, erection, and sensation.
7. Advise the patient that a gel-filled testicular prosthesis can be implanted that will preserve scrotal appearance and feel.
8. Refer the patient to a social worker or counselor as needed for problems and concerns with relationships, peers, or work life.

Patient Education and Health Maintenance

1. Teach all young men to perform monthly testicular self-examination; after orchiectomy, the patient should examine the remaining testicle monthly.
2. Review schedule for radiation treatments or chemotherapy; teach the patient and family possible side effects; discuss expectations for treatment period.
3. Provide information about retrograde ejaculation after retroperitoneal lymph node dissection and alternatives for fertility.

Cancer, Thyroid

Thyroid cancer is a malignant neoplasm of the gland that is especially likely to occur in patients who have received

C

radiation treatments to the head and neck in early life. Incidence increases with age; the average age at time of diagnosis is 45. Thyroid cancer occurs in several forms.

Papillary and well-differentiated adenocarcinoma is the most common type. It grows slowly and does not spread beyond the lymph nodes surrounding the thyroid. The cure rate is excellent after removal of involved tissues.

Follicular carcinoma is a rapidly growing, widely metastasizing cancer that occurs predominantly in middle-aged and elderly persons. Although x-ray treatments may temporarily retard this cancer, it has a high mortality rate.

Parafollicular or *medullary thyroid carcinoma* (MTC) is a rare, inheritable cancer that can be completely cured if detected early enough by radioimmunoassay for calcitonin.

◆ Assessment

1. Patient is usually asymptomatic, but hyperthyroidism may occur.
2. Palpation shows a firm, irregular, fixed, painless mass or nodule.

◆ Diagnostic Evaluation

1. A thyroid scan with ^{99m}-technetium pertechnetate differentiates between malignant "cold" nodules, which absorb little of the isotope, compared with nonmalignant nodules or uninvolved tissue.
2. Biopsy using fine-needle aspiration may be done.

◆ Collaborative Management

Therapeutic and Pharmacologic Interventions

1. Thyroid hormone is administered to suppress secretion of TSH after surgical intervention. Treatment is continued indefinitely and requires annual checkups.
2. For unresectable cancer, patient is referred for treatment with ^{131}I treatment or radiation therapy.

Surgical Interventions

1. Thyroidectomy is partial or complete, as required (see p. 840).

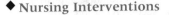

2. Postsurgical radiation therapy is often done to reduce chances of recurrence.
3. Follow-up includes periodic radioiodine uptake scan to detect evidence of recurrence.

◆ Nursing Interventions

Monitoring

1. Monitor the patient postoperatively for hemorrhage, tracheal compression caused by swelling, and laryngeal nerve damage.

Supportive Care

1. Provide all explanations in a simple, concise manner and repeat important information as necessary to reduce anxiety, which may interfere with the patient's ability to process information.
2. Reinforce the positive aspects of treatment and high cure rate as outlined by the health care provider.
3. Encourage support by significant other, clergy, social worker, nursing staff, etc.

Patient Education and Health Maintenance

1. Instruct the patient on the need for compliance with thyroid hormone replacement regimen.
2. Advise the patient regarding the need for follow-up to monitor replacement therapy and to check for recurrence of malignancy.
3. Supply the patient with additional information or suggest appropriate community resources dealing with cancer prevention and treatment.

Cancer, Uterine

Uterine cancer usually occurs as adenocarcinoma of the endometrium of the fundus or body of the uterus. Its cause is unknown, but it is linked to increased estrogen stimulation, as in obesity, late menopause, nulliparity, and unopposed estrogen replacement. Uterine cancer is the most common gynecologic cancer, and the fourth leading cancer in women. Most cases occur in women older than age 55 years. This cancer may spread to involve all pelvic structures and metastasizes to lungs, liver, bone, and brain.

◆ Assessment

1. Irregular bleeding before menopause or postmenopausal bleeding; anemia secondary to bleeding
2. Vaginal discharge—watery, usually malodorous
3. Pain, fever, and bowel and bladder dysfunctions are late signs.

◆ Diagnostic Evaluation

1. Pelvic examination detects enlarged uterus.
2. Endocervical aspirate—shows abnormal cells
3. Endometrial biopsy—may be false negative
4. Dilation and curettage (D&C)—most accurate diagnostic tool
5. Additional testing includes metastatic workup (x-ray studies and cystoscopy).

◆ Collaborative Management

Therapeutic Interventions

1. Radiation therapy is the usual treatment for all stages. Therapy is individualized according to the stage of disease and the patient's response to and tolerance of radiation.
2. Intracavitary radiation—radium via applicator in endocervical canal
   a. Applicator remains in place 24 to 72 hours.
   b. Complications include hemorrhagic cystitis, proctitis, vaginal stenosis, uterine perforation.
3. External radiation—via linear accelerator or cobalt
   a. External radiation over pelvis may supplement intracavitary to eliminate cancer spread via lymphatic system.
   b. Complications include bone marrow depression, bowel obstruction, fistula

Pharmacologic Interventions

1. Hormonal therapy (progestational agents) to alter receptor sites in endometrium for estrogen and thus decrease growth in metastatic disease

2. Chemotherapy is given for metastatic and recurrent disease; low response rate of short duration.

Surgical Interventions

1. Hysterectomy with bilateral salpingo-oophorectomy is treatment of choice.

◆ Nursing Interventions

Monitoring

1. Monitor the patient's response to pain control medications.
2. Observe for signs and symptoms of radiation sickness—nausea, vomiting, fever, diarrhea, abdominal cramping.
3. Monitor for complications of surgery—bleeding, infection.

Supportive Care

1. Administer pain medications and encourage use of relaxation techniques such as deep breathing, imagery, and distraction to help promote comfort.
2. Support the patient through the diagnostic process and reinforce information given by the health care provider about treatment options.
3. Prepare the patient for hysterectomy (see p. 495).
4. If indicated, prepare the patient for intracavitary radiation.
   a. Advise the patient that you will be administering an enema and vaginal douche and inserting an indwelling catheter before placement of the applicator in the operating room under anesthesia. X-ray confirms placement.
   b. Encourage the patient to bring diversional materials, because she will remain on bed rest during radiation treatment.
   c. Instruct the patient on radiation safety measures.
   d. Reassure the patient that radioactivity is monitored by specially trained personnel, that neither the patient nor secretions are radioactive, and that when applicators are removed, no radioactivity remains.
   e. Reinforce that help is readily available.
5. During radiation treatment, perform the following:

a. Maintain the patient on strict bed rest on her back with head of bed elevated 20 to 30 degrees. The patient may be log-rolled three to four times per day. Use egg-crate mattress.

b. Have the patient bathe her upper body. Perineal care and linen changes are done only when absolutely necessary.

c. Maintain the patient on a low-residue diet to prevent bowel movements, which could dislodge the apparatus. Encourage the patient to eat a variety of small servings.

d. Inspect indwelling catheter frequently to ensure proper drainage. A distended bladder may cause severe radiation burns.

e. Encourage fluids to prevent bladder infection.

f. Check the patient frequently to minimize anxiety, but minimize time spent at bedside to reduce radiation exposure.

6. During radiation removal, perform the following:

a. Ensure that sterile gloves, long forceps, and lead container are available.

b. Check number of tubes removed against number applied, should be noted in chart.

c. Practice radiation precautions in handling and returning source to radiation department.

d. Administer a cleansing enema and douche before the patient gets out of bed.

e. Provide assistance during ambulation because of postural hypotension from prolonged bed rest.

Patient Education and Health Maintenance

1. Explain the importance of reporting any postmenopausal bleeding.

2. Encourage keeping follow-up visits.

3. Explain that surgery or radiation treatment does not prevent satisfying sexual activity.

4. Refer the patient to a local cancer support group.

Cancer, Vulvar

Vulvar cancer most commonly occurs as squamous cell carcinoma of the labia majora or clitoris. Its cause is unknown, but it has been linked to viral infections such as human papilloma virus (HPV) or herpes simplex virus (HSV). It spreads primarily through the lymphatic system. Distant metastasis is rare. Vulvar cancer is most common in women older than age 60. Incidence is rising because of an increasingly elderly population, and the disease now represents approximately 4% of gynecologic cancers. If cancer is confined to the vulva, the 5-year survival rate after surgery is 90%.

C

◆ Assessment

1. Lesion present for several months; may be reddened, pigmented, white, or slightly elevated or ulcerated
2. Vulvar pruritus, pain
3. Discharge or bleeding; may be foul-smelling because of secondary infection
4. Dysuria caused by invasion of urethra with bacteria
5. Lymphadenopathy, edema of vulvar tissue

◆ Diagnostic Evaluation

1. Biopsy of lesion and lymph nodes to confirm diagnosis
2. If lesion is small, it may be excised at time of biopsy.

◆ Collaborative Management

Pharmacologic Interventions
1. Chemotherapy is primarily investigational. May shrink lesion so surgery can be less extensive.

Surgical Interventions
1. Noninvasive carcinoma is usually treated by simple vulvectomy.
   a. Postoperative complications include wound breakdown, lymphedema, leg cellulitis, and vaginal stenosis.
   b. Laser therapy also may be used.
2. Invasive carcinoma is treated by radical or modified radical vulvectomy with bilateral resection of groin lymph nodes. Pelvic nodes also may be removed if involvement is suspected.
3. Advanced carcinoma is treated by pelvic exenteration,

or surgery and radiation as a palliative measure. Radiation has a limited role because of tumor insensitivity and complications such as severe vulvitis.

◆ Nursing Interventions

Supportive Care

1. Emphasize the positive outcomes of the prescribed treatment plan; reinforce what the surgeon has already described to her.
2. Prepare the patient for surgery and describe to her the postoperative appearance of the wound, use of drains, urinary catheter, etc.
3. Administer an enema to evacuate intestinal tract before surgery; there will be no bowel movement for 2 to 3 days after surgery.
4. After surgery, maintain drainage and compression of tissues to remove fluid that could cause edema and prevent wound healing. Empty drains as needed (at least every 8 hours).
5. Provide meticulous wound care.
   a. Keep wound clean and dry.
   b. Change sterile dressings as prescribed.
   c. Apply heat lamp if prescribed to increase circulation and healing.
6. Perform perineal care or sitz baths after each bowel movement or voiding (after catheter removed).
7. Maintain patency of urinary catheter (about 10 days) to prevent wound contamination.
8. Encourage low Fowler's position to promote comfort and reduce tension on sutures.
9. Prevent straining with defecation by providing a low-residue diet initially, stool softeners later, as ordered.
10. While patient is on bed rest, administer mini-dose heparin, if prescribed, and encourage leg exercises to prevent thrombus or embolus formation.
11. Encourage careful ambulation the day after surgery while preventing perineal tension.
12. Inform the patient of changes that may occur because of surgery—loss of sexual arousal if clitoris is removed, shortening of vaginal, decreased lubrication.
    a. Tell the patient that if vagina is still intact, vaginal intercourse is still possible.

  b. Help the patient explore alternate methods of sexual intimacy and encourage her to discuss feelings with her partner.

Patient Education and Health Maintenance

1. Encourage follow-up visits for additional therapy if required.
2. Encourage regular health checkups and screening for cancer and other age-related illness.
3. Encourage early evaluation of any suspicious lesions, bleeding, or discharge.

Cardiac Dysrhythmias
See Dysrhythmias

Cardiac Surgery

Cardiac surgery, or open-heart surgery, is performed for coronary artery bypass grafting (CABG), valve replacement with prosthetic or biologic valves, and repair of congenital defects. The procedure requires temporary cardiopulmonary bypass (diversion of the blood from the heart and lungs for mechanical oxygenation and recirculation) to provide a dry, bloodless field during the operation. Table 3 gives additional cardiac procedures.

◆ **Potential Complications**

1. Cardiac dysrhythmias (common)
2. Cardiac tamponade
3. Myocardial infarction
4. Cardiac failure (low-output syndrome)
5. Persistent bleeding (blood clotting disturbance usually transient after cardiopulmonary bypass, but may be severe)
6. Hypovolemia, hypotension, renal insufficiency or failure
7. Embolization (common sites include lungs, coronary

(text continues on p. 170)

C

TABLE 3 Additional Cardiac Procedures

Procedure, Indications, Description	Nursing Considerations
Cardiac Catheterization To measure oxygen concentration, saturation, tension, and pressure in heart chambers; to detect shunts; provide blood samples for analysis; evaluate valvular function; and determine cardiac output and pulmonary blood flow **Description** Diagnostic procedure involves introducing a catheter or catheters into the heart chambers and blood vessels. Angiography is usually combined with catheterization to visualize coronary arteries.	**Preprocedure** 1. Withhold food and fluids for 6 hours to prevent vomiting and aspiration. 2. Get allergy history for any dyes. 3. Mark distal pulses for easy reference after procedure. 4. Warn patient of urge to cough and feeling of warmth during injection of contrast medium; also palpations as catheter is manipulated. 5. Remove dentures, administer medication as directed. **Postprocedure** 1. Monitor BP and apical pulase every 15 minutes until stable to detect dysrhythmias. 2. Check peripheral pulses in extremities and evaluate extremities to detect arterial insufficiency. 3. Monitor cutdown site for signs of bleeding/hematoma. 4. Maintain bed rest until following morning. 5. Assess for and report complaints of chest pain; may indicate MI, a serious complication. 6. Assess complaints of back pain, thigh, or groin pain; may indicate retroperitoneal bleeding.

7. Be alert for nausea, diaphoresis, hypotension, and bradycardia caused by vagal reaction; treat as directed with atropine and fluids.

Preprocedure

1. Explain the procedure and mark peripheral pulses for easy reference later.
2. Administer sedation so the patient will remain awake and be able to report chest pain if it occurs during procedure.
3. Maintain NPO status.

Postprocedure

1. Check vital signs every 15 minutes for 1 hour, every half hour for 2 hours, and then hourly until stable.
2. Continually evaluate for signs of restenosis—chest, jaw, back, or arm pain; nausea or abdominal distress; ECG changes.
3. Evaluate for excessive diuresis and hypokalemia caused by contrast media.
4. Watch for vasovagal response (bradycardia, hypotension) during removal of groin catheter 4–6 hours after procedure. Be prepared to place patient in Trendelenberg position and give atropine and fluids as directed.

Percutaneous Transluminal Coronary Angioplasty (PTCA)

To treat coronary artery disease by widening the lumen of a stenosed coronary artery, thereby improving blood flow below the lesion. Used in stable/unstable angina not responding to conventional therapy, in evolving MI (may be in conjunction with thrombolytic therapy) and to reopen obstructed coronary bypass grafts.

Description:

A balloon-tipped catheter is introduced through a guidewire into a coronary vessel with a noncalcified atheromatous lesion. Inflation of the balloon disrupts the atheroma to increase diameter of the vessel lumen. The balloon is inflated and deflated until best result is achieved. Restenosis may occur acutely within 24 hours, or within 6 months. Recent advanced techniques include laser-assisted PTCA, atherectomy using a rotating catheter head, and intracoronary stenting.

(continued)

C

TABLE 3 (Continued)

Procedure, Indications, Description	Nursing Considerations
	5. Maintain bed rest with head elevated no more than 30 degrees and affected extremity immobilized for 12–24 hours.
	6. Check pulses, color, sensation, and temperature of extremity and insertion site for bleeding and hematoma.
	7. Be aware that heparin is given during procedure and increases risk of bleeding. Report any signs of bleeding and apply direct pressure if bleeding occurs at insertion site.
	Preprocedure
	1. Explain that patient will remain awake and receive sedative and local anesthetic.
	2. Maintain NPO status.
	Postprocedure
Cardiac Pacing	1. Monitor vital signs, urine output, and alertness frequently to assure adequate cardiac output with paced rhythm.
To initiate and maintain natural heart rate when normal pacemaker cannot. Corrects a variety of brady-/tachydysrhythmias, and symptomatic heart blocks; also may be used prophylactically after acute MI, before/after cardiac surgery, and during certain cardiac function tests (including catheterization).	2. Analyze ECG strips every 4 hours and report dysrhythmias. Obtain 12-lead ECG daily as directed.
Description	
Pulse generator may be permanent (entire unit implanted subcutaneously) or temporary (attached externally to subcutaneous leads).	

C

Generator may stimulate atrium, ventricle, or both heart chambers in sequence and initiate electrical depolarization and cardiac contraction.

External cardiac pacing is also possible in emergency situations, using transcutaneous leads, and does not require surgery.

❖

NURSING ALERT:
If patient is to be moved, provide portable ECG monitoring and nurse. Patients with temporary pacemakers should never be placed in unmonitored areas.

3. Monitor for signs of hemothorax (hypotension, diaphoresis, restlessness); pneumothorax (acute dyspnea, cyanosis, chest pain, absent breath sounds); bleeding; lead migration (chest wall twitching or hiccups); or perforation of heart (chest pain, distant heart sound, pulsus paradoxus).

4. Report signs of infection at incision site or systemically.

5. Provide electrically safe environment—all equipment grounded, lead wires protected by plastic, no electric razor, MRI, etc.

(continued)

C

TABLE 3 (Continued)

Procedure, Indications, Description	Nursing Considerations
Automatic Implantable Defibrillator (AID) To control ventricular fibrillation/tachycardia not remedied by other means, or after survival of one incident of sudden cardiac death not associated with acute MI. **Description** Pulse generator is implanted in subcutaneous pocket in upper abdomen. Leads attached to heart muscle from generator detect lethal dysrhythmias and deliver 15–25 joules electric shock to terminate dysrhythmia. Nontermination results in sequence of up to 4 or 5 shocks of 30–32 joules.	**Preprocedure** 1. Explain surgical procedure and that patient will be under general anesthesia. 2. Explain that defibrillation will be experienced as a strong sensation in the chest if the patient is conscious during dysrhythmia. **Postprocedure** 1. Monitor vital signs until stable. 2. Monitor incision site for bleeding and infection, and monitor chest tube drainage if in place. 3. Maintain cardiac monitoring and expect to treat dysrhythmias as directed.

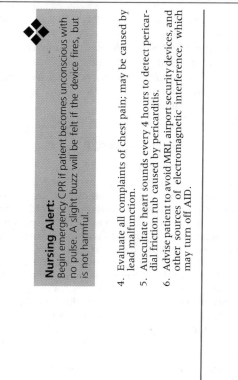

> ❖❖
> **Nursing Alert:**
> Begin emergency CPR if patient becomes unconscious with no pulse. A slight buzz will be felt if the device fires, but is not harmful.

4. Evaluate all complaints of chest pain; may be caused by lead malfunction.
5. Auscultate heart sounds every 4 hours to detect pericardial friction rub caused by pericarditis.
6. Advise patient to avoid MRI, airport security devices, and other sources of electromagnetic interference, which may turn off AID.

C

arteries, mesentery, extremities, kidneys, spleen, and brain)
8. Postpericardiotomy syndrome (unknown cause, may be related to anticardiac antibodies)
9. Postperfusion syndrome (characterized by fever, splenomegaly, lymphocytosis)
10. Febrile complications
11. Hepatitis

◆ **Collaborative Management**

Preoperative Care

1. Review the patient's condition to detect underlying problems such as history of cardiac dysrhythmias, chronic lung disease, depression, alcohol intake, and smoking that may impact postoperative recovery.
2. Obtain samples for preoperative laboratory studies, including complete blood count, electrolytes, lipids, renal and hepatic function tests, antibody screen, coagulation studies, and cultures for any underlying infection.
3. Evaluate the patient's drug history for drugs that may impact on surgery such as digitalis (may be stopped preoperatively to prevent toxicity associated with cardiopulmonary bypass); diuretics (may be associated with electrolyte imbalance); beta-adrenergic blockers (usually continued); psychotropic drugs (postoperative withdrawal may cause extreme agitation); reserpine (stopped in advance to allow norepinephrine repletion); anticoagulants (discontinued several days preoperatively); corticosteroids (if taken within the year before surgery, may be given in supplemental doses to mitigate surgical stress).
4. Improve underlying pulmonary disease and respiratory function to reduce risk of complications.
   a. Encourage the patient to stop smoking.
   b. Treat infection and pulmonary vascular congestion.

GERONTOLOGIC ALERT
Elderly and debilitated patients are at greater risk for postoperative respiratory complications. Close monitoring and aggressive coughing and deep breathing are indicated.

5. Prepare the patient and family for events in the postoperative period, including chest physical therapy procedures, pain management plan, and the loose restraint of hands for several hours after surgery to avoid risk of inadvertent removal of tubes and intravenous lines.
6. Evaluate the patient's emotional state and try to reduce anxieties.
7. Prepare the patient for the procedure:
   a. Shave anterior and lateral surfaces of trunk and neck; shave entire body down to ankles (for coronary bypass).
   b. Have the patient shower or bathe with Betadine soap.
   c. Give a sedative as directed before moving patient to the operating room.

Postoperative Care

1. Monitor and support respiratory status because respiratory insufficiency is common after open-heart surgery.
   a. Provide care while on mechanical ventilator (usually the first 24 hours); assist with weaning and extubation when indicated.
   b. Auscultate breath sounds for crackles, indicating pulmonary congestion, or decreased or absent breath sounds, indicating pneumothorax.
   c. Promote coughing, deep breathing, and turning to keep airways patent, prevent atelectasis, and facilitate lung expansion. Use chest physiotherapy if congestion develops.
   d. Suction as indicated; however, prolonged suctioning leads to hypoxia and possible cardiac arrest.
   e. Restrict fluids (per request) for first few days to reduce risk of pulmonary congestion from excessive fluid intake.
2. Monitor and support cardiac output through hemodynamic monitoring by blood pressure readings from intraarterial line, central venous pressure readings, left atrial line pressure, and pulmonary artery and capillary wedge pressures.
3. Also monitor for decreased urine output, cyanosis of the integument, and decreased level of responsiveness that reflect decreased cardiac output.

4. Be alert for signs of hypoxia—restlessness, headache, confusion, dyspnea, hypotension, and cyanosis.
5. Maintain adequate fluid volume and watch for signs of electrolyte imbalance.
   a. Hypokalemia—dysrhythmias, seeing halos around objects associated with digitalis toxicity, ECG changes, cardiac arrest. Treat with potassium supplement intravenously, as prescribed.
   b. Hyperkalemia—confusion, restlessness, nausea, weakness, and paresthesia of extremities. Be prepared to administer Kayexalate, which binds the potassium, by enema.
   c. Hyponatremia—weakness, fatigue, confusion, convulsions, and coma. Administer normal saline solution or higher concentration, as prescribed.
   d. Hypocalcemia—paresthesias, carpopedal spasm, muscle cramps, and tetany. Give calcium replacement intravenously, as directed.
   e. Hypercalcemia—dysrhythmias similar to digitalis toxicity. Institute treatment as directed—this condition may lead to asystole and death.
6. Keep intake and output flow sheet to track fluid balance and the patient's fluid requirements, including IV fluids and flush solutions as intake and postoperative chest drainage (should not exceed 200 mL/hr for first 4–6 hours) as output.
7. Provide adequate pain control; differentiate between incisional pain and anginal pain. Be alert to possible myocardial infarction after surgery.
8. Examine sternotomy incision and leg incisions for drainage, hematoma, signs of infection.
9. Monitor ECG continuously and be prepared to treat dysrhythmias.
   a. Institute cardiac pacing with temporary pacing wires from incision; wires usually pulled within 48 hours if rhythm is stable.
   b. Valvular and some other surgeries may cause swelling in the atrioventricular area, requiring pacing for 48 hours or so.
10. Assess for signs of cardiac tamponade, including hypotension, increasing central venous pressure, increasing left atrial pressure, muffled heart sounds, weak, thready pulse, neck vein distention, decreasing urinary output, and possible diminished drainage in

the chest-collection bottle; be prepared to assist with pericardiocentesis.

11. Be alert for excessive bleeding.
    a. Prepare to administer blood products, IV solutions or protamine sulfate, or vitamin K, as ordered.
    b. Prepare for possible return to surgery if bleeding persists (more than 300 mL/hour from chest tube) for 2 hours.

12. Evaluate and treat fever as indicated. Most common cause of fever within first 24 hours is atelectasis.
    a. Evaluate for respiratory, urinary tract, or wound infection.
    b. If infective endocarditis is suspected because of persistent fever, draw blood cultures.

13. Watch urine output, blood urea nitrogen, and serum creatinine levels to evaluate for renal insufficiency.

14. Encourage early ambulation to prevent embolic complications.

15. Promote perceptual and psychological orientation and watch for symptoms of postcardiotomy delirium (may appear after brief lucid period and may include delirium, transient perceptual distortions, visual and auditory hallucinations, disorientation, or paranoid delusions).
    a. Encourage interaction with family and communication about patient's experience.
    b. Maintain normal day/night pattern and limit environmental stimulation.
    c. Reassure patient that psychiatric disturbance after surgery is usually transient.

◆ Patient Education and Health Maintenance

Note: Guidelines vary among health care providers and institutions; check with patient's surgeon or cardiologist.

1. Instruct patient to increase activities gradually within limits. Avoid strenuous activities until after exercise stress testing.

2. Advise taking short rest periods, avoiding lifting more than 20 pounds, and participating in activities that do not cause pain or discomfort.

3. Advise increasing walking time and distance each

C

day. Stairs may be done one to two times daily the first week; increase as tolerated.

4. Tell patient to avoid large crowds initially, and driving until after first postoperative checkup.
5. Tell patient that sexual activities usually may be resumed 2 weeks after surgery. Avoid if tired or after a heavy meal. Consult health care provider if chest discomfort, difficulty breathing, or palpitations occur after intercourse.
6. Tell patient that work may be resumed after first postoperative checkup, as advised by health care provider.
7. Tell the patient to expect some chest discomfort from incision.
8. Advise about low-salt and low-fat diet as indicated. Tell patient to report weight gain of more than 5 pounds per week, which may indicate fluid retention.
9. Teach about medications, including one aspirin a day, antihypertensives, antilipid medications, and antidysrhythmics, as indicated. Label all medications and explain purposes and side effects.
10. Advise patients with prosthetic valves:
    a. Warfarin regimen may be continued indefinitely. Patients should watch for bleeding and should avoid use of aspirin (and many other drugs) that interfere with action of warfarin.
    b. Pregnancy should be avoided.
    c. Antibiotic prophylaxis is needed before dental and surgical procedures.
11. Encourage compliance with rehabilitation and exercise program after exercise stress testing.
12. Inform the patient whom to contact (and how) in case of an emergency.
13. Refer patient and family to community support groups: American Heart Association, Mended Hearts Society.

Cardiomyopathy

Cardiomyopathy refers to any disease of the heart muscle in which other cardiac structures are spared. Primary cardiomyopathies have no known causes; secondary cardiomyopathies have a known or suspected basis (eg, coronary artery disease can cause ischemic cardiomyopathy). The cardiomyopathies fall into three major groups (dilated, hypertrophic, and restrictive), according to variations in structural and functional abnormalities that can occur.

In *dilated cardiomyopathy,* both right and left ventricles enlarge (dilate) significantly, reducing the heart's ability to pump blood efficiently to the body. Causes include alcohol abuse, chemotherapy, chemical agents, pregnancy (third trimester, postpartum), and infections.

In *hypertrophic cardiomyopathy (HCM),* the ventricular septum is abnormally thickened. Other changes, such as patches of myocardial fibrosis, disorganization of myocardial fibers, and abnormalities of coronary microvasculature, also occur, leading to abnormal mitral valve function, filling, and contraction of the heart. This disorder has a genetic cause.

In *restrictive cardiomyopathy,* the heart muscle becomes infiltrated by various substances, resulting in severe fibrosis. The fibrotic muscle becomes stiff and nondistensible, causing inadequate ventricular filling. This disorder may be caused by myeloidosis and hemochromatosis (excessive iron deposition).

Complications of cardiomyopathy may include mural thrombus (caused by blood stasis in ventricles with dilated cardiomyopathy), severe heart failure, sudden cardiac death, and pulmonary embolism.

◆ Assessment

1. Exertional dyspnea, chest pain, and palpitations
2. Dysrhythmias—atrial/ventricular ectopic beats; sinus, atrial, and ventricular tachycardia
3. Decreased breath sounds caused by pericardial effusion in restrictive cardiomyopathy
4. Signs of congestive heart failure (see p. 393), and pulmonary edema (see p. 692)

◆ Diagnostic Evaluation

1. ECG and 24-hour Holter monitoring to detect dysrhythmias
2. Chest x-ray to detect cardiomegaly
3. Echocardiogram to evaluate wall motion abnormalities

4. Radionuclide imaging to evaluate ventricular function
5. Cardiac catheterization may be necessary to determine cause.

◆ Collaborative Management

Pharmacologic Interventions

1. In dilated cardiomyopathy:
   a. Provide effective management of heart failure (see p. 393).
   b. Administer oral anticoagulants, as indicated, especially in patients with atrial fibrillation, and to prevent thrombus and pulmonary embolus.

NURSING ALERT
Patients with dilated cardiomyopathy are susceptible to digoxin toxicity. Monitor the patient carefully for evidence of nausea, vomiting, "yellow vision" (yellow-green halos around visual images), and dysrhythmias.

2. In hypertrophic cardiomyopathy:
   a. Administer beta-adrenergic blockers to reduce the force of myocardial contraction, diminish obstructive pressure gradients, and decrease oxygen requirements.
   b. Administer calcium channel blockers, primarily to improve the heart's ability to relax, but also to help reduce the force of myocardial contraction, thereby providing symptom relief. Implemented when beta-adrenergic agents fail to control symptoms.
   c. Administer antidysrhythmics to prevent lethal dysrhythmias.

NURSING ALERT
Chest pain experienced by HCM patients is managed by rest and elevation of the feet (to improve venous return to the heart). Vasodilator therapy (nitroglycerin) may worsen chest pain by decreasing venous return to the heart and worsening obstruction of blood flow from the heart; agents that increase myocardial contractility (dopamine, dobutamine) should be avoided or used with extreme caution.

3. In restrictive cardiomyopathy:
   a. Therapy is palliative unless a specific underlying process is established.
   b. Institute fluid restrictions and diuretic therapy to control heart failure.
   c. Administer digoxin as indicated, to control atrial fibrillation.
   d. Administer oral anticoagulants to prevent embolization.

Surgical Interventions

1. Heart transplantation must be considered in the terminal phase of dilated cardiomyopathy.
2. Myotomy and myectomy—surgical resection of a portion of the septum—may be needed to reduce muscle thickness and provide symptom relief in hypertrophic cardiomyopathy.
3. Pacemakers and automatic internal defibrillators may be implanted to treat severe bradycardias and lethal tachycardias.

◆ Nursing Interventions

Monitoring

1. Monitor heart rate, rhythm, temperature, and respiratory rate frequently.
2. Institute continuous cardiac monitoring, as directed, if dysrhythmias occur.
3. Evaluate central venous pressure (CVP), pulmonary artery, and pulmonary capillary wedge pressures with a pulmonary artery catheter to assess progress and effect of drug therapy.
4. Calculate cardiac output, cardiac index, and systemic vascular resistance.
5. Observe for subtle changes in cardiac output, such as decreased BP, change in mental status, decreased urine output.
6. Monitor coagulation studies and observe for evidence of bleeding if anticoagulants used.
7. After cardiac catheterization, monitor blood pressure and apical pulse closely, check peripheral pulses in affected extremity, watch for hematoma formation at puncture site, assess for chest, back, thigh, or groin pain, and keep the patient in bed until the following morning.

Supportive Care

1. Orient the patient to the unit, purpose of equipment, and plan of care. Explain all procedures and treatments.
2. Encourage the patient to ask questions and ventilate fears and concerns.
3. Ensure that the patient and visitors understand the importance of adequate rest. Advise about visiting hours and institutional policy and who to contact for information.
4. Provide uninterrupted rest periods and assist with ambulation as ordered.
5. Assist the patient in identifying stressors and reducing their effect. (This is especially important for patients with hypertrophic cardiomyopathy, because stress worsens the outflow obstruction.) Teach the use of diversional activities and relaxation techniques to relieve tension.

Patient Education/Health Maintenance

1. Instruct the patient about taking medications such as digoxin.
   a. The patient should take the drug daily after taking a pulse. The patient should notify a health care provider if the pulse is below 60 beats/min (or other specified rate).
   b. Tell the patient to immediately report signs of digitalis toxicity: anorexia, nausea, vomiting, "yellow vision."
   c. Advise the patient that follow-up blood tests will be done to monitor serum drug levels.
2. Advise the patient to follow a low-sodium diet; teach how to read food labels.
3. Advise the patient to immediately report signs of heart failure: weight gain, edema, shortness of breath, increased fatigue.

COMMUNITY CARE CONSIDERATIONS
Ensure that family members know CPR because the patient is at risk for sudden cardiac arrest.

Cardiomyopathy in Children

Cardiomyopathy is an abnormality of the myocardium that impairs cardiac muscle contractility. Other heart structures are not usually involved, and in most cases the cause is unknown. This condition is rare in children; the type known as dilated congestive cardiomyopathy is most commonly seen. Complications of cardiomyopathy include intraatrial or intraventricular thrombi, systemic or pulmonary emboli, severe malignant arrhythmias, and sudden death.

◆ Assessment

1. Tachycardia, dyspnea
2. Fatigue, lethargy, exercise intolerance
3. Poor growth
4. Chest pain, syncope
5. Hepatosplenomegaly
6. Dysrhythmias, murmur

◆ Diagnostic Evaluation

1. 12-lead ECG is usually abnormal, with ST segment changes, dysrhythmias.
2. Chest x-ray shows cardiomegaly, congested lung fields.
3. Echocardiogram shows poor ventricular contractility, dilated left or right ventricle, asymmetric septal hypertrophy, increased left ventricular wall thickness with small left ventricular cavity.
4. Cardiac catheterization or angiography may be done to assist with diagnosis, identify possible infectious causes, and evaluate ventricular function.

◆ Collaborative Management

Pharmacologic Interventions

1. Correct underlying cause of the disease, although cardiomyopathy is usually not a reversible disease.
2. Decrease workload of the heart with drugs for arterial dilation and relaxation, such as calcium channel blocking agents.

3. Anticoagulants to prevent emboli
4. Diuretics to relieve pulmonary and venous congestion
5. Treatment is mostly palliative.

Surgical Interventions

1. Cardiac transplantation is considered in severe disease unresponsive to other treatment.

◆ Nursing Interventions

Monitoring

1. Employ continuous ECG monitoring; immediately report dysrhythmias.
2. Monitor electrolytes; imbalances may depress cardiac output and cause increased dysrhythmias.
3. Monitor intake and output, edema, and lung fields for crackles, all indicating heart failure (see p. 398).
4. Monitor prothrombin time for patient receiving oral anticoagulants.

Supportive Care

1. Provide supplemental oxygen therapy as required.
2. Observe bleeding precautions for patients on anticoagulants (ie, no IM injections, no rectal temperatures, urine and stool tests for blood).
3. Use mechanical ventilation to lessen the workload of the heart for severely ill and dyspneic children.
4. Maintain bed rest to lessen cardiac work load.
5. Provide frequent, small meals and high-calorie supplements, such as milkshakes.
6. Consider supplemental tube feedings if nutritional requirements not met, or infuse hyperalimentation as ordered.
7. Answer questions about available treatment options, including ventilatory support and cardiac transplantation.

Family Education and Health Maintenance

1. Teach about interactions with other medications, side effects, and special precautions such as bleeding precautions for child on anticoagulant therapy.
2. Advise on symptoms to report, such as worsening shortness of breath, fatigability, irregular pulse, syncope.
3. Teach CPR to caregivers.

4. Advise on frequent follow-up for prothrombin times and other testing to monitor condition.

Cataract

Cataracts are a gradual and painless clouding or opacifying of the creptalline lens of the eye. Cataracts have various causes. *Senile cataracts* commonly develop in elderly patients because of degenerative changes in lens proteins. *Congenital cataracts* occur in newborns as genetic defects or possibly from measles in the mother. *Traumatic cataracts* may occur after injury sufficient to force vitreous humor into the lens capsule.

If untreated, cataracts progress to blindness.

◆ Assessment

1. Gradual painless vision loss, blurred or distorted vision, excessive glare from bright lights
2. Pupil may appear milky or white.

◆ Diagnostic Evaluation

1. Complete ophthalmologic testing:
   a. Slit-lamp examination to provide magnification and confirm diagnosis of an opacity
   b. Tonometry, to determine if there is increased intra-ocular pressure
   c. Direct and indirect ophthalmoscopy to rule out disease of retina
   d. Perimetry, to detect any loss of visual field

◆ Collaborative Management

Surgical Interventions

1. Surgery is the only cure and is recommended when vision causes problems in daily activities. Extracapsular extraction is usually done by cryosurgery or phaco-emulsification under local anesthesia.
   a. Preoperative sedation is given to decrease response to pain and lessen motor activity.

b. Medications is given to reduce intraocular pressure.

2. An intraocular lens implant is usually inserted at the time of surgery, designed for distance vision.

3. Nonsteroidal antiinflammatory agents, antibiotic ointments, and possibly corticosteroids may be necessary after lens implantation to reduce inflammation on other eye structures and prevent infection.

4. If patient cannot tolerate lens implant, eyeglasses and contact lenses are used to correct vision.

◆ Nursing Interventions

Monitoring

1. Check the patient's vision regularly:
   a. Preoperatively to monitor the degree of visual impairment and determine when surgery can be performed
   b. Postoperatively to monitor results of surgery, detect any complications, and adjust postoperative medications and dosages

2. Monitor pain level postoperatively. Sudden onset may be caused by a ruptured vessel or suture and may lead to hemorrhage. Severe pain accompanied by nausea and vomiting may be caused by increased intraocular pressure (IOP).

3. Assess the patient's ability to ambulate and perform activities independently postoperatively.

Supportive Care and Patient/Family Education

1. Keep the patient comfortable and advise not to touch eyes.

PEDIATRIC ALERT
Administer sedation to the infant for 24 hours postoperatively to prevent crying and vomiting, which may increase intraocular pressure (IOP) and damage sutures.

---

2. If eye patch or shield is in place, advise using it for several days, as prescribed, to rest and protect eye, especially at night.

C

3. Caution the patient against coughing or sneezing, any rapid movement or bending from the waist to prevent increased IOP for first 24 hours. Should avoid contact sports for 2 weeks.

4. Advise the patient to increase activities gradually; can usually resume normal activity the day after the procedure.

5. Teach proper instillation of eye drops.

6. Encourage follow-up ophthalmologic examinations for corrective lenses and checking of intraoperative pressure. Adjustment to eyeglasses to correct vision may take weeks to months.

   a. Tell the patient that glasses will cause the perceived image to be approximately one third larger than that seen by the patient before cataract formation.

   b. Tell the patient that only one eye can be used at a time with glasses (if only one eye is operated for cataract), because the operated eye has a 30% increase in image size, and the unoperated eye still has "normal" sized images, which cannot be superimposed.

   c. Instruct the patient to look through the center of the corrective glasses and to turn head when looking to the side because peripheral vision is markedly distorted.

   d. Warn that it is necessary to relearn space judgment—walking, using stairs, reaching for articles on the table, pouring liquids.

7. If contact lenses are to be worn, teach the patient that:

   a. With contact lenses, magnification is only about 5% to 10% and peripheral vision is not distorted.

   b. Both eyes may be used together because the image difference between an aphakic (without lens) eye with a contact lens and the unoperated eye is only 8% to 10%. Spacial judgment presents little difficulty.

8. If the patient has a lens implant, magnification problems will be negligible. Both the operated eye and the unoperated eye can work together after cataract surgery with lens implantation.

   a. Advise use of sunglasses in bright lights because the pupil is not able to constrict completely after lens implant.

b. Advise that no eyeglasses may be required for distance but may be needed for reading and writing.
c. Advise not getting soap in the eyes.
d. Advise the patient to avoid tilting the head forward when washing hair, and to avoid vigorous head shaking, to prevent disruption of the lens until cleared by surgeon.

Cellulitis

Cellulitis is an inflammation of the subcutaneous tissue of the skin caused by infection with group A beta-hemolytic streptococci, *Staphylococcus aureus, Haemophilus influenzae,* or other organisms. The organisms usually enter through traumatized skin (eg, blunt trauma, needle stick, insect bite, or wound), and the resulting infection may spread rapidly through the lymphatic system. Untreated disease may lead to tissue necrosis and septicemia.

◆ Assessment

1. Tender, warm, erythematous, and swollen area that is well demarcated
2. Tender, warm, erythematous streak extending proximally from the area, indicating lymph vessel involvement
3. Possibly fluctuant abscess or purulent drainage
4. Possibly fever, chills, headache, malaise

◆ Diagnostic Evaluation

1. Gram stain and cultures to identify causative organism from drainage
2. Blood cultures may be helpful if septicemia develops.

◆ Collaborative Management

Pharmacologic Interventions

1. Oral antibiotics (penicillinase-resistant penicillins, cephalosporins, or quinolones) may be adequate to treat small localized areas of cellulitis of legs or trunk.

2. Parenteral antibiotics may be needed for cellulitis of the hands, face, or lymphatic spread.

NURSING ALERT

Diabetic patients and patients with peripheral vascular disease may require more intensive and longer-term therapy because of poor tissue penetration by antibiotic and slow healing.

Surgical Interventions

1. Drainage and debridement may be required for suppurative areas.

◆ Nursing Interventions

Supportive Care

1. Administer or teach self-administration of antibiotics as prescribed; teach dosage schedule and side effects.
2. Maintain IV infusion or venous access to administer IV antibiotics, if indicated.
3. Encourage comfortable position and immobilization of affected area.
4. Elevate affected extremity to promote drainage from area.
5. Use bed cradle to relieve pressure from bed covers.
6. Administer warm soaks to relieve inflammation and promote drainage.
7. Administer, or teach self-administration of, analgesics as prescribed; monitor for side effects.

Patient Education and Health Maintenance

1. Ensure that the patient understands dosage schedule of antibiotics and the importance of complying with therapy to prevent complications.
2. Advise the patient to notify a health care provider immediately if condition worsens; hospitalization may be necessary.
3. Outpatient-treated cellulitis should be observed within 48 hours of starting antibiotics, to determine adequacy of treatment.
4. Teach the patient with impaired circulation or sensation proper skin care and inspection of skin for trauma.

Cerebral Palsy

Cerebral palsy refers to a group of incurable nonprogressive disorders resulting from central nervous system damage that occurs before, during, or soon after birth, from such causes as infections, anoxia, or birth trauma. Although there are varying degrees and clinical manifestations of cerebral palsy, it is generally characterized by paralysis, weakness, or ataxia.

Three major clinical types of cerebral palsy are recognized: *spastic* (most common), *dyskinesic or athetoid* (25% of cases), and *ataxic* (10% of cases). In the spastic type, a defect in the cortical motor area or pyramidal tract causes abnormally strong tonus of certain muscle groups. Attempts at movement cause muscles to contract and block the motion, and permanent contractures develop without muscle training. In the dyskinetic type, lesions of the extrapyramidal tract and basal ganglia cause involuntary, uncoordinated, uncontrollable movements of muscle groups (athetosis). In the ataxic type, cerebellar involvement causes disturbances of balance, and gross or fine motor coordination is nearly impossible.

Cerebral palsy is a major cause of disability among children in the United States, occurring in approximately 2 per every 1,000 live births.

◆ Assessment

1. Early manifestations (soon after birth) may include one or more of the following:
   a. Asymmetric movements
   b. Listlessness or irritability
   c. Difficulty in feeding, swallowing, or poor sucking with tongue thrust
   d. Excessive, high-pitched, or feeble cry
   e. Poor head control
2. Late manifestations may include one or more of the following:
   a. Failure to follow normal pattern of motor development. Delayed gross motor development is a universal manifestation of cerebral palsy.
   b. Persistence of infantile reflexes

c. Weakness
d. Preference for one hand before the child is 12 to 15 months old
e. Abnormal postures
f. Delayed or defective speech
g. Evidence of mental retardation

◆ **Diagnostic Evaluation**

1. Thorough evaluation of prenatal, perinatal, and postnatal factors; APGAR scores
2. CT scanning and blood testing to rule out presence of toxins, infectious processes, neoplasms of central nervous system
3. Psychological testing may be done to determine cognitive functioning.

◆ **Collaborative Management**

Therapeutic Interventions
1. Orthopedic management of scoliosis, contractures, and dislocations with splints and surgery as needed
2. Developmental enrichment programs including prevocational, vocational, and socialization skills; emotional and behavioral counseling

Pharmacologic Interventions
1. Antispasticity medications such as dantrolene
2. Antireflux medications such as metoclopramide (for associated gastroesophageal reflux)

Surgical Interventions
1. Selective dorsal rhizotomy may be performed in an attempt to decrease spasticity.

◆ **Nursing Interventions**

Supportive Care
1. Carry out, and teach the parents to carry out, appropriate exercises under the direction of the physical therapist.
2. Use splints and braces to facilitate muscle control and improve body functioning.

3. Use assistive devices, such as adapted grooming tools, writing implements, and utensils, to enhance independence.

4. Encourage self-dressing with easy pull-on pants, large sweatshirts, and other loose clothing.

5. Use play, such as board games, ball games, peg boards, and puzzles, to improve coordination.

6. Maintain good body alignment to prevent contractures.

7. Provide adequate rest periods.

8. Evaluate the child's developmental level and then assist with tasks within that level.

9. Provide for continuity of care at home, day care, therapy centers, and the hospital.

10. During feeding, maintain a pleasant, distraction-free environment.
   a. Serve the child alone, initially. After the child begins to master the task of eating, encourage the child to eat with other children.
   b. Allow the child to hold the spoon, even if self-feeding is minimal.
   c. Use spoon and fork with special handles, plate and glass holders, and special feeding chair.
   d. Serve foods that stick to the spoon, such as thick applesauce or mashed potatoes.
   e. Encourage finger foods that the child can handle alone.

11. If the child must be fed, do so slowly and carefully. Be aware of any difficulty sucking and swallowing caused by poor muscle control.

12. Be alert for associated sensory deficits (hearing, speech, vision) that delay development and could be corrected. Report any squinting, failure to follow objects, or bringing objects very close to the face.

13. Evaluate the child's need for specific safety measures such as suction machine, safety helmet, or seizure precautions, and modify the environment as appropriate to ensure the child's safety.

14. Assist the parents to appraise the child's assets so that they may capitalize on these positive features.

15. Provide positive feedback for effective parenting skills and positive approaches to caring for the child.

16. Assist parents to find local resources to help in the

child's care, such as county social service agency, hospital social worker or discharge planner, local United Way, or Catholic Charities office.

Family Education and Health Maintenance

1. Instruct the parents in all areas of the child's physical care; their active participation in the rehabilitation program is the key to successful management of CP.
2. Encourage regular medical and dental evaluations.
   a. The child should receive all regular immunizations.
   b. Dental visits should occur every 6 months, starting at age 2 years.
3. Advise parents that the child needs discipline to feel secure and relaxed.
   a. Set realistic limits within which the child can function successfully.
   b. Be firm but not rejecting.
4. Refer parents to agencies such as:

> **The United Cerebral Palsy Association of America, Inc.**
> 1522 K St. NW
> Washington, DC 20005
> 800-872-5827

Cerebrovascular Accident

Cerebrovascular accident (CVA) or *stroke* results from sudden interruption of blood supply to the brain, which precipitates neurologic dysfunction lasting longer than 24 hours. Causes of stroke include partial or complete occlusion of a cerebral blood vessel caused by cerebral thrombosis or embolism, causing infarction; ischemia caused by reduced cerebral blood flow secondary to cardiac or metabolic disease; or hemorrhage that occurs outside the dura, beneath the dura mater, in the subarachnoid space, or within the brain substance itself.

Complications of CVA include aspiration pneumonia, contractures, deep vein thrombosis, pulmonary embolism, depression, and brain stem herniation.

C

◆ Assessment

1. Risk factors include: transient ischemic attacks (TIAs—warning sign of impending CVA), hypertension, arteriosclerosis, heart disease, elevated cholesterol, diabetes mellitus, obesity, carotid stenosis, polycythemia, and cigarette smoking.
2. Clinical manifestations of stroke depend on the vessel affected and the portion of the brain it perfuses.
   a. Sudden severe headache
   b. Numbness, (paresthesia), weakness (paresis), or loss of motor ability (plegia), on one side of the body
   c. Difficulty in swallowing (dysphagia)
   d. Speech or communication impairment (aphasia)
   e. Visual difficulties: loss of half of visual field, double vision, etc.
   f. Altered cognitive abilities and psychological effects
3. Tone of muscles and presence of deep tendon reflexes change from initial flaccid period to later spastic period
4. Dysfunction in cranial nerves, sensation, proprioception, and bladder control

◆ Diagnostic Evaluation

1. Carotid ultrasound—to detect carotid stenosis
2. Computed tomography—to determine cause and location of stroke.
3. Cerebral angiography—to determine extent of cerebrovascular insufficiency.
4. Positron emmission tomography (PET) and MRI scans may be done to localize ischemic damage.

◆ Collaborative Management

Therapeutic Interventions

1. In the acute phase (first 48–72 hours), maintain the patient's airway, breathing, oxygenation, and circulation.
2. Physical therapy and rehabilitation program are initiated as soon as medically stable.

Pharmacologic Interventions

1. During acute phase:
   a. Dextran or pentastarch to facilitate reperfusion and hemodilution

   b. Thrombolytics (tissue plasminogen activator or urokinase) to reverse occlusion in embolic CVA
   c. Diuretics to reduce cerebral edema, which peaks 3
to 5 days after infarction
   d. Calcium-channel blockers to reduce blood pressure
and prevent cerebral vasospasm

2. Provide additional treatment after the acute phase:
   a. Anticoagulants for nonhemorrhagic CVA
   b. Antiplatelet agents such as ticlopidine or aspirin
   c. Antispasmodic agents for spastic paralysis
   d. Antidepressants to treat poststroke depression

◆ Nursing Interventions

Monitoring

1. Maintain a neurologic flow sheet during the acute
phase (48–72 hours after onset of stroke).
2. Frequently assess the patient's respiratory status, vital
signs, heart rate and rhythm, to maintain and support
vital functions.
3. Monitor bowel and bladder function.
4. Frequently assess the patient's level of function and
psychosocial response to condition. Look for signs of
poststroke depression.
5. Monitor effectiveness of anticoagulation therapy.

> **NURSING ALERT**
> Prothrombin time levels are reported in International Normalized
> Ratios (INR). Anticoagulants are adjusted to maintain an INR at
> 2.0 to prevent stroke and the associated complication of intracra-
> nial and subdural hemorrhage. Report INRs that are elevated to
> reduce the risk of bleeding, or decrease levels to adjust therapy
> to be more effective.

Supportive Care

1. During the acute phase:
   a. Maintain bed rest with head of bed slightly elevated
and side rails in place.
   b. Administer oxygen as ordered to maximize cerebral
oxygenation.

C

    c. Perform intermittent or indwelling bladder catheterization.
2. Position the patient and align the extremities carefully, to prevent complications of immobility:
    a. Use a foot board during flaccid period after stroke to keep feet dorsiflexed; after spasticity develops, avoid using the board.
    b. Apply splints and braces as needed. Splints support flaccid extremities and can also be used on spastic extremities to decrease stretch stimulation and reduce spasticity.
    c. Place the patient in a prone position for 15 to 30 minutes daily; avoid having the patient sit up in a chair for long periods, to prevent knee and hip flexion contractures.
    d. Exercise the affected extremities passively through range of motion four to five times daily to maintain joint mobility and enhance circulation; encourage active range-of-motion exercise as able. Teach the patient to use unaffected extremity to move affected one.

COMMUNITY CARE CONSIDERATIONS
Hemiplegic deformities resulting from stroke commonly include "frozen" shoulder; adduction and internal rotation of arm with flexion of elbow, wrist, and fingers; and external rotation of the hip with flexion of the knee and plantar flexion of the ankle. Instruct the patient and family in range-of-motion exercises. Reinforce that these muscle and ligament deformities resulting from stroke can be prevented with daily stretching and strengthening exercises.

3. Prepare for ambulation cautiously. Check for orthostatic hypotension; assess the patient's standing balance. Help the patient begin walking as soon as standing balance is achieved; assure safety with a patient waist belt.
4. Participate in cognitive retraining program (reality orientation, visual imagery, cueing procedures) as outlined by occupational or rehabilitation therapist.
5. To facilitate communication, speak slowly, using visual

cues and gestures, be consistent and repeat as necessary. Allow the patient plenty of time to respond; reinforce correct responses. Minimize distractions. Alternatively, use nonverbal methods of communication.
6. Help restore the patient's feelings of independence.
   a. Teach the patient to use non-affected side for ADLs,
      but not to neglect affected side. To help the patient
      with visual deficits avoid injury, teach how to scan
      the environment.
   b. Encourage the family to provide clothing that is a
      size larger than the patient wears, with front clo-
      sures, Velcro, and stretch fabric; teach the patient
      to dress while sitting to maintain balance.
   c. Ensure that personal care items, urinal, commode,
      etc., are nearby and that the patient obtains assis-
      tance with transfers and other activities as needed.
7. Facilitate adequate oral intake:
   a. Help the patient relearn swallowing sequence.
   b. Make sure soft or puree diet is provided, based on
      the patient's ability to chew.
   c. Position the patient so he or she is sitting with 90
      degrees of flexion at the hips and slight flexion at
      the neck. Use pillows behind the back and along
      the weak side to achieve correct position.
   d. Maintain position for 30 to 45 minutes after the
      meal to prevent regurgitation and aspiration.
   e. Teach the family how to assist the patient with
      meals to facilitate chewing and swallowing.
8. Help the patient regain bladder control:
   a. The patient will have been catheterized during the
      acute stage. Once bladder tone returns, establish
      regular schedule of voiding (every 2 to 3 hours).
   b. Assist with standing or sitting to void (especially
      males).
9. To help the family cope with patient care, teach stress
   management techniques such as relaxation exercises,
   use of community and church support networks, respite program, or other available resources in area.

Patient Education and Health Maintenance
1. Teach the patient and family to adapt the home environment for safety and ease of use.
2. Emphasize importance of rest periods throughout day.

C

TABLE 4 Aphasia

Aphasia is an acquired disorder of communication resulting from brain damage due to stroke, head injury, brain tumors, or brain cysts. It may involve impairment of the ability to speak, understand the speech of others, read, write, calculate, and understand gestures. Most aphasic individuals have difficulty with expression and comprehension to varying degrees. Fatigue will have adverse effect on speech.

To enhance your communication with the aphasic patient, keep the environment simple and relaxed, minimize distractions, and use multiple sensory channels. Refer the family to: American Speech-Language-Hearing Association, 10801 Rockville Pike, Rockville, MD 20852.

Aphasia Syndromes	Specific Nursing Interventions
Fluent aphasia: patient retains verbal fluency but may have difficulty in understanding speech.	Speak at your normal rate and volume: the patient is not hard of hearing.
Wernicke's aphasia; patient speaks readily but speech lacks clear content, information, and direction; jargon frequently used	Allow plenty of time to answer.
	Do not ask questions that require complex answers.
	Rote phrases can be spontaneous.
Anomic or amnesic aphasia: speech is almost normal, but marred by word-finding difficulty	Provide pad and pen if the patient prefers and is able to write.
	Avoid forcing speech.
Conduction aphasia; comprehension of language is good but has difficulty repeating spoken material	Watch the patient for clues and gestures if his or her speech is jargon; make neutral statements.
	Allow plenty of time for response.
Nonfluent aphasia: speech is sparse and produced slowly and with effort and poor articulation; usually has a relative preservation of auditory comprehension.	Ask for minimal word response.
	Encourage patient to speak slowly.
	Expect frustration and anger at inability to communicate.
Global aphasia; severe disruption of all aspects of communication (verbal speech, written, reading, understanding).	Keep environment simple.
	Use gestures as well as language.
	Allow patient to manipulate objects for additional sensory input.

3. Reassure the family that it is common for post-stroke patients to experience emotional lability and depression; treatment can be given.
4. Assist family to obtain self-help aids for the patient.
5. Instruct the family in management of aphasia (Table 4).
6. Refer the patient and family for more information and support to agencies such as:

National Stroke Association
1420 Ogden St.
Denver, CO 80218
303-839-1992

Cervical Cancer
See Cancer, Cervical

Cholecystectomy

Cholecystectomy is the surgical removal of the gallbladder for acute and chronic cholecystitis. It is one of the most frequent surgical procedures, with more than 600,000 performed each year in the United States. The procedure may be done through open laparotomy or laparoscopy (gallbladder removed through a small incision just above the umbilicus assisted by a laparoscope). Laparoscopic method decreases recovery time and risk of complications. Following cholecystectomy, the bile ducts eventually dilate to accommodate the volume of bile once held by the gallbladder.

◆ Potential Complications

1. Hemorrhage
2. Incisional infection
3. Bile duct injury
4. Thrombophlebitis and pulmonary embolism (with laparotomy)

◆ Collaborative Management

Preoperative Care
1. Ensure that the patient knows reason for cholecystectomy, what the procedure involves, and what to expect postoperatively.
2. Patient must remain NPO from midnight the night before surgery, and must void before surgery.

3. Administer IV fluids to improve hydration status if the patient has been vomiting.
4. Administer antibiotics for acute cholecystitis, as ordered.

Postoperative Care

1. Assess vital signs, level of consciousness.
2. Administer prescribed pain medications or monitor patient-controlled analgesia.
3. Promote ambulation to prevent thromboembolus, facilitate voiding, decrease flatus and abdominal distention, and stimulate peristalsis.
4. Encourage splinting of incision when moving and coughing and deep breathing.
5. Assess wound dressings for any increased or purulent drainage.
6. Assess T-tube site for any drainage; note amount, color, and odor.
7. Assess bile drainage from T-tube; report any increase or decrease in drainage. Maintain T-tube patency and security.
8. Report right upper quadrant pain, abdominal distention, fever, chills, or jaundice indicating bile duct injury.
9. Administer antibiotics as prescribed.
10. Assess intake and output, including nasogastric and T-tube drainage.
11. Assess for nausea and vomiting and administer antiemetics as prescribed. Ensure adequate replacement of fluids.
12. Discontinue suction of nasogastric (NG) tube (if used) and monitor for bowel sounds when NG drainage decreases.
13. Encourage fluid intake and advance to regular diet as tolerated.
14. Clamp T-tube when ordered and assess tolerance of food and color of stools.

◆ Patient Education and Health Maintenance

1. Tell the patient to keep the incision or wound sites dry for 5 to 7 days and to report any signs of redness, pain, or drainage.

2. Instruct the patient that usual activities can usually be resumed within 7 to 10 days after laparoscopic chole-cystectomy or within 6 weeks of open cholecystec-tomy.
   a. Sexual activity may be resumed when pain has abated.
   b. Consult surgeon for specific instructions on heavy lifting, strenuous activity, showers and tub baths, and driving.
3. Advise patient that fats may not be well tolerated for 4 to 6 weeks, until bile ducts dilate.

Cholelithiasis, Cholecystitis, Choledocholithiasis

Cholelithiasis is the presence of stones in the gallbladder. *Cholecystitis* is acute or chronic inflammation of the gall-bladder. *Choledocholithiasis* is the presence of stones in the common bile duct.

Gallstones result from precipitation of cholesterol, bili-rubin pigment (or both) from bile, which predisposes to stone formation and inflammation. An estimated 25 mil-lion people in the United States have gallstones, with one million new cases diagnosed each year. Women are four times as likely to develop cholesterol stones as men, and the risk increases if they are older than age 40, multipa-rous, and obese. Other risk factors for cholesterol stones include use of estrogens and cholesterol-lowering drugs, bile acid malabsorption with gastrointestinal disease, bile fistula, gallstone ileus, carcinoma of the gallbladder, ileal resection or bypass, genetic predisposition, and rapid weight loss. Pigment stones occur when free bilirubin combines with calcium. These stones occur primarily in patients with cirrhosis, hemolysis, and biliary infections.

Acute cholecystitis is caused primarily by gallstone ob-struction of the cystic duct with edema, inflammation, and bacterial invasion. It may also occur in the absence of stones, as a result of major surgical procedures, severe trauma, or burns.

Chronic cholecystitis results from repeated attacks of

cholecystitis, presence of stones, or chronic irritation. The gallbladder becomes thickened, rigid, and fibrotic, and functions poorly.

Complications of gallbladder disease include cholangitis; necrosis, empyema, and perforation of gallbladder; biliary fistula through duodenum; gallstone ileus; and adenocarcinoma of the gallbladder.

◆ Assessment

1. Gallstones may be asymptomatic or cause biliary colic.
   a. Steady, severe aching pain or sensation of pressure in the epigastrium or right upper quadrant, which may radiate to the right scapular area or right shoulder
   b. Begins suddenly and persists for 1 to 3 hours until the stone falls back into the gallbladder or is passed through the cystic duct
2. Acute cholecystitis causes pain that persists more than 4 to 6 hours and increases with movement, including respirations.
   a. Also causes nausea and vomiting, low-grade fever, and possibly jaundice (with stones or inflammation in the common bile duct)
   b. Right upper quadrant guarding and Murphy's sign (inability to take a deep inspiration when examiner's fingers are pressed below the hepatic margin) are present.
3. Chronic cholecystitis causes heartburn, flatulence, and indigestion. Repeated attacks of symptoms may occur, resembling acute cholecystitis.

◆ Diagnostic Evaluation

1. Oral cholecystography, ultrasonography, and hepatobiliary scan (radiolabeled iminodiacetic acid [HIDA]) to visualize stones or inflammation
2. Endoscopic retrograde cholangiopancreatography (ERCP) and percutaneous transhepatic cholangiography (PTC) to visualize location of stones and obstruction
3. Elevated conjugated bilirubin levels caused by obstruction

◆ Collaborative Management

Therapeutic and Pharmacologic Interventions

1. Supportive management includes rest, IV fluids, nasogastric suction, pain management, and possibly antibiotics.
2. Oral therapy with chenodeoxycholic acid, ursodeoxycholic acid, or a combination of both may decrease the size of existing cholesterol stones or dissolve small ones.
   a. Indicated for patients at high risk for surgery because of age or systemic disease
   b. Major adverse effects include diarrhea, abnormal liver function tests, increases in serum cholesterol.
   c. Pigment stones cannot be dissolved.
3. Direct contact therapy, in which a local cholelitholytic agent is infused directly into the gallbladder via a percutaneous transhepatic catheter
   a. Indicated for symptomatic, high-risk patients whose gallbladder can be visualized on oral cholecystography
   b. Side effects include pain from the catheter, nausea, transient elevations of liver function tests and white blood count.
4. Intracorporeal lithotripsy is used to fragment stones in the gallbladder or common bile duct by ultrasound, pulsed laser, or hydraulic lithotripsy applied through an endoscope directly to the stones. The stone fragments are removed by irrigation and aspiration. A cholecystectomy may be performed later.

Surgical Interventions

1. Cholecystectomy, open or laparoscopic (see p. 195)
   a. Intraoperative cholangiography and choledochoscopy for common bile duct exploration
   b. Placement of a T-tube in the common bile duct to decompress the biliary tree and allow access into the biliary tree postoperatively.

◆ Nursing Interventions

Monitoring

1. Monitor temperature and white blood cell count for indications of infection or perforation.

2. Assess for signs of dehydration: dry mucous membranes, poor skin turgor, decreased urine output.

Supportive Care

1. Administer medications or monitor patient-controlled analgesia to control pain.
2. Assist the patient to position of comfort; maintain bed rest during acute illness.
3. Administer IV fluids and electrolytes as prescribed.
4. Administer antiemetics as prescribed to decrease nausea and vomiting.
5. Maintain nasogastric decompression until nausea and vomiting subside.
6. Begin food and fluids as tolerated, after acute symptoms subside or postoperatively when bowel sounds return.
7. Observe and record amount of T-tube drainage, if applicable.

Patient Education and Health Maintenance

1. Advise the patient to eat a low-fat diet to prevent contraction of gallbladder, which will aggravate symptoms.
2. Instruct the patient in care of any tubes or catheters that may be in place at discharge.
   a. Observe for bleeding or drainage around insertion site.
   b. Replace gauze dressing when it becomes wet or soiled.
   c. Report any change in drainage.
3. Review postoperative discharge instructions for activity, diet, medications, and postoperative follow-up.
4. Teach the patient to recognize and report symptoms of complications: pain, fever, jaundice, unusual drainage.
5. Encourage follow-up for further treatment as indicated.

Chronic Obstructive Pulmonary Disease (COPD)

Chronic obstructive pulmonary disease is a collective term for several conditions marked by continued increased resis-

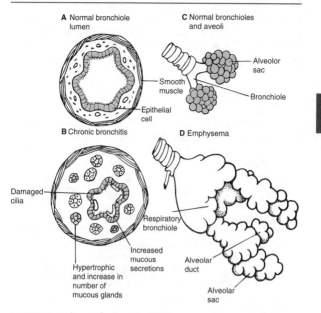

FIGURE 7 *Airway changes in COPD compared to normal.*

tance to expiratory airflow. COPD includes chronic bronchitis and pulmonary emphysema. Though sometimes included in COPD, *asthma* is a reversible disorder and is therefore considered elsewhere in this book.

Chronic bronchitis is chronic inflammation of the lower airways characterized by excessive secretion of mucus and recurring infection, progressing to narrowing and obstruction of airflow. Emphysema is the enlargement of air spaces distal to the terminal bronchioles, with loss of alveolar walls and loss of elastic recoil of the lungs (Fig. 7). The two conditions may overlap, resulting in subsequent derangement of airway dynamics (eg, obstruction to airflow). In pulmonary emphysema, lung function progressively deteriorates for many years before the illness becomes apparent.

Causes of COPD include cigarette smoking, air pollution, occupational exposure, allergy, autoimmunity, infection, genetic predisposition, and aging. Complications include respiratory failure, pneumonia or other overwhelming respiratory infection, right heart failure (cor pulmonale), dysrhythmias, and depression.

C

◆ Assessment

1. Symptoms of chronic bronchitis:
   a. Productive cough lasting at least 3 months during a year for 2 successive years
   b. Thick, gelatinous sputum (greater amounts produced during superimposed infections)
   c. Dyspnea and wheezing as disease progresses
2. Symptoms of emphysema (gradual in onset and steadily progressive):
   a. Dyspnea, decreased exercise tolerance
   b. Cough (may be minimal with mild sputum production, except with respiratory infection)
3. Use of accessory muscles of respiration and abdominal muscles during expiration. Note increase of anteroposterior diameter of chest (barrel chest).
4. Decreased/absent breath sounds, crackles, decreased heart sounds

NURSING ALERT
Recognize early manifestations of respiratory infection—increased dyspnea and fatigue; changes in color, amount, and character of sputum; low-grade fever; nervousness; irritability—so treatment can be started early.

◆ Diagnostic Evaluation

1. Chest x-rays to detect hyperinflation, flattened diaphragm, increased retrosternal space, decreased vascular markings, possible bullae (all in late stages)
2. Pulmonary function tests (PFT), to demonstrate airflow obstruction—reduced forced expiratory volume in 1 second (FEV_1), FEV_1 to forced vital capacity (FVC) ratio; increased residual volume to total lung capacity (TLC) ratio, possibly increased TLC
3. Arterial blood gases (ABGs), to detect decreased arte-

rial oxygen pressure (PaO_2), pH, and increased CO_2; and alpha$_1$-antitrypsin assay to detect genetic predisposition to emphysema
4. Sputum smears and cultures to identify pathogens

◆ Collaborative Management

Therapeutic Interventions

1. Low-flow oxygen to correct severe hypoxemia in a controlled manner and minimize CO_2 retention

NURSING ALERT
Normally, CO_2 levels in the blood stimulate respiration. However, in patients with COPD, chronically elevated CO_2 impairs this mechanism, so low O_2 levels in the blood stimulate respiration. Giving a high O_2 concentration may remove the hypoxic drive, leading to hypoventilation, respiratory decompensation, and the development of a worsening respiratory acidosis.

2. Home oxygen therapy, especially at night to prevent nocturnal oxygen desaturation
3. Pulmonary rehabilitation to reduce symptoms that limit activity

Pharmacologic Interventions

1. Bronchodilators to control bronchospasm and assist with raising sputum
   a. Sympathomimetics, such as metaproterenol, protect against bronchospasm; delivered by metered-dose inhalers, other hand-held devices, or nebulization
   b. Methylxanthines, such as theophylline, given orally as sustained-release form for chronic maintenance therapy
2. Corticosteroids by mouth, IV, or by inhaler to control inflammation in acute exacerbations
3. Antimicrobials to control secondary bacterial infections in the bronchial tree, thus clearing the airways.

C

◆ Nursing Interventions

Monitoring

1. Monitor for side effects of bronchodilators—tremulousness, tachycardia, cardiac dysrhythmias, central nervous system stimulation, hypertension.
2. Monitor condition after administration of aerosol bronchodilators to assess for improved aeration, reduced adventitious breath sounds, reduced dyspnea.
3. Monitor serum theophylline level, as ordered, to ensure therapeutic level and prevent toxicity.
4. Review ABGs; record values on a flow sheet so comparisons can be made over time.

NURSING ALERT
Watch for and report excessive somnolence, restlessness, aggressiveness, anxiety, or confusion; central cyanosis; and shortness of breath at rest, which frequently is caused by acute respiratory insufficiency and may signal respiratory failure.

Supportive Care

1. Eliminate all pulmonary irritants, particularly cigarette smoke. Smoking cessation usually reduces pulmonary irritation, sputum production, and cough. Keep the patient's room as dust-free as possible.
2. Use postural drainage positions to help clear secretions responsible for airway obstruction.
3. Teach controlled coughing.
4. Keep secretions liquid.
   a. Encourage high level of fluid intake (8–10 glasses; 2–$2\frac{1}{2}$ liters daily) within level of cardiac reserve.
   b. Give inhalations of nebulized water to humidify bronchial tree and liquefy sputum. Add moisture (humidifier, vaporizer) to indoor air.
   c. Avoid dairy products if these increase sputum production.
5. Encourage the patient to assume comfortable position to decrease dyspnea.

6. Instruct and supervise patient's breathing retraining exercises. Teach lower costal, diaphragmatic, and abdominal breathing, using a slow and relaxed breathing pattern to reduce respiratory rate and decrease work of breathing.

7. Use pursed lip breathing at intervals and during periods of dyspnea to control rate and depth of respiration and improve respiratory muscle coordination.

8. Discuss and demonstrate relaxation exercises to reduce stress, tension, and anxiety.

9. Maintain the patient's nutritional status:
   a. Obtain nutritional history, weight, and anthropometric measurements.
   b. Encourage frequent small meals if the patient is dyspneic; even a small increase in abdominal contents may press on diaphragm and impede breathing.
   c. Offer liquid nutritional supplements to improve caloric intake and counteract weight loss.
   d. Avoid foods producing abdominal discomfort.
   e. Advise good oral hygiene before meals to sharpen taste sensations.
   f. Encourage pursed-lip breathing between bites (or give supplemental oxygen, as directed) if the patient is very short of breath; allow rest after meals.
   g. Monitor body weight.

10. Reemphasize the importance of graded exercise and physical conditioning programs (enhances delivery of oxygen to tissues; allows a higher level of functioning with greater comfort).

   Encourage use of portable oxygen system for ambulation for patients with hypoxemia and marked disability.

11. Encourage the patient to carry out regular exercise program to increase physical endurance.

12. Train the patient in energy conservation techniques.

13. Assess the patient for reactive behaviors (anger, depression, acceptance). Allow the patient to express feelings and retain (within a controlled degree) the mechanisms of denial and repression.

14. Be aware that sexual dysfunction is common in pa-

tients with COPD; encourage alternate displays of affection to loved one.

Patient Education/Health Maintenance

1. Review with the patient the objectives of treatment and nursing management. Work with the patient to set goals (ie, stair climbing, return to work, etc.).

C

COMMUNITY CARE CONSIDERATIONS

Early in the patient's course, the issues of living will, advanced directives, and resuscitation status need to be addressed. It is better to have these discussions with the patient before crisis situations.

2. Advise the patient to avoid respiratory irritants.
3. Warn the patient to stay out of extremely hot/cold weather (or to shower in warm [not too hot or too cold] water) to avoid aggravating bronchial obstruction and sputum production.
4. Instruct the patient to humidify indoor air in winter; maintain 30% to 50% humidity for optimal mucociliary function.
5. Warn the patient to avoid persons with respiratory infections, and to avoid crowds and areas with poor ventilation.
6. Stress the importance of obtaining influenza and pneumococcal vaccines to guard against respiratory infections.
7. Teach the patient how to recognize and report evidence of respiratory infection *promptly*—chest pain, changes in character of sputum (amount, color, or consistency), increasing difficulty in raising sputum, increasing coughing and wheezing, increasing shortness of breath.
8. Tell the patient to use bronchodilators only as directed, and advise how to use metered-dose inhaler properly to maximize aerosol deposition in the bronchial tree. If the patient cannot use inhaler effectively, suggest using a spacer device.

COMMUNITY CARE CONSIDERATIONS
 Suggest a pulmonary rehabilitation program that is offered in most communities. Although studies show no appreciable difference in lung function as a result of such programs, there is a decrease in hospital admissions, decreased length of stay, and increase in the patient's sense of well-being. Contact the local American Lung Association or local hospitals for further information.

C

Cirrhosis, Hepatic

Cirrhosis of the liver is a chronic disease that causes cell destruction and fibrosis (scarring) of hepatic tissue. Fibrosis alters normal liver structure and vasculature, impairing blood and lymph flow and resulting in hepatic insufficiency and hypertension in the portal vein. Complications include bleeding esophageal varices, coagulopathy, spontaneous bacterial peritonitis, and hepatic encephalopathy.

 Cirrhosis is known in three major forms. In *Laennec's (alcohol-induced) cirrhosis*, fibrosis occurs mainly around central veins and portal areas. This is the most common form of cirrhosis and results from chronic alcoholism and malnutrition. *Postnecrotic cirrhosis* results from previous acute viral hepatitis or drug-induced massive hepatic necrosis. *Biliary cirrhosis* results from chronic biliary obstruction and infection (cholangitis), and is much rarer than the preceding forms.

◆ Assessment

1. Early complaints include fatigue, anorexia, edema of the ankles in the evening, epistaxis, bleeding gums, and weight loss.
2. In later disease look for:
   a. Chronic dyspepsia, constipation or diarrhea
   b. Dilated cutaneous veins around umbilicus (caput medusa); internal hemorrhoids, ascites, splenomegaly
   c. Fatigue, weakness, and wasting caused by anemia and poor nutrition

    d. Deterioration of mental function
    e. Estrogen-androgen imbalance causing spider angioma and palmar erythema; menstrual irregularities in women; testicular and prostatic atrophy, gynecomastia, loss of libido, and impotence in men
    f. Bleeding tendencies and hemorrhage
3. Enlarged, nodular liver

◆ Diagnostic Evaluation

1. Elevated serum liver enzyme levels, reduced serum albumin
2. Esophagoscopy to determine the presence of esophageal varices
3. Percutaneous transhepatic cholangiography to differentiate extrahepatic from intrahepatic obstructive jaundice
4. Paracentesis to examine ascitic fluid for cell, protein, and bacteria counts
5. Liver biopsy to detect cell destruction and fibrosis of hepatic tissue
6. Liver scan to show abnormal thickening and a liver mass
7. Scan to determine the size of the liver and its irregular nodular surface
8. Laparoscopy to allow direct visualization of the liver

◆ Collaborative Management

Therapeutic Interventions

1. Minimize further deterioration of liver function through the withdrawal of toxic substances, alcohol, and drugs.
2. Correct nutritional deficiencies with vitamins and nutritional supplements and a high-calorie and moderate- to high-protein diet.
3. Correct ascites and fluid and electrolyte imbalances.
    a. Restrict sodium and water intake, depending on amount of fluid retention.
    b. Bed rest to aid in diuresis

Pharmacologic Interventions

1. Provide symptomatic relief measures such as pain medication and antiemetics.

2. Diuretic therapy, frequently with spironolactone, a potassium-sparing diuretic that inhibits the action of aldosterone on the kidneys

3. IV albumin to maintain osmotic pressure and reduce ascites

4. Administration of lactulose for hepatic encephalopathy

Surgical Interventions

1. Abdominal paracentesis—to remove fluid and relieve symptoms of ascites; ascitic fluid may be ultrafiltrated and reinfused through a central venous access.

2. Peritoneovenous shunt may be performed in patients whose ascites is resistant to other forms of treatment. Complications include spontaneous bacterial peritonitis, shunt obstruction, and intravascular coagulopathies.

3. Orthotopic liver transplantation may be necessary.

◆ Nursing Interventions

Monitoring

1. Observe stools and emesis for color, consistency, and amount, and test each one for occult blood.

2. Be alert for symptoms of anxiety, epigastric fullness, weakness, and restlessness, which may indicate gastrointestinal bleeding.

3. Observe for external bleeding: ecchymosis, leaking needle stick sites, epistaxis, petechiae, and bleeding gums.

4. Monitor serum ammonia levels; restrict high-protein loads while serum ammonia is high to prevent hepatic encephalopathy.

5. Monitor fluid intake and output and serum electrolyte levels to prevent dehydration and hypokalemia (may occur with the use of diuretics), which may precipitate hepatic encephalopathy.

6. Assess daily weight and abdominal girth measurements for progression of ascites.

7. Assess level of consciousness and reorient the patient as needed.

C

NURSING ALERT

Avoid giving narcotics, sedatives, and barbiturates to a restless patient to avoid precipitating hepatic encephalopathy.

Supportive Care

1. Maintain some periods of bed rest with legs elevated to mobilize edema and ascites. Alternate rest periods with ambulation.
2. Encourage and assist with gradually increasing periods of exercise.
3. Encourage the patient to eat high-calorie, moderate-protein meals and supplementary feedings. Suggest small, frequent feedings.
4. Encourage oral hygiene before meals.
5. Administer or teach self-administration of medications for nausea, vomiting, diarrhea or constipation.
6. Note and record degree of jaundice of skin and sclera along with any skin trauma from scratching.
7. Encourage frequent skin care, bathing without soap, and massage with emollient lotions.
8. Keep the patient's fingernails short to prevent scratching from pruritus.
9. Keep the patient quiet and limit activity if signs of bleeding are evident.
10. Institute and teach measures to prevent trauma:
    a. Maintain safe environment.
    b. Blow nose gently.
    c. Use soft toothbrush.
11. Encourage eating foods with high vitamin C content.
12. Use small-gauge needles for injections and maintain pressure over injection site until bleeding stops.
13. Protect from sepsis through good handwashing and prompt recognition and management of infection.
14. Pad side rails and provide careful nursing surveillance to ensure the patient's safety.

Patient Education and Health Maintenance

1. Stress the necessity of giving up alcohol completely.
2. Urge joining a substance abuse program.
3. Emphasize the importance of rest, a sensible lifestyle,

and an adequate, well-balanced diet. Provide written dietary instructions.
4. Encourage daily weighing for self-monitoring of fluid retention or depletion.
5. Discuss side effects of diuretic therapy.
6. Involve the person closest to the patient, because recovery often is not easy and relapses are common.
7. Stress the importance of continued follow-up for laboratory tests and evaluation by the health care provider.

Cleft Lip and Palate

Cleft lip and palate deformities cause a variety of structural facial malformations that are usually apparent at birth. These defects originate during the second or third months of pregnancy for unknown reasons, but chromosomal abnormalities or hereditary predisposition may play a role.

Because the lip and palate develop independently, any combination of defects and degree of involvement can occur. Cleft lip varies from a notch in the lip to complete separation of the lip into the nose, and may be unilateral or bilateral. It appears in approximately 1 in 1000 births, and is more frequent in boys. Cleft palate may involve the uvula, soft palate, or both the soft and hard palates through the roof of the mouth, and also may be unilateral or bilateral. It appears in approximately 1 in 2500 births, and is more frequent in girls. Complications of cleft lip and palate deformities include impaired speech and hearing, improper tooth placement, and recurrent otitis media. Continuing therapy aims to ameliorate faulty social adjustment, poor self-concept, abnormal speech, and possible intellectual deficits.

◆ Assessment

1. Physical appearance of cleft lip or palate
   a. Incompletely formed lip
   b. Opening in roof of mouth felt with examiner's finger on palpation

2. Eating difficulty
   a. Suction cannot be created for effective sucking.
   b. Food returns through the nose.
3. Nasal speech

◆ **Diagnostic Evaluation**

1. Photography to document the abnormality
2. Serial x-rays are taken before and after treatment.
3. Magnetic resonance imaging (MRI) may be done to evaluate extent of abnormality before treatment.
4. Dental impressions are taken for expansion prosthesis in older child.

◆ **Collaborative Management**

Therapeutic Interventions
1. Speech therapy for older child postrepair

Surgical Interventions
1. The cleft lip is generally repaired before the palate defect.
   a. Immediate repair: Several hours to several weeks after birth is preferred by some surgeons.
   b. Intraoral or extraoral prosthesis to prevent maxillary collapse, stimulate bony growth, and aid in feeding and speech development; may be used before surgical repair
   c. Later repair when infant is 6 to 12 weeks old is often done; hemoglobin must be 10 g/dL and steady weight gain seen—10 lbs.
2. Cleft palate repair may be done anytime between 6 months and 5 years, based on degree of deformity, width of oropharynx, neuromuscular function of palate and pharynx, and surgeon's preference.
   a. Repair at 12 to 24 months may be preferred because speech patterns have not been set, yet growth of involved structures allows for improved surgical repair.
   b. If repair is delayed to age 4 or 5 years, a special denture palate is used to help occlude the cleft and aid in establishing speech patterns.

◆ Nursing Interventions

Monitoring

1. Observe for fever, irritability, redness, or drainage around cleft, and report these signs of infection promptly.
2. Monitor feeding pattern and weight both preoperatively and postoperatively.

Supportive Care

Preoperative Care

1. Administer gavage feedings if nipple feeding is to be delayed to prevent spread of a cleft lip.
2. If sucking is permitted, use a soft nipple with enlarged holes to facilitate feeding.
3. If sucking is ineffective because of inability to create a vacuum, try alternate oral feeding methods, such as regular nipple with enlarged holes or rubber-tipped asepto syringe or dropper.
4. Feed baby in an upright, sitting position to decrease possibility of fluid being aspirated or returned through the nose, or back to the auditory canal.
5. When feeding the infant with Pierre Robin syndrome (cleft palate, floppy tongue, and underdeveloped mandible), feed slowly and observe carefully for airway obstruction.
6. Advance diet as appropriate for age and needs of baby.
7. Encourage the mother to begin feeding the baby as soon as possible to enhance bonding. Assist mother with breast-feeding if this is preferred.
8. Clean the cleft after each feeding with water and a cotton-tipped applicator.
9. Support parents. Demonstrate acceptance of both the baby and the parents' feelings. Parents may be grieving about the infant's cosmetic imperfections and may harbor ambivalent feelings about this baby. Reassure them that successful reparative surgery can be done.
10. Prepare family for home feedings by providing several days to practice feeding and to become familiar with the baby's feeding pattern.
11. Suggest that about a week before scheduled admission for surgery, the mother begin using feeding tech-

niques preferred by surgeon for postoperative feeding.

12. Prepare the parents emotionally for the postoperative appearance of the child.

   a. Explain the use of the Logan bow (a curved metal wire that prevents stress on the suture line) and restraints.

   b. Encourage a parent to be with the child, especially when awakening from anesthesia, to offer security and comfort.

Postoperative Care

1. Postoperatively, apply elbow restraints to prevent child's hands from reaching the mouth while still allowing some freedom of movement.

2. Protect the suture line from tension.

   a. Check Logan bow, butterfly-type adhesive, or Band-Aid placed across top of lip to prevent lateral tension on cleft lip incision.

   b. Avoid wetting tape, or it will loosen.

   c. Observe for and report bleeding.

   d. Prevent the child from crying, blowing, sucking, talking or laughing.

3. Position the child on back or propped on side (eg, on infant seat) to keep from rubbing lip on the sheets. If only cleft palate was repaired, child may lie on abdomen.

4. Provide for appropriate diversional activity, hanging toys, mobiles, etc.

5. Monitor respiratory effort after cleft palate repair.

   a. Be aware that breathing with a closed palate is different from the child's customary way of breathing; the child must also contend with increased mucus production.

   b. Provide croup tent with mist to decrease occurrence of respiratory problems and provide moisture to mucus membranes that may become dry from mouth breathing.

6. Accomplish feeding without tension on the suture line for several days after lip repair.

   a. Use dropper or syringe with a rubber tip, and insert from the side to avoid suture line or to avoid stimulating sucking.

   b. Perform nasogastric gavage if needed.

   c. Advance slowly to nipple feeding as directed. The infant should be able to suck more efficiently with the lip repaired.

7. Clean suture line after every feeding; keep the mouth moist to promote healing and provide comfort.

8. After palate repair, feed the child in the manner used preoperatively (cup, side of spoon, or rubber-tipped syringe). Never use straw, nipple, or plain syringe.

   a. Diet progresses from clear liquids to full liquids to soft foods.

   b. Soft foods are usually continued for about 1 month after surgery, at which time a regular diet is started, excluding hard food.

9. Administer prophylactic antibiotics as prescribed because the mouth and suture line are constantly contaminated.

Family Education and Health Maintenance

1. Instruct on continued protection of the mouth after surgery. Child cannot put anything in mouth, including lollipops.

2. Demonstrate how to rinse mouth after eating.

3. Advise on increased risk of ear infections and need to seek medical attention for colds, ear pain, fever, or other signs and symptoms. Routine ear examinations and hearing tests should be done to reduce the risk of hearing deficits.

4. Stress the importance of speech therapy and the parents practicing exercises with the child as directed by speech therapist.

5. Help the parents realize that even though rehabilitation of the child is long and expensive, the child can live a normal life.

6. Advise the parents to discuss the child's problem with the school nurse, teacher, and other responsible adults who will have close contact with the child.

7. For additional information and support refer to:

   Prescription Parents Inc.
   P. O. Box 426
   Quincy, MA 02269
   617-479-2463

Clubfoot, Congenital

Clubfoot (talipes equinovarus) is a congenital anomaly in which the foot is plantar flexed at the ankle and subtalar joints, the hind foot is inverted, and the midfoot and forefoot are adducted and inverted. Contractures of the soft tissues maintain the malalignments. Clubfoot occurs bilaterally in 50% of cases. The exact cause of clubfoot is unknown, but hereditary factors are often involved. If there is no familial tendency, the anomaly may result from arrested development during the 9th and 10th weeks of gestation. Clubfoot occurs in 1 to 2 of every 1000 births and is twice as common in boys.

◆ Assessment

1. Deformity is usually obvious at birth, with varying degrees of rigidity and ability to correct position.

◆ Diagnostic Evaluation

1. Clinical presentation and physical examination are usually diagnostic.
2. X-ray determines bony anatomy and assesses treatment efficacy.

◆ Collaborative Management

Therapeutic Interventions

1. Treatment should begin as soon after birth as possible, to establish a functional, pain-free foot that can be fit with standard footwear.
   a. Initially, serial manipulations followed by immobilization in a plaster cast, taping, or strapping started at the time of diagnosis. Done daily as an inpatient or weekly as an outpatient.
   b. After the initial period (age 2–6 months), evaluation will determine the need to continue with manipulation and casting, proceeding to corrective shoes or solid ankle orthotics or a definitive surgical correction.
2. Corrective footwear consists of a reverse last or outflare

shoe with or without a Dennis-Browne bar or the more recent Wheaton brace or Bebax shoe.

Surgical Interventions

1. Usually performed at age 4 to 9 months so that the child is free of postoperative immobilization before the beginning of walking
2. The child who presents late or has a recurrent or residual deformity may require an aggressive surgical procedure to stabilize the bony structures and balance the muscle and tendons by a combination of fusions, releases, lengthenings, and transfers.
3. Postoperative routines usually include a period of cast immobilization of up to 12 weeks followed by a brace or corrective shoe for a period of 2 to 4 years.

◆ Nursing Interventions

Monitoring

1. Perform frequent neurovascular assessments after surgery, including color, warmth, sensation, capillary refill, pulses, and presence of pain.

Supportive Care

1. Discuss the deformity and expected treatment in terms the parents can understand. Respond to their questions and concerns.
2. Encourage parents to hold and play with child and participate in care.
3. Assess fit of cast, splint, orthotic device, or special shoes. Teach parents that, because of the rapid growth rate of the infant, device may need to be replaced to prevent blistering.
4. Assess and teach parents to assess for signs of excessive pressure on skin: redness, excoriations, foul odor from underneath cast, or pain.
5. Elevate the extremity to prevent edema.
6. Place ice packs over casts for the first 24 hours.
7. Stimulate movement of toes to promote circulation.
8. Assess for signs of discomfort such as irritability, crying, poor feeding and sleeping, tachycardia, increased blood pressure.
9. Administer analgesics regularly for 24 to 48 hours after surgery.

10. Provide comfort measures such as soft music, pacifier, or teething ring, rocking.

Family Education and Health Maintenance

1. Teach parents to remove cast by soaking in water and vinegar mixture at home before weekly manipulation and recasting. This avoids anxiety and possible abrasions from using cast saw.
2. Teach the parents when orthotic devices may be removed (usually for bathing). Stress that devices must be worn as prescribed.
3. Advise parents that infant's sleep may be disturbed initially because of wearing brace at night; may be irritable while awake because of fatigue.
4. Instruct parents on providing a safe environment for the ambulatory child.
5. Discuss the importance of long-term and frequent follow-up and obtain social work consult to assist the parents with special needs such as transportation, flexible appointment times, and financing orthotic equipment, as needed.

Colorectal Cancer
See Cancer, Colorectal

Congenital Heart Disease
See Heart Disease, Congenital

Congestive Heart Failure
See Heart Failure

Conjunctivitis

Conjunctivitis is inflammation or infection of the conjunctiva, the mucous membrane that lines the inner surface of the eyelids and the anterior portion of the eyeball. The disorder may be caused by bacteria, viruses, *Chlamydia*, fungi, allergens, chemical exposure, or trauma. Also known as "pinkeye," this disorder is easily spread by contact with infectious material. It is usually self-limiting, but some bacteria may cause extensive tissue damage and visual impairment.

◆ Assessment

1. Itching, burning, feeling of foreign body in eye, and possible photophobia
2. Redness, swelling, lacrimation, crusting of lids, and any discharge
   a. Purulent discharge if infected by *Neisseria gonorrhoeae*
   b. Abundant lacrimation with little discharge indicates viral infection
3. Visual acuity is usually not affected.

NURSING ALERT
A painful red eye should be evaluated promptly for evidence of herpesvirus infection or corneal damage.

◆ Diagnostic Evaluation

1. If indicated by purulent discharge, specimens for culture and sensitivity tests are collected to determine causative organism.

◆ Collaborative Management

Therapeutic Intervention
1. If foreign body is suggested, eye is irrigated with normal saline or prescribed solution to dislodge particles.
2. For common viral conjunctivitis, no treatment is usually indicated unless risk of secondary bacterial infection; then topical antibiotic is given.

Pharmacologic Interventions
1. Topical antibiotic drops or ointment for bacterial conjunctivitis.

2. A topical or systemic antiviral may be given for herpes conjunctivitis.
3. For allergic conjunctivitis, antiinflammatory, antihistamine, or mast cell stabilizer drops may be given.

PEDIATRIC ALERT
   One dose antibiotic ointment is given after delivery to prevent gonococcal or chlamydial conjunctivitis in newborns.

◆ Nursing Interventions

Family Education and Health Maintenance

1. Teach frequent handwashing, prompt disposal of contaminated tissues, and no sharing of washcloths and towels to prevent spread of infection.
2. Teach proper technique of instilling eyedrops or applying ointment.
3. Encourage use of warm compresses to remove crusting, or cold compresses to relieve redness and discomfort.
4. Encourage the patient to take medication for entire length of prescription.

Coronary Artery Disease

Coronary artery disease (CAD) is characterized by the accumulation of fatty deposits along the innermost layer of the coronary arteries. The fatty deposits may develop in childhood and progressively enlarge and thicken throughout the lifespan. The enlarged lesion (atheroma/plaque) can cause a critical narrowing of the coronary artery lumen, resulting in a decrease in coronary blood flow and an inadequate supply of oxygen to the heart muscle. Ischemia may be silent (asymptomatic but evidenced by ST depression of 1 mm or more on ECG) or may be manifested by angina.

Stable (effort) angina pectoris frequently results, with

chest pain precipitated by physical exertion or emotional stress. Increased oxygen demands are placed on the heart muscle, but the ability of the coronary artery to deliver blood to the muscle is impaired because of obstruction by a significant coronary lesion (75% narrowing of the vessel). Rest and nitroglycerin relieve the pain.

Unstable (preinfarction) angina pectoris may occur, with chest pain occurring at rest. No increase in oxygen demand is placed on the heart muscle, but an acute lack of blood flow to the muscle occurs because of coronary artery spasm aggravated by the presence of an enlarged plaque or hemorrhage/ulceration of a complicated lesion. Critical narrowing of the vessel lumen occurs abruptly in either instance.

◆ Assessment

CAD is manifested by angina, or chest pain.

1. *Character*—substernal chest pain, pressure, heaviness, or discomfort. Other sensations include a squeezing, aching, burning, choking, strangling, or cramping pain.
2. *Severity*—Pain may be mild or severe and typically presents with a gradual buildup of discomfort and subsequent gradual fading away.
3. *Location*—behind middle or upper third of sternum; the patient generally will make a fist over the site of the pain (positive Levine sign; indicates diffuse deep visceral pain), rather than point to it with fingers.
4. *Radiation*—usually radiates to neck, jaw, shoulders, arms, hands, and posterior intrascapular area. Pain occurs more commonly on the left side than the right; may produce numbness or weakness in arms, wrist, or hands.
5. *Duration*—usually lasts 1 to 5 minutes after stopping activity; nitroglycerin relieves pain within 1 minute.
6. *Precipitating factors*—physical activity, exposure to hot or cold weather, eating a heavy meal, and sexual intercourse increase the workload of the heart and therefore increase oxygen demand.
7. *Associated manifestations*—include diaphoresis, nausea, indigestion, dyspnea, tachycardia, and increase in blood pressure.
8. Signs of unstable angina

a. A change in frequency, duration, and intensity of stable angina symptoms
b. Angina pain lasts longer than 10 minutes, is unrelieved by rest or sublingual nitroglycerin, and mimics signs and symptoms of impending myocardial infarction (see p. 589).

C

> **NURSING ALERT**
> Unstable angina may cause sudden death or result in myocardial infarction. Early recognition and treatment are imperative.

9. Risk factors for CAD:
   a. Three major risk factors—elevated blood cholesterol levels, hypertension, cigarette smoking
   b. Unmodifiable risk factors—age, male sex, race, family history of CAD
   c. Other risk factors—diabetes mellitus, obesity, sedentary lifestyle, stress, type-A personality

◆ Diagnostic Evaluation

1. ECG may show ST segment changes indicative of ischemia.
2. Exercise stress testing with or without perfusion studies shows ischemia.
3. Cardiac catheterization shows blocked vessels.
4. Fasting blood levels of cholesterol, low-density lipoprotein (LDL), high-density lipoprotein (HDL), and triglycerides may be abnormal.

◆ Collaborative Management

Pharmacologic Interventions

1. Antianginal medications (nitrates, beta-blockers, calcium channel blockers) to promote blood flow to the heart muscle, thereby increasing oxygen supply
2. Antilipid medications to decrease blood cholesterol and triglyceride levels in patients with elevated levels

◆ Surgical Interventions

1. Percutaneous transluminal coronary angioplasty (PTCA) or intracoronary athrectomy, or placement of intracoronary stent. These procedures are performed through a catheter introduction through the femoral artery and into the coronary circulation to relieve obstruction.
2. Coronary artery bypass grafting (CABG) (see p. 163).

◆ Nursing Interventions

Monitoring

1. Monitor blood pressure, apical heart rate, and respirations every 5 minutes during an anginal attack.
2. Maintain continuous ECG monitoring or obtain a 12-lead ECG, as directed; monitor for dysrhythmias and ST elevation.
3. Assess response to nitroglycerin, rest, or other treatment.
4. Assess for headache, orthostatic hypotension, and change in heart rate and rhythm related to antianginal therapy.
5. Evaluate for development of heart failure (due to treatment with beta-blockers or calcium channel blockers).
   a. Obtain serial weights.
   b. Auscultate lung fields for crackles.
   c. Monitor for the presence of edema.
6. After cardiac catheterization, monitor blood pressure and apical pulse closely, check peripheral pulses in affected extremity, watch for hematoma formation at puncture site, assess for chest, back, thigh, or groin pain, and keep the patient in bed until the following morning.

Supportive Care

1. Place patient in comfortable position and administer oxygen, if prescribed, to enhance myocardial oxygen supply.
2. Identify specific activities patient may engage in that are below the level at which anginal pain occurs.
3. Reinforce the importance of notifying nursing staff whenever angina pain is experienced.

4. Encourage supine position for dizziness caused by anti-anginals (usually associated with a decrease in blood pressure; preload is enhanced by this mechanism, thereby increasing blood pressure). Be sure to remove previous nitrate patch or paste before applying new paste/pad (prevents hypotension).

5. Be alert to adverse reaction related to abrupt discontinuation of beta-blocker and calcium channel blocker therapy. These drugs must be tapered to prevent a "rebound phenomenon": tachycardia, increase in chest pain, hypertension.

Patient Education/Health Maintenance

1. Explain to the patient the importance of anxiety reduction to assist in control of angina. (Anxiety and fear put an increased stress on the heart, requiring the heart to use more oxygen.) Teach relaxation techniques.

2. Discuss measures to be taken when an anginal episode occurs.

   a. Place nitroglycerin under tongue at first sign of chest discomfort.

   b. Stop all effort/activity; sit, and take nitroglycerin tablet—relief should be obtained in a few minutes.

   c. Bite the tablet between front teeth and slip under tongue to dissolve if quick action is desired.

   d. Repeat dosage in a few minutes for total of 3 tablets if relief is not obtained.

   e. Go to the nearest health care facility if chest pain persists more than 15 minutes, is unrelieved by 3 nitroglycerin tablets, or is more intense and widespread than the usual angina episodes (Should not drive self).

   f. Keep a record of number of tablets taken—to evaluate any change in anginal pattern.

3. Review specific risk factors that affect CAD development and progression; highlight those risk factors that can be modified and controlled to reduce risk.

   a. Inform patient of methods of stress reduction such as biofeedback and relaxation techniques.

   b. Review information on low-fat/low-cholesterol diet with patient and person who shops/cooks in home. Suggest available cookbooks (American

Heart Association) that may assist in planning and preparing foods.

c. Have dietitian visit patient to design a menu plan for patient.

d. Inform patient of available cardiac rehabilitation programs that offer structured classes on exercise, smoking cessation, and weight control.

e. Avoid excessive caffeine intake (coffee, cola drinks) that can increase the heart rate and produce angina.

f. Do not use "diet pills," nasal decongestants, or any over-the-counter medications that can increase the heart rate or stimulate high blood pressure.

g. Avoid the use of alcohol or drink only in moderation (alcohol can increase hypotensive side effects of drugs).

h. Encourage follow-up for tight control of diabetes and hypertension.

4. Advise the patient on activity level to prevent angina.

a. Participate in a normal daily program of activities that do not produce chest discomfort, shortness of breath, and undue fatigue. Begin regular regimen of exercise as directed by health care provider.

b. Avoid activities known to cause anginal pain—sudden exertion, walking against the wind, extremes of temperature, high altitude, emotionally stressful situations; may accelerate heart rate, raise blood pressure, and increase cardiac work.

c. Refrain from engaging in physical activity for 2 hours after meals. Rest after each meal if possible.

d. Do not undertake activities requiring heavy effort (carrying heavy objects).

e. Try to avoid cold weather; dress warmly and walk more slowly. Wear scarf over nose and mouth when in cold air.

COMMUNITY CARE CONSIDERATIONS

Ensure that patient has enough medication until next follow-up appointment or trip to the pharmacy. Warn against abrupt withdrawal of beta- or calcium channel blockers to prevent rebound effect.

Craniotomy

Craniotomy is the surgical opening of the skull to gain access to intracranial structures. Surgical approach may be supratentorial (above the tentorium, or dural covering that divides the cerebrum from cerebellum) or infratentorial (below the tentorium, including the brain stem). Procedures include craniotomy by means of bur holes or body flap, craniectomy in which a portion of the skull is excised, cranioplasty in which a cranial defect is repaired, or transsphenoidal approach to the pituitary (see p. 668). Craniotomy is indicated for a variety of treatments, including removing a tumor or abscess, aspirating a hematoma, clipping an aneurysm, relieving intracranial pressure (ICP), stopping hemorrhage, or removing epileptogenic tissue.

◆ Potential Complications

1. Intracranial hemorrhage or hematoma
2. Cerebral edema
3. Infections (postoperative meningitis, pulmonary, wound, etc.)
4. Seizures
5. Cranial nerve dysfunction

◆ Collaborative Management

Preoperative Care

1. Reinforce the surgeon's explanation of diagnostic findings, surgical procedure, and expectations.
2. Assist the patient with presurgical shampoo with an antimicrobial agent; explain the extent of head shave.
3. Administer corticosteroids to reduce cerebral edema.
4. Administer anticonvulsants to reduce risk of seizures.
5. Explain use of intraoperative antibiotics to reduce risk of infection, and urinary catheterization to assess urinary volume during operative period.
6. Administer mannitol and a diuretic such as furosemide immediately before the procedure, as ordered, to reduce cerebral edema.

7. Evaluate and record the patient's neurologic baseline and vital signs for postoperative comparison.
8. Explain immediate postoperative care, and where the doctor will contact the family after surgery.
9. Provide supportive care to the patient with neurologic deficits.

Postoperative Care

1. Closely monitor level of consciousness, vital signs, pupillary response, and intracranial pressure, if indicated. Use Glasgow coma scale.
2. Assess respiratory status by monitoring rate, depth, and pattern of respirations. Maintain a patent airway.
3. Teach the patient to avoid activities that can raise intracranial pressure (ICP), such as excessive flexion or rotation of the head and Valsalva maneuver (coughing, straining at stool).
4. Administer corticosteroids and other medications as prescribed to reduce ICP.
5. Manage arterial and central venous or pulmonary artery lines for accurate manipulation of blood pressure and fluid status.
6. Prepare for computed tomography if patient status deteriorates.
7. Weigh the patient daily, and monitor intake and output.
8. Offer oral fluids only when patient is alert and swallow reflex and bowel sounds have returned.
9. Have suction equipment available at bedside. Suction only if necessary and carefully to prevent rise in ICP.
10. Elevate head of bed to maximum of order and patient comfort.
11. Use sterile technique for dressing changes, catheter care, and ventricular drain management to prevent infection.
12. Be aware of patients at higher risk of infection—those undergoing lengthy operations, those with ventricular drains left in longer than 48 to 72 hours, and those with operations of the third ventricle.
13. Assess surgical site for redness, tenderness, and drainage.
14. Watch for leakage of cerebrospinal fluid (CSF), which increases the danger of meningitis.

C

   a. Watch for sudden discharge of fluid from wound;
      massive leak requires surgical repair.
   b. Warn against coughing, sneezing, or nose blow-
      ing, which may aggravate CSF leakage.
   c. Assess for moderate elevation of temperature and
      nuchal rigidity.
   d. Note patency of ventricular catheter system.
15. Control incisional and headache pain with analgesics
    as prescribed. Darken room if patient is photophobic.
16. Employ measures to reduce periorbital edema such
    as cold compresses, or moist tea bags. Apply lubricant
    to eyelids.
17. After supratentorial craniotomy, anticipate the use
    of postoperative anticonvulsants. Position the patient
    on back or unoperative side with one pillow under
    head.
18. After an infratentorial operation, keep the patient on
    side and off back with only a small firm pillow under
    head.

◆ Patient Education and Health Maintenance

1. Reinforce need to prevent IICP for several weeks by not
   bending over, straining at stool, lifting heavy objects,
   engaging in vigorous sexual activity, and having prolonged coughing.
2. Advise reporting of fever or any new or worsening
   neurologic deficits after surgery.
3. Advise proper care and precautions to prevent injury
   for specific neurologic deficits.

Crohn's Disease

Crohn's disease (regional enteritis, granulomatous colitis)
is a chronic transmural inflammation of the bowel wall
that usually affects the small and large intestines. However, it can occur in any part of the alimentary canal.
Cause is unknown, but theories include viral or bacterial
infection, immune disorder, psychosomatic illness, ge-

netic predisposition, and dietary factors (chemical additives, milk products, heavy metals, low fiber).

Crohn's disease appears more often in persons of Jewish Eastern European ancestry and in persons between 15 and 35 years of age. The intestinal tissue thickens, first by edema and later by formation of scar tissues and granulomas. Inflammation and ulcers form in the bowel mucosa, producing a constant irritating discharge. In some patients, the inflamed intestine may perforate and form intraabdominal and anal abscesses.

Complications include stricture and fistulae formation (ischiorectal, perianal—even to bladder or vagina); hemorrhage; bowel perforation; mechanical intestinal obstruction. Incidence of colorectal cancer is higher in these patients.

◆ Assessment

1. Signs and symptoms are characterized by exacerbations and remissions; onset may be abrupt or insidious.
2. Crampy pain occurs after meals because of inability of the intestine to transport the contents of upper intestine through the constricted lumen.
   a. Cramps cause the patient to eat in small amounts or even to avoid eating, which then results in malnutrition, weight loss, and possible anemia (hypochromic or macrocytic).
   b. Milk products and chemically or mechanically irritating food may aggravate the problem.
3. Abdominal tenderness occurs, especially in right lower quadrant; may simulate acute appendicitis.
4. Chronic diarrhea caused by irritating discharge; usual consistency is soft or semiliquid. Bloody stools or steatorrhea (fatty stools) may occur.
5. Low-grade fever occurs if abscesses are present.
6. Lymphadenitis occurs in mesenteric nodes.

◆ Diagnostic Evaluation

1. Barium enema permits visualization of lesions of large intestine and terminal ileum; needs to be scheduled before upper GI to prevent interference by barium passing through colon.

2. Upper GI barium studies to show classic "string sign" at terminal ileum that suggests constriction of a segment of intestine
3. Proctosigmoidoscopy to note ulceration, possibly rule out ulcerative colitis, and obtain tissue biopsy specimen for definitive diagnosis
4. Increased white blood cells count and sedimentation rate; decreased hemoglobin; and possibly decreased potassium, magnesium, and calcium

◆ Collaborative Management

Therapeutic Interventions

1. Diet low in residue, fiber, and fat, and high in calories, protein, and carbohydrates, with vitamin supplements (especially vitamin K)
2. During exacerbation, hyperalimentation to maintain nutrition while allowing the bowel to rest
3. During remission, regular balanced diet to maintain ideal body weight

Pharmacologic Interventions

1. Sulfasalazine to inhibit inflammatory process; effective only for colonic disease
2. Mesalamine; usually given by enema or suppository and only effective in colon; mechanism unclear, but seems to have topical rather than systemic effect
3. Corticosteroids to reduce inflammation; orally or IV, depending on severity of disease
4. Metronidazole to treat infection in perianal disease or fistula formation
5. Antidiarrheal agents to control diarrhea related to malabsorption of bile salts

Surgical Interventions

1. Surgery is indicated only for complications. Roughly 70% of Crohn's disease patients eventually require one or more operations for obstruction, fistulae, fissures, abscesses, toxic megacolon, or perforation. Also see p. 350.
   a. Because the goal is palliation, minimal resection, bypass, and stricture-plasty may be done to preserve bowel.

b. Kock pouch and ileal reservoir anal anastomosis are contraindicated in Crohn's disease because disease can develop within the pouches.

2. Other surgical options include:
   a. Bowel resection with anastomosis
   b. Partial colectomy; temporary end ileostomy and Hartmann's pouch, or ileorectal anastomosis (spares rectum)
   c. Total proctocolectomy with end ileostomy for severe disease in colon and rectum

C

◆ **Nursing Interventions**

Monitoring

1. Monitor frequency and consistency of stools to evaluate volume losses and effectiveness of therapy.
2. Monitor dietary therapy; weigh the patient daily.
3. Monitor electrolytes, especially potassium. Monitor intake and output. Monitor acid–base balance because diarrhea can lead to metabolic acidosis.
4. Monitor for distention, increased temperature, hypotension, and rectal bleeding; all signs of obstruction caused by inflammation.
5. Observe and record changes in pain—frequency, location, characteristics, precipitating events, and duration.
6. Watch for cardiac dysrhythmias and muscle weakness caused by loss of electrolytes.

Supportive Care

1. Offer understanding, concern, and encouragement—patient is often embarrassed about frequent and malodorous stools, and often fearful of eating.
2. Have patient participate in meal planning to encourage compliance and increase knowledge.
3. Encourage patient's usual support persons to be involved in management of the disease.
4. Provide small frequent feedings to prevent distention of the gastric pouch.
5. Provide fluids as prescribed to maintain hydration (1,000 mL/24 hours is minimum intake to meet body fluid needs).
6. Clean rectal area and apply ointments as necessary to decrease discomfort from skin breakdown.
7. Facilitate supportive counseling, if appropriate.

C

Patient Education and Health Maintenance

1. Instruct patient on prescribed medications to encourage compliance and understanding of management.
2. Review dietary changes such as increased fiber content and fluid intake and their importance in improving bowel function.
3. Instruct postoperative patient regarding wound care or ostomy care if applicable to promote healing and self-confidence.
4. Explain signs and symptoms of postoperative complications to report—elevated temperature, nausea or vomiting, abdominal distention, changes in bowel function and stool consistency, hemorrhage.
5. Assess the need for home health follow-up and initiate appropriate referrals if indicated.

Cryptorchidism

Cryptorchidism is a congenital disorder in which one or both testes fail to descend through the inguinal canal to their normal position in the scrotum. The cause is unknown, but hormonal factors thought to be involved in the mechanism of testicular descent may play a role. Mechanical lesions or, possibly, endocrine disorders also may be involved.

Cryptorchidism primarily affects premature male newborns. If cryptorchidism is not corrected before puberty, impaired spermatogenesis and infertility result because abdominal temperatures are higher than in the scrotum. In addition, the risks of testicular torsion, associated hernias, emotional disturbances, and testicular malignancy are significantly increased.

◆ Assessment

1. Physical examination discloses absence of one or both testes within the scrotum.

◆ Diagnostic Evaluation

1. Ultrasonography shows undescended testis.
2. Serum testosterone measurements may be decreased.

◆ Collaborative Management

Pharmacologic Interventions

1. Administration of human chorionic gonadotropin has produced descent of the testes in some children. Testes may have descended spontaneously in many of these cases.

Surgical Interventions

1. Orchiopexy is performed to achieve permanent fixation of the testis in the scrotum. Surgery should be performed when the child is between the ages of 1 and 3 years to prevent damage to the tissues and to lessen emotional concerns related to body image.
2. Plastic surgery may be performed in patients with an absent testis.

◆ Nursing Interventions

Supportive Care

1. Encourage the parents to express their concerns about the condition and ask questions about surgery.
2. Monitor vital signs after surgery and ensure that child voids.
3. Prevent contamination of the suture line by changing diapers frequently, and keep operative site clean.
4. Administer antibiotics as prescribed to prevent infection.
5. Maintain traction on the testicle.
   a. A suture is placed in the lower portion of the scrotum and is attached to a rubber band that is fastened to the upper aspect of the inner thigh by a piece of adhesive.
   b. This traction anchors the testis to the scrotum and is removed in 5 to 7 days.
6. Administer analgesics as needed.

Family Education and Health Maintenance

1. Encourage family to follow-up to ensure proper fixation of testicle in scrotum.
2. Explain that sexual function should not be impaired with treatment.

Cushing's Syndrome

Cushing's syndrome results from excessive secretion of one or all of the adrenocortical hormones: the glucocorticoid *cortisol* (predominant type), the mineralocorticoid *aldosterone,* and the *androgenital corticoids.* Types of Cushing's syndrome include:

Pituitary Cushing's syndrome (Cushing's disease) is the most common cause of Cushing's syndrome, and stems from hyperplasia of both adrenal glands caused by overstimulation by adrenocorticotropic hormone (ACTH), usually from pituitary adenoma. The syndrome affects mostly women between the ages of 20 and 40 years.

Adrenal Cushing's syndrome is associated with adenoma or carcinoma of the adrenal cortex. The disease may recur after surgery.

Ectopic Cushing's syndrome results from autonomous ACTH secretion by extrapituitary tumors (such as the lung) producing excess ACTH.

Iatrogenic Cushing's syndrome is caused by exogenous glucocorticoid administration.

◆ Assessment

1. Signs and symptoms of excess glucocorticoid (cortisol) secretion:
   a. Weight gain or obesity
   b. Heavy trunk; thin extremities
   c. Fat pad (Buffalo hump) in neck and supraclavicular area
   d. Rounded face (moon face); plethoric, oily complexion
   e. Skin—fragile and thin; striae and ecchymosis, acne
   f. Musculoskeletal—muscle wasting caused by excessive catabolism; osteoporosis; characteristic kyphosis, backache
   g. Mental disturbances—mood changes, psychosis
   h. Increased susceptibility to infections
2. Manifestations of excess mineralocorticoid (aldosterone) secretion:
   a. Hypertension
   b. Hypernatremia, hypokalemia

c. Weight gain
d. Expanded blood volume
e. Edema
3. Manifestations of excess androgens:
   a. Females experience virilism (masculinization) with hirsutism (excessive growth of hair on the face and midline of trunk); atrophied breasts; enlarged clitoris; masculinized voice; loss of libido; hermaphroditism (if exposed in utero)
   b. Males—loss of libido

◆ Diagnostic Evaluation

1. Excessive plasma cortisol levels
2. Increased blood glucose levels and glucose intolerance
3. Decreased serum potassium level
4. Reduced eosinophils
5. Elevation of plasma ACTH in patients with pituitary tumors
   a. Very low plasma ACTH levels with adrenal tumor
   b. Loss of normal diurnal variation of plasma cortisol levels
6. Elevated urinary 17-hydroxycorticoids and 17-ketogenic steroids
7. Overnight dexamethasone suppression test, possibly with cortisol urinary excretion measurement, to check for:
   a. Unsuppressed cortisol level in Cushing's *syndrome* caused by adrenal tumors
   b. Suppressed cortisol level in Cushing's *disease* caused by pituitary tumor
8. Skull x-rays to detect erosion of the sella turcica by a pituitary tumor; CT scan and ultrasonography to locate tumor

◆ Collaborative Management

Pharmacologic Interventions

1. In patients unable to undergo surgery, cortisol synthesis–inhibiting drugs may be used. These include:
   a. Mitotane, an agent toxic to the adrenal cortex (DDT derivative), known as "medical adrenalectomy."

Side effects include nausea, vomiting, diarrhea, somnolence, and depression.
  b. Metyrapone is given to control steroid hypersecretion in patients who do not respond to mitotane.
  c. Aminoglutethimide is given to block cortisol production. Side effects include gastrointestinal disturbances, somnolence, and skin rashes.

Surgical Interventions

1. Pituitary surgery to treat pituitary Cushing's syndrome
   a. Transsphenoidal adenomectomy or hypophysectomy (see p. 226)
   b. Transfrontal craniotomy may be necessary when a pituitary tumor has enlarged beyond the sella turcica (see p. 226).
2. Bilateral adrenalectomy is used to treat adrenal causes.
3. Radiation therapy also may be used to treat pituitary or adrenal tumors.
4. Postoperative hormone replacement therapy is necessary.
   a. Adrenalectomy patients require lifelong replacement therapy with glucocorticoids and mineralocorticoids.
   b. After pituitary irradiation or hypophysectomy, the patient may require adrenal replacement plus thyroid, posterior pituitary, and gonadal hormone replacement therapy.
   c. After transsphenoidal adenomectomy, the patient needs hydrocortisone replacement therapy for 12 to 18 months, and additional hormones if excessive loss of pituitary function has occurred.
   d. Protein anabolic steroids may be given to facilitate protein replacement; potassium replacement is usually required.

◆ Nursing Interventions

Monitoring

1. Monitor intake and output, daily weights, and serum glucose and electrolytes.
2. Monitor for signs of infection because risk is high.
3. Monitor for skin changes and bone pain related to osteoporosis.

4. After hypothysectomy, monitor for diabetes insipidus (p. 259), hypothyroidism (p. 491), and other endocrine changes.

5. After adrenalectomy, monitor for adrenal crisis (p. 9).

Supportive Care

1. Assess the skin frequently to detect reddened areas, skin breakdown, or tearing, excoriation, infection, or edema.

2. Handle skin and extremities gently to prevent trauma; protect from falls by use of siderails.

3. Avoid using adhesive tape on the skin to reduce trauma on its removal.

4. Encourage the patient to turn in bed frequently or ambulate to reduce pressure on bony prominences and areas of edema.

5. Assist the patient with ambulation and hygiene when weak and fatigued. Use assistive devices during ambulation to prevent falls and fractures.

6. Help the patient to schedule exercise and rest. Advise the patient how to recognize signs and symptoms of excessive exertion.

7. Instruct the patient in correct body mechanics to avoid pain or injury during activities.

8. Provide foods low in sodium to minimize edema, and provide foods high in potassium (bananas, orange juice, tomatoes) and administer potassium supplement as prescribed to counteract weakness related to hypokalemia.

9. Report edema and signs of fluid retention.

10. Encourage the patient to verbalize concerns about illness, changes in appearance, and altered role functions.

NURSING ALERT
Observe for evidence of depression, which may progress to suicide. Alert health care provider of mood changes, sleep disturbance, change in activity level, change in appetite, or loss of interest in visitors or other experiences.

11. Refer the patient for counseling, if indicated.

12. Explain to the patient who has benign adenoma or hyperplasia that, with proper treatment, evidence of masculinization can be reversed.

Patient Education and Health Promotion

1. Teach the patient about lifelong hormone replacement therapy and the need for regular follow-up visits to determine if dosage is appropriate or to detect side effects.
2. Instruct the patient in proper skin care and stress prompt reporting of trauma or infection.
3. Teach the patient to monitor urine or blood glucose or report for blood glucose tests as directed to detect hyperglycemia.
4. Help the patient prevent hyperglycemia and obesity by teaching a low-calorie, low–concentrated carbohydrate and fat diet and to increase activity as tolerated.
5. Encourage diet high in calcium (dairy products, broccoli) and weight-bearing activity to prevent osteoporosis caused by glucocorticoid replacement.

CVA

See Cerebrovascular Accident

Cystic Fibrosis

Cystic fibrosis (CF) is an inherited disorder of the exocrine glands, in which their secretions, normally free-flowing, become abnormally viscous and liable to obstruct glandular ducts. Cystic fibrosis primarily affects pulmonary and gastrointestinal function.

The disease is most common in Caucasians (1 in every 1600 to 2500 births). The average life expectancy for the CF patient is currently about 30 years. Death may occur because of pneumonia, emphysema, or atelectasis. Other complications include esophageal varices, diabetes, chronic sinusitis, pancreatitis, rectal polyps, intussusception, growth retardation, and infertility.

◆ Assessment

1. Meconium ileus is found in newborn; usually occurs before age 6 months but may occur at any age.
2. Parents report salty taste when skin is kissed.
3. Cough (dry and hacking to loose and productive); wheezing
4. Vomiting after coughing
5. Recurrent pulmonary infections
6. Failure to gain weight or grow in the presence of a good appetite
7. Frequent, bulky, and foul-smelling stools (steatorrhea); excessive flatus
8. Protuberant abdomen, pot belly
9. Wasted buttocks
10. Clubbing of fingers in older child
11. Increased anteroposterior chest diameter (barrel chest)
12. Decreased exertional endurance
13. Hyperglycemia, glucosuria with polyuria, and weight loss

◆ Diagnostic Evaluation

1. Sweat chloride test to measure sodium and chloride level in sweat
   a. Chloride level of more than 60 mEq/L is virtually diagnostic
   b. Chloride level of 40 to 60 mEq/L is borderline and should be repeated
2. Diagnosis is made when a positive sweat test is seen in conjunction with one or more of the following:
   a. Positive family history for cystic fibrosis
   b. Typical chronic obstructive lung disease
   c. Documented exocrine pancreatic insufficiency
3. Duodenal secretions: low trypsin concentration is virtually diagnostic.
4. Stool analysis:
   a. Reduced trypsin and chymotrypsin levels—used for initial screening for cystic fibrosis
   b. Increased stool fat concentration
   c. BMC (Boehringer-Mannheim Corp.) meconium

strip test for stool includes lactose and protein content; used for screening
5. Chest x-ray may be normal initially; later shows increased areas of infection, overinflation, bronchial thickening and plugging, atelectasis, and fibrosis
6. Pulmonary function studies (after age 4) show decreased vital capacity and flow rates and increased residual volume or increased total lung capacity.

◆ Collaborative Management

Therapeutic Interventions

1. Chest physical therapy for bronchial drainage, especially during acute exacerbations.
   a. Postural drainage
   b. Coughing and deep breathing exercises
2. Some centers employ bronchopulmonary lavage to treat atelectasis and mucoid impaction using large volumes of saline.
3. Increased carbohydrates, protein, and fat (possibly as high as 40%) for growth and repair, infection, the work of breathing, and energy expenditure for coughing, malabsorption, and physical activity.
4. Ensure adequate fluid and salt intake.

Pharmacologic Interventions

1. Antimicrobial therapy as indicated for pulmonary infection
   a. Oral or IV antibiotics as required
   b. Inhaled antibiotics, such as gentamicin (Garamycin) or tobramycin (Nebcin), may be used for severe lung disease or colonization of organisms. Recently, some practitioners advocate using nebulized antibiotics earlier in therapy.
2. Bronchodilators and vasoconstrictors to relieve bronchospasm
3. Aerosols, expectorants, and mucolytic agents as prescribed to decrease viscosity of secretions
4. Pancreatic enzyme supplements with each feeding
   a. Favored preparation is pancrelipase
   b. Occasionally antacid is helpful to improve tolerance of enzymes.
   c. Favorable response to enzymes is based on tolerance of fatty foods, decreased stool frequency, ab-

sence of steatorrhea, improved appetite, and lack of abdominal pain.

5. Administration of aerosolized recombinant human deoxyribonuclease has been tried to reduce viscosity of sputum, thereby facilitating its removal and decreasing the incidence of infection. Early trials show improvement in forced vital capacity (FVC) and forced expiratory volume (FEV).

Surgical Interventions

1. Lobectomy (resection of symptomatic lobar bronchiectasis) may be done to retard progression of lesion to total lung involvement.
2. Heart–lung, double-lung, or single-lung transplantation has been tried for end-stage lung disease.
3. Gene therapy, in which recombinant DNA containing a corrected gene sequence is introduced into the diseased lung tissue, is in clinical trials.

◆ Nursing Interventions

Monitoring

1. Monitor weight at least weekly to assess effectiveness of nutritional interventions.
2. Monitor respiratory status and sputum production, to evaluate response to respiratory care measures.

Supportive Care

1. To promote airway clearance, employ intermittent aerosol therapy three to four times a day when the child is symptomatic.
   a. Use before postural drainage.
   b. Administer bronchodilators and other medications, diluted in normal saline, in aerosol form to penetrate respiratory tract.

NURSING ALERT

Mist tent therapy is no longer recommended because water droplets may cause bronchospasm in some patients, and the equipment required to deliver the therapy is frequently contaminated with opportunistic organisms.

2. Perform chest physical therapy three to four times a day after aerosol therapy; perform more frequently if infection is present.
3. Help the child to relax to cough more easily after postural drainage.
4. Suction the infant or young child when necessary, if not able to cough.
5. Teach the child breathing exercises using pursed lips to increase duration of exhalation.
6. Provide good skin care and position changes to prevent skin breakdown in malnourished child.
7. Provide frequent mouth care to reduce chances of infection since mucous is present.
8. Restrict contact with people with respiratory infection.
9. Encourage diet composed of foods high in calories and protein and moderate to high in fat because absorption of food is incomplete.
10. Administer fat-soluble vitamins (A, D, E, K) in water-miscible solution in 2 to 3 times the normal dose, as prescribed, to counteract malabsorption.
11. Administer pancreatic enzymes with each meal and snack. Withhold enzymes, as ordered, if child is only taking clear liquid diet or enteral feedings.
12. Increase salt intake during hot weather, fever, or excessive exercise to prevent sodium depletion and cardiovascular compromise.
13. To prevent vomiting, allow ample time for feeding because of irritability if not feeling well and coughing.
14. To reassure the child and promote self-esteem, explain each procedure, medication, and treatment to the child as appropriate for age.
15. Encourage older child to take responsibility for treatments and be involved in care plan.
16. Encourage regular exercise and activity to foster sense of accomplishment and independence and improve pulmonary function.
17. Provide opportunities for parents to learn all aspects of care for the child.

Family Education and Health Maintenance

1. Teach parents about dietary regimen and special need for calories, fat, and vitamins. Encourage consultation with a dietitian, as needed.

2. Discuss need for salt replacement, especially on hot summer days or when fever, vomiting, and diarrhea occur.
3. Help the parents to become skilled at chest physical therapy and other pulmonary treatments.
4. Help the family to schedule care for the child within the framework of family life.
5. Help the parents to provide emotional support for their child. The child needs love, understanding, and security—not overprotection.
6. Inform the family about genetic counseling and support them through the process.
7. Impress on the parents the importance of regular medical follow-up care and immunizations.
8. Discuss with parents limitations and expectations for the child. School nurse and teachers should be involved.
9. Refer families for additional information and support to agencies such as:

> **Cystic Fibrosis Foundation**
> 6931 Arlington Rd.
> Bethesda, MD 20814-3205
> 800-FIGHT CF.

Cystocele and Urethrocele

Cystocele is a downward displacement (protrusion) of the bladder into the vagina. *Urethrocele* is a downward displacement of the urethra into the vagina. These conditions may result from obstetric trauma to pelvic muscles, fascia, and ligaments during childbirth or hysterectomy. Impaired muscular support often becomes apparent years later, when genital atrophy associated with aging occurs. Some cases may result from a congenital defect. Complications include urinary incontinence and infection.

◆ Assessment

1. Pelvic pressure or heaviness or backache aggravated by coughing, sneezing, standing for long periods, and obesity, which increase intraabdominal pressure. Relieved by resting or lying down.
2. Urgency, frequency, incontinence, incomplete emptying

3. Observe perineum while the patient bears down, or observe the patient in upright position for telltale bulge in vagina

◆ Diagnostic Evaluation

1. Pelvic examination to identify condition
2. Urine specimens for urinalysis and culture to rule out infection

◆ Collaborative Management

Therapeutic and Pharmacologic Interventions

1. Vaginal pessary to insert into vagina to temporarily support pelvic organs
   a. Prolonged use may lead to necrosis and ulceration.
   b. Should be removed and cleaned every 1 to 2 months
2. Estrogen therapy after menopause may decrease genital atrophy.

Surgical Interventions

1. If cystocele is large and interferes with bladder functioning, may perform anterior vaginal colporrhaphy (repair of anterior vaginal wall).
2. Complications of surgery include urinary retention, bleeding (requires vaginal packing).

◆ Nursing Interventions

Supportive Care

1. Encourage periods of rest with legs elevated to relieve strain on pelvis.
2. Advise use of mild analgesics as necessary.
3. Provide postoperative care:
   a. Encourage voiding every 2 to 4 hours to reduce pressure so that no more than 150 mL will accumulate in bladder.
   b. Catheterize as necessary.
   c. Administer perineal care to the patient after each voiding and defecation.
   d. Employ a heat lamp to help dry the incision line and enhance the healing process.

e. Use available sprays for anesthetic and antiseptic effects.
f. Apply an ice pack locally to relieve congestion and discomfort.
4. Teach the patient Kegel pelvic floor exercises to regain muscle tone and control incontinence.
   a. Practice while voiding by stopping the flow of urine for 3 to 5 seconds, then releasing for 5 seconds.
   b. Patient can then tighten pelvic floor muscle at any time, repeat 10 times, three times a day, increase as able.
5. Encourage the patient to void frequently, respond to the urge to void promptly.
6. Warn the patient to avoid straining to prevent incontinence.
7. Encourage fluids to decrease bacterial flora in the bladder.

Patient Education and Health Maintenance

1. Teach women to avoid straining, remain active, avoid weight gain, and perform Kegel exercises to minimize pelvic relaxation in older years.
2. Encourage the patient to recognize and report symptoms of urinary tract infection (dysuria, frequency, foul-smelling urine).

Delirium, Dementia, and Amnesic Disorder

Delirium, dementia, and amnesic disorder are classed by the *Diagnostic and Statistical Manual, 4th Edition* as cognitive impairment disturbances, in which psychological or behavioral dysfunction results from temporary or permanent neuronal damage.

Delirium is a disturbance of consciousness and a change in cognition that develops over a brief period. It can be caused by numerous pathophysiologic conditions. Some of the major possibilities include head trauma; hypertensive encephalopathy; seizures; brain tumors; hypothyroidism; hypoxemia; hypothermia or hyperthermia; intoxication, abstinence and withdrawal states; poisoning due to metals, toxins, or drugs; diabetic ketoacidosis; hypoglycemia; acid–base imbalances; hepatic encephalopathy; thiamine deficiency; and psychosocial stressors such as relocation, sensory deprivation or overload, sleep deprivation, and immobilization. Delirium is reversible if the underlying cause is treated.

Dementia is a disturbance involving multiple cognitive deficits, including memory impairment. Primary dementias are degenerative disorders that are progressive, irreversible, and not attributable to any other condition. Basic types are dementia of the Alzheimer's type and vascular (formerly multi-infarct) dementia. Secondary dementias are also permanent and accompany many disorders, such as infections (acquired immunodeficiency syndrome, chronic meningitis, syphilis); degenerative disorders (Parkinson's disease); head trauma; brain tumors; inflammatory conditions; toxins; and metabolic disorders.

Amnesic disorder is characterized by memory impairment in the absence of other significant cognitive impairments. Amnesia is most commonly caused by head trauma. Other causes include stroke, neoplasms, anoxic or hypoglycemic states, herpes simplex encephalitis, epileptic seizures, electroconvulsive therapy, or substance abuse. Amnesia is often reversible.

◆ Assessment

1. Delirium
   a. Acute onset, usually brief course (1 week)
   b. Fearfulness, anxiety, irritability
   c. Auditory, visual, tactile hallucinations; illusions
   d. Impaired short-term memory
   e. Slurred speech, confabulation
   f. Fluctuating levels of awareness

    g. Confusion and disorientation
    h. Altered sleep–wake cycle
    i. EEG changes
2. Dementia
    a. Slow, insidious onset, progresses over years
    b. Labile mood; personality traits accentuated
    c. Hallucinations not a prominent feature
    d. Impaired short-term memory followed by impaired long-term memory
    e. Progressive aphasia and confabulation
    f. Deterioration of cognitive abilities (judgment, abstract thinking)
    g. Personality changes
    h. Absent or slow EEG changes
3. Amnesic disorder
    a. Sudden onset, may be transient or chronic
    b. Apathy, agitation, emotional blandness
    c. Impaired short- and long-term memory
    d. Impaired ability to learn new information
    e. Confabulation
    f. Remote memory is better preserved.

◆ Diagnostic Evaluation

1. Basic laboratory examination to determine underlying cause, including complete blood count with differential, chemistry panel (including blood urea nitrogen, creatine, and ammonia), arterial blood gases, chest x-ray, toxicology screen, thyroid function tests, and serologic tests for syphilis
2. Other tests include computed tomography, magnetic resonance imaging, lumbar puncture, and positron-emission tomography.
3. Mental status examination (Folstein scale, mini-mental)
4. Blessed Dementia Scale
5. Physical examination, vital signs, and review of medications

◆ Collaborative Management

Therapeutic Interventions
1. Safe, structured environment to prevent disorientation, accidents, or violence toward self, others, or property

D

2. Treatment of specific causes of delirium
3. Family involvement in therapy

Pharmacologic Interventions

1. Benzodiazepines are used for abstinence withdrawal states.
2. Neuroleptics (eg, haloperidol) for agitation or psychosis
3. Combined intravenous administration of haloperidol and lorazepam for agitated and psychotic symptomatology
4. Antidepressants for depression
5. Ergoloid mesylates (Hydergine) for cognitive dysfunction
6. Hypertension management in vascular dementia

◆ Nursing Interventions

Monitoring

1. Monitor food and fluid intake; weigh patient weekly.
2. Monitor functional capacity and self-care ability.
3. Closely observe the patient if he or she is smoking.

Supportive Care

1. Speak slowly and use short, simple words and phrases.
2. Consistently identify yourself, and address the person by name at each meeting.
3. Focus on one piece of information at a time. Review what has been discussed with the patient.
4. If the patient has vision or hearing disturbances, have the patient wear prescription eyeglasses or a hearing device.
5. Maintain a well-lighted environment.
6. Use clocks, calendars, and familiar personal effects in the patient's view.
7. If the patient becomes verbally aggressive, identify and acknowledge how he or she is feeling.
8. If the patient becomes aggressive, shift the topic to a safer, more familiar one. Respond calmly and do not raise your voice.
9. If the patient becomes delusional, acknowledge his or her feelings and reinforce reality. Do not attempt to challenge the content of the delusion.

10. Remove objects that might be used to harm self or others.
11. Identify stressors that increase agitation.
12. Distract the patient when an upsetting situation develops.
13. Use clothing with elastic and Velcro closures. Label clothes with the patient's name, address, and telephone number.
14. Remain with the patient during mealtime to determine the level of need for assistance or cueing in the ability to eat.
15. Initiate a bowel and bladder training program early in the disease process to maintain continence and prevent constipation or urinary retention.
16. Give the patient a card with simple instructions (address and phone number) in case he or she is lost. Also provide a medical alert bracelet.
17. Encourage participation in simple, familiar group activities, such as singing, reminiscing, and painting.
18. Encourage participation in simple activities that promote the exercise of large muscle groups.

Patient Education and Health Maintenance

1. Instruct the family about the disease process.
2. Instruct the family about safety measures to be used when the patient is at home or in the hospital.

COMMUNITY CARE CONSIDERATIONS

Assess the patient's home for safety: remove throw rugs, label rooms, and keep the house well lit, including nightlights. Advise installing complex safety locks and alarm devices on doors to outside or basement; install safety bars in bathroom. Assess community for safety, and, if the patient tends to wander, alert neighbors about wandering behavior; alert police and have current pictures taken.

3. Instruct and refer family members to community-based groups (adult day care centers, senior assessment centers, home care, respite care, and family support groups).

4. For additional information and support, refer to:

Alzheimer's Association
919 N. Michigan Ave.
Suite 1000
Chicago, IL 60611-1676
800-272-3900

Depressive Disorders

Depressive disorders include major depressive disorder and dysthymic disorder. These are categorized as mood disorders, in which a disturbance of mood (sustained emotion) is overly intense and prolonged; in severe cases it ultimately interferes with interpersonal or occupational functioning. Depression is much more than just sadness; it affects the way one feels about the future and can alter basic attitudes about the self. A depressed individual can become so despairing as to express hopelessness and may contemplate suicide.

Depressive disorders have multiple causes that are not fully understood. Factors that play a role include genetic predisposition; neurotransmitter abnormalities involving serotonin, norepinephrine, and dopamine; hyperactivity of the limbic-hypothalamic-pituitary-adrenal axis; sleep abnormalities; and psychosocial factors such as preexisting personality disorders, severe personal loss, or relationship problems.

◆ Assessment

1. Major depressive disorder occurs over a 2-week period, and impairs social and occupational functioning. Five or more of the following signs and symptoms occur nearly every day for most waking hours:
   a. Depressed mood
   b. Anhedonia—inability to express pleasure
   c. Significant weight loss or gain (more than 5% of body weight per month)
   d. Insomnia or hypersomnia
   e. Increased or decreased motor activity

   f. Anergia (fatigue or loss of energy)

   g. Feelings of worthlessness or inappropriate guilt (may be delusional)

   h. Decreased concentration or indecisiveness

   i. Recurrent thought of death or suicidal ideation (with or without plan)

2. Depression is further classified by the following specifiers:

   a. Severity

   b. Psychotic features

   c. Remission—chronic

   d. Seasonal affective disorder related to either winter or summer

   e. Catatonic features

   f. Melancholic features

   g. Atypical features

   h. Postpartum onset

3. Dysthymic disorder occurs over a 2-year period (1 year for children and adolescents) with depressed mood, but still retaining social and occupational functioning. Some of the following signs and symptoms are present:

   a. Decreased or increased appetite

   b. Insomnia or hypersomnia

   c. Anergy or chronic fatigue

   d. Anhedonia

   e. Decreased self-esteem

   f. Poor concentration or difficulty making decisions

   g. Perceived inability to cope with routine responsibilities

   h. Feelings of hopelessness or despair

   i. Pessimistic about the future, brooding over the past, or feeling sorry for self

   j. Recurrent thoughts of death or suicide

4. "Masked depression" may be evidenced by:

   a. Hypochondriasis

   b. Psychosomatic disorders

   c. Compulsive gambling

   d. Compulsive overwork

   e. Accident proneness

   f. Eating disorders

   g. Addictive illnesses

D

◆ Diagnostic Evaluation

1. Rating scales used to determine presence and severity of depression:
   a. Zung Self-Rating Scale
   b. Raskin Severity of Depression Scale
   c. Hamilton Depression Scale
   d. Beck Depression Inventory
2. Laboratory studies:
   a. Thyroid function tests and thyrotropin-releasing hormone stimulation test detect underlying hypothyroidism, which may cause depression.
   b. Dexamethasone suppression test evaluates depression that may be responsive to antidepressant or electroconvulsive therapy (ECT).
   c. Twenty-four-hour urinary 3-methoxy-4-hydroxyphenylglycol (MHPG) levels may be slightly lower in unipolar depression than in bipolar depression.
3. Polysomography detects an increase in the overall amount of REM sleep and shortened REM latency period in patients with major depression.
4. Additional diagnostic tests to evaluate physical conditions include computed tomography or magnetic resonance imaging, complete blood count, chemistry panel, serologic test for syphilis, human immunodeficiency virus test, electroencephalogram, vitamin B_{12} and folate levels, toxicology studies.

◆ Collaborative Management

Therapeutic Interventions

1. Inpatient treatment is required for those with the following conditions:
   a. Suicidal
   b. Severely disabled
   c. In crisis
   d. Require a complex diagnostic evaluation
   e. Require high-risk treatments
   f. Require ECT
2. Goals of treatment for depression are symptom reduction, improved function, and recurrence prevention
3. Psychotherapy styles include:
   a. Interpersonal psychotherapy

b. Cognitive therapy
c. Behavioral therapy
d. Marital therapy
e. Family therapy
4. Additional somatic therapies
   a. ECT
   b. High-intensity artificial light therapy
   c. Sleep deprivation therapy
5. Exercise program

Pharmacologic Interventions

1. Antidepressant therapy includes:
   a. Tricyclic antidepressants such as amitriptyline
   b. Serotonin reuptake inhibitors such as fluoxetine
   c. Monoamine oxidase (MAO) inhibitors such as iso-carboxazid
   d. Bicyclic agents such as venlafaxine
   e. Other antidepressants such as bupropion and trazo-done

◆ Nursing Interventions

Monitoring

1. Monitor patient's response to antidepressant therapy; some medications may lower seizure threshold.
2. If indicated, implement appropriate level of observation based on a focused suicide assessment (eg, constant observation or 15-minute checks); explain observation precautions to the patient.

Supportive Care

1. Initiate interaction with the patient at a regularly scheduled time.
2. Be clear and honest about your own feelings related to the patient's behavior.
3. Encourage verbal expression of feelings.
4. Validate feelings that are appropriate to the situation.
5. Explore with the patient what is producing and maintaining the feeling of depression.
6. Assess real, significant losses the patient has experienced.
7. Identify cultural and social factors that may contribute to how the patient copes with loss and feelings.

D

8. Assess the patient's support network.
9. Assess current suicide risk.
10. Remove harmful objects from the patient's possession, and assess environmental safety of the patient's room and unit.
11. Encourage the patient to negotiate a no self-harm/no suicide agreement with the staff.
12. Provide additional structure by keeping the patient involved in therapeutic and psychorehabilitative activities.
13. Collaborate with occupational and physical therapists to determine patient's functional capacity to accomplish activities of daily living (ADLs).
14. If patient is unable to accomplish ADLs independently, provide hygienic activities in collaboration with patient.
15. Acknowledge and reinforce the patient's efforts to maintain appearance; do not rush the patient when self-care is slow.
16. Reinforce what the patient can do rather than what he or she cannot do without assistance.
17. Remain with the patient during mealtime to determine the level of need for assistance or cuing in the ability to eat.
18. Determine the patient's past and current sleep patterns and sleep hygiene. Reinforce patient's successful sleep strategies.
19. Consider decreasing the amount of daytime sleep by encouraging participation in an activity.
20. Discuss alternative methods for facilitating sleep:
    a. Avoid caffeine.
    b. Avoid emotionally charged or upsetting discussions before bedtime.
    c. Avoid exercise $\frac{1}{2}$ to 1 hour before bed.
    d. Increase physical activity within functional limits.
    e. Use relaxation techniques.
    f. Try a warm bath or warm milk.

Family Education and Health Maintenance

1. Instruct patient and family members about biologic symptoms of depression.
2. Instruct patient and family members about purpose of antidepressant medication, effects, side effects and

their management, and how to recognize early signs and symptoms of relapse:

a. Do not drink alcoholic beverages if taking tricyclic antidepressants.

b. Avoid foods containing caffeine, tryptophan, or tyramine, if taking MAO inhibitors. (Examples are cheese, beer, chianti, sherry, coffee, cola drinks, liver, raisins, bananas, avocados, fava beans.)

3. Provide patient and family members with written material on coping with depression.

4. Provide patient and family members with information about appropriate community-based programs and support groups, such as:

National Foundation for Depressive Illness
P.O. Box 2257
New York, NY 10116
800-248-4344

Dermatitis, Atopic

Atopic dermatitis (eczema) is a chronic or chronically relapsing inflammatory response in the skin in those with personal or family history of atopy (asthma, allergic rhinitis, atopic dermatitis). Skin changes include dryness, lowered threshold for pruritus to minor irritants, lichenification (leathery thickening), rash, and frequent colonization with *Staphylococcus aureus*. Atopic dermatitis usually starts in infancy or young childhood and may or may not last into adulthood. Cause is unknown, but there is a familial tendency and histamine is thought to play a role.

◆ Assessment

1. Infantile (2 months to 2 years)—half of patients have spontaneous resolution by age 2 or 3
   a. Intense itching, erythema, papules, vesicles, oozing, and crusting

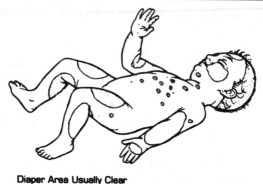

Diaper Area Usually Clear

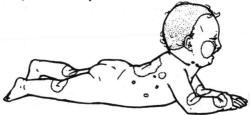

FIGURE 8 *Infantile atopic eczema occurs primarily on the face, but may develop on symmetrical areas of the body (From Sauer, GC. Manual of Skin Diseases. 6th ed. Philadelphia, JB Lippincott, 1991).*

    b. Begins on cheeks, forehead, or scalp and extends to the trunk or extremities in scattered, often symmetrical patches

    c. Perioral and perinasal areas are spared (Fig. 8).

2. Childhood (4–10 years)—may resolve completely; stop, then recur in adulthood; or progress with little relief

    a. Dry, papular, circumscribed, scaly patches

    b. Chronic rash with lichenification

    c. Involves face (not perioral or perinasal), neck, antecubital and popliteal fossae, wrists, and ankles

3. Adult (puberty to old age)

    a. Dry, thick, confluent papular lesions and lichenified plaques

    b. Weeping and crusting may occur as result of irritation or infection
4. Classified into three stages based on appearance of lesions
    a. Acute—moderate to intense erythema, vesicles, wet surface, and severe itching
    b. Subacute—faint erythema and scaling, dry surface, indistinct borders, pruritus
    c. Chronic—thickened lesions with prominent skin markings, dry surface, well-defined borders, moderate to intense itching

D

◆ Diagnostic Evaluation

1. Skin biopsy may be done if diagnosis cannot be made by clinical presentation

◆ Collaborative Management

Therapeutic Interventions

1. Open wet dressings for 1 to 3 days during acute stage to reduce inflammation
2. Prevention of drying of skin in subacute and chronic stages through decreased bathing, use of mild soap and hydrophilic lotions, use of emollients, tar preparations in baths, and increased environmental humidity
3. Avoidance of known allergens and skin irritants
4. Hypoallergenic diet trial for severe, recalcitrant atopic dermatitis

Pharmacologic Interventions

1. Topical corticosteroids applied three times a day
2. Oral antipruritics such as hydroxyzine
3. Oral antibiotics to manage secondary infection

◆ Nursing Interventions

Supportive Care

Perform or teach the family to perform the following:
1. Apply lightweight, nonfibered cloth dressings (such as sheeting) saturated in lukewarm water to lesions for 20 minutes, three to four times a day during acute stage.

2. Discourage long, hot tub baths; instead use lukewarm water and mild soap such as Neutrogenia. Rinse well and pat dry with towel.
   a. If bath water stings, add 1 cup of table salt.
   b. Prepare tar bath as directed for soaking 15 to 20 minutes daily, preferably in the evening. Tar can stain skin and clothes and cause photosensitivity of skin.
   c. If bathing must be avoided, cleanse skin with a hydrophilic lotion such as Cetaphil. Apply without water until foam occurs, then remove with soft cotton cloth.
3. Monitor for response to treatment.
   a. Overuse of topical corticosteroids may cause striae, cutaneous atrophy, telangectasia, and acne.
   b. Warn patient of sedation caused by antipruritics.
4. Apply an unscented emollient cream or ointment (not lotion) such as Eucerin or Lubriderm to the skin within 3 minutes of bathing.
5. If hypoallergenic diet is prescribed, avoid cow's milk, eggs, tomatoes, citrus fruits, chocolate, wheat products, spiced foods, fish, nuts, and peanut butter.
   a. Begin with a minimal diet as prescribed, composed of milk substitute, rice cereal, 2 fruits, 2 vegetables, beef, and a multivitamin.
   b. Add a new food every 3 to 5 days and note response.
   c. Foods causing no response are added to diet, and those causing reactions are eliminated.
6. Report any discharge, oozing, or crust formation that may indicate secondary infection and administer antibiotics as directed. Loosen crusts with water or wet dressings.

Family Education and Health Maintenance

1. Teach about possible exacerbating factors:
   a. Excessive heat or cold, windy weather, and rapidly changing temperatures
   b. Wearing wool or occlusive synthetic fabrics
   c. Strenuous athletic activity that provokes sweating
   d. Emotional stress
   e. Soaps, bubble baths, detergents, cleaning preparations and other chemicals
2. Advise using a humidifier, especially in the winter.

Diabetes Insipidus

Diabetes inspidus (DI) is failure of the body to conserve water because of lack of antidiuretic hormone (ADH, vasopressin), which is secreted by the kidneys, or because of inability of the kidneys to respond to ADH. The condition may be temporary or chronic and results from one of several causes. Deficiency of ADH (central DI), which may be congenital or acquired, is caused by CNS defects, head trauma, infection, brain tumor, or is idiopathic. Decreased renal sensitivity to ADH (nephrogenic DI) is usually attributable to chronic renal disease, or suppression of ADH secondary to excessive ingestion of fluids (primary polydipsia).

D

◆ Assessment

1. Sudden onset of excessive thirst and polyuria
2. In infants:
   a. Excessive crying—quieted with water more than milk feeding
   b. Rapid weight loss—caloric loss due to water preference over feedings
   c. Constipation
   d. Growth failure—failure to thrive
   e. Sunken fontanel with dehydration
3. In children:
   a. Excessive thirst and drinking; child may even drink from toilet bowls or pet dishes
   b. Polyuria with nocturia and enuresis
   c. Pale dry skin with reduced sweating
   d. Fever, increased pulse
   e. Listlessness or irritability
   f. Weight loss

◆ Diagnostic Evaluation

1. Urinalysis shows decreased specific gravity, decreased osmolality, and decreased sodium.
2. Elevated serum osmolality (greater than 295 mOsm)
3. Elevated serum sodium
4. Serum ADH is low in conjunction with high serum osmolality.

5. Water deprivation test (potentially dangerous) to distinguish central DI from nephrogenic DI
   a. Fluids are restricted, and the urinary volumes and concentrations are monitored hourly, along with the patient's weight.
   b. Test is terminated if patient loses more than 3% to 5% of body weight. Posttest serum sodium and osmolality are high; urine osmolality remains lower.
   c. Test is completed by giving a dose of ADH, which should stop the abnormal diuresis. If it does not, the child may have nephrogenic DI.
6. Magnetic resonance imaging or computed tomography scans may be done to examine hypothalamic-pituitary region (high incidence of associated anterior pituitary disorders).

◆ Collaborative Management

Pharmacologic Interventions

1. Daily replacement of vasopressin using desmopressin acetate (DDAVP), a synthetic analogue
2. Available as a metered nasal spray or a measured insufflation (nasal) tube. In children with cleft lip and palate, sublingual administration has been shown to be effective.
3. In nephrogenic DI, chlorpropamide or thiazide diuretics may be of value.

◆ Nursing Interventions

Monitoring

1. Monitor intake and output and urine specific gravity to adjust medication dosage if needed.
2. Monitor for signs of water intoxication while on DDAVP therapy.

❖

NURSING ALERT
Watch for and report signs of water intoxication due to excess free water and hyponatremia—drowsiness, listlessness, headache, confusion, anuria, weight gain. Hold DDAVP to prevent seizures, coma, and death.

3. Monitor infant's length, weight, and developmental milestones periodically.

Supportive Care

1. Assess for and teach parents assessment of dehydration.
2. Administer IV fluids as ordered if acutely dehydrated.
3. Maintain and teach parents to maintain liberal intake of fluids in child. Free access of water should be available. Reduced output may require restriction of fluids if overdosage of DDAVP is suspected.
4. Calculate rough estimate of total daily fluid requirements based on body size to assess fluid replacement versus excess: 100 mL/kg for first 10 kg body weight, 50 mL/kg for second 10 kg body weight, 20 mL/kg for each additional kilogram.
5. Stress to parents or caregivers the importance of providing nutritional requirements with fluids to ensure meeting caloric demands for growth.
   a. For infant feeding, ensure that adequate formula is ingested between bottles of plain water.
   b. For older child, provide liquid nutritional supplements.
   c. Consult with dietitian about need for vitamins or other supplements.
6. Administer and teach proper administration of DDAVP. Proper management should eliminate symptoms. Ensure adequate evening dose to prevent nighttime water craving and enuresis.
7. Suggest use of diapers at night and plastic padding on bed to make bedwetting easier until condition is adequately managed, or ensure easy access to toilet or commode for older child during night.

Family Education and Health Maintenance

1. Teach family about administration of medication.
   a. Demonstrate insufflation method for infants and young children; inhalation for older children and adults.
   b. Nostrils should be as clear as possible before administration of dose.
   c. Advise that medication must remain cool or refrigerated.

    d. If dose is thought to be swallowed, **do not** readminister, because of potential for overdosage. Split the dose into both nares if swallowing is occurring.

2. Advise use of medical alert bracelets.
3. Advise parents to notify school personnel about the child's condition and symptoms needing attention.
4. Advise routine follow-up; treatment may be temporary or life-long, depending on cause.

Diabetes Mellitus

Diabetes mellitus is a metabolic disorder characterized by hyperglycemia, and results from defective insulin production, secretion, or utilization. Insulin is a hormone secreted by the beta cells of the islets of Langerhans in the pancreas. It is key to glucose use in cellular metabolism and to protein and fat metabolism as well. Absolute or relative insulin deficiency or resistance causes several forms of diabetes.

In *insulin-dependent diabetes mellitus (IDDM, type I)*, the pancreas produces little or no endogenous insulin, and must be treated with injections of insulin to control the diabetes and prevent ketoacidosis. Cause may be related to autoimmunity, viral infection, and genetics.

In *non–insulin-dependent diabetes mellitus (NIDDM, type 2)*, disease results from a defect in insulin manufacture and release from the beta cells and from insulin resistance in the peripheral tissues. NIDDM has a strong genetic component and is often associated with obesity.

In *impaired glucose tolerance,* glucose levels are abnormal, but the disorder is usually asymptomatic. It may be a risk factor for hypertension, coronary artery disease, and hyperlipidemia.

In *gestational diabetes,* carbohydrate intolerance occurs during pregnancy but usually disappears after delivery. It occurs in 3% of all pregnancies, and these women are at higher risk for developing diabetes later. Risk of fetal morbidity is increased.

Complications include diabetic ketoacidosis (DKA), which occurs primarily in IDDM during times of severe insulin deficiency or illness (see p. 274); hyperglycemic hyperosmolar nonketotic syndrome (HHNKS), which affects patients with NIDDM (see p. 467); and chronic complications, occurring both in NIDDM and IDDM (Table 5).

◆ **Assessment**

1. Onset is usually abrupt with IDDM, insidious with NIDDM.
2. Symptoms of hyperglycemia include polyuria, polydipsia, polyphagia, weight loss, fatigue, blurred vision.
3. Signs of altered tissue response: poor wound healing and recurrent infections, particularly of the skin

◆ **Diagnostic Evaluation**

1. Elevated serum glucose levels
   a. Fasting blood sample (FBS)—glucose greater than 140 mg/dL on two occasions confirms DM.
   b. Random blood sample—glucose greater than 200 mg/dL in presence of classic symptoms (polyuria, polydipsia, polyphagia, and weight loss) confirms DM.
   c. Two-hour postprandial blood sample evaluates glucose metabolism, assists with control.

NURSING ALERT
Capillary blood glucose values obtained by fingerstick samples tend to be higher than in venous samples.

2. Glucose tolerance test (GTT) may be indicated.
   a. FBS is obtained before ingestion of 50 to 200 g glucose load, and blood samples are taken at $\frac{1}{2}$, 1, 2, 3, and possibly 4 and 5 hours.
   b. Diagnostic blood values are: FBS less than 140 mg/dL and the 2-hour result and one other value greater than 200 mg/dL after a 75-g glucose load.
3. Glycosylated hemoglobin measures glycemic control over 60- to 120-day period; fructosamine assay measures control over 20 days.

TABLE 5 Chronic Complications of Diabetes Mellitus

Complication	Manifestations
Macroangiopathy	
Cerebrovascular disease Increased risk of stroke and TIA	Hypertension, change in mental status, hemiparesis, aphasia, other focal neurologic symptoms
Coronary artery disease Multiple vessels may be affected in diabetics and higher incidence of silent myocardial infarction	May be asymptomatic with only ECG changes; or pain in neck, jaw, or epigastric area
Peripheral vascular disease Intermittent claudication, ischemic gangrene; accounts for 50% of nontraumatic amputations	Decreased lower-leg hair, decreased pedal pulses, poor capillary refill, pale and cool extremity
Microangiopathy	
Retinopathy: After 10 years of IDDM, 60% are affected: about 20% of NIDDM present with it at time of diagnosis, and after 15 years, 60%–85% are affected.	Floaters, flashing lights, blurred vision indicate hemorrhage or retinal detachment; may progress to blindness
Background retinopathy: Hard exudates, blot hemorrhages, and microaneurysms on retinal background; progress to proliferative retinopathy with neovascularization.	
Nephropathy: Glomerulosclerosis occurs; higher incidence in native Americans, Hispanics, and African Americans	Asymptomatic; microalbuminuria is first sign, followed by proteinuria, elevated BUN and creatinine
Peripheral Neuropathy	
Affects 60% of diabetic patients, most commonly in lower extremities; occurs as acute painful neuropathy, small-fiber, and large-fiber neuropathy	Decreased light touch, vibratory, and temperature sensation; loss of foot proprioception, followed by ataxia and gait disturbance; diminished ankle reflex; hypersensitivity and dysesthesia, followed by hypestheia and anesthesia
Autonomic Neuropathy	
Gastroparesis: Delayed gastric emptying, prolonged pylorospasms	Nausea, vomiting, early satiety, bloating, poor glucose absorption
Diarrhea: Frequent watery stools, steatorrhea, may alternate with constipation	Often occurs without warning during night or after meals, may cause incontinence
Sexual dysfunction: Changes in erection, ejaculation, libido	Men may experience absence of early morning erection; females may have vaginal dryness and dyspareunia
Orthostatic hypotension: Lack of increased heart rate and peripheral vascular resistance that should occur with posture change	Syncope, weakness, visual impairment with postural changes; decrease in systolic pressure of 30 mm Hg or diastolic pressure of 10 mm Hg with change from lying to standing

◆ Collaborative Management

Therapeutic Interventions
1. Weight reduction is a primary goal for NIDDM.
2. Dietary control with caloric restriction of carbohydrates and saturated fats to maintain ideal body weight and control blood glucose and lipid levels.
3. Regular exercise promotes utilization of carbohydrates, assists with weight control, enhances the action of insulin, and improves cardiovascular fitness.

Pharmacologic Interventions
1. Oral hypoglycemic agents for patients with NIDDM who do not achieve glucose control through diet and exercise.
   a. First- or second-generation sulfonylureas that stimulate secretion of insulin by beta cells, decrease hepatic glucose production, and increase peripheral sensitivity to insulin.
   b. Second-generation agents such as glipizide and glyburide have fewer adverse reactions and longer duration of action than first-generation agents.
   c. A distinctly different agent, metformin, may be used alone or in combination with sulfonylureas to decrease hepatic glucose production and triglyceride levels.
   d. An alpha-glucosidase inhibitor, acarbose, has recently been approved for use alone or in combination with sulfonylureas. It works locally in the small intestine to slow carbohydrate breakdown and glucose absorption.
2. Insulin therapy for patients with IDDM and those with NIDDM who do not respond to diet, exercise, and oral agents
   a. Hypoglycemia and rebound hyperglycemia (Somogyi effect) may result.
   b. Regimens are based on glycemic control, provider preference, and patient motivation. They include NPH insulin only once or twice a day; NPH and regular combination to better control postprandial glucose elevations; intensive insulin therapy with multiple injections related to meals and physical ac-

D

tivity; sliding scale therapy; continuous subcutaneous insulin infusion (insulin pump therapy); and combination oral agent and insulin therapy.

◆ Nursing Interventions

Monitoring

1. Closely monitor glucose levels by fingerstick or serum specimens to detect hyperglycemia and hypoglycemia.
2. Monitor serum cholesterol and triglycerides.
3. Monitor and report signs and symptoms of hypoglycemia.
   a. Adrenergic—sweating, tremor, pallor, tachycardia, palpitations, nervousness from the release of adrenaline when blood glucose falls rapidly
   b. Neurologic—headache, lightheadedness, confusion, irritability, slurred speech, lack of coordination, staggering gait from depression of central nervous system as glucose progressively falls
4. Monitor for microvascular, macrovascular, and neuropathic complications by performing repeated physical assessments.

Supportive Care

1. Advise patient on the importance of an individualized meal plan in meeting weekly weight loss goals, and assist with compliance.
2. Assess patient for cognitive or sensory impairments, which may interfere with ability to accurately administer insulin.
3. Demonstrate and explain thoroughly the procedure for insulin self-injection. Help patient to achieve mastery of technique by taking a step-by-step approach.

GERIATRIC ALERT
Assess elderly patients for sensory deficits such as impaired vision, hearing, and fine touch, and tremors that may impact on learning and ability to self-administer insulin. Suggest use of an insulin pen or magnifying glass to assist with drawing up insulin. Discourage the practice of prefilling syringes, because insulin my be absorbed by the plastic syringe and alter dosage.

4. Review dosage and time of injections in relation to meals, activity, and bedtime based on patient's individualized insulin regimen.
5. Instruct patient in the importance of accuracy in insulin preparation and meal timing to avoid hypoglycemia.
6. Treat hypoglycemia promptly with 10 to 15 g fast-acting carbohydrates.
   a. Give orally one-half cup (4 oz) juice, three glucose tablets, four sugar cubes, or five to six pieces of hard candy.
   b. Provide glucagon 1 mg SC or IM if the patient cannot ingest a sugar treatment. A family member or care provider must administer injection.
   c. Give IV bolus of 50 mL 50% dextrose solution if the patient fails to respond to glucagon within 15 minutes.
7. Encourage the patient to carry a portable treatment for hypoglycemia at all times.

COMMUNITY CARE CONSIDERATIONS

A small tube of Cake Mate glossy decorating gel can be easily carried in a pocket or purse, contains about 15 g of glucose, and can be easily squirted in the mouth for fast absorption during a hypoglycemic attack.

8. Explain the importance of exercise in maintaining or reducing body weight.
9. Advise patient to assess blood glucose level before strenuous exercise and to eat a carbohydrate snack before exercising to avoid hypoglycemia.
10. Advise patient that prolonged strenuous exercise may require increased food at bedtime to avoid nocturnal hypoglycemia.
11. Instruct patient to avoid strenuous exercise whenever blood glucose levels exceed 250 mg/d and urine ketones are present, to prevent lactic acidosis.
12. Advise the patient to inject insulin into the abdominal site on days when arms or legs are exercised.
13. Assess feet and legs for skin temperature, sensation, soft tissue injuries, corns, calluses, dryness, hammer

toe or bunion deformation, hair distribution, pulses, deep tendon reflexes.

14. Maintain skin integrity by protecting feet from breakdown.
    a. Use of heel protectors, special mattresses, foot cradles for patients on bed rest
    b. Avoidance of drying agents to skin (eg, alcohol)
    c. Application of skin moisturizers to maintain suppleness and prevent cracking, fissures
15. Advise the patient who smokes to stop smoking or reduce if possible, to reduce vasoconstriction and enhance peripheral blood flow.

Patient Education and Health Maintenance

1. For newly diagnosed patients or those undergoing stressful circumstances that preclude more in-depth education, focus on skills management related to insulin/oral agents, hypoglycemia treatment, blood glucose monitoring, and basic dietary information.
2. For ongoing education, include advanced skills and rationales for treatment and management. Focus on lifestyle management issues such as sick day management, exercise adjustments, travel preparations, foot care guidelines, intensive insulin management, and dietary considerations for dining out.
3. For additional information and support, refer to agencies such as:

American Diabetes Association, Inc.
1660 Duke St.
Alexandria, VA 22314
703-549-1500

American Dietetic Association
216 West Jackson Blvd.
Chicago, IL 60606-6995
800-366-1655

Diabetes Mellitus, Juvenile

Diabetes mellitus is a disorder of glucose intolerance caused by a deficiency in insulin production and action resulting in hyperglycemia and abnormal carbohydrate, protein, and fat metabolism. More than 98% of juvenile cases are type I or insulin-dependent diabetes mellitus (IDDM). In this disorder, the pancreas produces little or no endogenous insulin, which must be treated with insulin injections to control the diabetes and prevent ketoacidosis. IDDM may be caused by autoimmunity, viral and genetic components. The disease affects 15 of every 100,000 persons younger than age 20.

Diabetic ketoacidosis (DKA), also known as diabetic coma, is the most important acute complication (see p. 274). Diabetic ketoacidosis occurs primarily in IDDM during times of severe insulin deficiency or illness, producing severe hyperglycemia, ketonuria, dehydration, and acidosis. It accounts for 70% of diabetes-related deaths in children younger than 10 years of age. However, if treated promptly, DKA is reversible. Chronic complications of diabetes include skeletal and joint abnormalities; growth failure and delayed sexual maturation caused by under-insulinization; and, rarely, retinopathy, neuropathy, nephropathy, and cardiac disease.

D

◆ Assessment

1. Onset in children usually more rapid than in adults (usually over a few weeks)
2. Major symptoms include increased thirst and appetite, frequent urination, enuresis, weight loss, and fatigue.
3. Minor symptoms include dry skin, skin infections, poor wound healing, and (in adolescent girls) monilial vaginitis.
4. Manifestations of DKA
   a. Drowsiness, dry skin, cherry-red lips, hyperpnea, acetone odor to the breath, abdominal pain (may mimic appendicitis), nausea, vomiting
   b. Child in coma manifests severe hyperpnea (Kussmaul's respirations), sunken eyeballs, abdominal rigidity, rapid, weak pulse, reduced temperature and blood pressure.
   c. Circulatory collapse and renal failure may follow, resulting from combination of lowered pH, electrolyte deficiency, and dehydration.

◆ Diagnostic Evaluation

1. Random blood glucose higher than 200 mg/dL.
2. Glycosuria on routine examination
3. Ketonuria
4. Metabolic acidosis (pH less than 7.3 and bicarbonate less than 14 mEq/L)

◆ Collaborative Management

Therapeutic Interventions

1. Diet therapy
   a. The diet plan eliminates concentrated sweets and follows recommended allowances from the four basic food groups, but otherwise does not usually require measuring or rigidity.
   b. The diet should be composed of approximately 55% carbohydrate (mostly complex carbohydrates), 30% fat, and 15% protein. It may be based on the exchange method recommended by the American Diabetes Association.
   c. Foods are distributed throughout the day to accommodate varying peak action of insulins. Distribution may be adjusted to amount of exercise.

Pharmacologic Interventions

1. Insulin therapy used to reduce hyperglycemia, inhibit lipolysis and ketogenesis
   a. Subcutaneous insulin may be given twice a day at a dose usually of a 2:1 ratio of NPH to regular, and a 2:1 ratio for morning to evening dose.
   b. Dosage needs are based on the child's size, diet, and level of activity. Dosages are adjusted through daily monitoring of blood glucose levels.
   c. More rigorous regimens include continuous insulin infusion therapy through an implanted pump and four-times-a-day blood glucose monitoring with regular insulin coverage.

◆ Nursing Interventions

Monitoring

1. Monitor intake and output, blood pressure, serum electrolyte results, and daily weights.

2. Monitor for potential cerebral edema (diminished level of consciousness) when fluid replacement is initiated.
3. Monitor for tachycardia with dehydration and arrhythmias related to potassium imbalances.
4. Monitor urine for ketones if the child is ill or if glucose is greater than 240 mg/100 mL.
5. Observe for hypoglycemia caused by overtreatment of insulin.
6. Review blood glucose diaries for level of control and need for insulin adjustments (check for appropriate adjustments of insulin made by parents).
7. Monitor insulin injection sites.
   a. Watch for signs of lipohypertrophy (localized tissue buildup from giving injections in the same site).
   b. Observe for signs of irritation; avoid injection site for several weeks if these occur.
   c. Observe skin for signs of hypersensitivity reaction to insulin and notify doctor immediately.

Supportive Care

1. Administer IV fluids as ordered during periods of dehydration.
2. Provide an adequate diet for the child and teach the family about the diet.
3. Develop a systematic plan for giving insulin injections that emphasizes rotation of sites. Give serial injections subcutaneously, about 2.5 cm (1 in) apart (Fig. 9).
   a. Arms: begin below the deltoid muscle and end one hand breadth above the elbow. Begin at the midline and progress outward laterally, using the external surface only.
   b. Thighs: begin one handbreadth below the hip and end one handbreadth above the knee. Begin at the midline and progress outward laterally, using only the outer, anterior surface.
   c. Abdomen: avoid the beltline and 1 inch around the umbilicus.
   d. Buttocks: use the upper outer quadrant of the buttocks.
4. Help child control fear of injections through interactive play and participation in the procedure.

D

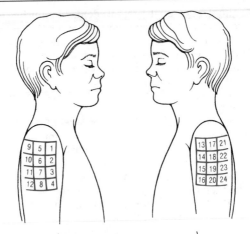

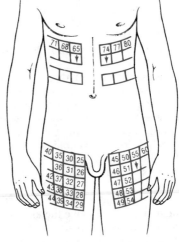

FIGURE 9 Rotating injection sites for insulin in the pediatric patient.

5. Be aware of factors that influence insulin therapy, especially exercise and infection:
   a. Exercise tends to lower blood sugar level; encourage normal activity, regulated in amount and time.
   b. Infection or illness increases insulin requirement (insulin still administered during illness). Be alert for signs of infection and dehydration.
6. Teach child and parents the chosen method for blood glucose monitoring:
   a. Blood glucose measurements are usually made four times a day, before meals and at bedtime. May be more frequent during hypoglycemic episodes or other problem situations.
   b. Help child to understand how disease is controlled by teaching the child to test own blood, record results, and report information to health care provider and parents.
7. Have glucagon available if hypoglycemic reaction occurs. Administer 0.5 to 1 mg intramuscularly or subcutaneously and assess response.
8. Explain to child that he or she did not cause the disease to occur; young children often blame themselves for "bad" things that happen to them. Help the child understand that good management is the key to participating in all usual activities. The perspective should be that he or she is a "child with diabetes," not a "diabetic child."

Family Education and Health Maintenance

1. Teach parents about influence of exercise, emotional stress, and other illnesses on both insulin and diet needs.
2. Teach parents to recognize the symptoms of insulin shock and DKA and review related emergency management.
3. Teach family the causes, signs and symptoms, and treatment for hypoglycemia.
   a. Watch for a pattern of activity or time of day that precedes hypoglycemic reactions, and work with the family to alter behavior to prevent reactions.
   b. If prescribed, teach the child and family how to use an emergency glucagon injection kit.

D

COMMUNITY CARE CONSIDERATIONS

Suggest a simple, convenient source of sugar that can be easily carried by the child or parents in a pocket, purse, or backpack to have available for hypoglycemic symptoms. A good example is cake decorating gel that comes in a tube, such as Cake Mate.

4. Instruct parents regarding prevention of infection.
   a. Attend to regular body hygiene with special attention to foot care.
   b. Report any breaks in the skin; treat promptly.
   c. Use only properly fitted shoes; do not wear vinyl or plastic, which lack ventilation. Take measures to prevent calluses and blisters.
   d. Dress the child appropriately for the weather.
   e. Ensure that the child receives regular dental checkups and maintenance every 6 months.
   f. Follow routine immunizations according to the recommended schedule.
5. Have the child carry a medical alert card or bracelet.
6. Have the family discuss the child's disease with the school nurse and with other responsible adults who are in close contact with the child.
7. Advise parents that vials of insulin should be kept on one's person when traveling because baggage may be subjected to extreme temperatures and pressures incompatible with the stability of insulin. If necessary, a thermos can be used to keep the insulin at appropriate temperature.
8. For additional information and support, refer to agencies such as:

   Juvenile Diabetes Foundation
   120 Wall St.
   New York, NY 10005
   800-JDF-CURE

Diabetic Ketoacidosis

Diabetic ketoacidosis (DKA) is an acute complication of diabetes mellitus (usually type I) characterized by hyperglycemia, ketonuria, acidosis, and dehydration. It is caused by inadequate levels of endogenous and/or exogenous insulin to control hypoglycemia. DKA frequently occurs from failure to increase the insulin dose during periods of stress (eg, infection, surgery, pregnancy). It may also occur in previously undiagnosed or untreated diabetics.

◆ Assessment

1. Early manifestations include polydipsia, polyuria, fatigue, malaise, drowsiness, anorexia, nausea, vomiting, abdominal pain, and muscle cramps.
2. Later signs include Kussmaul (deep) respirations, acetone breath (fruity, sweet odor), hypotension, weak pulse, stupor, and coma.

◆ Diagnostic Evaluation

1. Serum glucose: usually elevated over 300, may be as high as 1,000 mg/dL.
2. Serum and urine ketone bodies present
3. Serum bicarbonate and pH decreased because of metabolic acidosis, and arterial partial pressure of carbon dioxide (pCO_2) decreased as a respiratory compensation mechanism
4. Serum sodium and potassium may be low, normal, or high because of fluid shifts and dehydration, despite total body depletion.
5. Serum BUN, creatinine, hemoglobin, and hematocrit elevated because of dehydration.

NURSING ALERT
Severity of DKA cannot be determined by serum glucose levels; acidosis may be prominent with glucose of 200 or less.

6. Urine glucose present in high concentration and specific gravity increased, reflecting osmotic diuresis

◆ Collaborative Management

Therapeutic and Pharmacologic Interventions

1. IV fluids to replace losses from osmotic diuresis and vomiting.

NURSING ALERT
Too-rapid infusion of IV fluids in cases of severe dehydration can cause cerebral edema and death.

2. Short-acting IV insulin drip to increase glucose utilization and decrease lipolysis
   a. Premature discontinuation of IV insulin can result in prolongation of DKA.
   b. Failure to institute subcutaneous insulin injections before discontinuation of IV insulin can result in extended hyperglycemia.
3. Replace electrolytes:
   a. Sodium chloride and phosphate as required
   b. Potassium chloride IV up to 10 mEq/hour
   c. Magnesium sulfate up to 2 mEq/kg every 4 hours

NURSING ALERT
Electrolyte levels may not reflect the total body deficit of potassium and sodium (to a lesser extent) caused by compartment shifts and fluid volume loss. Replacement is necessary despite normal to high serum values.

◆ Nursing Interventions

Monitoring

1. Monitor for symptoms of hypokalemia: fatigue, anorexia, nausea, vomiting, muscle weakness, decreased bowel sounds, parasthesias, dysrhythmias, flat T waves, ST segment depression.
2. Monitor intake and output every hour for fluid balance.
3. Monitor urine specific gravity to assess fluid changes.
4. Monitor capillary blood glucose frequently.
5. Monitor serum glucose, bicarbonate, and pH levels periodically.
6. Monitor blood pressure and heart rate frequently, depending on patient's condition; check skin turgor and temperature.

Supportive Care

1. Reassure the patient about improvement of condition and that correction of fluid imbalance will help reduce discomfort.
2. Replace fluids and electrolytes as ordered through peripheral IV line.

NURSING ALERT

Any interruption in insulin administration may result in reaccumulation of ketone bodies and worsening acidosis. Glucose will normalize before acidosis resolves so IV insulin is continued until bicarbonate levels normalize and subcutaneous insulin takes effect and the patient starts eating.

---

3. Administer regular insulin drip through peripheral or central IV. Flush the entire IV infusion set with solution containing insulin and discard the first 50 mL, because plastic bags and tubing may absorb some insulin—thereby reducing insulin concentration of initial solution.

Patient Education and Health Maintenance

1. To prevent further episodes of DKA, teach patient to identify and report early signs and symptoms of DKA.
2. Help patient to identify and avoid precipitating events to DKA.
3. Instruct the patient in sick day guidelines.
   a. Never omit dose of insulin when sick.
   b. When blood glucose is greater than 240 mg/dL, test urine for ketones.
   c. Drink 6 to 8 ounces of fluid every hour.
   d. If unable to eat, drink fluids with carbohydrates.

Diarrhea in Children

Diarrhea refers to excessive loss of water and electrolytes that occurs with passage of unformed stools. It is a symptom of many conditions and may be caused by many diseases. Organisms causing diarrhea in infants and young children include: bacteria (*Escherichia coli; Salmonella, Shigella, Yersinia enterocolitica,* and *Campylobacter fetus*); viruses (echo viruses, adenoviruses, human reovirus-like agent, and rotaviruses); fungi (*Candida*); and parasites (*Giardia*). Diarrhea may also result from other disorders such as celiac disease; food allergies; mechanical obstruction; and congenital anomalies.

Acute diarrhea is characterized by a sudden change in frequency and quality of stools. It is usually self-limiting, but can result in dehydration. Chronic diarrhea lasts more than 2 weeks. Uncontrolled diarrhea may lead to severe dehydration, acid–base derangements with acidosis, and shock.

D

COMMUNITY CARE CONSIDERATION
Infants and young children in day care centers may be at increased risk for diarrhea due to *Shigella, Salmonella,* rotavirus, endopathogenic *E. coli,* and giardiasis. This is known as "day care diarrhea," and handwashing is the major preventative measure.

◆ Assessment

1. Loose and fluid consistency stools that are greenish or yellow-green color and may contain mucus, pus, or blood. Frequency varies from 2 to 20 per day. Stools are expelled with force and may be preceded by pain.

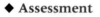

PEDIATRIC ALERT:
   Severe diarrhea with sudden onset in the infant carries a high risk of mortality.

2. General appearance indicates dehydration in severe cases.
   a. Little to extreme loss of subcutaneous fat
   b. Up to 50% total body weight loss
   c. Poor skin turgor and dry skin
   d. Pallor

e. Sunken fontanelles and eyes
3. Fever (low-grade to 41.1°C [106°F]), anorexia, and vomiting may occur.
4. Behavioral changes
   a. Crying or legs drawn up to abdomen usually indicates pain.
   b. Irritability and restlessness
   c. Weakness
   d. Extreme prostration
   e. Stupor and convulsions
   f. Flaccidity

◆ **Diagnostic Evaluation**

1. Serum electrolytes, blood urea nitrogen, and creatinine are performed to evaluate fluid and electrolyte balance and kidney function.
2. Serum CO_2, arterial pH, and arterial CO_2 may be abnormal because of acid–base imbalance.
3. Complete blood count can determine plasma volume by hematocrit; white blood cell count WBC and differential can detect infection.
4. Sedimentation rate is elevated in infection and inflammation.
5. Blood cultures can rule out septicemia.
6. Serologic studies can detect viruses.
7. Stool and rectal swab cultures, stool for ova and parasites can detect specific pathogens.
8. Stool pH, reducing substances—decreased pH may indicate various noninfectious causes; acid stool containing sugar is characteristic of disaccharide intolerance.
9. Breath hydrogen test can determine carbohydrate malabsorption and bacterial overgrowth.

NURSING ALERT
Follow universal precautions when handling specimens, and transport to laboratories in appropriate containers per hospital policy.

◆ Collaborative Management

Therapeutic Interventions

1. Prevent spread of disease: suspect disease to be communicable until proven otherwise. Use enteric isolation precautions.
2. Maintain hydration and electrolyte balance through oral or IV fluids. Oral electrolyte rehydrating solution may be used for mild to moderate diarrhea.

Pharmacologic Interventions

1. Specific antimicrobial therapy against causative organism.
2. Antidiarrheal medications are seldom used.

◆ Nursing Interventions

Monitoring

1. Monitor volume and rate of IV fluid therapy.
   a. Check flow rate and amount absorbed hourly and totally.
   b. Follow prescribed volume carefully when oral feedings are given in conjunction with IV fluid.
   c. Observe for signs of fluid overload: edema, increased blood pressure, bounding pulse, labored respirations, and crackles in lung fields.
2. Check IV site for infiltration or improper flow so site can be changed as necessary.
3. Weigh the infant or child daily to guide fluid needs and patient status.
4. Monitor urine output and keep accurate intake and output record, including vomitus and liquid stools.

Supportive Care

1. Provide frequent mouth care and nonnutritive sucking with a pacifier if food and fluids are being restricted. Continue to bubble infant to expel air swallowed while crying or sucking.
2. Give oral rehydrating solution based on number of stools.
   a. Resume previous diet once fluid and electrolytes are replaced. If diarrhea was severe, advance slowly from clear liquids to half-strength formula to regular diet. Older child may advance more rapidly.

b. If infant or young child is well hydrated, regular formula may not be omitted.

c. As diet is advanced, note any vomiting or increase in stools and report it immediately. Oral feedings should not be resumed too early or advanced too rapidly, because diarrhea may recur.

d. Advise family to avoid milk products and lactose-containing formulas for at least a week for children with severe diarrhea.

e. Breast-feeding may be resumed once electrolytes are replaced.

D

NURSING ALERT
Diluted fruit juices and soft drinks are not recommended because their high carbohydrate content aggravates diarrhea by osmotic effect.

3. To prevent spread of infection, ensure adherence to good handwashing and gown technique protocols for all persons having contact with enteric secretions.

4. Dispose of diapers carefully, following institution policy.

5. Implement measures to prevent skin irritation or breakdown.

a. Avoid commercial baby wipes, which contain alcohol and may sting inflamed or excoriated diaper area. Use mild soap and water or place infant in tub of water for cleaning.

b. Prevent scratching or rubbing of irritated area.

c. Use protective barrier creams, such as zinc oxide or karaya powder; completely remove after each bowel movement for thorough cleansing.

d. Leave diaper area open to air until thoroughly dried.

6. Explain to family that intermittent abdominal cramps may be painful, and provide support.

7. Provide some means of pleasant stimulation, entertainment, or diversion, especially while child remains in bed.

Family Education and Health Maintenance

1. Teach good hygiene measures to older child and parents.

COMMUNITY CARE CONSIDERATION

Assess home sanitation and hygiene practices for overcrowding; number of working toilets per number of people; availability of working sinks with soap and towels in the bathrooms and their proximity to food preparation areas; disposal of diapers; and handwashing practices of caregivers and children.

2. After the cause of the diarrhea is determined, it may be necessary to teach proper hygiene, formula or food preparation, handling, and storage.
   a. Use handwashing before bottle and food preparation.
   b. Use disposable bottles, or sterilize or use dishwasher for reusable bottles.
   c. Refrigerate reconstituted formula and all other fluids between uses. Milk may become contaminated within 1 hour if left out at room temperature; juice becomes contaminated within several hours.
   d. Discard small amounts of food or fluid from containers already used.
3. Explain the fecal–oral mode of transmission of infectious diarrheal illnesses.
4. Explain the early symptoms of a diarrheal illness and of dehydration, which requires notification of the health care provider.

Disseminated Intravascular Coagulation

Disseminated intravascular coagulation (DIC) is an acquired thrombotic and hemorrhagic syndrome involving abnormal activation of the clotting cascade together with accelerated fibrinolysis. This causes widespread clotting in small blood vessels with consumption of clotting factors and platelets, so that bleeding and thrombosis occur simultaneously.

For unknown reasons, DIC occurs as a complication of a wide variety of underlying disorders or events, such as overwhelming infections (bacterial sepsis), massive tissue injury (burns, trauma, fractures, major surgery, fat embolism); obstetrical complications (abruptio placentae, eclampsia, amniotic fluid embolism, retention of dead fetus); vascular and circulatory collapse; shock; hemolytic transfusion reaction; and malignancies, particularly of the lung, colon, stomach, and pancreas.

Clotting may lead to pulmonary embolism, cerebral myocardial, splenic or bowel infarction, acute renal failure, tissue necrosis or gangrene; hemorrhage may lead to cerebral hemorrhage, which is the most common cause of death in DIC.

D

◆ Assessment

1. Abnormal clotting: coolness and mottling of extremities; acrocyanosis (cold, mottled extremities with clear demarcation from normal tissue); dyspnea, adventitious breath sounds; altered mental status; decreased urine output; pain of extremities, abdomen, chest, etc., related to infarction
2. Abnormal bleeding: oozing, bleeding from sites of procedures, IV catheter insertion sites, suture lines, mucous membranes, orifices; hematuria; internal bleeding leading to changes in vital organ function, altered vital signs.

◆ Diagnostic Evaluation

1. Platelet count—diminished
2. Prothrombin time and partial thromboplastin time—prolonged
3. Fibrinogen level—decreased
4. Fibrin split products—increased
5. Arterial blood gases, BUN, creatinine and other laboratory tests to monitor functioning of vital organs

◆ Collaborative Management

Therapeutic Interventions

1. Treat underlying disorder.
2. Supportive measures, including fluid replacement, ox-

ygenation, maintenance of blood pressure and renal perfusion

Pharmacologic Interventions

1. Replacement therapy for serious hemorrhaging:
   a. Fresh frozen plasma, to replace clotting factors
   b. Platelet transfusions
   c. Cryoprecipitate—replaces clotting factors
2. Heparin therapy (controversial) to inhibit clotting component of DIC

D

◆ Nursing Interventions

Monitoring

1. When administering blood products, monitor for signs and symptoms of allergic reactions, anaphylaxis, and volume overload.
2. Monitor cardiac rhythm, level of consciousness, respiratory status, and urine output for dysfunction of vital organs caused by ischemia.
3. Evaluate fluid status and bleeding by frequently measuring vital signs, central venous pressure, intake and output.

NURSING ALERT
Be aware that all seriously ill patients are at risk for DIC; monitor closely.

Supportive Care

1. Institute bleeding precautions—avoid use of plain razor, hard toothbrush or floss, IM injections, tourniquets, rectal procedures or suppositories; administer stool softeners as necessary to prevent constipation.
2. Monitor pad count and amount of saturation during menses; administer hormones to suppress menstruation, as ordered.
3. Avoid dislodging clots. Apply pressure to sites of bleeding for at least 20 minutes; use topical hemostatic agents. Use tape cautiously.
4. Maintain bed rest.

5. If internal bleeding is suspected, assess bowel sounds and abdominal girth.
6. To promote tissue perfusion, keep patient warm, avoid systemic or topical vasoconstrictive agents, and change patient's position frequently. Perform range-of-motion exercises.

Patient Education and Health Maintenance

1. Reassure the patient and family by explaining the syndrome and its management. Answer all questions.

Dissociative Disorders

See Anxiety, Somatoform, and Dissociative Disorders

Diverticular Disease

Diverticular disease has three clinical forms: prediverticular disease, diverticulosis, and diverticulitis. In prediverticular disease, the colonic musculature is weakened and degenerated, and the bowel lumen is narrowed. In diverticulosis, there are multiple diverticula, or saccular dilatations at weak points of the colonic wall where nutrient blood vessels penetrate (Fig. 10). In diverticulitis, one or more of the pouches become inflamed and may perforate the thin diverticular wall, because of a fecalith plug and accumulating bacteria. If the diverticulum perforates, local abscess or peritonitis may occur. Uninflamed or minimally inflamed diverticula may erode adjacent arterial branches, causing acute massive rectal bleeding.

The cause of diverticular disease is unclear, but a low-residue diet is a contributing factor. Diverticulosis occurs more often in persons older than 60 years. Complications include hemorrhage, bowel obstruction, fistula formation, and septicemia.

◆ **Assessment**

1. Prediverticular disease—intermittent or chronic abdominal pain, worsening after eating or before bowel

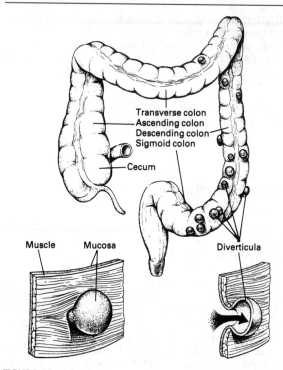

FIGURE 10 Diverticula are most common in the sigmoid colon; they diminish in number and size as the colon approaches the cecum. Diverticula are rarely found in the rectum.

movements; constipation or diarrhea; may be asymptomatic

2. Diverticulosis—crampy abdominal pain; bowel irregularity; periodic abdominal distention; possible sudden massive hemorrhage; or may be asymptomatic

3. Mild diverticulitis—bouts of soreness, mild lower abdominal cramps; bowel irregularity; mild nausea, gas, low-grade fever

4. Severe diverticulitis—crampy left lower quadrant pain; low-grade fever and chills; signs of peritonitis or massive hemorrhage if rupture; stool in the urine or vagina if fistula

5. Peritonitis and sepsis:
    a. Increasing abdominal pain, rigidity
    b. Guarding, rebound tenderness
    c. Abdominal distention, nausea and vomiting
    d. Fever, hypotension

◆ Diagnostic Evaluation

1. WBC and differential may show leukocytosis with shift to the left; hemoglobin and hematocrit may be low with chronic or acute bleeding.
2. X-rays of abdomen, ultrasonography, and CT scan may show free air under diaphragm with perforation into the abdominal cavity.
3. Sigmoidoscopy, and possible colonoscopy, to rule out carcinoma
4. After infection subsides, barium enema to visualize diverticular sacs, narrowing of colonic lumen, partial or complete obstruction, or fistulae

NURSING ALERT
In patients with acute diverticulitis, a barium enema may rupture the bowel.

◆ Collaborative Management

Therapeutic Interventions

1. In prediverticular disease, a high-fiber diet with additional bran or psyllium products to counteract tendency toward constipation
2. In diverticulosis:
    a. High-fiber diet with possible avoidance of large seeds or nuts, which may clog diverticular sac
    b. Bran supplements, psyllium preparations, or stool softeners to avoid constipation
    c. For abdominal pain, switch to a liquid or low-residue diet and stool softeners to relieve symptoms, minimize irritation, and slow progression to diverticulitis.
3. In diverticulitis, bed rest, liquid or low-residue diet, and stool softeners are indicated. IV therapy, nasogas-

tric intubation, and NPO status are indicated if peritonitis or massive bleeding occur.

Pharmacologic Interventions

1. Broad-spectrum antibiotic to control infection with diverticulitis
2. Analgesics and anticholinergics to control pain and spasms in diverticulitis
3. Vasopressin and blood replacement for massive bleeding

Surgical Interventions

1. Bowel resection and possible temporary colostomy if there is little response to medical treatment, or if severe complications develop

◆ Nursing Interventions

Monitoring

1. Monitor for shock and dehydration caused by hemorrhage
2. Monitor dietary intake and weight to determine nutritional status.

Supportive Care

1. Evaluate pain control regimen for effectiveness.
2. Auscultate bowel sounds to monitor bowel motility.
3. Encourage patient to follow prescribed diet that is high in soft residue and low in sugar to provide bulk and more consistency to the stool. Refer to nutritionist as indicated.
4. Encourage fluids to promote bowel stimulation if patient is constipated.
5. Advise patient to establish regular bowel habits to promote regular and complete evacuation.
6. Observe color, consistency, and frequency of stools and record.

Patient Education and Health Maintenance

1. Explain the disease process to the patient and its relationship to diet.
2. Inform patient that bran products will add bulk to the stool and can be taken with milk or sprinkled over cereal.

3. Have the patient continue periodic medical supervision and follow-up; report problems and untoward symptoms.

Down Syndrome

Down syndrome (trisomy 21) is a genetic disorder that usually results from formation of three copies of chromosome 21 instead of the normal two, because of impaired chromosome separation during meiosis. If the fertilized embryo survives, it has 47 chromosomes instead of 46. Two other causes of Down syndrome, translocation of chromosome 21 and mosaicism involving two cell lines that develop after conception, are rare.

This disorder is the most common identifiable cause of mental retardation and is often associated with heart defects and other congenital anomalies. Down syndrome occurs in 1 of every 700 births. Incidence increases with parental age; risk at maternal age 25 is 1 in 1,350; at age 35, 1 in 384; and at age 45, 1 in 28.

The most common life experience of a child with Down syndrome is to live with the family, participate in infant stimulation and preschool programs, and attend school while receiving some support for special education. Adults with Down syndrome can function in supported employment programs, and live in small groups. Their life expectancy depends on the presence of medical complications; where there are no complications, it is slightly shorter than average.

◆ Assessment

1. Physical signs of Down syndrome are usually apparent at birth, and include:
   a. Brachycephaly (flattened head)
   b. Upward slanting eyes with prominent epicanthal folds
   c. Brushfield spots (small white spots on iris of each eye)
   d. Flat nasal bridge
   e. Small mouth with protruding tongue
   f. Small, low-set ears

    g. Clinodactyly (small little finger that curves inward)
    h. Simian crease (single transverse palmar crease)
    i. Hypotonia
    j. Dry, scaly skin
2. Other clinical manifestations include:
    a. Heart defects (eg, atrial or ventricular septal defects, tetralogy of Fallot)—40% of patients
    b. Gastrointestinal malformations (eg, pyloric stenosis, duodenal atresia, tracheoesophageal fistula)—12% of patients
    c. Hypothyroidism—10% to 20% of patients
    d. Visual defects—refractive errors (70%), strabismus (50%), nystagmus (35%), cataracts (3%)
    e. Hearing defects (60%–90% of patients)—mild to moderate conductive hearing loss, chronic middle ear infections, enlarged adenoids, sleep apnea
    f. Hypotonia of infants
    g. Atlanto-occipital and atlanto-axial subluxation (dislocation of upper spine caused by joint laxity)—15% of patients
    h. Gait abnormalities—15% of patients
    i. Short stature—100% of patients
    j. Obesity—50% of patients
    k. Malocclusions—60% to 100% of patients
    l. Mental retardation (mild to moderate)—100% of patients

◆ Diagnostic Evaluation

1. Amniocentesis may be done for prenatal diagnosis; recommended for pregnant women past age 34 even with negative family history.
2. Chromosome analysis may be done to rule out other chromosomal aberrations.
3. Echocardiogram to check for heart defects—usually done during newborn period on all infants with Down syndrome
4. Radiographic studies to demonstrate congenital GI abnormalities
5. An interdisciplinary and multispecialty team is essential to evaluate physiologic and psychosocial functioning.
6. Vision screening to demonstrate deficits
7. Auditory brain stem response assesses hearing in in-

fants; sound field testing is done for children older than 1 year.

8. Spinal x-rays at age 2 and then every 5 years during childhood, to document alignment of skull and vertebrae for possible correction to avoid compression and neurologic damage.

9. Hip x-rays can document dislocation or subluxation in gait abnormalities.

10. TSH, T_4 assays in newborn screening to detect hypothyroidism; done biannually thereafter

◆ Collaborative Management

D

Therapeutic Interventions

1. Hypotonia in infants requires physical therapy. Adaptive equipment gives extra support to head and neck when handling newborn.

2. Physical therapy to correct gait abnormalities

3. Special education and training for mental retardation

Pharmacologic Interventions

1. Thyroid hormone replacement in hypothyroidism

2. Possible use of human growth hormone to correct short stature (controversial)

Surgical Interventions

1. Correction of congenital heart defects, gastrointestinal malformations

2. Myringotomy tubes, adenoidectomy for severe hearing defects

3. Correction of severe upper spine dislocation through fusion of cervical vertebrae and occiput

4. Orthopedic procedures sometimes required to correct gait abnormalities

◆ Nursing Interventions

Monitoring

1. Monitor hypotonic infant for feeding and head control; should be placed on abdomen periodically while being observed for potential for suffocation.

2. Assess for potential cardiac defects:
   a. Color, pulse, and respiratory rate changes at rest and with stress
   b. Early tiring or frequent interruptions in feeding

3. Observe for coughing or vomiting, with or after feeding, indicating gastrointestinal defects.
   a. Bile-stained vomitus suggests lower tract problem, partially digested contents suggest upper tract problem.
   b. Observe bowel movements and for abdominal distention.
4. Monitor growth on Down syndrome growth chart.
5. Monitor for failure to thrive:
   a. Check feedings for length of feeding, feeding schedule, loss of feeding by vomiting or poor seal on nipple.
   b. Monitor type of formula and caloric content.

Supportive Care

1. Allow the parents access to the baby at all possible times to promote bonding when parents appear ready.
2. Focus on the positive aspects of the baby and serve as a role model for handling and stimulating.
3. Be aware of the grieving process (loss of the "normal child") that families experience when a diagnosis is made, and be aware that spouses can be at different stages.
4. Accept all questions and reactions nonjudgmentally, and offer verbal and written explanations.
5. Provide the family a quiet place to discuss their questions with each other and someone knowledgeable about the condition (primary care provider, clinical nurse specialist) to support them in grieving, understanding of the condition, and their ability to cope.
6. Offer the family the option to take advantage of counseling, eg, with a social worker or psychologist.

PEDIATRIC ALERT
Children with developmental disabilities and chronic illness are at greater risk of experiencing divorce, child abuse, and neglect than the general population.

---

7. For those parents concerned with their ability to care for a child, explore with them their options of adoption or institutionalization in a nonjudgmental manner.

8. Demonstrate proper feeding positioning with head elevated and encourage the parents to always hold the infant during feedings with head elevated and supported in arms.
   a. Investigate alternative positions and nipples for feeding caused by weak sucking reflex and large, protruding tongue.
   b. The head must be elevated for at least 1 hour after meals.
   c. Allow adequate time for feeding and increase frequency of feedings if infants tires easily.
   d. Offer support and guidance for breast-feeding.

9. When handling the infant, provide adequate support with a firm grasp because infant may be very floppy because of poor muscle tone.

10. Position the infant so that if vomiting should occur aspiration will be prevented.
    a. Prop infant with a diaper roll so that position will be maintained.
    b. Change position frequently because this infant is not usually very active.

11. Continuously check environment for safety needs for this child.

COMMUNITY CARE CONSIDERATIONS
Teach caregivers to base safety needs on the developmental rather than chronologic age of the child.

12. Demonstrate and encourage play with the child at the appropriate level to provide stimulation, and work toward achieving developmental milestones.

13. Use appropriate behavior modification techniques such as extinction, time-out, and reward to achieve cooperation and success.

Family Education and Health Maintenance

1. Remind the parents to recognize the child's routine health care needs and maintain regular follow-up with a primary care provider:
   a. Immunizations
   b. Regular dental checkups beginning at age 2
   c. Visual and hearing examinations—should be seen by an ophthalmologist at 1 year of age

2. Teach parents to provide a therapeutic home environment:
   a. Maintain regular sleeping, eating, working, and playing routines.
   b. Divide tasks and expectations into small, manageable parts. Give only one or two instructions at a time.
   c. Set firm but reasonable limits on behavior and carry through with consistent discipline.
   d. Provide energy outlet through physical activity, vocal outlet, and outdoor play.

3. Advise parents to teach habits to older children that are essential to later vocational life, such as getting to places on time, cooperating, focusing on the task at hand, and establishing acceptable interpersonal relationships.

4. Tell family about genetic counseling, which supplies information on risk in subsequent pregnancies (parents), or risk to offspring (patient).

5. Refer to local parent support group or

> **National Down Syndrome Society**
> 666 Broadway, Suite 810
> New York, NY 10012
> 800-221-4602; 212-460-9330

Dysrhythmias

Cardiac dysrhythmias are disturbances in regular heart rate or rhythm caused by change in electrical conduction or automaticity. Dysrhythmias may arise from the SA node (sinus bradycardia or tachycardia) or anywhere within the atria or ventricles (known as ectopic beats). Some may be benign and asymptomatic, whereas others are life-threatening.

◆ Assessment

1. Detect dysrhythmias by a change in pulse or heart rate or rhythm by auscultation.
2. Obtain a 12-lead ECG and rhythm strip, as directed.
3. Institute continuous cardiac monitoring for potentially life-threatening dysrhythmias.

4. Analyze ECG strip (Fig. 11):
   a. Determine the rate for bradycardia or tachycardia.
   b. Determine the rhythm for regularity.
   c. Assess P waves for their relationship to QRS complex and their similarity to each other.
   d. Measure the P–R interval for prolongation.
   e. Assess the QRS complexes for their appearance, length, and similarity to each other.
   f. Assess T waves for presence after each QRS and their configuration.
5. Assess that pulse reflects ECG reading, as well as other vital signs and level of consciousness to see if cardiac output is affected by dysrhythmia.

D

NURSING ALERT
Be prepared to begin CPR if pulselessness develops.

◆ Collaborative Management

1. Recognition and treatment of underlying cause such as hypoxia, metabolic acidosis, electrolyte imbalance, myocardial ischemia or infarction, valvular disease, congestive heart failure, digitalis toxicity, illicit drug overdose, or other cardiac or systemic disorders
2. Paroxysmal atrial tachycardia (PAT)—adenosine, a beta-adrenergic blocker, or a calcium channel blocker administered IV; cardioversion may be effective
3. Atrial fibrillation—no treatment unless ventricular response is greater than 100 or of recent onset; digoxin is drug of choice, if ineffective, quinidine, beta-adrenergic blocking agent, or calcium channel blocker may be used; cardioversion if patient is unstable
4. Atrial flutter—calcium channel blocker, digoxin, quinidine, or beta-adrenergic blocking agent; cardioversion if drugs unsuccessful
5. Premature ventricular contractions (PVC)—treated when they occur at a rate exceeding 6 per minute, occur as 2 or more consecutively, fall on T wave, or are of varying configurations; lidocaine is drug of choice, procainamide or bretyllium also used

(text continues on p. 299)

D

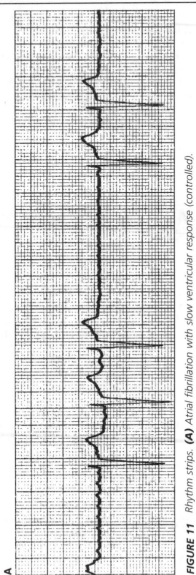

FIGURE 11 Rhythm strips. **(A)** Atrial fibrillation with slow ventricular response (controlled).

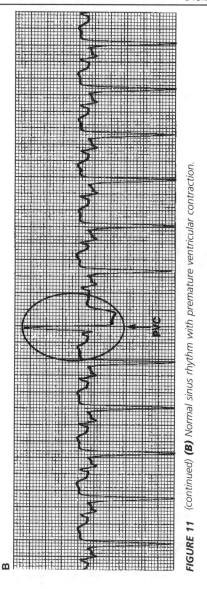

FIGURE 11 *(continued)* *(B)* *Normal sinus rhythm with premature ventricular contraction.*

B

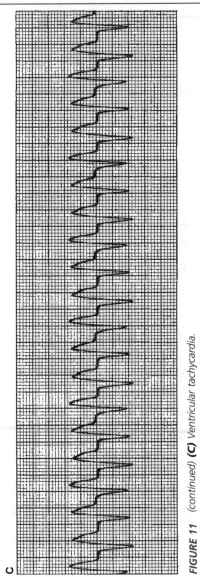

FIGURE 11 (continued) **(C)** Ventricular tachycardia.

6. Ventricular tachycardia (VT)—lidocaine if patient is conscious and not decompensated; cardioversion if lidocaine ineffective and patient remains alert; precordial blow if unconscious and event was witnessed; defibrillation if consciousness and pulse lost; surgery for long-term management; magnesium sulfate for torsades de pointes

NURSING ALERT
Torsades de pointes is an atypical VT characterized by a Q–T interval greater than 0.06 seconds, varying R–R, and polymorphous QRS complexes. It may be caused by quinidine toxicity. Lidocaine is to be avoided because this will prolong the Q–T. Treatment is magnesium sulfate 1 g IV.

E

7. Ventricular fibrillation (VF)—defibrillation at 200 watt/second, then 200 to 300, then 360 if not responsive; after third shock, begin CPR and administer epinephrine to reverse lactic acidosis and make the heart more responsive to defibrillation.
8. Atrioventricular block—no treatment necessary for first-degree AV block; atropine temporarily until pacemaker can be inserted

Eating Disorders

The two major eating disorders are *anorexia nervosa* and *bulimia nervosa*. Anorexia nervosa is characterized by self-induced weight loss greater than 15% of minimally normal weight for age and height. Periods of starvation may be mixed with gorging and purging. This leads to a semistarvation state with glucose and protein sparing, fat utilization, endocrine changes, and fluid and electrolyte disturbances. Psychological components include a distorted body image, fear of gaining weight, and loss of self-esteem.

In contrast to anorexia, bulimia nervosa is marked by recurrent episodes of binge eating at least twice a week for 3 months. The patient feels a lack of control over eating behavior during these episodes, and later tries to prevent weight gain by self-induced vomiting, excessive use of laxatives, diuretics, fasting or excessive exercise. Self-induced vomiting may result in electrolyte imbalance (hypokalemia, hyponatremia, hypochloremia, elevated bicarbonate), or esophageal tears or gastric rupture. Starvation and its physiologic effects may or may not be evident as they are in anorexia nervosa. Bulimia is linked to a personal or family history of obesity, substance abuse, depression, anxiety, or mood disorders.

Most patients with an eating disorder are between ages 14 and 24, in the middle and upper socioeconomic levels, and 90% are women. Anorexia and bulimia may occur simultaneously.

◆ Assessment

1. In anorexia look for:
   a. Loss of adipose tissue and weight loss of greater than 15% of ideal body weight
   b. Bradycardia, hypotension, cold intolerance, hypothermia
   c. Dry skin, thinning scalp hair, lanugo hair
   d. Amenorrhea for 3 consecutive months, decreased libido
   e. Constipation and abdominal pain
   f. Perfectionistic or obsessive–compulsive behavior with high performance expectations
   g. Anxiety, increased exercise activity, inhibited or destructive social interactions, sleep disturbance
   h. Depression, diminished sexual interest
2. In bulimia look for:
   a. Callouses or skin changes on hands and fingers
   b. Loss of dental enamel, swollen lymph nodes, and bad breath or mouthwash smell on breath because of self-induced vomiting
   c. Endocrine changes such as amenorrhea

   d. Weight is often maintained within normal range, or may be significantly elevated or decreased.

   e. Depression, anxiety, personality disorder, abnormal eating behaviors, history of family dysfunction

◆ Diagnostic Evaluation

1. May be severely decreased chloride, potassium, phosphate, magnesium, zinc, albumin
2. Increased BUN, creatinine, liver function tests, bicarbonate, amylase
3. Hormone studies may show decreased LH, FSH, estrogen, testosterone (in men), and thyroid hormone, and decreased response to LHRH.
4. CBC may show decreased white blood cells and hematocrit, indicating starvation's effect on immunity and anemia.
5. ECG should be done to detect dysrhythmias or other signs of electrolyte imbalance.
6. Urinalysis may show ketonuria.

E

◆ Collaborative Management

Therapeutic and Pharmacologic Interventions

1. Develop a nutritional plan to accomplish weight goal (gain or loss) and achieve normal eating habits.
2. Assist in setting up an exercise program.
3. Psychological counseling and support
   a. Assist anorexic or bulimic patient to develop insight into behavior and a more realistic body image.
   b. Assist the patient to develop effective coping strategies and problem-solving mechanisms.
4. Enteral or parenteral feeding may be necessary if prescribed diet cannot be maintained by anorexic patient and physical status warrants.
5. Antidepressants may be tried as well as other pharmacologic agents for associated psychiatric problems.

◆ Nursing Interventions

Monitoring

1. Monitor daily dietary intake and daily weights.
2. Monitor intake and output and serum electrolytes.
3. Monitor urine for ketones.

Supportive Care

1. Assess bowel function. Promote fluids and activity to prevent constipation in anorexia.
2. Assist the patient to select well-balanced diet and maintain appropriate eating habits.
   a. Encourage small frequent meals or snacks of high-calorie foods and beverages in anorexia, with liquid nutritional supplements, as tolerated.
   b. Educate the patient to choose low-fat foods in small portions to gain control of calorie intake in bulimia.
   c. Encourage the patient to keep a food log and eat only at mealtime in bulimia.
3. Provide positive reinforcement for improved intake and weight control.
4. Establish a trusting relationship and provide for the patient's safety and security needs.
5. Be alert for lying and manipulation the patient may display to preserve control.
6. Involve the patient in the treatment plan, offering choices to increase the patient's sense of control. Set limits to give a sense of externa control.
7. Encourage the patient to verbalize feelings about body image, self-concept, fears and frustrations.
8. Stress the importance of counseling, stress management, assertiveness training, and other therapies.
9. Teach the patient the risks associated with abnormal eating behavior and benefits of maintaining healthful nutritional and exercise habits.
10. Encourage the patient to set realistic goals for weight and appearance.

Patient Education and Health Maintenance

1. Teach principles of nutrition and healthful diet and eating habits. Discuss food matter-of-factly to avoid feeding into the patient's preoccupation with food.
2. Teach the impact of starvation on both physiologic and psychological functioning.
3. Involve the patient's family and significant others in the treatment plan as appropriate.
4. Describe the dangers of using laxatives and diuretics in weight control, such as electrolyte imbalances, dehydration, and bowel atony.

5. Stress the importance of maintaining follow-up and counseling.

Eczema
See Dermatitis, Atopic

Encephalitis

Encephalitis is an inflammation of cerebral tissue caused by an infectious agent or other toxin. Common causes are viruses such as rabies virus, enteroviruses, and herpesvirus. The disease, which is often fatal, causes lymphocytic infiltration of the brain, which leads to cerebral edema, basal ganglia degeneration, and diffuse nerve cell destruction. Complications include coma and death.

E

◆ Assessment

1. Fever, headache, nausea and vomiting, mental status changes
2. Meningeal signs—nucchal rigidity (stiff neck), photophobia
3. Seizures
4. May be history of recent infection, or mosquito, tick, or animal bite

◆ Diagnostic Evaluation

1. Lumbar puncture to evaluate cerebrospinal fluid for increased cell count
2. Electroencephalogram (EEG) may reveal abnormalities.
3. Magnetic resonance imaging (MRI) and computed tomography (CT) detect diffuse pattern of inflammation.
4. Blood cultures rarely identify causative organism.

◆ Collaborative Management

Pharmacologic Interventions
1. Antiviral agent acyclovir for herpes simplex virus
2. Anticonvulsants to treat seizures

3. Corticosteroids to reduce cerebral edema
4. Sedatives and analgesics as supportive therapy

◆ Nursing Interventions

Monitoring

1. Monitor temperature and vital signs frequently.
2. Monitor the patient's response to medications and observe for adverse reactions.
3. Monitor neurologic status closely. Watch for subtle changes such as behavior or personality changes, weakness, or cranial nerve involvement. Notify health care provider if changes occur.
4. Monitor fluid intake and output to ensure adequate hydration.

Supportive Care

1. Maintain quiet environment and provide care gently, to avoid excessive stimulation and agitation, which may cause increased intracranial pressure.
2. Maintain seizure precautions: pad side rails of bed, have airway and suction equipment available at bedside.
3. Administer antipyretics and other cooling measures as indicated.
4. Provide fluid replacement through IV lines as needed.
5. Reorient patient frequently.
6. Provide supportive care if coma develops; may last several weeks.
7. Encourage significant others to interact with patient even while in coma and to participate in care to promote rehabilitation.

Family Education and Health Maintenance

1. Encourage follow-up for evaluation of deficits and rehabilitation potential.
2. Educate others about the signs and symptoms of encephalitis if epidemic is suspected.
3. Urge rabies prophylaxis if patient was bitten by an unvaccinated animal.

Endocarditis, Infective

Infective endocarditis (IE, bacterial endocarditis) is an infection of the inner lining of the heart caused by direct invasion of bacteria or other organisms leading to deformity of the valve leaflets. When the inner lining of the heart (endocardium) becomes inflamed, a fibrin clot (vegetation) forms, which may become colonized by pathogens during transient episodes of bacteremia resulting from invasive procedures (venous/arterial cannulation, dental work causing gingival bleeding, gastrointestinal or genitourinary tract surgery, liver biopsy, sigmoidoscopy, etc.), indwelling catheters, urinary tract infections, and wound/skin infections.

Common organisms include *Streptococcus viridans* (after dental work or upper respiratory infection), *Staphylococcus aureus* (after cardiac surgery or parenteral drug abuse), *Enterococci* (penicillin-resistant group D streptococci), which usually occurs in elderly with genitourinary tract infection, fungi such as *Candida albicans* and *Aspergillus*, and Rickettsiae.

Increased risk for infective endocarditis exists with rheumatic heart disease, congenital defects, abnormally vascularized valves, and mechanical/biologic heart valves.

Infective endocarditis may be acute or subacute, depending on the microorganisms involved. Acute IE manifests rapidly with danger of intractable heart failure and occurs more commonly on normal heart valves. Additional complications include uncontrolled/refractory infection, embolic episodes (ischemia or necrosis of extremities and organs), conduction disturbances.

Subacute IE manifests a prolonged chronic course with a lesser chance of complications and occurs more commonly on damaged/defective valves.

◆ Assessment

1. Fever, chills, sweats, anorexia, weight loss, weakness, cough, back and joint pain, headache
2. Characteristic skin and nail manifestations:
   a. Petechiae of conjunctiva and mucous membranes

E

    b. Splinter hemorrhages in nail beds
    c. Osler's nodes—painful red nodes on pads of fingers and toes; usually late sign of infection and found with a subacute infection
    d. Janeway's lesions—light pink macules on palms or soles, nontender, may change to light tan within several days, fade in 1 to 2 weeks. Usually an early sign of IE.
3. New pathologic or changing murmur—no murmur with other signs/symptoms may indicate right heart infection.
4. Additional findings may include splenomegaly, altered mental status, aphasia, hemiplegia, cortical sensory loss, Roth's spots on fundi, pulmonary involvement.

◆ Diagnostic Evaluation

1. Laboratory tests include sedimentation rate and CBC to detect infection; a series of blood cultures from well-cleansed venipuncture site to isolate bacteria or fungi; and additional blood tests to evaluate kidney function.
2. Baseline ECG is usually normal.
3. Echocardiography to identify vegetations and assess location and size of lesions

◆ Collaborative Management

Pharmacologic Interventions

1. IV antimicrobial therapy based on sensitivity of causative agent, usually penicillin, vancomycin, or an aminoglycoside, alone or in combination for 4 to 6 weeks. Obtain repeat blood cultures to assess efficacy of drug therapy.
2. Antipyretics and analgesics

Surgical Interventions

1. Surgery is necessary in the event of:
    a. Acute destructive valvular lesion—excision of infected valves or removal of prosthetic valve
    b. Hemodynamic impairment
    c. Recurrent emboli
    d. Infection that cannot be eliminated with antimicrobial therapy

e. Drainage of abscess/empyema—for patient with localized abscess or empyema
f. Repair of peripheral or cerebral mycotic aneurysm

◆ Nursing Interventions

Monitoring

1. Monitor for signs of decreased cardiac output caused by heart failure such as third heart sound, decreasing blood pressure, increasing pulse, pulsus alternans, decreased pulse pressure, jugular venous distention, crackles of lung fields.
2. Monitor intake and output and daily weights.
3. Monitor temperature every 2 to 4 hours and record on graph.
4. Watch for signs of embolic episodes such as altered mentation, aphasia, loss of muscle strength, loss of vision, hemoptysis, hematuria, complaints of pain, and report promptly.
5. Monitor for therapeutic antibiotic blood levels.
6. Monitor for signs of renal toxicity, such as changes in urinalysis, BUN, and creatinine, caused by antibiotic therapy.

Supportive Care

1. Position patient frequently to prevent skin breakdown and pulmonary complications associated with bed rest.
2. Observe basic principles of asepsis, good handwashing techniques, and continuity of patient care by primary nurse.
3. Employ meticulous IV care for long-term antibiotic therapy.
4. Provide cooling measures such as cool compresses and cooling blanket as directed.
5. Provide blankets and temperature-controlled comfortable environment if patient has shaking chills; change bed linens as necessary.
6. Observe patient for a general "sense of well-being" within 5 to 7 days after initiation of therapy.
7. Promote adequate hydration, as diaphoresis and increased metabolic rate may cause dehydration.
   a. Encourage oral fluid intake.

E

b. Administer IV fluids as directed.

c. Observe skin turgor, urine specific gravity, and mucous membranes.

8. Promote adequate nutrition through small meals and snacks throughout the day to meet the body's needs in fighting infection.

9. Encourage diversional activities appropriate for patient's age such as television, reading, and quiet games.

10. Coordinate home care nursing and IV therapy for outpatient antibiotic treatment, as indicated.

Patient Education and Health Maintenance

For all patients at risk for IE

1. Discuss endocarditis, the mode of entry of infection, and early signs and symptoms.

2. Indicate that antibiotic prophylaxis is recommended for persons with:

   a. Congenital heart defects, prosthetic/biologic heart valves, idiopathic hypertrophic subaortic stenosis (IHSS)

   b. History of endocarditis

   c. Mitral valve prolapse with insufficiency

   d. Rheumatic heart disease and valvular dysfunction

3. Identify procedures most likely to cause bacteremia (dental procedures causing gingival bleeding, surgery on or instrumentation of GI tract, and certain genitourinary procedures, etc.).

4. Identify individual steps necessary to prevent infection:

   a. Good oral hygiene, regular tooth brushing, and flossing

   b. Notification to health care personnel of any history of congenital heart disease or valvular disease

   c. Importance of carrying emergency identification with information of medical history at all times

   d. Take temperature if infection is suspected and notify health care provider of elevation.

   e. Early treatment of symptoms of illness indicating bacteremia—injuries, sore throats, furuncles, etc.

5. Encourage susceptible individuals to receive pneumococcal vaccine and influenza vaccine.

6. Teach women in childbearing years the risks of using

IUDs for birth control (source of infection) and that antibiotic therapy is not necessary for individuals having normal deliveries.

For individuals who have had endocarditis, regarding possible relapse:

1. Discuss importance of keeping follow-up appointments after hospital discharge (infection can recur in 1–2 months).
2. Teach individual to inspect soles of feet for Janeway's lesions indicative of possible relapse.
3. Advise family to allow child to resume activities gradually, and to ensure adequate rest periods throughout the day.

E

Endometriosis

Endometriosis is an abnormal proliferation of uterine endometrial tissue outside the uterus. Although it most commonly occurs in the pelvic area, ectopic endometrial tissue may occur elsewhere in the body; an intact uterus is not needed for endometriosis to occur. This ectopic tissue is sensitive to ovarian hormones and bleeds during menstruation, resulting in accumulated blood and inflammation and subsequent adhesions and pain. It also regresses during amenorrhea (ie, pregnancy and menopause) and with oral contraceptive and androgen use.

Endometriosis is most common in women aged 25 to 45, but may occur at any age. It is more likely to occur in women with shorter menstrual cycles and longer duration of flow; in siblings; in whites more than blacks; and in women who do not exercise and are obese. Complications include infertility and rupture of endometrial cysts.

◆ Assessment

May be asymptomatic or cause pain based on site of implantation:

1. Pelvic pain—especially during or before menstruation
2. Flank pain, hematuria, dysuria—if bladder involved
3. Painful defecation—if sigmoid colon or rectum are involved

4. Dyspareunia (painful sexual intercourse)
5. Rupture of endometrial cysts mimics ruptured appendix.
6. Abnormal uterine bleeding and infertility often occur.

◆ Diagnostic Evaluation

1. Pelvic and rectal examinations reveal tender, fixed nodules or ovarian mass or uterine retrodisplacement. (Nodules may not be palpable.)
2. Laparoscopy is done to view ectopic implants and determine extent of disease.
3. Other studies, include ultrasound, CT, and barium enema to determine extent of organ involvement

◆ Collaborative Management

Pharmacologic Interventions
Drug treatment may include one or more of the following:
1. Danazol—most commonly used drug; synthetic androgen suppresses endometrial growth. Contraindicated in pregnancy
2. Progestins—create a hypoestrogenic environment
3. Gonadotropin-releasing hormone antagonist (Lupron) injections over a 6-month period—create hypoestrogenic environment
4. Oral contraceptives—use small amount of estrogen, maximum amount of progestin and androgen effect to decrease ectopic implant size

Surgical Interventions
1. Laparoscopic surgery—preferred procedure to remove implants and lyse adhesions; not curative; high recurrence rate
2. CO_2 laser laparoscopy—for minimal to moderate disease; vaporizes tissue; may be done at same time as diagnosis; good pregnancy rate
3. Laparotomy—for severe endometriosis or persistent symptoms
4. Presacral neurectomy—to decrease central pelvic pain; preserves fertility
5. Hysterectomy—if fertility is not desired and symptoms are severe; ovaries are preserved if not affected

E

◆ **Nursing Interventions**

Supportive Care

1. Teach the use of analgesics and other medications, as prescribed, along with side effects
2. Encourage the patient to use a heating pad for painful areas, as needed.
3. Teach the patient relaxation techniques to control pain, such as deep breathing, imagery, and progressive muscle relaxation.
4. Encourage the patient to try position changes for sexual intercourse if experiencing dyspareunia.
5. Include the patient in treatment planning; answer questions about drug and surgical treatment so she can make informed choices.
6. Encourage adequate rest and nutrition.
7. Provide emotional support and encourage the patient to discuss treatment of infertility with her health care provider.

Patient Education and Health Maintenance

1. Instruct the patient in the side effects of prescribed medication. For example, danazol may cause voice changes, increased facial hair, acne, weight gain, decreased breast size, and vasomotor reactions.
2. Refer the patient to support groups such as:

> **Endometriosis Association**
> 8585 North 76th Place
> Milwaukee, WI 53223
> 800-992-3636

Esophageal Atresia With Tracheoesophageal Fistula

Esophageal atresia is failure of the esophagus to form a continuous passage from the pharynx to the stomach during embryonic development. Tracheoesophageal fistula (TEF) is an abnormal connection between the trachea and esophagus. The two conditions usually occur together, and may be accompanied by other anomalies such as congenital heart disease and imperforate anus. For unknown reasons, the esophagus and trachea fail to properly differentiate during the fourth and fifth weeks of gestation.

Esophageal atresia is classified into five types (Fig. 12). Type III is most common (80%–90% of cases) and will be discussed further in this entry. The proximal segment of the esophagus has a blind end, whereas the distal segment connects with the trachea via a fistula. In type I atresia, which comprises most of the remaining cases, both proximal and distal segments of the esophagus are blind, with no connection to the trachea.

In TEF, the child is unable to swallow effectively, and saliva or formula may be aspirated into the airway; air entering the lower esophagus through the fistula may cause gastric distention and respiratory distress. Aspiration pneumonia and dehydration are the greatest complications. Other congenital defects occur in 40% to 50% of infants. Esophageal atresia occurs in approximately 1 in every 3,500 births, often in association with prematurity and low birth weight.

E

◆ Assessment

1. Excessive secretions, constant drooling, large amount of secretions from nose
2. Intermittent unexplained cyanosis
3. Laryngospasm caused by aspiration of accumulated saliva in blind pouch
4. Abdominal distention
5. Violent response after first or second swallow of feeding; infant coughs and chokes as fluid returns through nose and mouth; cyanosis occurs
6. Infant is often premature, and pregnancy may have been complicated by hydramnios (excessive amniotic fluid in sac).

◆ Diagnostic Evaluation

1. Inability to pass a stiff, radiopaque size 8 to 10 French catheter into stomach through nose or mouth
2. X-ray flat plate of abdomen and chest may show presence of gas in stomach and tip of catheter in blind pouch.

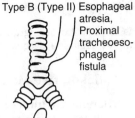

Type B (Type II) Esophageal atresia, Proximal tracheoesophageal fistula

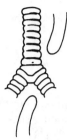

Type a (Type I) Esophageal atresia

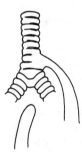

Type C (Type III) Esophageal atresea, Distal tracheoesophageal fistula

Type D (Type IV) Esophageal atresia, Proximal and distal tracheoesophageal fistula

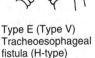

Type E (Type V) Tracheoesophageal fistula (H-type)

FIGURE 12 *Types of esophageal atresia: Esophageal atresia and tracheoesophageal fistula (TEF).*

E

3. Ultrasound scans may show TEF in utero with some infants.
4. ECG and echocardiograms may be done because of the high correlation with cardiac anomalies.

◆ **Collaborative Management**

Therapeutic Interventions

1. Immediate treatment consists of propping infant at 30-degree angle to prevent reflux of gastric contents; suctioning of upper esophageal pouch with Replogle tube or sump drain; gastrostomy to decompress stomach and prevent aspiration (later used for feedings); nothing by mouth, fluids given IV.
2. Appropriate treatment of any coexisting pathologic processes, such as pneumonitis or congestive heart failure
3. Supportive therapy includes meeting nutritional requirements, IV fluids, antibiotics, respiratory support, and maintaining a thermally neutral environment.

Surgical Interventions

1. Prompt primary repair: division of fistula followed by esophageal anastomosis of proximal and distal segments if infant is greater than 2,000 g (4.4 lb) and is without pneumonia
2. Short-term delay (subsequent primary repair): to stabilize infant and to prevent deterioration when the infant cannot tolerate immediate surgery
3. Staging: initially, fistula division and gastrostomy are performed with later secondary esophageal anastomosis. Approach may be used with a very small, premature infant or a very sick neonate, or when severe congenital anomalies exist.
4. Circular esophagomyotomy may be performed on proximal pouch to gain length and allow for primary anastomosis at initial surgery.
5. Cervical esophagostomy (artificial opening in neck that allows for drainage of the upper esophagus) may be done when ends of esophagus are too widely separated; esophageal replacement with segment of intestine is done at 18 to 24 months of age.

6. Postoperative complications (occur in 5% to 10% of cases):
   a. Leak at anastomosis site
   b. Recurrent fistulas
   c. Esophageal strictures
   d. Gastroesophageal reflux and esophagitis
   e. Tracheomalacia
   f. Feeding problems with the older child

◆ **Nursing Interventions**

Monitoring

1. Preoperatively be alert for indications of respiratory distress: retractions, circumoral cyanosis, restlessness, nasal flaring, increased respiration and heart rate.
2. Monitor vital signs frequently for changes in blood pressure and pulse, which may indicate dehydration or fluid volume overload.
3. Record intake and output, including gastric drainage (if gastrostomy tube for decompression is present).
4. Monitor for abdominal distention.
5. Monitor for signs or symptoms that may indicate additional congenital anomalies or complications.
6. Postoperatively, assess for leak at the anastomosis causing mediastinitis and pneumothorax: look for saliva in chest tube, hypothermia or hyperthermia, severe respiratory distress, cyanosis, restlessness, weak pulses.
7. Continue to monitor for complications during the recovery process:
   a. Stricture at the anastomosis: difficulty in swallowing, vomiting or spitting up of ingested fluid, refusing to eat, fever (secondary to aspiration and pneumonia)
   b. Recurrent fistula: coughing, choking, and cyanosis associated with feeding; excessive salivation; difficulty in swallowing associated with abnormal distention; repeated episodes of pneumonitis; general poor physical condition (no weight gain)
   c. Atelectasis or pneumonitis: aspiration, respiratory distress

E

Supportive Care

Preoperative

1. Position the infant with head and chest elevated 20 to 30 degrees to prevent or reduce reflux of gastric juices into the tracheobronchial tree. Turn the infant frequently to prevent atelectasis and pneumonia.
2. Perform intermittent nasopharyngeal suctioning or maintain indwelling Replogle tube (double lumen tube) or sump tube with constant suction to remove secretions from esophageal blind pouch.
   a. Ensure that indwelling tube is kept patent and changed as needed and at least once every 12 to 24 hours (by the health care provider); alternate nostrils. Prevent necrosis of nostrils from pressure by catheter.
   b. Suction mouth to keep clear of secretions and prevent aspiration.
3. If gastrostomy placed prior to definitive surgery, maintain tube to straight gravity drainage, and do not irrigate before surgery.
4. Place the infant in an Isolette or under a radiant warmer with high humidity.
   a. Aids in liquefying secretions and thick mucus
   b. Maintains the infant's temperature in thermoneutral zone and ensures environmental isolation to prevent infection
5. Administer oxygen as needed.
6. Maintain nothing by mouth and administer parenteral fluids and electrolytes as prescribed, to prevent dehydration.
7. Be available and recognize need for emergency care or resuscitation.
8. Explain procedures and necessary events to parents as soon as possible. Orient them to hospital and intensive care nursery environment.
9. Allow family to hold and assist in caring for infant.
10. Offer reassurance and encouragement to family frequently. Provide for additional support by social worker, clergy, or counselor as needed.

Postoperative

1. Maintain airway patency. Suction frequently, at least every 1 to 2 hours; may be needed every 5 to 10 minutes.

    a. Ask the surgeon to mark a suction catheter to indicate how far the catheter can be safely inserted without disturbing the anastomosis.

    b. Observe for signs of obstructed airway.

2. Administer chest physiotherapy as prescribed.

    a. Change the infant's position by turning; stimulate crying to promote full expansion of lungs.

    b. Elevate head and shoulders 20 to 30 degrees.

    c. Use mechanical vibrator 2 to 3 days postoperatively (to minimize trauma to anastomosis), followed by more vigorous chest physical therapy after the third day.

E

❖❖

NURSING ALERT

Avoid hyperextending the neck, which places stress on the operative site.

3. Continue use of Isolette or radiant warmer with humidity.

4. Continue to have emergency equipment available, including suction machine, catheter, oxygen, laryngoscope, endotracheal tubes in varying sizes.

5. Administer IV solutions until gastrostomy feedings can be started.

6. Begin gastrostomy feedings as soon as ordered, because adequate nutrition is an important factor in healing.

    a. Gastrostomy is generally attached to gravity drainage for 3 days postoperatively, then elevated and left open to allow for air escape and passage of gastric secretions into the duodenum for a time before feedings are begun.

    b. Give the infant a pacifier to suck during feedings, unless contraindicated.

    c. Prevent air from entering the stomach and causing gastric distention and possible reflux.

    d. Continue gastrostomy feedings until the infant can tolerate full feedings orally.

7. Maintain patency of chest drainage.

    a. If a break occurs in closed drainage system, immediately clamp tubing close to the infant to prevent pneumothorax.

8. If infant has had cervical esophagostomy:
   a. Keep the area clean of saliva and place an absorbent pad over the area.
   b. As soon as possible, allow the infant to suck a few milliliters of milk at the same time gastrostomy feeding is being done.
   c. Advance the infant to solid foods as appropriate if esophagostomy is maintained for a few months.

9. May begin oral feedings 10 to 14 days after anastomosis
   a. Use demand feedings rather than strictly scheduled feeding.
   b. Do not allow the infant to become overtired at feeding time. Note cardiac rate.

10. Try to make each feeding a pleasant experience for the infant. Use a consistent approach and patience. Encourage parental involvement.

11. Encourage parents to cuddle and talk to the infant.

12. Provide for visual, auditory, and tactile stimulation as appropriate for the infant's physical condition and age.

13. Help to develop a healthy parent–child relationship through flexible visiting, frequent phone calls, and encouraging physical contact between child and parents.

Family Education and Health Maintenance

1. Teach all procedures to be done at home. Watch return demonstration of the following:
   a. Gastrostomy feedings and care
   b. Esophagostomy care with feeding technique
   c. Suctioning
   d. Identifying signs of respiratory distress

2. Help the parents understand the psychological needs of the infant for sucking, warmth, comfort, stimulation, and affection. Suggest that activity be appropriate for age.

3. Encourage the parents to continue close medical follow-up and help them learn to recognize possible problems:

a. Eating problems may occur, especially when solids are introduced.

b. Repeated respiratory tract infection should be reported.

c. Occurrence of stricture at site of anastomosis weeks to months later may be indicated by difficulty in swallowing, spitting of ingested fluid, and fever.

d. Dilatation of esophagus may be necessary to treat stricture at the site of the anastomosis.

e. Signs of fistula leakage are dusky color or choking with feeding.

4. Help the parents understand the need for good nutrition and the need to follow the diet regimen suggested by the health care provider.

5. Reassure parents that an infant's raspy cough is normal and will gradually diminish as the infant's trachea becomes stronger over 6 to 24 months (most infants have some tracheomalasia).

6. Teach parents to prevent the child from swallowing foreign objects.

E

Esophageal Cancer
See Cancer, Esophageal

Esophageal Varices, Bleeding

Esophageal varices are dilated tortuous veins that occur in the submucosa of the lower esophagus, and sometimes extend to the stomach or the upper esophagus. Varices usually result from portal hypertension, which commonly results from obstruction of the portal venous circulation and cirrhosis of the liver.

Mortality is high because of further deterioration of liver function with hepatic coma, and complications such as massive recurrent hemorrhage, aspiration pneumonia, sepsis, and renal failure.

◆ **Assessment**

1. Hematemsis—vomiting of bright red blood
2. Melena—passage of black, tarry stools

3. Possible bright red rectal bleeding caused by bowel hypermotility
4. Blood loss may be sudden and massive, causing shock.

◆ Diagnostic Evaluation

1. Upper gastrointestinal endoscopy to identify the cause and site of bleeding
2. Liver function tests, including ammonia level (elevated)

◆ Collaborative Management

Therapeutic and Pharmacologic (Emergency) Interventions

1. Administer blood and IV fluids to restore circulation and blood volume; give vitamin K to enhance clotting.
2. Administer vasopressin IV to reduce portal venous pressure and increase clotting and hemostasis.
3. Administer iced saline gastric lavage to remove blood from the gastrointestinal tract, vasoconstrict esophageal and gastric blood vessels, and enhance visualization for endoscopic examination.
4. Esophageal balloon tamponade (using Sengstaken-Blakemore tube), whereby balloons are inflated in the distal esophagus and the proximal stomach to collapse the varices and induce hemostasis

Surgical (Nonurgent) Interventions

1. Endoscopic sclerotherapy, whereby a sclerosing agent is injected directly into the varix with a flexible fiberoptic endoscope to control bleeding and reduce frequency of subsequent variceal hemorrhages. Repeated treatments may be required.
2. Administer parenteral feedings as ordered to allow the esophagus to rest.
3. Other surgical interventions include:
   a. Ligation of varices to tie off blood vessels at the site of bleeding
   b. Esophageal transection and devascularization to separate bleeding site from portal system
   c. Shunts to bypass liver, thereby lowering portal pressure: portal–systemic, splenorenal, mesocaval.

Care is similar to that of any abdominal surgery (see p. 350). Severe cirrhosis is a possible complication.

◆ Nursing Interventions

Monitoring

1. Monitor vital signs and respiratory function. Assess blood pressure, heart rate, skin condition, and urine output for signs of hypovolemia and shock.
2. Monitor infusion of blood products.
3. If the patient is receiving vasopressin, monitor for possible complications, including hypertension, bradycardia, esophageal ulceration or perforation, aspiration pneumonitis, abdominal cramps, chest pain, worsening variceal hemorrhage, water intoxication, and cardiac ischemia in patients with preexisting cardiac disease.
4. If the patient is receiving esophageal balloon therapy, monitor for possible complications, including esophageal necrosis, perforation, aspiration, asphyxiation, or stricture.
5. Check all gastrointestinal secretions and feces for occult and frank blood.

Supportive Care

1. Try to prevent straining, gagging, or vomiting; these increase pressure in the portal system and increase risk of further bleeding.
2. Note and report occurrence of signs of obstructed airway or ruptured esophagus from the esophageal balloon: changes in skin color, respirations, breath sounds, level of consciousness, or vital signs; presence of chest pain.
3. Check location and inflation of esophageal balloon; maintain traction on tubes if applicable.
4. Have scissors readily available. Cut tubing and remove esophageal balloon immediately if the patient develops acute respiratory distress.
5. Keep head of bed elevated to avoid gastric regurgitation and aspiration of gastric contents.
6. When using the Sengstaken-Blakemore esophageal balloon tube, ensure removal of secretions above the esophageal balloon: position nasogastric tube in the

esophagus for suctioning purposes; or provide intermittent oropharyngeal suctioning.

7. Inspect nares for skin irritation; cleanse and lubricate frequently to prevent bleeding.

8. Remain with the patient or maintain close observation and place call bell within the patient's reach.

9. Provide alternate means of communication if tubes or other equipment interfere with the patient's ability to talk.

10. Use protective restraints to prevent dislodging of tubes in confused, combative patient.

Patient Education and Health Maintenance

1. Discuss signs and symptoms of recurrent bleeding and the need to seek emergency medical treatment if these occur.

2. Instruct the patient to avoid behaviors that increase portal system pressure: straining, gagging, Valsalva maneuvers.

3. Warn the patient against effects of high protein diets and alcohol consumption in causing further complications.

4. Encourage joining a support organization such as Alcoholic Anonymous.

Esophagitis and Gastroesophageal Reflux

Esophagitis is acute or chronic inflammation of the esophageal mucosa caused by repeated or prolonged contact with acid gastric or duodenal contents. This condition most commonly results from gastroesophageal reflux associated with an incompetent lower esophageal sphincter (LES). Other causes include impaired gastric emptying from gastroparesis or partial gastric outlet obstruction; mechanical obstruction caused by esophageal cancer, hiatal hernia, peptic stricture, or Schatzki's (esophageal) ring; prolonged nasogastric intubation; gastric or duodenal surgery; certain medications (NSAIDs, potassium chloride pills, quinidine, and antibiotics); repeated vomiting (common in persons with bulimia); trauma; infections by viruses (herpes simplex or CMV) or fungi (*Candida*); ingestion of corrosive alkalis or acids; or motility disorders (achalasia, scleroderma, esophageal spasm).

Complications include stricture, ulceration and possible fistula, aspiration pneumonia, Barrett's esophagus (presence of columnar epithelium above gastroesophageal junction), which increases risk of adenocarcinoma.

◆ Assessment

1. Signs and symptoms of gastroesophageal reflux:
   a. Heartburn, most often occurring 30 to 60 minutes after meals and with reclining positions
   b. Complaints of spontaneous regurgitation of sour or bitter gastric contents into the mouth
   c. Dysphagia is less common.
   d. Patient may have substernal chest pain.
2. Signs and symptoms of infectious esophagitis:
   a. Oral thrush may occur with 50% of patients with candida esophagitis. Oral ulcers are common with herpes simplex esophagitis.
   b. Patient may report dysphagia (difficulty or discomfort in swallowing) and odynophagia (sharp substernal pain on swallowing) which may limit oral intake.
   c. Substernal chest pain may occur.
3. Signs and symptoms of corrosive esophagitis:
   a. Severe burns of mucosa
   b. Chest pain
   c. Gagging, dysphagia, and drooling
   d. Stridor and wheezing occur with aspiration.
4. Pain characteristic of motility disorders or mechanical lesions—dysphagia occurring with solids or liquids; chronic heartburn or chest pain
5. Characteristics of pill-induced esophagitis—severe retrosternal chest pain, odynophagia, dysphagia several hours after swallowing a pill

◆ Diagnostic Evaluation

1. Endoscopy to visualize inflammation, lesions, strictures, or erosions; obtain biopsy specimen; and dilate strictures, if necessary
2. Barium swallow (esophagography) to diagnose mechanical and motility disorders
3. Additional tests may include:
   a. Cineradiographic esophagogram to identify mass

E

lesions, strictures, and abnormalities in peristalsis and esophageal clearing

b. Esophageal manometry to measure esophageal sphincter tone

c. Acid perfusion test to evaluate response after ingestion of dilute hydrochloric acid and saline. Onset of symptoms is considered positive.

d. Ambulatory 24-hour pH monitoring to determine the amount of gastroesophageal acid reflux

◆ Collaborative Management

Therapeutic Interventions

1. Bland antireflux diet: avoid garlic, onion, alcohol, fatty foods, chocolate, coffee (even decaffeinated), citrus juices, colas, and tomato products, all of which reduce LES pressure.
2. Smoking cessation to help increase LES pressure
3. Prevent overeating, which induces esophageal sphincter relaxation.
4. Avoid tight-fitting clothes, which increase intraabdominal pressure.

Pharmacologic Interventions

1. Antacids PRN to treat heartburn. Provides symptomatic relief but does not heal esophageal lesions
2. Histamine$_2$-receptor antagonists to decrease gastric acid secretions and provide symptomatic relief. Therapy may be lifelong. Corrosive esophagitis requires higher doses.

NURSING ALERT
With chemical esophagitis—maintain airway, give IV fluids and analgesics. NG lavage and oral antidotes are not used because they risk causing further damage. Surgery may be indicated.

3. Proton pump inhibitor to suppress gastric acid (such as omeprazole) for a patient with corrosive esophagitis who does not respond to H$_2$-receptor antagonists.
4. Prokinetic agents, such as cisapride to raise LES pressure and improve gastric emptying
5. In candidal esophagitis, give antifungals by topical, oral or IV route.

6. In CMV esophagitis, give ganciclovir; in herpetic esophagitis, give acyclovir.
7. In pill-induced esophagitis, may give sucralfate with H_2-blockers; drug provides a protective coating against gastric acids.

Surgical Interventions

1. Surgery may be indicated when patient not responsive or noncompliant to other approaches. Procedures include:
   a. Fundoplication for reflux to throat and severe stricture. May be combined with vagotomy–pyloroplasty if esophagitis is associated with gastroduodenal ulcer.
   b. Stricture may need to be resected, and an esophagogastrostomy may be required.
2. For strictures, mechanical dilatation may be necessary several times.

◆ Nursing Interventions

Supportive Care and Patient Education

1. Raise the head of the bed 15 to 20 cm (6–8 in.) to reduce incidence of nighttime reflux.
2. Advise the patient not to lie down for 3 hours after eating (period during which greatest reflux may occur).
3. Teach the patient about prescribed medications and side effects, and when to notify the health care provider.
4. Inform the patient regarding medications that may exacerbate symptoms.

NURSING ALERT
Anticholinergics may further impair functioning of the lower esophageal sphincter, allowing reflux; antihistamines, antidepressants, antihypertensives, antispasmodics, and some neuroleptics and antiparkinson drugs decrease saliva production, which may decrease acid clearance from the esophagus.

5. Advise the patient to sit or stand when taking any solid medication (pills, capsules): emphasize the need to follow the drug with at least 100 mL liquid.

E

TABLE 6 Other Types of Eye Injuries

Type and Causes	Signs and Symptoms	Treatment
Hyphema Presence of blood in anterior chamber in front of the iris, caused by torn ciliary body and iris. Blood may be reabsorbed in 72 hours; if not, secondary glaucoma and loss of vision in affected eye may result.	Pain; blood partially or completely filling anterior chamber; increased intraocular pressure; patient may report seeing reddish coloration.	Keep patient on bed rest; provide eye shield. Monitor blood level in anterior chamber; continued bleeding may require paracentesis of anterior chamber.
Orbital Fracture Fracture and dislocation of walls of the orbit, orbital margins, or both	Pain, swelling around orbit, rhinorea, diplopia. Check for signs and symptoms of head injury.	Injury may heal on its own if there is no displacement of other structures. Otherwise may require surgery.
Foreign Body May occur on the cornea (25% of all ocular injuries) and conjunctiva. Intraocular particles may penetrate sclera, cornea, or globe.	Severe pain, lacrimation, foreign body sensation, photophobia, redness, swelling. Wood or plant parts may cause severe infection within hours.	Requires immediate medical attention. Removal by irrigation, cotton-tipped applicator, magnet, or possibly surgery.
Laceration, Perforation Cutting or penetration of tissue may occur. May affect any part of eye—eyelid, conjunctiva, cornea, sclera, globe	Pain, bleeding, lacrimation, photophobia	Requires immediate medical attention. Topical or systemic antibiotics may be given. Surgical repair depends on severity of injury.

E

Ruptured Globe
Concussive injury to globe with tearing of ocular coats (usually the sclera). May be caused by sharp penetrating object or high-velocity projectile.

Pain, altered intraocular pressure; limited gaze in field of rupture; hyphema; hemorrhage (poor prognostic sign)

Requires immediate medical attention. Antobiotics or steroids may be given. Surgery includes vitrectomy, scleral buckle, enucleation.

Burns
Caused by chemicals such as lye, cleaning fluids, acid; thermal burns from fire or intense heat; ultraviolet burns from excessive sunlight, sunlamp, or welding

Pain, burning, lacrimation, photophobia; fluid blisters with thermal burns; symptoms may occur later with ultraviolet burns. Ultraviolet burns are usually self-limiting.

Requires immediate medical attention. Determine causative agent; irrigate affected area until pH is 7.0 (neutral). Administer antibiotics and protective patch. Leave blisters intact. Severe scarring may require keratoplasty.

Corneal Abrasion
Loss of epithelial layers of cornea; may result from overwear of contact lenses. Corneal ulcer (keratitis) is inflammation and loss of entire depth of cornea.

Pain, lacrimation, photophobia, redness, positive fluorescein staining

Topical antibiotics and patching; abrasion usually heals in 24–48 hours; ulcer may require frequent around-the-clock drops or IV antibiotics and corticosteroids.

6. Teach the patient and family what foods and activities to avoid: fatty foods, garlic, onions, alcohol, coffee and chocolate; straining, bending over, tight-fitting clothes, smoking.
7. Encourage a weight-reduction program, if the patient is overweight, to decrease intraabdominal pressure.

Eye Injuries

Eye injuries refer to damage to the eyes resulting from a wide variety of causes, including blunt injuries (contusion); laceration or perforation; foreign bodies; orbital fracture; hyphema; ruptured globe; and burns. Complications include infection, retinal detachment, increased intraocular pressure, cataract formation, and disfigurement. Blunt trauma is considered here; refer to Table 6 for other types of eye trauma.

◆ Assessment

1. Obtain history of injury.
2. Assess the eyes for signs and symptoms of blunt trauma.
   a. Tissue swelling, discoloration
   b. Bleeding into tissues and eye structures
   c. Blurred or double vision
   d. Loss of portion of visual field

◆ Diagnostic Evaluation

1. Visual acuity tests to detect altered vision
2. Ophthalmoscopy to detect changes in cornea, vitreous, choroid, and retina
3. Possibly, tonometry to evaluate intraocular pressure

◆ Collaborative Management

Therapeutic Interventions
1. Measures to reduce tissue swelling
2. Administer analgesics as needed
3. Surgery may be indicated to repair retinal detachment or other eye or orbital structures.

◆ **Nursing Interventions**

Supportive Care and Family Education

1. Apply cool compresses to relieve discomfort and swelling.
2. Provide eye patch and instill medications, as ordered.
3. Maintain safe environment if visual acuity is affected.
4. Be alert for and report signs of complications: increased swelling or pain, worsening visual acuity, development of fever or drainage, neurologic deterioration.
5. Encourage follow-up ophthalmologic examinations.

F

Fractures

A fracture is a break in the continuity of bone. A fracture occurs when the stress placed on a bone is greater than the bone can absorb. The stress may be mechanical (trauma) or related to a disease process (pathologic). Muscles, blood vessels, nerves, tendons, joints, and body organs may be injured when fracture occurs. In elderly persons, osteoporosis is a major fracture risk, particularly for hip and vertebral compression fractures.

Complications of fractures include problems associated with immobility (muscle atrophy, joint contracture, pressure sores); infection; shock; venous stasis and thromboembolism; pulmonary emboli and fat emboli; and bone union problems.

◆ **Assessment**

1. Pain—usually progressive, localized, deep throbbing, persistent, unrelieved by immobilization and medications; increased on passive stretch, movement

2. Swelling, tenderness, deformity, and ecchymosis
3. Crepitus (grating sensation) and loss of function
4. Signs of shock with fractures causing overt hemorrhage through open wound or with femoral fracture or pelvic fracture

NURSING ALERT
Change in behavior or cerebral functioning may be an early indicator of cerebral anoxia from shock or pulmonary or fat emboli.

◆ **Diagnostic Evaluation**

1. Radiograph and other imaging studies such as bone scan to determine integrity of bone
2. Complete blood count, serum electrolytes if blood loss and extensive muscle damage have occurred; may show decreased hemoglobin and hematocrit
3. Arthroscopy to detect joint involvement
4. Angiography if associated with blood vessel injury
5. Nerve conduction and electromyograms to detect nerve injury

◆ **Collaborative Management**

(See Table 7)

Therapeutic Interventions
1. Emergency management includes splinting fracture above and below site of injury, applying cold, and elevating limb to reduce edema and pain.
2. Control bleeding and provide fluid replacement to prevent shock, if necessary.
3. Traction used for fractures of long bones
   a. Skin traction—force applied to the skin using foam rubber, tapes, etc.
   b. Skeletal traction—force applied to the bony skeleton directly, using wires, pins, or tongs placed into or through the bone
4. External fixation to stabilize complex and open fracture with use of a metal frame and pin system

(text continues on p. 339)

F

TABLE 7 Fractures of Specific Sites

Site and Mechanism	Management	Nursing Interventions
Clavicle Fall on shoulder	Closed reduction and immobilization with clavicular strap, figure 8 bandage or sling Open reduction and internal fixation (ORIF) for marked displacement, severely comminuted fracture, and extensive soft tissue injury.	1. Pad axilla to prevent nerve damage from pressure of immobilizer. 2. Assess neurovascular status of arm. 3. Teach shoulder exercises through full range of motion as prescribed, to prevent frozen shoulder.
Proximal Humerus Fall on outstretched arm Osteoporosis is predisposing factor.	Many of these fractures remain in alignment and are supported by a sling and swathe or Belpeau bandage for comfort. If displaced, treat with reduction under x-ray control, open reduction, or replacement of humeral head with prosthesis.	1. Place a soft pad under the axilla to prevent skin maceration. 2. Encourage shoulder range-of-motion exercises after specified period of immobilization to prevent frozen shoulder. 3. Instruct patient to lean forward and allow affected arm to abduct and rotate.

F

(continued)

TABLE 7 *(Continued)*

Site and Mechanism	Management	Nursing Interventions
Shaft of Humerus Direct fall, blow to arm, or auto injury. Damage to radial nerve may occur.	Immobilize with sling and swathe, splint, or hanging cast. A hanging cast is applied for its weight to correct displaced fractures with shortening of the humeral shaft. ORIF for associated vascular injury or pathologic fracture, followed by support in sling.	1. Hanging cast must remain unsupported to maintain traction. Patient should sleep in upright position to maintain 24-hour traction. 2. Encourage exercise of fingers immediately after application of cast. 3. Teach pendulum exercises of arm as prescribed to prevent frozen shoulder.
Elbow and Forearm Fall on elbow, outstretched hand, or direct blow (sideswipe injury)	Treatment depends on nature of fracture—ORIF, arthroplasty, external fixation, casting Closed drainage system may be used to decrease hematoma formation and swelling.	1. Assess neurovascular status of forearm and hand. 2. If radial pulse weakens or disappears, report immediately to prevent irreversible ischemia. 3. Elevate arm to control edema. 4. Encourage finger and shoulder exercises.

F

Wrist

Colles' fracture is common (1.2–2.5 cm above the wrist with dorsal displacement of lower fragment). Caused by fall on outstretched palm. Often associated with osteoporosis

Closed reduction with splint or cast support

Percutaneous pins and external fixator or plaster cast

1. Elevate arm above level of heart for 48 hours after reduction to promote venous and lymphatic return and reduce swelling.
2. Watch for swelling of fingers and check for constricting bandages or cast.
3. Teach finger exercises to reduce swelling and stiffness.
4. Encourage daily prescribed exercises to retore full extension and supination.

Hand

Caused by numerous injuries

Splinting for undisplaced fractures of fingers

Debridement, irrigation, and Kirchner wire fixation for open fractures

Reconstructive surgery may be necessary for complex injuries

1. Provide aggressive care and encouragement with rehabilitation plan to regain maximal hand function.

F

(continued)

TABLE 7 (Continued)

Site and Mechanism	Management	Nursing Interventions

Hip (Proximal Femur)
Occur frequently in older adults, women with osteoporosis, and with falls
	1. Hip fracture identified by shortening and external rotation of affected leg; pain in hip or knee; inability to move leg
	2. Immobilization with Buck's extension traction until surgery
	3. Surgery as soon as medically stable; choice depends on location, character, and patient factors
	   a. Internal fixation with nail, nail–plate combination, multiple pins, screw, or sliding nails
	   b. Femoral prosthetic replacement
	   c. Total hip replacement
		1. Provide constant monitoring and nursing care to reduce the risk of complications, eg, pneumonia, thrombophlebitis, fat emboli, dislocation of prosthesis, infection, and pressure sores.
		2. Administer aspirin, warfarin, or low-dose subcutaneous heparin as ordered.
		3. Use sequential compression devices as ordered.
		4. Provide meticulous skin care to prevent breakdown, and use trapeze to assist with position changes.
		5. Keep affected leg in abduction and neutral rotation.
		6. Teach quadriceps setting exercise to prevent muscle atrophy of affected leg.

F

Femoral Shaft
Falls from height, motor vehicle accidents with high impact

Closed reduction and stabilization with skeletal traction—Thomas leg splint with Pearson attachment; followed by use of orthosis (cast-brace) to allow weight bearing
Open reduction with hardware or with bone grafting may be necessary
External fixator may be used

1. Marked concealed blood loss may occur; watch for signs of shock initially and anemia later.
2. Examine skin under the ring of the Thomas splint for signs of pressure.

Knee
Direct blow to knee area; involve distal shaft of femur (supracondylar), articular surfaces, or patella.

Closed reduction or immobilization through casting, traction, braces, splints
ORIF
Goal is to preserve knee mobility

1. Elevate extremity by raising foot gatch of bed.
2. Evaluate for effusion—report and loosen pressure dressing if pain is severe; prepare for joint aspiration.
3. Teach quadriceps setting exercises and limited weight-bearing as prescribed.

F

(continued)

TABLE 7 (Continued)

Site and Mechanism	Management	Nursing Interventions
Tibia and Fibula/Ankle Distal tibia or fibula, malleoli, or talus fractures generally result from forceful twisting of ankle and often are associated with ligament disruption. Also high incidence of open fractures of tibial shaft, because tibia lies superficially beneath the skin	Closed reduction and toe-to-groin cast for closed fractures, later replaced by short leg cast or orthosis ORIF may be necessary for some closed fractures External fixator for open fracture	1. Elevate lower leg to control edema. 2. Avoid dependent position of extremity for prolonged periods. 3. Prepare patient for long immobilization period, because union is slow (12–16 weeks, longer for open and comminuted fractures). 4. Prepare patient for stiff ankle joint after immobilization.
Foot Metatarsal fracture caused by crush injuries of foot	Immobilization with cast, splint, or strapping	1. Encourage partial weight bearing as allowed. 2. Elevate foot to control edema.

F

Thoracic and Lumbar Spine

Trauma from falls, contact sports, or auto accidents or excessive loading may cause fracture of vertebral body, lamina, spinous and transverse processes.

Usually stable compression fractures

Suspected with pain that is worsened by movement and coughing and radiates to extremities, abdomen, or intercostal muscles; and presence of sensory and motor deficits.

Bed rest on firm mattress and pain relief followed by progressive ambulation and back strengthening to treat stable fractures; takes about 6 weeks to heal

ORIF with Harrington rod, body cast, or laminectomy with spinal fusion may be necessary for unstable or displaced fractures

1. Use log roll technique to change positions.
2. Monitor bowel and bladder dysfunction, because paralytic ileus and bladder distention may occur with nerve root injury.
3. Assist patient to ambulate when pain subsides, no neurologic deficit exists, and x-rays show no displacement.
4. Teach proper body mechanics and back-preservation techniques.
5. Encourage weight reduction.
6. Teach patient with osteoporosis the importance of safety measures to avoid falls.

F

(continued)

F

TABLE 7 (Continued)

Site and Mechanism	Management	Nursing Interventions
Pelvis Sacrum, ilium, pubic, ischium, coccyx fractures may occur from auto accidents, crush injuries, and falls. Most are stable fractures that do not involve the pelvic ring and have minimal displacement.	Emergency management to treat multiple trauma, shock from intraperitoneal hemorrhage, and injury to internal organs is necessary. Bed rest for several days followed by progressive weight-bearing for stable fracture Prolonged bed rest, external fixation, ORIF, skeletal traction, or pelvic sling are options for unstable fracture	1. Monitor and support vital functions as indicated. 2. Observe urine output for blood, indicating genitourinary injury. 3. Do not attempt to insert urethral catheter until patency of urethra is known; incidence of urethral injury in men is high with anterior fractures. 4. Fold pelvic sling back over buttocks to enable patient to use bedpan. Reach under sling to give skin care; line sling with sheepskin. Loosen sling only as directed.

Pharmacologic Interventions

1. Local anesthetic, narcotic analgesic, muscle relaxant, or sedative are given to assist the patient during closed reduction procedure.
2. Anesthesia may be given instead.
3. Analgesics are given as directed to control pain postoperatively.

Surgical Interventions

1. Reduction to restore bone continuity
   a. Closed reduction: bony fragments are brought into apposition (ends in contact) by manipulation and manual traction—restores alignment. Cast or splint is applied to immobilize extremity and maintain reduction.
   b. Open reduction with internal fixation (ORIF): Bone fragments are directly visualized. Internal fixation devices are used to hold bone fragments in position until solid bone healing occurs; they may be removed when bone is healed. After wound closure, splints or casts may be used for additional stabilization and support.
2. Endoprosthetic replacement
   a. Replacement of a fracture fragment with an implanted metal device
   b. Used when fracture disrupts nutrition of the bone or treatment of choice is bony replacement

◆ **Nursing Interventions**

Monitoring

1. Monitor for hemorrhage and shock in patients with severe fractures.
   a. Check vital signs as frequently as clinical condition indicates, observing for hypotension, elevated pulse, cold clammy skin, restlessness, pallor.
   b. Watch for evidence of hemorrhage on dressings or in drainage containers.
2. Monitor for any sudden or progressive changes in respiratory status that may indicate pulmonary embolus.
3. Monitor neurovascular status for compression of nerve, diminished circulation, development of compartment syndrome.

NURSING ALERT ❖❖

Monitoring the neurovascular integrity of the injured extremity is essential. Development of *compartment syndrome* (palpable tightness of muscle compartment and elevated measured tissue pressure causing anoxia) leads to permanent loss of function in 6 to 8 hours. This condition must be identified and managed promptly.

4. Monitor for development of thrombophlebitis with pain and tenderness in calf, increased size, and warmth of calf.
5. Monitor for development of infection.

Supportive Care

1. Administer prescribed fluids and blood products to maintain circulating volume in hemorrhage and shock.
2. Position the patient to enhance respiratory effort.
3. Encourage coughing and deep breathing to promote lung expansion and diminish pooling of pulmonary secretions.
4. Administer oxygen as prescribed.
5. Reduce swelling:
   a. Elevate injured extremity (unless compartment syndrome is suspected; may contribute to vascular compromise).
   b. Apply cold to injury if prescribed.
6. Relieve pressure caused by immobilizing device as prescribed (such as bivalving cast, rewrapping elastic bandage, or splinting device).
7. Relieve pressure on skin to prevent development of pressure sore; employ frequent repositioning, skin care, special mattresses.
8. Prevent development of thromboembolism.
   a. Encourage active and passive ankle exercises.
   b. Use elastic stockings and sequential compression devices as prescribed.
   c. Elevate legs to prevent stasis, avoiding pressure on blood vessels.
   d. Encourage mobility; change position frequently; encourage ambulation.
   e. Administer anticoagulants as prescribed.

F

GERONTOLOGIC ALERT
Older adults with fractures, trauma, immobility, obesity, or history of thrombophlebitis are at high risk for developing thromboembolism.

9. Evaluate the patient for proper body alignment and pressure from equipment (casts, traction, splints, appliances) that may cause pain.
10. Encourage nonpharmacologic measures for pain reduction, such as cutaneous stimulation, distraction, guided imagery, transcutaneous electrical nerve stimulation (TENS), and biofeedback.
11. Administer prescribed medications as indicated. Encourage use of less potent drugs as severity of discomfort decreases.
12. Cleanse, debride, and irrigate open fracture wound as prescribed as soon as possible, to minimize chance of infection. Use sterile technique during dressing changes.
13. Administer antibiotic therapy as prescribed.
14. Assist with activities of daily living as needed.
15. Teach family how to assist the patient while promoting independence in self-care.
16. Perform active and passive exercises to all nonimmobilized joints.
17. Encourage patient participation in frequent position changes, maintaining supports to fracture during position changes.
18. Minimize prolonged periods of physical inactivity, encouraging ambulation when prescribed.
19. Teach and encourage isometric exercises to diminish muscle atrophy and prevent development of disuse syndrome.
20. Help the patient move through phases of posttraumatic stress (outcry; denial; intrusiveness; working through; completion).
21. Encourage the patient to participate in decision making to reestablish control and overcome feelings of helplessness.
22. Teach relaxation techniques to decrease anxiety.

F

23. Refer the patient to support group or psychotherapy as needed.

Patient Education and Health Maintenance

1. Explain basis for fracture treatment and need for patient participation in therapeutic regimen.
2. Promote adjustment of usual lifestyle and responsibilities to accommodate limitations imposed by fracture.
3. Instruct the patient to actively exercise joints above and below the immobilized fracture at frequent intervals.
   a. Isometric exercises of muscles covered by cast—start exercise as soon as possible after cast application.
   b. Increase isometric exercises as fracture stabilizes.
4. After removal of immobilizing device, have the patient start active exercises and continue with isometric exercises.
5. Instruct on exercises to strengthen upper extremity muscles if crutch walking is planned.
6. Instruct in methods of safe ambulation—walker, crutches, cane.
7. Emphasize instructions concerning amount of weight bearing that will be permitted on fractured extremity.
8. Discuss prevention of recurrent fractures; review safety considerations, avoidance of fatigue, proper footwear.
9. Encourage follow-up medical supervision to monitor for bone union problems.
10. Teach the patient to recognize and report symptoms needing attention such as numbness, decreased function, increased pain, elevated temperature.
11. Encourage adequate balanced diet to promote bone and soft tissue healing.

F

Gallbladder Surgery
See Cholecystectomy

Gallstones
See Cholelithiasis, Cholecystitis, Choledocholithiasis

Gastric Cancer
See Cancer, Gastric

Gastroesophageal Reflux
See Esophagitis and Gastroesophageal Reflux

G

Gastroesophageal Reflux in Children

Gastroesophageal reflux is a malfunction of the lower esophageal sphincter (LES), a physiologic rather than an anatomic segment of the distal esophagus that forms an antireflux barrier. Failure of this barrier—caused by an incompetent LES or excessive gastric pressure—allows acidic stomach or duodenal contents to flow back up into the esophagus. Predisposing factors include physiologic immaturity; esophageal surgery; prolonged orogastric or nasogastric feeding; supine chest physical therapy positioning; medications such as theophylline; and coughing and wheezing from disorders such as cystic fibrosis, bronchopulmonary dysplasia, or asthma.

Recurrent gastroesophageal reflux may lead to complications such as chronic esophagitis, recurrent pulmonary disease, aspiration pneumonia, failure to thrive, anemia, apnea, and near-miss sudden infant death syndrome. Gastroesophageal reflux is a common problem during the first year of life and occurs in approximately 3% of newborns. It is more common in males than females.

◆ Assessment

1. In an infant:
   a. Unexplained vomiting occurs immediately after feeding, especially when placed in prone position.
   b. Usually regurgitation rather than projectile vomiting
   c. Onset usually soon after birth
   d. Weight loss or failure to gain weight; rumination
   e. Dehydration
   f. Recurrent pulmonary symptoms
   g. Colic, excessive crying
   h. Sleep disturbances
2. In an older child:
   a. Substernal burning, upper abdominal discomfort, pressure or "squeezing" feeling
   b. Persistent pulmonary problems
   c. Dysphagia as evidenced by irritability during eating
   d. Anemia
   e. Hematemesis or melena (blood in stools)

◆ Diagnostic Evaluation

1. Upper GI barium esophagography with fluoroscopy to show reflux into esophagus
2. Monitoring of pH in esophagus over 18 to 24 hours (appears to be most useful procedure)
3. Laboratory studies:
   a. Calcium: may be decreased
   b. pH: pH greater than 7.45 (alkalosis)
   c. Hemoglobin and hematocrit: may be decreased
4. Fiberoptic esophagoscopy may be done to show presence of gastric folds above the diaphragm and obtain esophageal biopsy

◆ Collaborative Management

Therapeutic Interventions

1. Positional therapy: based on premise that gravity will help reduce amount of reflux; should be maintained as much as possible

    a. Infants younger than 6 months: prone with head elevated, positioned in harness at 30 degrees, held upright. If positioned in infant seat, infant will probably slump, causing increased intraabdominal pressure and increased reflux.

    b. Older infant—placement in a walker with parental instruction about safety and continuous monitoring of infant

    c. Older child—head of bed raised with blocks to maintain 30- to 45-degree angle

2. Feeding

    a. Infant—thickened feedings, such as dry rice cereal or commercial thickening agent; small, frequent feedings followed by proper positioning

    b. Older child—nothing to eat 2 hours before bedtime; possible avoidance of certain foods; should remain upright while awake

Pharmacologic Interventions

1. Administration of medications to stimulate lower esophageal sphincter pressure (tone) and increase peristaltic wave amplitude and clearance rate, such as metoclopramide and bethanechol; given before meals and at hour of sleep

2. Histamine 2 (H_2) blockers, such as cimetidine, when esophagitis has been documented

3. Antacid between feedings if esophagitis is present (forms a floating barrier)

Surgical Interventions

1. Surgical reconstruction of esophagogastric junction (fundoplication) may be necessary if conservative management does not improve condition, or if recurrent severe respiratory disease and apnea or refractory esophagitis with stricture occur

2. Gastropexy, surgical fixation of stomach in the abdomen below the diaphragm

3. Temporary gastrostomy may be performed to decompress the stomach, avoiding gastric distention.

4. Complications include retching with feeding, watery diarrhea, growth retardation, small bowel obstruction, and dumping syndrome

5. Nursing care is similar to care of child after surgery for pyloric stenosis (p. 704).

G

◆ Nursing Interventions

Monitoring

1. Use cardiac and apnea monitors for infants and children with severe reflux.
   a. Observe for apnea episodes lasting longer than 20 seconds or accompanied by cyanosis, pallor, or bradycardia.
   b. Document apnea episodes, associated symptoms, and recovery efforts.
2. Monitor weight frequently to evaluate infant's progress.
3. Monitor vital signs and assess skin turgor for signs of dehydration.
4. Observe and record urinary output.
5. Monitor serum electrolytes and replace sodium and potassium as ordered.
6. Monitor for dumping syndrome after surgery: usually occurs 30 minutes after meal and includes symptoms such as diaphoresis, palpitations, weakness, syncope, abdominal fullness, nausea, and diarrhea.

Supportive Care

1. Observe careful positioning with infants at all times.

NURSING ALERT
Do not allow infant or child to slouch, because this may change angle of esophagus in relation to stomach, increase intraabdominal pressure, and facilitate reflux of stomach contents.

2. Use infant "antireflux" saddle—covered, padded wedges with a sling designed for infant to straddle face down at elevated angle.
   a. Observe for lower leg edema, flattening of parietal skull, and torticollis (muscle contraction of neck).
   b. Turn infant's head frequently.
   c. Elevate infant's legs before eating or bathing.
3. Thicken formula for each feeding; enlarge nipple hole so that formula can be more easily extracted. Use caution, however, because this reduces number of episodes of reflux but may increase their duration, thus increasing the risk of complications.

4. Provide comfort measures to reduce crying before and after meals to avoid increased intraabdominal pressure and swallowing of air.
5. Use a pacifier for nonnutritive sucking after eating only when infant is seated upright because use of pacifier while prone increases reflux.
6. Bubble infant frequently during and after feeding.
7. Accurately record infant feeding activity:
   a. Amount of food taken: whether retained
   b. Emesis: estimated amount, type, occurrence in relation to feeding
   c. Any change in behavior as a result of feeding technique
8. If breast-feeding, teach mother to express milk and thicken with cereal.
9. Ensure that older children avoid caffeine-containing food and beverages (such as chocolate) to reduce gastric acid production. Also maintain a low-fat diet because fat delays gastric emptying; discourage eating 2 to 4 hours before bedtime.

Family Education and Health Maintenance

1. Teach parents how to handle and care for the infant. Ensure that they have proper equipment for propping the infant; inform parents that it is not necessary to keep infant in infant seat or propped up at all times.
2. Help parents to understand that reflux is often self-limiting; symptoms usually disappear within 12 months.
3. If a temporary gastrostomy is done, teach parents about tube use and care.
4. Encourage follow-up for monitoring weight gain and development.
5. Instruct parents and caregivers in CPR training before discharge of infant, if indicated.
6. Provide written and verbal instructions regarding prescribed medications and side effects.

Gastrointestinal Bleeding

Gastrointestinal bleeding is a symptom of many upper or lower gastrointestinal disorders. It may be obvious (in emesis or stool) or occult (hidden). Such bleeding may result from trauma anywhere along the GI tract; erosions or ulcers; esophageal or gastric varices; esophagitis, gastritis, inflammatory bowel disease; bacterial infection; diverticulosis; neoplasms; ischemic bowel or aortoenteric fistula; Mallory-Weiss syndrome; or anal disorders such as hemorrhoids or fissures. Untreated GI bleeding may progress to hemorrhage, shock, and death.

◆ Assessment

1. Changes in bowel patterns or in stool color (dark black, red, or streaked with blood); hematemesis
2. Nausea, abdominal pain or tenderness, or rectal pain
3. Intermittent melena or "coffee ground" emesis to large amount of melena with clots or bright red hematemesis
4. Rapid pulse, drop in blood pressure, and signs of shock may occur with significant blood loss.
5. Pallor, weakness, dizziness, and shortness of breath may occur as anemia develops.
6. Stool or emesis will test positive for occult blood.
7. Characteristics of blood help determine site of origin:
   a. Bright red hematemesis—vomited from high in esophagus
   b. Bright red flow or coating stool—from rectum or distal colon
   c. Dark red blood mixed with stool—higher up in colon and small intestine
   d. Shades of black ("coffee ground") emesis—vomited from esophagus, stomach, and duodenum
   e. Tarry stool (melena)—occurs when excessive blood accumulates in the stomach

◆ Diagnostic Evaluation

1. Complete blood count to detect decreased hematocrit and hemoglobin; coagulation studies to evaluate prothrombin time
2. Nasogastric intubation and irrigation as a diagnostic and possibly therapeutic measure (controversial)
3. Endoscopy, to visualize the GI mucosa and site of bleeding

◆ Collaborative Management

Therapeutic Interventions

1. If life-threatening bleeding occurs, treat shock and administer blood replacement.
2. Placement of long tube (Miller-Abbott, Harris, Cantor) for upper GI bleeding to control bleeding by placing pressure against the bleeding site
3. Electrocoagulation and laser photocoagulation via endoscopy may be the treatment of choice. Instilling topical thrombin to clot blood at the bleeding site may be used as adjuvant therapy.

> **NURSING ALERT**
> Because of the action of topical thrombin, it is used only on the surface of bleeding tissue and never is injected into the bloodstream, where intravascular clotting could take place.

4. Surgery may be necessary to treat some causes of bleeding.

Pharmacologic Interventions

1. For upper GI bleeding, histamine 2 (H_2)-blockers IV to block the acid-secreting action of histamine. Antacids or cytoprotective agent such as sucralfate also may be used.
2. If peptic ulcer disease is the cause, an antiulcer drug is prescribed, along with lifestyle change and dietary modifications.
3. Discontinue any medications such as nonsteroidal antiinflammatory agents or antibiotics that may be causing bleeding.

◆ Nursing Interventions

Monitoring

1. Monitor intake and output and vital signs to evaluate fluid status.
2. Observe for changes indicating shock, such as tachycardia, hypotension, increased respirations, decreased urine output, changes in mental status.
3. Monitor all stools and NG drainage for blood.

Supportive Care

1. Maintain patient on NG tube and NPO status to rest GI tract and evaluate bleeding.
2. Administer IV fluids and blood products as ordered to maintain volume and treat anemia. Provide oxygen therapy as directed.
3. Begin liquids when patient is no longer NPO. Advance diet as tolerated. Diet should be high caloric, high protein. Frequent, small feedings may be indicated.
4. Weigh daily to monitor nutritional status.

Patient Education and Health Maintenance

1. Discuss the cause and treatment of GI bleeding with patient.
2. Instruct patient to report signs and symptoms of GI bleeding: melena, emesis that is bright red or "coffee ground" color; rectal bleeding; weakness, fatigue, shortness of breath.
3. Instruct patient on how to test stool or emesis for occult blood if applicable.
4. Encourage compliance with abstinence if alcohol use has caused bleeding.

G

Gastrointestinal or Abdominal Surgery

Gastrointestinal surgeries are operative procedures performed to aid in diagnosis and treatment of many types of gastrointestinal disorders. Procedures include stomach surgeries (total or partial gastrectomy, gastrostomy); hernia surgeries (herniorrhaphy, hernioplasty); bowel surgeries (appendectomy, various types of small and large bowel resections, total or partial colectomies), and, finally, ostomy surgeries (ileostomy, colostomy, Kock pouch). Some of these procedures require creating an artificial outlet, or *stoma*. A stoma is a part of the small or large intestine that is brought above the abdominal wall to serve as the outlet for discharge of intestinal contents. The term "stoma" is often used interchangeably with "ostomy."

Cholecystectomies, hernia repairs, and appendectomies are routinely done through laparoscopy, and additional procedures are being done through this approach.

Advantages include shorter hospital stay and recuperation time, less cost, less pain, and better cosmetic outcome. Abdominal surgeries may also include surgery to pelvic organs, the urologic system, adrenal glands, and other structures.

◆ Potential Complications

1. Paralytic ileus or obstruction
2. Peritonitis or sepsis
3. Anastomotic leakage which may result in peritonitis
4. For ostomy surgery:
   a. Mucocutaneous separation (between skin and stoma)
   b. Stomal ischemia
   c. Stomal stricture or stenosis
   d. Stomal prolapse
   e. Peristomal hernia
   f. Peristomal skin breakdown
5. General postoperative complications: hemorrhage, infection, thromboembolism, pneumonia, atelectasis, wound dehiscence and evisceration

◆ Collaborative Management

Preoperative Care

1. Explain all diagnostic tests and procedures to promote the patient's cooperation and relaxation.
2. Describe the reason for and type of surgical procedure, as well as postoperative care (ie, IV, patient-controlled analgesia [PCA] pump, NG tube, surgical drains, incision care, possibility of ostomy).
3. Explain the rationale for deep breathing and teach the patient how to turn, cough, deep breathe, use the incentive spirometer, and splint the incision. These measures will minimize postoperative complications.
4. Administer IV fluids or hyperalimentation before surgery, as ordered, to improve fluid and electrolyte balance and nutritional status. Before an ostomy procedure, give large quantities of replacement fluids, as ordered, to accommodate expected increased output during the postoperative phase.
5. Send blood samples, as ordered, for preoperative laboratory studies and monitor results.

6. Explain that bowel cleansing will be initiated 1 to 2 days before surgery for better visualization. Preparation may include diet modifications, such as liquid or low residue; oral laxatives; suppositories; enemas; or polyethylene glyco-electrolyte solution (CoLyte, Go-LYTELY).

7. Administer antibiotics, as ordered, to decrease bacterial growth in the colon.

8. Coordinate consultation with the enterostomal therapy nurse if patient is scheduled for an ostomy, to initiate early understanding and management of postoperative care. Tell the patient that the abdomen will be marked by the enterostomal therapist or surgeon to assure proper positioning of the stoma.

9. Explain that the patient may not have anything by mouth after midnight the night before surgery. Medications may be withheld, if ordered.

Postoperative Care

1. Assess vital signs frequently for signs of shock and infection—hypotension, tachycardia, fever, increased respirations.

2. Assess abdomen and report increased pain, distention, rigidity, and rebound tenderness because because they may indicate postoperative complications. Abdominal distention also causes reduction in blood flow to a stoma through mesenteric tension.

3. Administer prescribed pain medications and provide instructions if using PCA pump, to keep patient comfortable:

   a. Assess the effectiveness of the pain medications. If ordered, phenergan can potentiate the effectiveness of narcotic.

   b. Provide diversion and teach relaxation techniques as needed.

4. Encourage and assist patient with turning, coughing, deep breathing, and incentive spirometry every 2 hours.

   a. Assess breath sounds for decrease (atelectasis) or crackles (pneumonia).

   b. Assist patient to dangle legs at bedside the night of surgery and attempt ambulation the first postoperative day, unless ordered otherwise.

5. Apply antiembolism stockings to reduce risk of thromboembolism.

6. Maintain NG tube, if ordered. To maintain patency, irrigate the tube with 30 mL normal saline every 2 hours and as needed. If there are large amounts of NG output, IV replacement may be necessary.

> **NURSING ALERT**
> Because of the type of abdominal surgery and location of the suture line, the health care provider may order not to irrigate or manipulate the NG tube.

7. Monitor intake and output frequently to determine fluid retention, dehydration, or shock. Include all drains in evaluating output.
8. Weigh patient daily to ensure fluid balance and adequate calorie intake.
9. Assess bowel sounds frequently. Maintain NPO status until return within several days after surgery.
10. Advance diet as ordered, after presence of bowel sounds indicates GI tract has regained motility. The usual diet progression is ice chips, sips of water; clear liquids; full liquids; soft or regular diet.
11. Assess wound for signs of erythema, swelling, and purulent drainage, which may indicate infection.
    a. Change surgical dressings every 24 hours and as needed to protect skin from drainage and decrease risk of infection.
    b. Apply gauze on skin to protect against leaking from drains or stomas.
12. Assess ostomy patient's stoma every shift for color and record findings:
    a. Normal color—pink-red
    b. Dusky—dark red; purplish hue (ischemic sign)
    c. Necrotic—brown or black; may be dry (notify health care provider to determine extent of necrosis)
13. Select a pouching system based on type of ostomy and condition of stoma and skin:
    a. Apply pouching system with ⅛″ clearance to prevent stomal constriction, which contributes to edema.

G

    b. Empty pouch when ⅓ to ½ full to avoid overfilling, which interferes with pouch seal.

14. Treat peristomal skin breakdown as needed:
    a. Dust with skin barrier powder.
    b. Seal powder with water or skin sealant.
    c. Allow skin to dry before applying a pouching system.

15. Encourage early ambulation, but while in bed, turn patient frequently or encourage position changes to prevent skin breakdown at pressure areas.

16. Monitor for passage of stool from rectum or ostomy (Fig. 13). Note frequency, amount, and consistency.
    a. Administer stool softener, laxative, as ordered, to promote comfort with elimination.
    b. Encourage diet with adequate fiber, fluid content for natural laxative effect.
    c. Encourage and assist with ambulation to promote peristalsis.

G

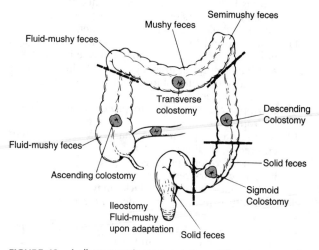

FIGURE 13   A diagrammatic representation of the placement of fecal ostomies and nature of discharge at these sites.

◆ **Patient Education and Health Maintenance**

1. Review signs and symptoms of wound infection so early intervention may be instituted.
2. Explain signs and symptoms of other postoperative complications to report—elevated temperature, nausea or vomiting, abdominal distention, changes in bowel function and stool consistency.
3. Instruct patient on turning, coughing, deep breathing, use of incentive spirometer, ambulation. Discuss purpose and continued importance of these maneuvers during the recovery period.
4. Review dietary changes such as increased fiber content and fluid intake and their importance in improving bowel function.
5. Inform ostomy patient about gas-forming foods, such as beans or cabbage, and eliminate when appropriate. It takes about 6 hours for gas to travel from mouth to colostomy. Advise avoiding foods that stimulate elimination, such as nuts, seeds, and certain fruits.

G

COMMUNITY CARE CONSIDERATION
A person who has undergone a total gastrectomy needs lifelong parenteral administration of vitamin B_{12} to prevent pernicious anemia.

6. Assess the need for home health follow-up and initiate the appropriate referrals if indicated.
7. Instruct patient regarding wound care or ostomy care if applicable to promote healing and self-confidence.
8. Teach colostomy irrigation procedure, if appropriate.
9. Involve the enterostomal therapist in ostomy teaching and reinforce information, including lifestyle modifications.
10. Teach about periostomy skin care, odor and gas control.
11. Teach ostomy patient about activities of daily living:
    a. Advise resumption of normal bathing habits (tub or shower) with or without pouching system on.

Suggest waterproof tape on edges of pouching system as it may be helpful with bathing or swimming.

b. Inform that clothing modifications are usually minimal. Girdles and panty hose can be worn.

c. Suggest carrying an ostomy supply kit during work or travel in case of an emergency.

d. Remind the patient with an ostomy that participation in sports is possible; however, caution must be exercised with contact sports. During vigorous sports, a belt or binder may provide extra security.

12. Help ostomy patient achieve sexual well-being:

a. Encourage patient and significant other to express feelings about the ostomy.

b. Discuss ways to conceal pouch during intimacy, if desired: pouch covers, special ostomy underwear. May use small-capacity pouch (mini-pouch or cap) for short period.

c. Recommend different positions for sexual activity to decrease stoma friction and skin irritation.

d. Review that an ostomy in a woman does not prevent a successful pregnancy.

e. Recommend counseling as needed.

13. Inform the patient about the United Ostomy Association, a self-help group for ostomates and other interested persons. The national headquarters is located at:

United Ostomy Association, Inc.
36 Executive Park, Suite 120
Irvine, CA 92714-6744
714-660-8624

Glaucoma

Glaucoma is a condition marked by high intraocular pressure (IOP) that damages the optic nerve. Glaucoma occurs in two major forms: *acute (angle-closure)* and *chronic (open-angle)*. Acute glaucoma results when the angle between the iris and the cornea becomes narrowed, restricting or blocking the drainage of aqueous humor through the trabecular network and canal of Schlemm. This causes IOP to increase suddenly. Acute angle closure may result from trauma, stress, or any process that pushes the iris forward against the inside of the cornea.

Chronic glaucoma results from the gradual deterioration of the trabecular network, which, as in the acute form, blocks drainage of aqueous humor and causes IOP to increase. Chronic glaucoma is the most common form of the disorder, affecting about 2% of Americans older than age 35. This may result from long-term corticosteroid use, ocular tumors or infection, eye surgery, for systemic disease. Glaucoma may also occur in neonates and children because of a congenital abnormality or acquired obstruction.

Glaucoma is one of the leading causes of blindness. There is a genetic predisposition and incidence is higher among African Americans.

◆ **Assessment**

1. Acute glaucoma:
   a. Severe pain, occurring in and around the eyes due to increased IOP (often above 75 mm Hg); transitory attacks
   b. Cloudy, blurred vision; rainbow of color around lights
   c. Red eye, dilated pupils
   d. Nausea and vomiting may occur.

NURSING ALERT
Acute angle closure glaucoma is a medical emergency and requires immediate treatment. Untreated, it can result in blindness in less than a week.

2. Chronic glaucoma:
   a. Mild, bilateral discomfort (tired feeling in eyes)
   b. Slow loss of peripheral vision—central vision remains unimpaired; in later stages, progressive loss of visual field
   c. Increased IOP causes halos to appear around lights

PEDIATRIC ALERT

Glaucoma presents in infants and children as haziness of the cornea, photophobia, excessive tearing, and decreased visual acuity.

◆ Diagnostic Evaluation

1. Tonometry shows elevated IOP in acute and chronic disease
2. Gonioscopy to study the angle of the anterior chamber of the eye in acute disease.
3. Ophthalmoscopy may show a pale optic disk (acute disease); or signs of clipping and atrophy of the disk (chronic disease).

COMMUNITY CARE CONSIDERATIONS

All persons older than 35 and those at risk for developing glaucoma (family history, diabetic, previous eye trauma or surgery) should have periodic examination and tonometry by an ophthalmologist. Early detection and treatment will prevent blindness.

◆ Collaborative Management

Pharmacologic Interventions

1. In acute glaucoma, emergency drug management is initiated to decrease eye pressure.
   a. Parasympathomimetics may be used as miotics to cause the pupil to contract and draw the iris away from the cornea, thus enlarging the angle and allowing aqueous humor to drain.

NURSING ALERT

Dilatation of pupils is avoided if the anterior chamber is shallow to avoid worsening of condition. This is determined by oblique illumination of the anterior segment of the eye.

b. Sympathomimetics or carbonic anhydrase inhibitors to depress aqueous humor production

c. Beta-blockers, which may reduce aqueous humor or facilitate its drainage

d. Hyperosmotics increase blood osmolarity and diurese the aqueous humor

2. In chronic glaucoma, a combination of miotic agent and carbonic anhydrase inhibitor is usually given. Follow-up is continued at 3- to 6-month intervals to control IOP.

Surgical Interventions

1. Surgery is indicated if IOP is not maintained within normal limits by pharmacotherapy and if there is progressive visual field loss with optic nerve damage.

2. Types of surgery for acute glaucoma include peripheral iridectomy (treatment of choice) or trabeculectomy (necessary if peripheral anterior adhesions have developed because of repeated glaucoma attacks).

3. Types of surgery for chronic glaucoma include laser trabeculoplasty (treatment of choice if IOP unresponsive to medical regimen); iridencleisis (to bypass blocked meshwork and allow aqueous humor to be absorbed into conjunctival tissues); cyclodiathermy or cyclocryotherapy (depresses secretion of aqueous humor by ciliary body); and corneoscleral trephine (rarely done—a permanent drainage opening is made at the junction of the cornea and sclera through the anterior chamber).

G

◆ Nursing Interventions

Monitoring

1. Monitor visual acuity and for any pain or visual changes.

2. Monitor the patient's compliance with medications and lifetime follow-up care.

Supportive Care and Patient/Family Education

1. Explain the importance of medications and the proper procedure for administration of drops.

2. After surgery:
   a. Elevate head of the bed to promote drainage of aqueous humor after a trabeculectomy.
   b. Administer medications (steroids and cycloplegics) as prescribed after peripheral iridectomy to decrease inflammation and to dilate the pupil.
   c. Use an eye patch or shield in children for several days to protect the eye.
3. Alert the patient to avoid, if possible, circumstances that may increase IOP:
   a. Prolonged coughing or vomiting
   b. Emotional upsets—worry, fear, anger
   c. Exertion such as snow shoveling, pushing, heavy lifting
4. Instruct the patient to seek immediate medical attention if signs and symptoms of increased IOP should recur.
5. Recommend the following:
   a. Moderate use of the eyes
   b. Exercise in moderation to maintain general well-being
   c. Fluid intake is not restricted: alcohol and coffee may be permitted unless they are noted to cause increased IOP in the particular patient.
   d. Maintenance of regular bowel habits to decrease straining
   e. Wearing a medical identification tag indicating the patient has glaucoma

Glomerulonephritis, Acute

Acute glomerulonephritis (poststreptococcal glomerulonephritis [PSGN]) is an inflammation of the glomeruli that occurs when antigen–antibody complexes become trapped in the glomerular capillary membranes. Eventual scarring and loss of glomerular filtering surface may lead to renal failure. The disease occurs 1 to 2 weeks after onset of an upper respiratory infection (typically, pharyngitis from group A beta-hemolytic streptococci), skin infection, or systemic infection (hepatitis B, endocarditis).

Acute glomerulonephritis affects males more than females (2:1) and can occur at any age, but frequently occurs in early school age and is rare in children younger than age 2 years. Complications are rare but include hypertension, congestive heart failure, uremia, anemia, endocarditis, hypertensive encephalopathy, and end-stage renal disease.

◆ Assessment

1. Oliguria, proteinuria, hematuria
2. Edema—periorbital or generalized and dependent; weight gain
3. Hypertension (in more than 50% of patients)—usually mild, but can be moderate or severe
4. Malaise, mild headache, anorexia and vomiting

◆ Diagnostic Evaluation

1. Urinalysis:
   a. Hematuria (microscopic or gross)
   b. Proteinuria (3+ to 4+)
   c. Sediment: Red cell casts, WBCs, renal epithelial cells
   d. Specific gravity: moderately elevated
2. Blood studies:
   a. Serum complement and C3 decreased
   b. BUN and creatinine elevated
   c. DNA-ase B antigen titer elevated
   d. Erythrocyte sedimentation rate (ESR) elevated
   e. Albumin decreased
   f. Antistreptolysin-O titer (ASO) increased
3. Needle biopsy of the kidney to show obstruction of glomerular capillaries and confirm diagnosis

◆ Collaborative Management

Therapeutic Interventions

1. Restrict fluid intake, potassium and sodium.
2. Moderate protein restriction with oliguria and elevated BUN; more drastic restriction if acute renal failure develops
3. Increased carbohydrates to provide energy and reduce protein catabolism

G

Pharmacologic Interventions

1. Antihypertensives and diuretics to control hypertension and edema
2. Cation-exchange resin to control hyperkalemia secondary to renal insufficiency, if necessary
3. H_2 blockers to prevent stress ulcers in acute illness
4. Phosphate-binding agents to reduce phosphate and elevate calcium levels
5. Antibiotics if infection is still present
6. Therapy for rapidly progressive glomerulonephritis may include:
   a. Plasma exchange
   b. Immunosuppressive therapy with corticosteroids or cyclophosphamide
   c. Dialysis may be considered if fluid retention and uremia cannot be controlled.

◆ Nursing Interventions

Monitoring

1. Monitor vital signs and intake and output during acute phase of the disease.
2. Carefully monitor fluid balance with central venous pressure or pulmonary artery pressure readings as indicated, and weigh the patient daily.
3. Monitor for signs and symptoms of congestive heart failure: distended neck veins, tachycardia, gallop rhythm, enlarged and tender liver, increasing edema, crackles at bases of lungs.
4. Monitor neurologic status for signs of encephalopathy or seizure activity secondary to hypertension.

NURSING ALERT
Hypertensive encephalopathy is a medical emergency; treatment must reduce blood pressure without impairing renal function. Monitor vasodilator therapy closely.

Supportive Care

1. Encourage bed rest during the acute phase until the urine clears and BUN, creatinine, and blood pressure normalize. Rest also facilitates diuresis.

2. For children on fluid restriction, offer small amount of desired fluids in appropriate size cup at regular intervals during day. Give fluids after, rather than with meals.
3. Suggest age-appropriate nonexertional diversional activities while on bed rest.
4. Ensure adequate fluid replacement once diuresis phase begins (usually 1–2 weeks after onset of symptoms) through oral fluid intake.

Family Education and Health Maintenance

1. Encourage evaluation of all family members for sore throats to prevent recurrence.
2. Advise that tonsillectomy or oral surgery is not recommended for several months after glomerulonephritis to prevent endocarditis.
3. Explain that the patient must have follow-up evaluations of blood pressure, urinalysis, and BUN concentrations to check for exacerbation of the disease. Microscopic hematuria and proteinuria may persist for many months.
4. Explain that prognosis is good, with 90% of patients regaining normal renal function within 60 days.
5. Advise reporting any signs of decreasing renal function and obtaining treatment immediately.

Gout

Gout is a disorder of purine metabolism characterized by elevated uric acid levels with deposition of urate crystals in joints and other tissues. High uric acid levels result from decreased excretion of uric acid (90% of cases) or overproduction of the acid (10% of cases) due to a wide variety of causes. The disorder may progress from an asymptomatic stage through acute gouty arthritis, to chronic tophaceous gout. Complications include erosive deforming arthritis and uric acid kidney stones and urate nephropathy caused by hyperuricemia.

◆ Assessment

1. Acute gouty arthritis:
   a. Generally affects one joint—often the first metatarsophalangeal joint (podagra).

b. Other joints can be affected, such as ankle, tarsals, knee. Upper extremities less commonly involved.
c. Warm erythema and swelling of tissue surrounding the affected joint
d. Pain—sudden onset, severe intensity
e. Duration of symptoms is self-limiting; lasts approximately 3 to 10 days without treatment

2. Chronic tophaceous gout:
a. Tophi (deposits of uric acid) in and around joints, cartilage and soft tissues, such as pinnae, olecranon bursa, Achilles tendon
b. Arthritis more chronic in nature, with discrete attacks less common; can produce bone erosions and subsequent bony deformities that can resemble rheumatoid arthritis

◆ Diagnostic Evaluation

1. Synovial fluid for analysis:
a. Identification of monosodium urate crystals under polarized microscopy
b. Synovial WBC count can range from 2,000 to 100,000/mm^3.
c. Culture to rule out infection
2. Uric acid level decreased on 24-hour urine specimen with underexcretion; increased with overproduction
3. Elevated serum uric acid level with overproduction
4. Elevated erythrocyte sedimentation rate.
5. X-rays of affected joints show changes consistent with gout.

◆ Collaborative Management

Therapeutic Interventions
1. Avoidance of obesity
2. Avoidance of alcohol
3. Low-purine diet (obtains small reduction of serum uric acid levels)

Pharmacologic Interventions
1. Nonsteroidal antiinflammatory drugs (NSAIDs) to relieve pain and swelling of acute attacks
2. Colchicine to prevent as well as treat acute attacks

G

   a. IV for acute attacks
   b. PO at onset of attack, given hourly until first signs of toxicity (diarrhea)
3. Corticosteroids given intraarticularly if attack is confined to a single joint; or orally in short tapering course if other treatments contraindicated or if attack involves many joints
4. Urate-lowering agents to prevent renal disease progression of gout:
   a. Uricosurics such as probenecid interfere with tubular reabsorption of uric acid
   b. Allopurinol interferes with conversion of hypoxanthine and xanthine to uric acid
   c. Give cautiously to patients with renal disease.

◆ Nursing Interventions

Monitoring

1. Monitor skin surrounding affected joint because it is prone to break down.
2. Monitor for side effects of allopurinol, including skin rash (including exfoliative rashes), hypersensitivity syndrome (fever, eosinophilia, leukocytosis, worsening renal failure, hepatocellular injury, rash) bone marrow depression.

Supportive Care

1. Administer and teach self-administration of pain-relieving medications as prescribed.
2. Encourage adequate fluid intake to assist with excretion of uric acid and decrease likelihood of stone formation.
3. Reinforce importance of taking prescribed medications consistently because interruption of therapy can precipitate acute attacks.
4. Elevate and protect affected joint during acute attack.
5. Assist with activities of daily living.
6. Encourage exercise and maintenance of routine activity in chronic gout, except during acute attacks.
7. Protect draining tophi by covering and application of antibiotic ointment as needed.
8. Avoid thiazide diuretics, low-dose aspirin and the anti-

G

tubercular agent pyrazinamide, which may increase uric acid levels in these patients.

Patient Education and Health Maintenance

1. Instruct the patient and family in nature of disease.
   a. Generally acute attacks are followed by periods of remission.
   b. Once need for chronic treatment has been determined, it will generally be lifelong.
2. Encourage the patient to avoid alcohol, which can precipitate acute attack.
3. Instruct the patient to avoid rapid weight loss by fasting or crash diets. Explain that rapid weight loss results in production of chemicals that compete with uric acid for excretion from the body, causing increased uric acid levels.
4. Advise prompt treatment of acute attacks to reduce joint damage associated with repeated attacks.
5. Teach the patient to recognize and report signs and symptoms of allopurinol hypersensitivity syndrome.
6. Review foods containing purines (eg, sardines, anchovies, shellfish, organ meats) if low-purine diet has been advised.

Graves' Disease
See Hyperthyroidism

Growth Hormone Insufficiency

Growth hormone insufficiency is a form of hypopituitarism in which impaired secretion of growth hormone (GH) by the anterior pituitary gland slows the rate of growth and bone maturation. A child with this condition has short stature but normal body proportions. Causes include tumors, intracranial cysts, head trauma, infection, radiation therapy, birth trauma, or genetic predisposition. Classic GH insufficiency occurs in 1 of every 3,500 births. Complications include hypoglycemia, causing seizures and death in the newborn.

◆ Assessment

1. Growth velocity usually less than the 5th percentile for chronologic age
2. Delayed skeletal maturation—bone age at least 1 year behind chronologic age
3. "Pudgy," where the weight age (50% for weight) exceeds the height age (50% for height)
4. Delayed eruption of primary and secondary teeth (not as severe as in hypothyroidism)
5. Delayed or absent sexual development

COMMUNITY CARE CONSIDERATION
The school nurse who measures the child on an annual basis is the best source for detecting a growth disorder. Height percentiles should accompany absolute measurements. Changes in percentiles on consecutive measurements indicate need for a closer evaluation of growth.

G

◆ Diagnostic Evaluation

1. Rule out organic, nonendocrine causes of short stature (eg, chronic illness, nutritional deficiencies, genetic disorders, psychosocial factors).
2. Calculate growth velocity to determine if growth pattern parallels or deviates from the growth curve.
3. Assess bone age by x-ray to ascertain age of physical development; usually delayed.
4. Thyroid function tests may be done to rule out hypothyroidism.
5. Growth hormone secretion laboratory indicators: insulin-like growth factor I (IGF-I), IGF binding protein 3 are decreased.
6. Subnormal secretion of GH in provocative testing.
7. In the newborn with hypoglycemia, GH release is reduced at time of documented hypoglycemia.
8. Computed tomography or magnetic resonance imaging may be done to rule out central nervous system lesions.

◆ Collaborative Management

Pharmacologic Interventions

1. Replacement of deficiency uses recombinant DNA-derived GH (somatrem) given as subcutaneous injection.
2. Typical dose is 0.2 to 0.3 mg/kg per week divided in 3, 6 or 7 doses weekly until final height is achieved.
3. Use cautiously in patients with active underlying intracranial lesion.

NURSING ALERT
Observe for signs of glucose intolerance and hyperglycemia during growth hormone therapy.

◆ Nursing Interventions

Supportive Care

1. Teach the child through written and verbal instructions how to inject GH. Give demonstration and encourage return demonstration.
2. Encourage rotation of sites in the subcutaneous tissue of the upper arms or thighs if irritation occurs.
3. Document growth at regular intervals.
4. Encourage the child to verbalize feelings regarding short stature. Help the child understand that friendships and social value are based on personality traits rather than physical height.
5. Suggest involvement in activities that do not use height as an advantage, such as music, art, and gymnastics.
6. Help child and parents to identify age-appropriate behaviors and develop a plan for maintaining consistent behaviors both in the home and socially.
7. Make sure parents have realistic expectations of child; encourage use of positive feedback rather than punishment.

Family Education and Health Maintenance

1. Teach that growth catch-up to peers usually occurs when peers have stopped growing. After initial startup of treatment, growth rate should be at 2 to 3 inches per year.
2. Stress that treatment is not to make child tall—it is

to restore normal growth that is reflected in height achievement.
3. Review medication dosage and injection techniques periodically.
4. Tell family to think of GH as a replacement rather than a medication; therefore, it should always be given regardless of illness or other medication therapies.
5. Encourage regular follow-up for growth evaluation and maintenance of therapy.

Guillain-Barré Syndrome

Guillain-Barré syndrome (polyradiculoneuritis) is an acute inflammatory polyneuropathy of the peripheral sensory and motor nerves and nerve roots. Affected nerves are demyelinated with possible axonal degeneration. Although its exact cause is unknown, Guillain-Barré syndrome is believed to be an autoimmune disorder that may be triggered by viral infection, immunization, or other precipitating event. The syndrome is marked by acute onset of symmetrical progressive muscle weakness, most often beginning in the legs and ascending to involve the trunk, upper extremities, and facial muscles. Paralysis may develop. Complications may include respiratory failure, cardiac dysrhythmias, and complications of immobility; however, recovery is spontaneous and complete in about 95% of patients.

◆ Assessment

1. Muscle weakness and fasciculation
2. Reduced or absent deep tendon reflexes, position and vibratory perception
3. Paresthesia and painful sensations
4. Possible hypoventilation due to chest muscle weakness
5. Difficulty with swallowing, chewing, speech, and gag, indicating fifth (trigeminal) and ninth (glossopharyngeal) cranial nerve involvement

◆ Diagnostic Evaluation

1. Lumbar puncture to obtain cerebrospinal fluid samples, which reveal low cell count, high protein levels

G

2. Nerve conduction studies, which show decreased conduction velocity of peripheral nerves due to demyelination

◆ Collaborative Management

Therapeutic Interventions

1. Plasmapheresis may be tried to temporarily reduce circulating disease-related antibodies.
2. Continuous cardiac monitoring to monitor for dysrhythmias, indicating thoracic spinal nerve involvement
3. If respiratory paralysis develops, intubation, mechanical ventilation, and support of vital functions

Pharmacologic Interventions

1. Analgesics and muscle relaxants to control painful sensations and fasiculations

◆ Nursing Interventions

Monitoring

1. Monitor respiratory status through vital capacity measurements, rate and depth of respirations, breath sounds.
2. Monitor level of muscle weakness as it ascends toward respiratory muscles. Watch for breathlessness while talking, a sign of respiratory fatigue.
3. Monitor the patient for signs of impending respiratory failure; heart rate >120 or <70; respiratory rate > 30 breaths/min; prepare to intubate.

Supportive Care

1. Position the patient with the head of bed elevated to provide for maximum chest excursion.
2. Avoid giving narcotics and sedatives that may depress respirations.
3. Position the patient correctly and provide range of motion exercises.
4. Assess for complications such as contractures, pressure sores, edema of lower extremities, and constipation.
5. Ensure adequate nutrition without the risk of aspiration.
6. Auscultate for bowel sounds; if bowel sounds are absent, hold feedings to prevent gastric distention.

7. Encourage physical and occupational therapy exercises to help the patient regain strength during rehabilitation phase.

8. Provide assistive devices as needed (cane or wheelchair) to maximize independence and activity.

9. During rehabilitation period, encourage a well-balanced, nutritious diet using small, frequent feedings with vitamin supplement if indicated. Weigh weekly.

10. If verbal communication is possible, discuss the patient's fears and concerns. Reassure the patient that complete recovery is probable.

11. If the patient cannot speak, use mechanical speech aids or a communication board. Provide some type of patient call system.

12. Encourage speech therapy during rehabilitation phase.

13. Provide adjunct pain management therapies such as therapeutic touch, massage, diversion, imagery.

14. Provide choices in care to give the patient a sense of control.

Patient Education and Health Maintenance

1. Advise the patient and family that the acute phase of the syndrome lasts 1 to 4 weeks, then the patient stabilizes and rehabilitation can begin; however, convalescence may be lengthy, from 3 months to 2 years.

2. Instruct the patient in breathing exercises or use of an incentive spirometer to reestablish normal breathing patterns.

3. Teach the patient to wear good supportive and protective shoes while out of bed to prevent injuries due to weakness and paresthesias.

4. Instruct the patient to check feet routinely for injuries because trauma may go unnoticed due to sensory changes.

5. Urge the patient to maintain normal weight; additional weight will further stress motor function.

6. Encourage scheduled rest periods to avoid fatigue.

7. Refer the patient and family to agencies such as:

The Guillain-Barré Syndrome Foundation, International
PO Box 262
Wynnewood, PA 19096
610-667-0131

Head Injury

Head injury, also known as brain injury, is the disruption of normal brain function due to trauma (blunt or penetrating injury). Neurologic deficits result from shearing of white matter, ischemia and mass effect from hemorrhage, and cerebral edema of surrounding brain tissue. Types of brain injuries include *concussion, cerebral contusion, brain stem contusion, epidural hematoma, subdural hematoma,* and *skull fracture.*

◆ Assessment

1. Signs of increased intracranial pressure (IICP)—altered level of consciousness, abnormal pupil responses, vomiting, widened pulse pressure, bradycardia, hyperthermia
2. Headache, vertigo, confusion, possibly coma, resulting from IICP or intracranial bleeding
3. Respiratory irregularities (Cheyne-Stokes respirations, periods of apnea)
4. Cerebrospinal fluid leakage at ears and nose, which may indicate skull fracture
5. Contusions about eyes and ears or other signs of injury
6. Possible cranial nerves, motor, sensory, or deep tendon reflex dysfunction
7. Decreased consciousness or behavioral alterations, such as agitation, restlessness, impulsivity, uninhibited aggression, emotional lability

NURSING ALERT
Regard every patient who has a brain injury as having a potential spinal cord injury. Many patients are under the influence of alcohol at the time of injury, which may mask the nature and severity of the injury.

◆ Diagnostic Evaluation

1. Computed tomography or magnetic resonance imaging to identify and localize lesions, cerebral edema, bleeding
2. Skull and cervical spine x-rays to identify fracture, displacement
3. Neuropsychological tests during rehabilitation phase to determine cognitive deficits

◆ Collaborative Management

Pharmacologic Interventions

1. Management of IICP—osmotic diuretics, corticosteroids, mechanical hyperventilation, barbiturates to induce coma
2. Antibiotics to prevent infection in open skull fractures or penetrating wounds

Surgical Interventions

1. Surgery may be necessary for evacuation of intracranial hematomas, debridement of penetrating wounds, elevation of skull fractures or repair of CSF leaks.

◆ Nursing Interventions

Monitoring

1. Maintain intracranial pressure monitoring, as indicated, and report abnormalities.
2. Monitor for signs of meningitis or ventriculitis as a result of skull fracture, and for respiratory, urinary tract, or systemic infection caused by immobility.
3. Monitor results of serial serum and urine electrolyte and osmolality studies to maintain the level of dehydration ordered to reduce cerebral edema.
4. Monitor hemodynamic measurements to guide fluid replacement.
5. Monitor urinary output.
6. Monitor respiratory rate, depth, and pattern of respirations; report any abnormal pattern such as Cheyne-Stokes respirations or periods of apnea.
7. Maintain constant vigilance of agitated patient confined to bed and avoid restraints if possible.

H

Supportive Care

1. Maintain a patent airway.
2. Restrict fluid intake if needed to avoid increased ICP.
3. Administer IV solutions slowly to avoid overhydration and cerebral edema.
4. Insert urethral catheter to measure urinary output.
5. Assist with intubation and ventilatory assistance if needed.
6. To facilitate respirations, turn the patient every 2 hours and encourage coughing and deep breathing.
7. Suction the patient as needed; hyperventilate the patient before suctioning to prevent hypoxia.
8. Feed the patient as soon as possible after a head injury and administer histamine 2 (H_2) blocking agents to prevent gastric ulceration and hemorrhage from gastric acid hypersecretion.
9. If the patient is unable to swallow, provide hyperalimentation, then enteral feedings once bowel sounds have returned.
10. Elevate the head of the bed after feedings and check residuals to prevent aspiration.

H

❖

NURSING ALERT
Caloric needs of the head-injured patient are similar to those of a patient with 30% body burns. Consult your dietitian to institute hyperalimentation within the first 2 to 3 days after injury to support the recovery process.

11. During rehabilitation, recognize the dysphagic patient and encourage oral feeding of soft or pureed foods. Refer to speech or physical therapist as indicated for feeding difficulties.
12. Provide stimulation of all sensory avenues. Orient the patient to time and place.
13. Observe the patient for fatigue or restlessness from overstimulation.
14. Involve the family in sensory stimulation program; refer the patient for cognitive retraining if appropriate.
15. Warn the family regarding restlessness and combat-

iveness that may occur during recovery from brain injury.

16. Pad side rails, and wrap hands in mitts if the patient is agitated.
17. Investigate for physical sources of restlessness such as uncomfortable position, signs of urinary tract infection (UTI), or pressure sores.
18. Provide adequate light if the patient is hallucinating.
19. Perform passive range-of-motion exercises to release muscle tension from inactivity.
20. Avoid sedatives to avoid medication-induced confusion and altered states of cognition.
21. Refer the family to social worker and community support services such as respite care.

COMMUNITY CARE CONSIDERATIONS
Observe for signs of postconcussion syndrome (PCS), which include headache, decreased concentration, irritability, dizziness, insomnia, restlessness, diminished memory, anxiety, easy fatigability, and alcohol intolerance. Be aware that persistence of these symptoms can interfere with relationships and employability of the patient. Encourage the patient and family to report these symptoms and obtain additional support and counseling as needed. PCS may persist as long as 1 to 2 years.

H

Patient Education and Health Maintenance

1. Review with the family the signs of increased ICP.
2. Teach the family therapeutic use of touch, massage, and music to calm the agitated patient.
3. Refer the patient and family to agencies such as:

National Brain Injury Foundation
1776 Massachusetts Ave. NW
Washington, DC 20036
202-296-6443

Headache

Headache is one of the most common human ailments. Tension and vascular headaches are the most common types. Tension headaches result from irritation of sensitive nerve endings in the head, jaw, and neck caused by prolonged muscle contraction and often are related to prolonged or abnormal posture, or teeth clenching. Vascular headaches (including migraine and cluster headaches) are thought to result from genetically based serotonin abnormalities. In these headaches, pain and other phenomena result from constriction and dilation of intracranial and extracranial arteries. Other types of headache result from infection (sinusitis) or inflammation caused by an underlying disorder (temporal arteritis).

◆ Assessment

1. *Tension headache:* Pain and pressure in the back of the head and neck, across forehead, bitemporal areas; dull, persistent ache; tender spots of head or neck
2. *Migraine headache:* Preceded by sensory, motor, or mood alterations. Scintillating scotoma, hemianopsia, and paresthesias may occur with classic migraine; nausea, vomiting, and photophobia may occur with common migraine. Gradual onset of severe unilateral, throbbing pain that may become bilateral occurs. May be triggered in women by hormonal fluctuations (menses, pregnancy)
3. *Cluster headache:* Pain is severe, unilateral, always occurs on the same side, and occurs suddenly at the same time of day, sometimes at night; occurs in clusters of 2 to 8 weeks followed by periods of remission. Associated with unilateral excessive tearing, redness of the eye, facial swelling, flushing, and sweating. Attacks last 20 minutes to 2 hours. Several attacks may occur in 1 day.
4. *Sinus headache:* Pain is usually felt over sinus areas; above the eyes, along the side of the nose, and in the cheeks. May be accompanied by fever, nasal drainage, erythema, swelling and tenderness of the sinus areas with acute sinusitis
5. *Temporal arteritis:* Unilateral or bilateral pain is particularly severe at night with tender temporal areas.

◆ Diagnostic Evaluation

1. Skull and sinus x-rays may be done to rule out headache-related lesions or sinusitis.

2. Computed tomography or magnetic resonance imaging to rule out lesions or hemorrhage
3. Erythrocyte sedimentation rate (ESR) elevated in temporal arteritis

◆ Collaborative Management

Therapeutic Interventions

1. Nonpharmacologic management includes relaxation techniques, such as distraction, imagery, and progressive muscle relaxation, as well as biofeedback to control pain
2. Avoidance of tyramine-containing foods (eg, cheese or chocolate) to prevent migraines
3. Inhalation of 100% oxygen to abort a cluster headache

Pharmacologic Interventions

1. Aspirin, acetaminophen, and nonsteroidal antiinflammatory drugs for mild to moderate pain of tension, sinus, or mild vascular headaches
2. Antihistamines and decongestants for sinus headaches
3. Drugs to terminate vascular headaches at their onset, including methysergide, a serotonin antagonist; ergotamine, a vasoconstrictor; or sumatriptan, a 5-HT agonist.
4. Beta-adrenergic blocking agents, calcium channel blockers, or antidepressants as prophylaxis against recurrent migraines
5. Corticosteroids for temporal arteritis
6. Narcotic analgesics, muscle relaxants, and antianxiety agents for severe pain of any headache

◆ Nursing Interventions

Supportive Care

1. Reduce environmental stimuli such as light, noise, movement.
2. To relieve tension headaches:
   a. Suggest light massage of tight muscles in neck, scalp, and back.
   b. Apply warm, moist heat to areas of muscle tension.
   c. Teach progressive muscle relaxation.

H

3. Encourage the patient to lie down and attempt to sleep. Encourage adequate rest once headache is relieved to recover from fatigue of the pain.
4. Encourage the patient to become aware of triggering factors and early symptoms of headache, so it can be prevented or promptly treated.
5. Encourage adequate nutrition, rest and relaxation, and avoidance of stress and overexertion to better cope with headaches.
6. Review coping mechanisms and strengthen positive ones.

Patient Education and Health Maintenance

1. Teach proper administration of medications:
   a. Sumatriptan, given subcutaneously with autoinjector for quick relief, or given orally.
   b. Ergotamine given through metered dose inhaler.
   c. Take pain medications at onset of headache and repeat as prescribed.
2. Teach side effects of headache medications. Reportable adverse effects include:
   a. Numbness, coldness, parasthesias, and pain of extremities with ergot derivatives
   b. Chest pain, wheezing, or flushing with sumatriptan
   c. Lightheadedness and hypotension with beta-blockers and calcium channel blockers. (Warn the patient using beta-blockers to arise slowly, adhere to prescribed dosage, and avoid abrupt withdrawal of the drug.)
3. Warn the patient to avoid alcohol, which can aggravate headaches.
4. Teach the patient with migraines to avoid foods high in tyramine.

Heart Disease, Congenital

Congenital heart disease (CHD) refers to a variety of structural malformations of the heart or great vessels, which are present at birth but not necessarily diagnosed at that time. An individual heart defect or a combination of defects may be present. The exact cause of CHD is unknown in approximately 90% of cases. In general, it results from abnormal embryonic development or the persistence of fetal structure beyond the time of normal involution.

Congenital heart disease is the most common form of heart disease in children; 8 of every 1,000 live births. Children with CHD are more likely to have extracardiac defects, such as tracheoesophageal fistula, renal agenesis, and diaphragmatic hernia. Complications include congestive heart failure (see p. 398), infective endocarditis, sudden death, and stroke caused by embolus.

Congenital cardiac anomalies are generally classified by the presence or absence of cyanosis. However, there may be variations in the clinical presentation because of the degree of defect and individual response. Acyanotic congenital heart disease includes:

1. Obstructive lesions (normal pulmonary blood flow)
   a. Aortic valvular stenosis
   b. Pulmonic stenosis
   c. Coarctation of the aorta
2. Left-to-right shunts (increased pulmonary blood flow)
   a. Patent ductus arteriosus (PDA)
   b. Atrial septal defect (ASD)
   c. Ventricular septal defect (VSD)

Cyanotic congenital heart disease includes:

1. Right-to-left shunts (decreased pulmonary blood flow)
   a. Tetralogy of Fallot
   b. Tricuspid atresia
2. Mixed blood flow
   a. Transposition of great arteries
   b. Total anomalous pulmonary venous return
   c. Truncus arteriosus
   d. Hypoplastic left heart syndrome

See Table 8 for Assessment and Collaborative Management

◆ Diagnostic Evaluation

1. Chest x-ray may show cardiomegaly.
2. Electrocardiogram may show hypertrophy and axis deviation.

(text continues on p. 390)

H

TABLE 8 Congenital Heart Abnormalities

Description	Assessment	Management
Aortic Valvular Stenosis Occurs when there is obstruction to the left ventricular outflow at the level of the valve; accounts for 6% of all congenital heart defects Causes left ventricular hypertrophy, left heart failure, and pulmonary edema	Rarely symptomatic during infancy; may be evidence of decreased cardiac output, such as faint peripheral pulses; pale, gray, cool skin, in infants with severe cases Chest pain, dyspnea, fatigue, and shortness of breath with exertion in older children. Narrow pulse pressure Fainting spells Exercise intolerance Harsh, low-pitched systolic ejection murmur, maximal at the second right intercostal space, radiates to apex, back, neck	1. Treat congestive heart failure. 2. Restrict exercise. 3. Institute precautions against bacterial endocarditis. 4. Surgical management with aortic valvulotomy, prosthetic valve replacement, or balloon dilatation

Pulmonic Stenosis

Refers to any lesion that obstructs the flow of blood from the right ventricle. It accounts for 8% of congenital heart defects; 90% of obstruction occurs at the level of the pulmonary valve. Right ventricular pressure increases and can cause right ventricular hypertrophy and eventual right-sided heart failure in severe cases.

Generally asymptomatic, may be decreased exercise tolerance with fatigue and dyspnea

With severe obstruction, may have dyspnea and cyanosis

Older child may complain of precordial pain

Systolic ejection murmur over pulmonic area

1. Treat CHF.
2. Institute precautions against bacterial endocarditis.
3. Administer prostaglandin E_1 (PGE_1) to maintain patency of ductus arteriosus until surgical correction.
4. Asymptomatic children with moderate pulmonic stenosis should be evaluated at regular intervals for progression of the lesion
5. Valvulotomy, balloon dilatation, or shunt (palliative) for symptomatic cases.

H

(continued)

TABLE 8 (Continued)

Description	Assessment	Management
Coarctation of the Aorta Refers to a narrowing or constriction of the aorta at any point (usually just distal to origin of the left subclavian artery near ductus arteriosus). Left ventricular pressure and workload are increased; collateral vessels bypass the constriction and maintain circulation to lower extremities. Accounts for 6% of congenital heart defects.	Usually asymptomatic in childhood—growth and development are normal Child may demonstrate fatigue, headache, dizziness, nosebleeds, leg cramps, cold feet Absent or greatly reduced femoral pulsations; full bounding carotid pulses; wide pulse pressure Hypertension in upper extremities and diminished blood pressure in lower extremities Severe anomalies cause symptoms in infants, including poor feeding, growth failure, tachypnea, dyspnea, peripheral edema, acidosis, and severe CHF Nonspecific systolic murmur heard along the left sternal border	1. Treat CHF. 2. Administer prostaglandin E_1 (PGE_1) infusion to maintain ductal patency and maintain blood flow below the coarctation. 3. Surgical management indicated for infants who present in the first 6 months of life with heart failure and recommended for children aged 2–4 years with significant coarctation.

H

Patent Ductus Arteriosus
Refers to persistence of a fetal connection (ductus arteriosus) between the pulmonary artery and the aorta, resulting in a left-to-right shunt. PDA accounts for 10% of congenital heart defects. 15% of infants with PDA have other heart defects.

Small PDA: Usually asymptomatic

Large PDA: May develop symptoms in very early infancy: slow weight gain, feeding difficulties, decreased exercise tolerance, frequent respiratory infections, dyspnea

May have a wide pulse pressure or bounding posterior tibial and dorsalis pedis pulses

Continuous machinery-like murmur at the left intraclavicular area is heard in most older children. Neonates with PDA have a variety of murmurs.

1. Treat CHF.
2. Indomethacin appears to trigger the natural closing of the ductus. Treatment of choice for preterm infants
3. Surgical division of the PDA (closed heart surgery through lateral thoracotomy incision to ligate the ductus) may be done in early infancy if CHF develops and cannot be controlled; or may be done electively by age 1–2 years.

H

(continued)

TABLE 8 (Continued)

Description	Assessment	Management
Atrial Septal Defect Refers to an abnormal opening in the septum between the left atrium and the right atrium. In general, left-to-right shunting occurs. If pulmonary vascular resistance produces pulmonary hypertension, shunt is reversed, causing cyanosis. ASD accounts for 9% of congenital heart defects. Two main types: Ostium secundum (most common—due to abnormal development of septum secundum) Ostium primum (due to abnormal development of septum primum) Spontaneous closure occurs in a small percentage of patients.	Ostium secundum type is generally asymptomatic even when this defect is large Ostium primum type is generally asymptomatic, although the following may occur: low weight gain, fatigability, dyspnea with exertion, frequent respiratory infections, CHF, hypertension related to pulmonary edema Systolic, medium-pitched ejection murmur heard best at the second left interspace. Fixed widely split-second sound	1. Treat CHF. 2. Institute precautions for bacterial endocarditis. 3. Closure may be achieved by open heart surgery through medial sternotomy incision, with cardiopulmonary bypass by suture or patch.

H

Ventricular Septal Defect

Refers to an abnormal opening in the septum between the right and left ventricles. It may vary in size from very small defects to very large defects and may occur in either the membranous or the muscular portion of the ventricular septum. Left-to-right shunting occurs. If pulmonary vascular resistance produced pulmonary hypertension, shunt is reversed, causing cyanosis.

VSD accounts for 25%–29% of all congenital heart defects

Small VSDs: usually asymptomatic (many close spontaneously)

Large VSDs: may develop symptoms as early as age 1–2 months

Slow weight gain, failure to thrive

Feeding difficulties; increased fatigue

Pale, delicate-looking, scrawny appearance

Frequent respiratory infections

Tachypnea, excessive sweating, CHF

Harsh holosystolic murmur is heard best at the fourth interspace to the left of the sternum.

1. Treat CHF if this occurs in early infancy.

2. Surgical patch closure if CHF resists medical management.

3. Early pulmonary artery banding to decrease pulmonary blood flow and control CHF in patients with pulmonary hypertension to avoid irreversible pulmonary bed changes. Later, debanding and patch closure

4. Surgery is contraindicated if shunt is reversed.

H

(continued)

TABLE 8 (Continued)

Description	Assessment	Management
Tetralogy of Fallot Refers to a cyanotic heart defect consisting of four abnormalities 1. pulmonary stenosis 2. ventricular septal defect 3. overriding (dextraposition) of the aorta 4. right ventricular hypertrophy Right-to-left shunting occurs by ventricular septal defect directly into aorta, causing ventricular hypertrophy and shunting of unoxygenated blood back through the body. Most common defect causing cyanosis in children surviving past 2 years, accounting for 6%–10% of all congenital heart defects.	Cyanosis—onset and severity varies Clubbing of the fingers and toes Squatting (used after exertion once they can walk) Slow weight gain; failure to thrive Dyspnea on exertion Hypoxic spells ("tet" spells); transient cerebral ischemia Systolic ejection murmur at the second and third interspaces to the left of the sternum. Prominent ejection click immediately after the first heart sound	1. Management of tet spell—immediately place child in knee–chest position with head of bed elevated, administer oxygen by mask. 2. Palliative surgery: Blalock–Taussig shunt or Waterston shunt 3. Corrective surgery (treatment of choice): removal of shunt if previously performed with cardiopulmonary bypass. VSD is repaired with patch closure, and right ventricular outflow obstruction is relieved.

H

Transposition of the Great Arteries

TGA occurs when the pulmonary artery originates posteriorly from the left ventricle and the aorta originates anteriorly from the right ventricle. Causes 2 separate circulations: right heart manages systemic circulation (unoxygenated) and left heart manages pulmonary circulation (oxygenated). The two must be linked by an abnormal defect to sustain life. TGA accounts for 5%–10% of congenital heart defects.

Cyanosis, usually developing shortly after birth (degree depends on the type of associated malformations)

Low Apgar score at birth

Fatigability

Slow weight gain, although birth weight normal or above normal

Clubbing of the fingers and toes

Coexistence of CHF, manifested by tachypnea, cardiomegaly, hepatomegaly

Murmurs possibly absent in infancy; may be a murmur of an associated defect

1. Treat CHF vigorously.
2. Palliative procedures to allow improved interatrial mixing
   a. Rashkind procedure: creation of an atrial septal defect with a balloon catheter during cardiac catheterization
   b. Blalock–Hanlon procedure: surgical creation of an ASD
   c. Medical use of PGE to keep PDA open
3. Complete correction (redirection of blood flow assisted by cardiopulmonary bypass): Mustard procedure, Senning procedure, Rastelli procedure, newer procedures for correcting TGA by direct contraposition of the transposed vessels

(continued)

H

TABLE 8 *(Continued)*

Description	Assessment	Management
Tricuspid Atresia Refers to a condition in which there is 1. atresia of the tricuspid valve which disconnects the right atrium and right ventricle 2. interatrial septal defect (or patent foramen ovale 3. a small right ventricle Blood from the systemic circulation is shunted from right atrium through an ASD to the left atrium and then to the left ventricle. The lungs may receive blood through a PDA, bronchial circulation, or VSD.	Severe cyanosis in neonatal period Respiratory distress on exertion Clubbing Hypoxic spells Delayed weight gain Possible right heart failure Fatigability Pansystolic murmurs audible along left sternal border	1. Treat CHF. 2. PGE_1 infusion maintains ductal patency. 3. Palliative procedures to increase pulmonary blood flow: balloon septostomy, Waterston shunt, Glenn procedure, Blalock–Taussig shunt 4. Complete correction: Fontan procedure or placement of tubular conduit with valve between right atrium and main pulmonary artery

H

Hypoplastic Left Heart Syndrome

Refers to a condition in which there is

1. mitral atresia or stenosis
2. a diminutive or absent left ventricle
3. failure of the aortic valve to develop, resulting in aortic atresia, a severe hypoplastic ascending aorta, and aortic arch (severe coarctation of aorta).

The right ventricle must pump blood through both pulmonary and systemic circulations. Death occurs in more than half of the cases in the first few months of life.

May appear normal at birth; signs increase shortly afterward

CHF, dyspnea, hepatomegaly

Low cardiac output—pallor, mild to moderate cyanosis or a grayish color, weak peripheral pulses, decreased blood pressure

Nondescript systolic murmur

1. Treat CHF.
2. PGE; infusion maintains ductal patency until surgery.
3. Norwood procedure (staged approach) to establish systemic and pulmonary circulations
4. Fontan procedure, arterial switch, or cardiac transplantation also may be done.

H

3. Echocardiography, Doppler study, and color flow mapping show characteristic changes.
4. Cardiac catheterization may be done for further evaluation.

◆ Nursing Interventions

Monitoring

1. Assess and document growth and development parameters (including weight, length, head circumference, motor coordination, muscular development, cognitive abilities, and psychosocial skills).
2. Monitor exercise tolerance.
   a. Observe child at play and watch for squatting (characteristic position assumed by cyanotic child when resting after exertion).
   b. Be alert for infant who may stop feeding to rest or may fall asleep during feeding. Assess pulse and respirations during feeding.
3. Monitor skin and mucous membranes for color and temperature changes.
   a. Color changes vary from pink, dusky, mottled to cyanotic.
   b. Mucous membranes are vascular and indicate color changes quickly.
   c. Circumoral cyanosis is good indicator of central cyanosis.
4. Assess for clubbing of fingers, especially the thumbnails—may occur in cyanotic children by age 2 to 3 months.
5. Monitor for increased respiratory rate, grunting, retractions, nasal flaring, irregularity of respirations, weak cry.
   a. Infants—respirations greater than 60 breaths/min indicate respiratory difficulty.
   b. Young children—respirations greater than 40 breaths/min indicate respiratory difficulty.
6. Monitor pulses in all extremities.

PEDIATRIC ALERT
Radial or dorsalis pedis is difficult to feel in the newborn. Femoral pulsations are easily felt in the inguinal region and can be compared with brachial pulsations.

H

7. Monitor heart sounds to evaluate rhythm and any murmurs.
8. Monitor vital signs (apical pulse, blood pressure, respirations). Record which extremity is used for blood pressure measurement. Make sure that blood pressure cuff is the appropriate size for the child.
9. Monitor serum drug levels of digoxin and watch for signs of digoxin toxicity—bradycardia, nausea, vomiting, anorexia.

Supportive Care

1. To facilitate breathing, position the infant or child at a 45-degree angle (orthopnic position) to decrease pressure of the viscera on the diaphragm and increase lung volume.
   a. Tilt the infant's or child's head back slightly.
   b. Pin diapers loosely; provide loose-fitting pajamas for older children.
   c. Feed slowly to avoid risk of aspiration. Observe for abdominal distention, which may increase respiratory difficulty.
2. Suction the nose and throat if the child is unable to adequately cough up secretions.
3. Provide oxygen therapy as indicated.
4. Restrict fluids as ordered and maintain strict intake and output.
5. To improve cardiac output, organize nursing care to provide periods of uninterrupted rest.
   a. Avoid unnecessary activities such as frequent, complete baths and clothing changes; avoid excessive handling.
   b. Prevent excessive crying in infant; anticipate needs.
   c. Avoid temperature excesses; maintain normothermia.
6. Provide diversional activities for child that require limited expenditures of energy; provide passive play.
7. Try to prevent constipation with stool softeners or glycerin suppositories as ordered.
8. Provide small, frequent feedings; provide foods easy to chew and digest.
   a. Feeding should generally be completed within 45

H

minutes or sooner if the infant tires. Use soft nipples with large holes.

  b. Provide foods that have high nutritional value. Include foods high in iron and potassium levels, if needed.

 9. Maintain adequate hydration in the cyanotic child when vomiting, has diarrhea or fever, or is exposed to high environmental temperatures, because polycythemia predisposes to thrombosis.

10. To avoid infection, prevent exposure to children with upper respiratory infections, diarrhea, wound infections, and other contagious disorders.

11. Report temperature elevation, diarrhea, vomiting, and upper respiratory symptoms promptly.

Family Education and Health Maintenance

1. Instruct the family in necessary measures to maintain the child's health:
   a. Complete immunization
   b. Adequate diet and rest
   c. Prevention and control of infections
   d. Regular medical and dental checkups. The child should be given prophylactic antibiotics to prevent infective endocarditis when undergoing certain dental or genitourinary procedures.
   e. Regular cardiac checkups

2. Teach the family about the cardiac defect and its treatment, and any complications.
   a. Recognize and report signs and symptoms of complications, signs of infection, dehydration.
   b. Emergency precautions related to hypoxic attacks, pulmonary edema, cardiac arrest (if appropriate)
   c. Special home care equipment, monitors, and oxygen

3. Encourage the parents and other persons (teachers, peers, etc.) to treat the child in as normal a manner as possible.

4. Initiate home nursing referral and refer the family to appropriate resources, for example, social worker, organized support groups, and the

   American Heart Association
   772 Greenville Ave.
   Dallas, TX 75231
   214-373-6300

Heart Failure

Heart failure, also known as congestive heart failure (CHF), is a clinical syndrome that results from the heart's inability to pump sufficient oxygenated blood to meet the body's metabolic requirements. Compensatory mechanisms of increased heart rate, vasoconstriction, and hypertrophy eventually fail, leading to the characteristic syndrome of heart failure: elevated ventricular/atrial pressures, sodium and water retention, decreased cardiac output, and circulatory and pulmonary congestion. The left ventricle may fail initially, but in time, the right ventricle fails because of the additional workload. Combined left and right ventricular failure is common.

Causes of CHF include disorders of heart muscle that reduce cardiac contractility, such as myocarditis, pericarditis, myocardial infarction, congenital or acquired valvular disease, hypertension, and cardiomyopathy.

Complications of CHF include refractory heart failure leading to death, cardiac dysrhythmias, myocardial failure, pulmonary infarction, pneumonia, and emboli.

H

◆ Assessment

1. Manifestations of left-sided heart failure (forward failure):
   a. Shortness of breath, dyspnea on exertion, paroxysmal nocturnal dyspnea (caused by reabsorption of dependent edema that has developed during the day), orthopnea, cough (may be dry, unproductive; often occurs at night), fatigability, insomnia, restlessness
   b. Pulmonary edema (see p. 692)
2. Manifestations of right-sided heart failure (backward failure):
   a. Edema of ankles and feet (pitting edema is obvious only after retention of at least 4.5 kg or 10 lbs. of fluid), unexplained weight gain, upper abdominal pain (caused by liver congestion), anorexia and nausea (caused by hepatic and visceral engorgement, nocturia, weakness)

   b. Distended neck veins; pleural effusion, ascites, and other abnormal fluid accumulations
3. Cardiovascular findings in both left- and right-sided failure:
   a. Cardiomegaly—detected by displaced position of maximal impulse (PMI)
   b. S3 ventricular gallop by auscultation
   c. Rapid heart rate
   d. Pulsus alternans (alternating weak and strong beats)
4. History of precipitating stressor that may have overwhelmed compensatory mechanisms:
   a. Infection, fever
   b. Surgery, anesthesia
   c. Transfusions, IV infusions
   d. Pregnancy
   e. Anemia, hemorrhage
   f. Physical and emotional stress
   g. Excessive sodium intake

◆ Diagnostic Evaluation

1. 12-lead ECG will show ventricular hypertrophy and strain.
2. Chest x-ray will show cardiomegaly and possible pleural effusion and pulmonary vascular congestion.
3. Echocardiography will detect hypertrophy, dilation of chambers, and abnormal contraction.
4. Arterial blood gas analysis may be done to detect hypoxemia.
5. Liver function tests may be elevated with hepatic congestion.
6. Digoxin level, serum electrolytes, and kidney function tests also may be done to monitor condition.

◆ Collaborative Management

Pharmacologic Interventions

1. Diuretics eliminate excess body water and decrease ventricular pressures. Institute a low-sodium diet and fluid restrictions to complement this therapy.
2. Positive inotropic agents such as digoxin improve myo-

cardial contractility and increase the heart's ability to pump more effectively.

3. Vasodilators decrease cardiac workload by dilating peripheral vessels, thus reducing ventricular filling pressures (preload) and volumes, and reducing impedance to left ventricular ejection and thus improving stroke volume.

4. Angiotensin-converting enzyme (ACE) inhibitors such as captopril inhibit angiotensin II, a potent vasoconstrictor, thus decreasing left ventricular afterload, which reduces heart rate and cardiac workload, thereby increasing cardiac output.

◆ Nursing Interventions

Monitoring

1. Monitor for lowering of systolic pressure, narrowing of pulse pressure, and pulsus alternans, indicating progression of left ventricular failure.

❖

NURSING ALERT
Watch for sudden unexpected hypotension, which can cause myocardial ischemia and decrease perfusion to vital organs.

H

2. Auscultate heart sounds frequently, noting appearance of a new gallop or irregular heart beat.

3. Observe for signs/symptoms of reduced peripheral tissue perfusion: cool temperature of skin, pallor, and poor capillary refill of nailbeds.

4. Auscultate lung fields every 4 hours for crackles and wheezes in dependent lung fields. Mark with water-soluble ink the level on the patient's back where adventitious breath sounds are heard; use markings for comparative assessment over time.

5. Observe for increased rate of respirations (may indicate falling arterial pH) and Cheyne-Stokes respirations (may occur in elderly because of a decrease in cerebral perfusion).

6. Monitor intake and output and daily weight to determine adequate kidney perfusion and fluid balance.

7. Monitor potassium levels while patient is on diuretic therapy and observe for symptoms of hypokalemia: fatigue, anorexia, nausea and vomiting, muscle weakness, and dysrhythmias.

8. Monitor digoxin levels as indicated, and watch for signs of digitalis toxicity: fatigue, muscle weakness, anorexia, nausea, and yellow-green halos around objects.

Supportive Care

1. Place the patient at physical and emotional rest to reduce cardiac workload. Offer careful explanations and answers to the patient's questions. Avoid situations that tend to promote anxiety/agitation.

   a. Provide rest in semirecumbent position or in armchair in air-conditioned environment. (Recumbency also promotes diuresis by improving renal perfusion.)

   b. Provide a bedside commode, to reduce effort of toileting.

   c. Assist the patient with self-care activities early in the day to avoid fatigue.

2. Position the patient to minimize dyspnea.

   a. Raise the head of the bed 20 to 30 cm (8–10 in.) to reduce venous return to the heart and lungs and alleviate pulmonary congestion.

   b. Support lower arms with pillows to reduce the burden on the shoulder muscles.

   c. Have an orthopneic patient sit on the side of the bed with feet supported by a chair, head and arms resting on an over-the-bed table, and lumbosacral area supported with pillows.

   d. Reposition the patient every 2 hours (or encourage the patient to change position frequently) to help prevent atelectasis and pneumonia.

3. Administer oxygen as directed.

4. Encourage deep-breathing exercises every 1 to 2 hours to avoid atelectasis.

5. Use "egg-crate" mattress and sheepskin to prevent pressure sores (poor blood flow and edema increase susceptibility).

6. Offer small, frequent feedings to avoid excessive gastric filling, abdominal distention, and reduced lung capacity. To prevent hypokalemia from diuretic therapy, en-

H

courage foods or juices high in potassium, such as apricots, bananas, or tomatoes.

7. Caution patients to avoid added salt in food and foods with high sodium content.
8. Increase the patient's activities gradually. Alter or modify activities to keep within the limits of cardiac reserve.
9. Relieve nighttime anxiety and provide for rest and sleep. Give appropriate sedation to relieve insomnia and restlessness.

Patient Education/Health Maintenance

1. Explain the disease process to the patient; the term "failure" may have terrifying implications. Explain the difference between "heart attack" and congestive heart failure.
2. Teach the signs and symptoms of recurrence.
   a. Advise the patient to weigh self at same time daily to detect any tendency toward fluid retention and to report a weight gain of more than 2 to 3 pounds (0.9–1.4 kg) in a few days.
   b. Advise the patient to report swelling of ankles, feet, or abdomen; persistent cough; tiredness; loss of appetite; and frequent urination at night.
3. Review the patient's medication regimen.
   a. Teach the patient to take and record pulse rate and blood pressure.
   b. If the patient is taking oral potassium solution, it may be diluted with juice and taken after a meal.
   c. Explain major side effects and signs of toxicity that should be reported.
4. Review the patient's activity program. Instruct the patient to increase walking and other activities gradually, provided they do not cause fatigue and dyspnea. In general, the patient can continue at whatever activity level can be maintained without the appearance of symptoms.
5. Encourage a weight reduction program until optimal weight is reached.
6. Advise avoidance of extremes in heat and cold—which increase the work of the heart; air conditioning may be essential in a hot, humid environment.

H

7. Urge the patient to keep regular appointments with a health care provider or clinic.
8. Educate the patient to restrict dietary sodium, as indicated.
   a. Teach the patient that sodium is present in antacids, cough remedies, laxatives, pain relievers, estrogens, and other drugs. Advise the patient to examine all labels to ascertain sodium content.
   b. Teach the patient to rinse the mouth well after using tooth cleansers and mouthwashes—some of these contain large amounts of sodium. Water softeners are to be avoided.
   c. Encourage use of flavorings, spices, herbs, and lemon juice.
   d. If the patient has renal disease, warn against using potassium chloride–containing salt substitutes.

Heart Failure in Children

Heart failure, also called congestive heart failure (CHF), occurs when cardiac output is inadequate to meet the metabolic demands of the body. Compensatory mechanisms (increased heart rate, vasoconstriction, and hypertrophy) eventually fail, leading to the characteristic syndrome of heart failure: elevated ventricular/atrial pressures, sodium and water retention, decreased cardiac output, and circulatory and pulmonary congestion. The left ventricle may fail initially, but in time, the right ventricle fails because of the additional workload. Combined left and right ventricular failure is common.

Underlying causes of CHF include congenital heart disease, especially left-to-right shunts (the primary cause in the first 3 years of life); acquired heart disease (eg, rheumatic heart disease, endocarditis, myocarditis); and noncardiovascular causes such as acidosis, pulmonary disease, various metabolic diseases, and anemia.

Complications of CHF include pneumonia, pulmonary edema, pulmonary emboli, refractory heart failure, and myocardial failure.

◆ Assessment

1. Manifestations of left-sided heart failure (congestion occurs mainly in the lungs from backing up of blood into pulmonary veins and capillaries):
   a. Dyspnea, tachypnea, orthopnea
   b. Nonproductive, irritative cough
   c. Retractions, nasal flaring, grunting, cyanosis
2. Manifestations of right-sided heart failure (mainly signs and symptoms of elevated pressures and congestion in systemic veins and capillaries):
   a. Hepatomegaly/abdominal discomfort
   b. Peripheral, orbital, scrotal edema
   c. Neck vein distention
   d. Weight gain, oliguria
3. Manifestations of impaired myocardial function in both left- and right-sided failure:
   a. Tachycardia, restlessness
   b. Weak cry, easy fatigability
   c. Pallor, cool extremities, diaphoresis
   d. Decreased urine output
   e. Feeding difficulties or anorexia
   f. S3 gallop, possible murmur, lung field crackles (uncommon in infants)

H

◆ Diagnostic Evaluation

1. Chest x-ray shows cardiomegaly, pulmonary congestion.
2. Laboratory data—increased sodium (dilutional), decreased chloride, increased potassium
3. 12-lead ECG will show ventricular hypertrophy and strain.

◆ Collaborative Management

Pharmacologic Interventions

1. Digoxin to slow conduction through the atrioventricular node and increase cardiac contractility
2. Medications such as vasodilators and angiotensin-converting enzyme (ACE) inhibitors to reduce afterload and thus decrease cardiac workload
3. Diuretics to reduce intravascular fluid volume

◆ Nursing Interventions

Monitoring

1. Monitor digoxin levels as indicated and watch for signs of digitalis toxicity: anorexia, bradycardia, dysrhythmias, nausea, vomiting, diarrhea, fatigue, muscle weakness, altered emotional status ("digitalis blues"— not as evident in young children).
2. Monitor serum electrolytes. Hypokalemia may cause weakened myocardial contractions and may precipitate digitalis toxicity.

NURSING ALERT

Hypokalemia can contribute to the development of digitalis toxicity even in the presence of low serum digoxin levels. Hypomagnesemia and hypercalcemia also may aggravate digitalis toxicity.

---

3. Monitor the child's response to diuretic therapy.
4. Monitor vital signs and auscultate heart and lungs frequently.
5. Observe for signs and symptoms of reduced peripheral tissue perfusion: cool temperature of skin, facial pallor, and poor capillary refill of nailbeds.
6. Monitor intake and output and daily weight to determine kidney perfusion and fluid balance. Record urine specific gravity.

Supportive Care

1. Carefully calculate digoxin dosage *daily,* based on child's daily weight; digoxin is given to infants and children in very small amounts.
   a. Count apical pulse for 1 full minute before administering.

PEDIATRIC ALERT

Be aware of the heart rate at which the health care provider wants digoxin withheld (usually 90–100 beats/min for infants and 70 beats/min for older children). Contact health care provider if 2 consecutive doses are held.

---

b. Report vomiting, which may occur after administration of digoxin, to determine if health care provider desires dose to be repeated.

c. Observe for the development of premature ventricular contractions when digoxin is initially started; report this to health care provider.

2. Administer afterload-reduction medications cautiously.

a. Check blood pressure before and after administering.

b. Hold medication according to blood pressure parameters ordered by health care provider.

c. Notify health care provider if 2 consecutive doses are held.

d. Watch for hypotension.

3. Weigh the child at least daily to observe response to diuretic therapy (same time of day, same scale, same attire).

4. Encourage foods such as fruit juices, bananas, and tomatoes, which have a high potassium content, to prevent potassium depletion associated with many diuretics.

5. Administer oral potassium supplements as ordered when a child is on diuretics for an extended period.

6. Restrict sodium intake, as directed. Infants may require low-sodium formulas.

7. Restrict fluid intake; remember to count fluids used for medication administration in intake.

8. Administer oxygen therapy as directed to improve tissue oxygenation and relieve respiratory distress.

9. Anticipate the infant's needs to prevent excessive crying and reduce energy expenditure.

10. Provide diversional activities for child that require limited expenditure of energy.

11. To reduce danger of infection that could overwhelm compensatory mechanisms, avoid exposure to other children with upper respiratory infections, diarrhea, etc.

12. Report changes such as temperature elevation, diarrhea, vomiting, and upper respiratory symptoms promptly.

13. To support nutritional needs, provide foods that the

H

child enjoys in small amounts, because child may have a poor appetite because of liver enlargement.

14. For infant feeding, feed frequently in small amounts.
    a. Supplement oral feedings with gavage feeding if the infant is unable to take an adequate amount of formula by mouth. Consider tube feeding during sleeping hours.

15. To reduce anxiety, correct misinterpretations about treatment and allow parents and child to ask questions and express concerns.

Family Education and Health Maintenance

1. Teach signs and symptoms of CHF.
2. Teach home medications, including side effects, with holding parameters, toxic effects. Reinforce need to maintain schedule.
3. Teach home management if signs and symptoms develop (ie, oxygen therapy, fluid restriction, extra dose of diuretics as ordered by health care provider).
4. Reinforce appropriate time to seek medical help. Teach home CPR.
5. Explain dietary or activity restrictions.
6. Explain methods to prevent infection.
7. Initiate a community health nursing referral if indicated.
8. Stress need for continued follow-up care.

H

Heart Surgery
See Cardiac Surgery

Heat Exhaustion and Heat Stroke

Heat exhaustion is the inadequacy or the collapse of peripheral circulation caused by volume and electrolyte depletion. Untreated heat exhaustion may progress to *heat stroke*, which is a life-threatening medical emergency. A combination of hyperpyrexia (40.6°C or 105°F) and neurologic symptoms, heat stroke is caused by failure of the heat-regulating mechanisms of the body. The heat stroke patient should be admitted to an intensive care unit; death may occur from complications such as heart failure, cardiovascular collapse, hepatic failure, renal failure, disseminated intravascular coagulation, and rhabdomyolysis.

◆ Assessment

1. With heat exhaustion expect the patient to be alert without significant cardiorespiratory or neurologic compromise.
   a. Symptoms include headache, fatigue, dizziness, muscle cramping, and nausea.
   b. Skin is usually pale, ashen, and moist.
   c. Hypotension, orthostatic changes
   d. Tachycardia, tachypnea
   e. Temperature may be normal, slightly elevated, or as high as 104°F (40°C).
2. In heat stroke, initially the patient may exhibit bizarre behavior or irritability. This may progress to confusion, combativeness, deliriousness, and coma.
   a. Other central nervous system disturbances include tremors, seizures, fixed and dilated pupils, and decerebrate or decorticate posturing.
   b. Temperature greater than 40.6°C or 105°F
   c. Hypotension, tachycardia, tachypnea
   d. Skin may appear flushed and hot. In early heat stroke, skin may be moist, but as heat stroke progresses, skin becomes dry as the body loses its ability to sweat.

◆ Diagnostic Evaluation

1. Laboratory tests show hemoconcentration (increased hematocrit) and hyponatremia (if sodium depletion in the primary problem) or hypernatremia (if water depletion is the primary problem).
2. Electrocardiogram may show dysrhythmias without evidence of infarction.
3. Arterial blood gas analysis shows metabolic acidosis in heat stroke.
4. As condition progresses, laboratory tests reflect renal failure and other complications.

H

◆ Collaborative Management

Therapeutic Interventions

1. Rapid body cooling is treatment of choice in exhaustion or stroke. In heat stroke, the core (internal) temperature should be reduced to 39°C (102°F) as rapidly as possible.

> **NURSING ALERT**
> Once the diagnosis of heat stroke is made or suspected, rapid reduction of the temperature is imperative.

2. In heat stroke, oxygen therapy is begun to supply tissue needs that are exaggerated by the hypermetabolic condition. Use 100% nonrebreather mask or intubate the patient if necessary to support a failing cardiorespiratory system.
3. Fluid replacement is begun to support circulation and facilitate cooling.
   a. Oral rehydrating solutions such as Gatorade may be used in heat exhaustion if patient is fully conscious and vital signs are stable.
   b. Otherwise, initial IV therapy is Ringer's lactate or normal saline until electrolyte results are confirmed.
   c. With heat stroke, at least one intravenous line should be a central line.
   d. Amount of fluid replacement is based on the patient's response and laboratory results.

> **GERONTOLOGIC ALERT**
> Vigorous fluid replacement in the elderly or those with underlying cardiovascular disease may cause pulmonary edema.

4. CPR may be necessary at any time if cardiorespiratory arrest occurs.

Pharmacologic Interventions

1. Diuretics to promote diuresis
2. Anticonvulsant agents to control seizures

3. Potassium for hypokalemia and sodium bicarbonate to correct metabolic acidosis, depending on laboratory results

4. Antipyretics are not useful in treating heat stroke. They may contribute to the complications of coagulopathy and hepatic damage.

5. Intense shivering may be controlled by diazepam (Valium). Shivering will generate heat and increase the metabolic rate.

6. Patients with depleted clotting factors may be treated with platelets or fresh frozen plasma.

◆ Nursing Interventions

Monitoring

1. In heat exhaustion, monitor for changes in cardiac rhythm and vital signs. Take vital signs at least every 15 minutes until the patient is stable.

2. In heat stroke, monitor and record the core temperature continually during cooling process to avoid hypothermia; also, hyperthermia may recur spontaneously within 3 to 4 hours.

3. Monitor vital signs continuously, including cardiac rhythm, central venous pressure, blood pressure, pulse, and respiratory rate, for possible ischemia, infarction, and dysrhythmias.

4. Perform neurologic assessment every 30 minutes.

5. Monitor urinary output at least hourly to detect acute tubular necrosis.

6. Monitor for development of seizures and provide a safe environment in case of seizures.

Supportive Care

1. Move the patient to a cool environment and remove all clothing.

2. Position the patient supine with the feet slightly elevated.

3. If the patient complains of nausea or vomiting, do not give fluids by mouth.

4. Provide fans and cool sponge baths as cooling methods.

5. In heat stroke, spray tepid water on the skin as electric fans blow continuously over the patient to augment heat dissipation.

H

   a. Apply ice packs to neck, groin, axillae, and scalp (areas of maximal heat transfer).
   b. Soak sheets or towels in ice water and place on the patient, using fans to accelerate evaporative cooling rate.
   c. Immerse the patient in cold water (controversial because it may result in peripheral vasoconstriction and may decrease the body's heat loss).
6. If the temperature fails to decrease, initiate core cooling: iced saline lavage of stomach, cool fluid peritoneal dialysis, cool fluid bladder irrigation, or cool fluid chest irrigations.
7. Place the patient on a hypothermia blanket.
8. Discontinue active cooling when the temperature reaches 39°C (102°F). In most cases, this will reduce the chance of overcooling because the body temperature will continue to decrease after cessation of cooling.

Patient Education and Health Maintenance

1. Advise the patient to avoid immediate re-exposure to high temperatures; the patient may remain hypersensitive to high temperatures for a considerable length of time.
2. Emphasize the importance of maintaining an adequate fluid intake, wearing loose clothing, and reducing activity in hot weather.
3. Advise athletes to monitor fluid losses, replace fluids, and use a gradual approach to physical conditioning, allowing sufficient time for acclimatization.

H

COMMUNITY CARE CONSIDERATIONS
Identify persons at increased risk for heat exhaustion and heat stroke so that preventive measures can be taken. Risk factors include underlying conditions such as cardiovascular disease, alcohol abuse, malnutrition, diabetes, skin diseases and major burn scarring; very young or very old age; drugs such as anticholinergics, phenothiazines, diuretics, antihistamines, antidepressants, and beta-blockers; and behaviors such as working outdoors, wearing inappropriate clothing, inadequate fluid intake, and living in poor environmental conditions.

Hemophilia

Hemophilia is usually an inherited, congenital bleeding disorder marked by a deficiency of specific blood clotting factors in the intrinsic phase of the coagulation cascade. The deficiency prevents formation of a stable fibrin clot.

There are three forms: a person with hemophilia A, or classic hemophilia, has a deficiency of factor VIII (80%–85% of patients), and a person with hemophilia B, or Christmas disease, has a deficiency of factor IX (15%–20% of patients). Factor XI deficiency or hemophilia C is quite rare. Spontaneous mutations may cause the condition when the family history is negative for the disease (approximately 20% of patients). As an X-linked recessive trait, hemophilia appears in males but is transmitted by females. Hemophilia affects 1 of every 5,000 males, in all ethnic groups.

Poor clotting may result in death from exsanguination after any serious hemorrhage in intracranial, airway, or other highly vascular areas, and a number of complications can arise from bleeding into body structures (degenerative joints, intestinal obstruction, compartment syndrome). Infection with human immunodeficiency virus is also a complication for many who received contaminated platelet transfusions before 1985. However, as a result of advances in replacement therapy (viral inactivation of human plasma, derived factor concentrates, and new recombinant factor VIII concentrate), a normal life span is now possible for many persons with hemophilia.

◆ Assessment

1. Hemophilia is seldom diagnosed in infancy unless excessive bleeding is observed from the umbilical cord or after circumcision. It is usually diagnosed after the child becomes active.
2. Severity of disease depends on the plasma level of the coagulation factor involved.
   a. A patient with less than 1% of normal often demonstrates severe clinical bleeding with a tendency for spontaneous bleeds.
   b. A patient in the 1%-to-5% range may be free of

H

spontaneous bleeding and may not manifest severe
bleeding until after trauma or during surgery.

   c. A patient in the 6% to 30% range is mildly afflicted
and usually leads a normal life and bleeds only on
severe injury or surgery.

3. Signs and symptoms of abnormal bleeding include:

   a. History of prolonged bleeding episodes, such as
after circumcision

   b. Easily bruised

   c. Prolonged bleeding from the mucous membranes
of the nose and mouth from lacerations

   d. Spontaneous soft tissue hematomas

   e. Hemorrhages into the joints (hemarthrosis)—especially elbows, knees, and ankles, causing pain,
swelling, limitation of movement, contractures, atrophy of adjacent muscles

   f. Spontaneous hematuria

   g. Gastrointestinal or rectal bleeding

   h. Black, tarry stools

   i. Cyclic bleeding episodes may occur, with periods of
slight bleeding followed by periods of severe
bleeding.

   j. Intracranial hemorrhage from head trauma

◆ Diagnostic Evaluation

1. Prothrombin time (PT) and bleeding time: normal
2. Partial thromboplastin time (PTT): prolonged
3. Prothrombin consumption: decreased
4. Thromboplastin: increased
5. Factor VIII or IX assays: abnormal
6. Gene analysis may be done to detect carrier state, for
prenatal diagnosis.

◆ Collaborative Management

Therapeutic Interventions

1. Physical therapy may be required to prevent contractures and muscle atrophy in hemarthrosis. This includes exercise, whirlpool baths, and application of ice.
Casting may be necessary.
2. Orthopedic appliances may be employed to prevent

injury to affected joints and help to resolve hemorrhages.

Pharmacologic Interventions

1. Bleeding is resolved by replacement of deficient coagulation factors (VIII or IX) through IV administration of type-specific coagulation concentrates during bleeding episodes.
2. Persons with mild and moderate factor VIII–deficient hemophilia may respond to desmopressin, which causes the release of factor VIII from endothelial stores.
3. Antifibrinolytics such as aminocaproic acid are given as adjunctive therapy for mucosal bleeding to prevent clot breakdown by salivary proteins.
4. Activated prothrombin complex concentrates that have activated factors VII, X, and IX are used when inhibitors (autoantibodies) to infused factor VIII and IX replacements have developed. In the case of factor VIII inhibitors, porcine factor VIII may also be given.
5. NSAIDs are used to decrease inflammation and arthritic-like pain associated with chronic hemarthroses. Must be used with caution because some types and higher doses interfere with platelet adhesion. Short courses of corticosteroids may be necessary to relieve inflammation.

Surgical Interventions

1. Orthopedic surgery (synovectomy) may be done to remove damaged synovium in chronically involved joints, through open procedure, arthroscopy, or instillation of a radionucleotide.

◆ Nursing Interventions

Monitoring

1. Monitor vital signs; treat for shock if child becomes hypotensive.

Supportive Care

1. Provide emergency care for bleeding.
   a. Apply pressure and cold on the area for 10 to 15 minutes to allow clot formation. This should be done especially after any venipuncture or injection.
   b. Place fibrin foam or absorbable gelatin foam in the wound.

409

    c. Suturing and cauterization should be avoided.

2. Immobilize the affected part and elevate above the level of the heart.

3. Avoid rapid administration of coagulation factors to minimize the possibility of transfusion reaction; usually 2 to 3 mL per minute; consult package inserts. Stop the transfusion if hives, headaches, tingling, chills, flushing, or fever occur.

4. Apply fibrinolytic agents to wound for oral bleeding.

5. Keep child quiet during treatment to decrease pulse and rate of bleeding.

6. Provide protection against bleeding.
    a. Avoid taking rectal temperatures.
    b. Avoid injections; give medications orally whenever possible.
    c. If injection is necessary, use subcutaneous rather than intramuscular route. Apply pressure to injection site for 10 to 15 minutes, then apply pressure dressing with self-adhesive gauze.

NURSING ALERT
Children with hemophilia should not receive aspirin or compounds containing aspirin because this medication affects platelet function and prolongs bleeding time.

7. Maintain a safe environment and teach parents safety measures, eg, padding crib or bed rails, inspecting toys for sharp or rough edges, etc.

COMMUNITY CARE CONSIDERATIONS
Perform or encourage parents to perform a home-safety survey to identify potential hazards to the hemophiliac child such as cluttered furniture the child may bump into, sharp edges on furniture or other objects, loose rugs that promote falls, slippery tub or floor surfaces, rocks or holes in backyard, or concrete play areas.

8. Be aware that increased pain usually means that there is continuing bleeding, and further replacement therapy may be needed.

9. Assess pain level and manage through analgesics and nonpharmacologic measures such as hypnosis, biofeedback, relaxation techniques, and transcutaneous electrical nerve stimulation (TENS).

10. Provide emotional support to the child and family. Encourage the parents to allow the child to participate in as many normal activities as possible within the realm of safety.

Family Education and Health Maintenance

1. Review safety measures to prevent or minimize trauma.

2. Encourage parents to educate teachers, babysitters, and others involved in child's care so that they can respond in an emergency.

3. Advise wearing a medical alert bracelet.

4. Remind parents not to administer aspirin to the child.

5. Teach emergency treatment for hemorrhage.

6. Encourage regular medical and dental supervision.
    a. Preventive dental care is important. Soft-bristled or sponge-tipped toothbrushes should be used to prevent bleeding. Factor replacement therapy is necessary for extensive dental work and extractions.
    b. Hepatitis B vaccine is necessary to protect against hepatitis from blood transfusions.

7. Teach healthy diet to avoid overweight, which places additional strain on the child's weight-bearing joints and predisposes to hemarthroses. Also, teach child to avoid sharp utensils, hard candy, suckers, and other foods with sharp edges that may cause mucosal lacerations.

8. Assist the parents in teaching the child to understand the exact nature of the illness as early as possible. Special attention should be given to the signs of hemorrhage, and the child should be told of the need to report even the slightest bleeding to an adult immediately.

9. Provide teaching and referrals to initiate a home care program for infusion therapy at home when hemorrhage begins.

10. Advise families that genetic counseling and family

H

planning are available for parents and adolescent patients.

11. Educate regarding hepatitis B and C and HIV disease, and risks of treatment.

12. For additional information and support, refer to:

National Hemophilia Foundation
104 East 40th St., Suite 506
New York, NY 10016
212-682-5510

Hemorrhoids

Hemorrhoids are vascular masses that protrude into the lumen of the lower rectum or perianal area. They result when increased intraabdominal pressure causes engorgement in the vascular tissue lining the anal canal. Loosening of vessels from surrounding connective tissue occurs with protrusion or prolapse into the anal canal. There are two main types of hemorrhoids: External hemorrhoids appear outside the external sphincter, and internal hemorrhoids appear above the internal sphincter. When blood within the hemorrhoids becomes clotted because of obstruction, the hemorrhoids are referred to as being thrombosed.

Predisposing factors include pregnancy, prolonged sitting or standing, straining at stool, chronic constipation or diarrhea, anal infection, rectal surgery or episiotomy, genetic predisposition, alcoholism, portal hypertension (cirrhosis), coughing, sneezing, or vomiting, loss of muscle tone attributable to old age, and anal intercourse. Complications include hemorrhage, anemia, incontinence of stool, and strangulation.

Hemorrhoids are the most common of a variety of anorectal disorders, which are briefly described in the accompanying table (Table 9).

◆ Assessment

1. Pain (more so with external hemorrhoids), sensation of incomplete fecal evacuation, constipation, anal itch-

(text continues on p. 416)

H

TABLE 9 Anorectal Disorders

Condition	Signs and Symptoms	Interventions
Anal Fissure Linear laceration of anal epithelium. May result from abrasion by hard stool or perineum strain during childbirth	Painful defecation, bright red blood on stools, possibly spasm of anal canal	Bran, psyllium, stool softeners, suppositories to promote regular soft-bowel movements Silver nitrate or gentian violet solution to lesion Warm sitz baths, anesthetic ointment to relieve pain High-fiber diet with fluids to prevent constipation Fissurectomy may be necessary
Anorectal Abscess Localized area of pus from inflammation of anorectal tissue. May result from abrasion by foreign object with subsequent bacterial infection, Crohn's disease	Persistent, throbbing rectal pain with walking, sitting, and defecation; reddened bulge or swelling near anus; may be purulent	Incision and drainage Warm sitz baths Analgesics Ensure postoperative bowel movements

(continued)

H

TABLE 9 *(Continued)*

Condition	Signs and Symptoms	Interventions
Anal Fistula Abnormal tubelike passage from skin near anus into anal canal. May result from rupture of anal abscess; may be associated with inflammatory bowel disease, foreign body, or cancer	Purulent perianal discharge; itching and pain	Bowel rest to allow fistula to heal; possible temporary fecal diversion Possible fistulotomy or fistulectomy Analgesics Ensure postoperative bowel movements
Anal Condylomas (Warts) Caused by human papilloma virus; usually sexually transmitted. Must be differentiated from condylomata lata of syphilis	Small, soft, pink or flesh-colored growths in perianal region. Thrive in moist, macerated regions. Often recur. Commonly seen in homosexual men	Liquid nitrogen or 25% podophyllum resin in tincture of benzoin; wash off solution after 2–4 hours Electrofulguration Good anal hygiene, frequent use of talc powder Monitor for recurrence
Proctitis Acute or chronic inflammation of rectal mucosa. Commonly caused by *Neisseria gonorrhoeae*, chlamydiae, herpesvirus, syphilis	Anorectal pain, purulent or blood discharge, constipation, tenesmus. Often seen in homosexual men	Antimicrobial treatment Keep stool soft to allow rectum to heal.

H

Anorectal Stricture Narrowing of anorectal lumen, preventing dilation of sphincter. Usually caused by scarring after anorectal surgery or inflammation; may follow irradiation of pelvic area	Itching, constipation, ribbonlike stools, painful defecation; may not completely evacuate stools	Treat cause of inflammation Dilatation therapy In severe stenosis, plastic surgery to anal canal Postoperative care includes stool softeners, warm sitz baths, wound care; and continued prevention of anal stenosis
Rectal Prolapse Mucosal membrane protrudes through anus. Caused by muscular weakness, neurologic disorders, chronic diseases, aging	Associated with constipation and straining; rectal fullness; blood diarrhea; rectal ulcer secondary to intussusception	Injection of sclerosing agent may fix rectum in place Surgery may include sphincter repair or resection of prolapsed tissue High-fiber diet and fluids to avoid constipation; perineal strengthening exercises

H

ing. Sudden rectal pain may occur if external hemorrhoids are thrombosed.
2. Bleeding may occur during defecation; bright red blood on stool caused by injury of mucosa covering hemorrhoid
3. Visible and palpable masses at anal area

◆ Diagnostic Evaluation

1. External examination with anoscope or proctoscope shows hemorrhoid or hemorrhoids.
2. Barium enema or sigmoidoscopy to rule out more serious colonic lesions causing rectal bleeding, such as polyps

◆ Collaborative Management

Therapeutic Interventions
1. High-fiber diet to keep stools soft
2. Warm sitz baths to ease pain and combat swelling
3. Reduction of prolapsed external hemorrhoid manually by nurse or patient

Pharmacologic Interventions
1. Stool softeners to keep stools soft and relieve symptoms
2. Medications such as soothing anal suppositories 2 to 3 times daily or witch-hazel compresses to reduce itching

Surgical Interventions
1. Injection of sclerosing solutions to produce scar tissue and decrease prolapse
2. Cryodestruction (freezing) of hemorrhoids
3. Surgery may be indicated in presence of prolonged bleeding, disabling pain, intolerable itching, and general unrelieved discomfort.
   a. Barron ligation with a rubber band is treatment of choice. Internal hemorrhoid is encircled at the base. After a period, the hemorrhoid sloughs away.
   b. Dilatation of the anal canal and lower rectum may be performed under general anesthesia. This procedure is not advocated for patients whose main complaints are prolapse or incontinence. It also is not

H

recommended for aging patients with weak sphincters.

c. An acutely thrombosed hemorrhoid may be incised to remove clot.

d. Hemorrhoidectomy may be used to remove internal and external hemorrhoids.

◆ Nursing Intervention

Supportive Care

1. After thrombosis or surgery, assist with frequent positioning using pillow support for comfort.

2. Provide analgesics, warm sitz baths, or warm compresses to reduce pain and inflammation.

3. Apply witch-hazel dressing to perianal area or anal creams or suppositories, if ordered, to relieve discomfort.

4. Observe anal area postoperatively for drainage and bleeding; report if excessive.

5. Administer stool softener or laxative to assist with bowel movements soon after surgery, to reduce risk of stricture.

Patient Education and Health Maintenance

1. Teach anal hygiene and measures to control moisture to prevent itching.

2. Encourage regular exercise, high-fiber diet, and adequate fluid intake (8–10 glasses per day) to avoid straining and constipation, which predisposes to hemorrhoid formation.

3. Discourage regular use of laxatives; firm, soft stools dilate the anal canal and decrease stricture formation after surgery.

4. Tell patient to expect a foul-smelling discharge for 7 to 10 days after cryodestruction.

5. Determine the patient's normal bowel habits and identify predisposing factors to educate patient about preventing recurrence of symptoms.

H

Hepatitis, Viral

Hepatitis is a viral infection of the liver associated with a broad spectrum of clinical manifestations from asymptomatic infection through icteric hepatitis to hepatic necrosis. Currently, five forms of viral hepatitis have been identified, as follows:

Type A hepatitis (HAV) is caused by an RNA virus of the enterovirus family. It spreads primarily by the fecal–oral route, usually through the ingestion of infected food or liquids. It also may be spread by person-to-person contact, and rarely, by blood transfusion. Type A hepatitis occurs worldwide, especially in areas with overcrowding and poor sanitation.

Type B hepatitis (HBV) is caused by a double-shelled virus containing DNA. A related viral protein (HBeAg) circulates in the blood independently of the HBV virus particle. Type B hepatitis spreads primarily through blood (percutaneous and permucosal route). It can also spread via saliva, breast-feeding, or sexual activity (blood, semen, saliva, or vaginal secretions). Male homosexuals are at high risk for infection. Worldwide, HBV is the main cause of cirrhosis and hepatocellular carcinoma.

Type C hepatitis (HCV), also called non-A, non-B hepatitis, usually spreads through blood or blood product transfusion, usually from asymptomatic blood donors. It commonly affects IV drug users and renal dialysis patients and personnel. HCV is the most common form of post-transfusion hepatitis. Approximately 50% of cases develop chronic liver disease, and at least 20% progress to cirrhosis.

Type D hepatitis (HDV), or delta hepatitis, is caused by a defective RNA virus that requires the presence of hepatitis B—specifically, hepatitis B surface antigen (HBsAg)—to replicate. Hence, HDV occurs along with HBV or may superinfect a chronic HBV carrier, and cannot outlast a hepatitis B infection. Occurs primarily in IV drug abusers or multiply transfused patients in the United States, but the highest incidence is in the Mediterranean, Middle East, and South America. HDV causes approximately 50% of cases of fulminant hepatitis, which has an extremely high mortality rate.

Type E hepatitis (HEV) is caused by a nonenveloped, single-strand RNA virus. It is transmitted by the fecal–oral route, but is hard to detect because it is inconsistently shed in the feces. Occurrence is primarily in India, Africa, Asia, or Central America. Not much is yet known about HEV.

H

Fulminant hepatitis is a rare but severe complication of hepatitis, which may require liver transplantation.

◆ Assessment

1. Type A hepatitis (incubation period, 3–5 weeks)
   a. Prodromal symptoms: fatigue, anorexia, malaise, headache, low-grade fever, nausea, vomiting. Highly contagious at this time, usually 2 weeks before onset of jaundice
   b. Icteric phase: jaundice, tea-colored urine, clay-colored stools, right upper quadrant pain and tenderness
   c. Symptoms often milder in children
2. Type B hepatitis (incubation period, 2–5 months)
   a. Prodromal symptoms (insidious onset): fatigue, anorexia, transient fever, abdominal discomfort, nausea, vomiting, headache
   b. May also have myalgias, photophobia, arthritis, angioedema, urticaria, maculopapular rash, vasculitis
   c. Icteric phase occurs 1 week to 2 months after onset of symptoms.
3. Type C hepatitis (incubation period, 1 week to several months)
   a. Similar to HBV but less severe
4. Type D hepatitis (unclear incubation period)
   a. Similar to HBV but more severe
5. Obtain a patient history. Ask about IV drug use, blood transfusions, contact with infected persons (including sexual activity), travel to endemic areas, and ingestion of possible contaminated food or water to help determine cause of hepatitis.

◆ Diagnostic Evaluation

1. All forms of hepatitis: elevated serum transferase levels (AST, ALT)
2. HAV: Radioimmunoassay detects IgM antibodies to hepatitis A virus in the acute phase.
3. HBV: Radioimmunoassays detect HBsAg, anti-HBc, anti-HBsAg in various stages of hepatitis B infection.
4. HCV: Hepatitis C antibody may not be detected for 3

H

to 6 months after onset of illness; antigen tests to HCV are being developed that will confirm diagnosis sooner.

5. HDV: Anti-delta antibodies in the presence of HBsAg, or detection of IgM in acute disease and IgG in chronic disease.

6. Hepatitis E antigen (with HCV ruled out)

7. If indicated, prepare the patient for liver biopsy to detect chronic active disease, track progression, and evaluate response to therapy.

◆ Collaborative Management

Therapeutic Interventions

1. Provide adequate rest according to the patient's level of fatigue.

2. Hospitalization for protracted nausea and vomiting or life-threatening complications. Universal and enteric precautions are maintained.

3. Provide small frequent feeding of a high-calorie, low-fat diet. Proteins are restricted when the liver cannot metabolize protein by-products, as demonstrated by symptoms.

4. After jaundice has cleared, encourage gradual increase in physical activity. This may require many months.

Pharmacologic Interventions

1. Vitamin K injected subcutaneously if prothrombin time is prolonged

2. IV fluid and electrolyte replacements as indicated

3. Antiemetic for nausea

4. Long-term beta-interferon therapy may produce at least temporary remission in HCV patients.

◆ Nursing Interventions

Monitoring

1. Monitor hydration through intake and output.

2. Monitor prothrombin time and for signs of bleeding.

3. In severe infection, monitor for signs of encephalopathy—lethargy, confusion, excitability, asterixis (irregular flapping of forcibly dorsiflexed outstretched hands).

H

Supportive Care

1. Encourage the patient to eat meals in a sitting position to reduce pressure on the liver.
2. Encourage pleasing meals in an environment with minimal noxious stimuli (odors, noise, interruptions).
3. Administer or teach self-administration of antiemetics as prescribed. Avoid phenothiazines such as chlorpromazine (Thorazine), which have a cholestatic effect and may cause or worsen jaundice.
4. Encourage frequent oral fluids or administer IV fluids, as indicated.
5. Encourage rest during symptomatic phase, according to level of fatigue.
6. Encourage diversional activities when recovery and convalescence are prolonged.
7. Encourage gradual resumption of activities and mild exercise during convalescent period.
8. Stress importance of proper public and home sanitation and proper preparation and dispensation of foods.
9. Encourage specific protection for close contacts.
    a. Immune globulin as soon as possible to household contacts of HAV patients
    b. Hepatitis B immune globulin as soon as possible to blood or body fluid contacts of HBV patients, followed by HBV vaccine series
10. Explain precautions about transmission and prevention of transmission to others to the patient and family.
    a. Good handwashing and hygiene after using bathroom
    b. Avoidance of sexual activity (especially for HBV) until free of HBsAg
    c. Avoidance of sharing needles, eating utensils, and toothbrushes to prevent blood or body fluid contact (especially for HBV)
11. Report all cases of hepatitis to public health officials.
12. Warn the patient to avoid trauma that may cause bruising; limit invasive procedures, if possible, and maintain adequate pressure on needle stick sites.

H

Patient Education and Health Maintenance

1. Identify individuals or groups at high risk, such as IV drug abusers or their sexual contacts, and those living in crowded conditions with potentially poor hygiene or sanitation, and teach them proper hygiene, waste disposal, food preparation, use of condoms, not sharing needles, and other preventive measures.

2. Encourage vaccination for HBV with series of three shots (at 0, 1, and 6 months) for high-risk individuals such as health care workers or institutionalized patients.

3. Instruct all patients who have received a blood transfusion to avoid donating blood for 6 months (the incubation period of HBV). After hepatitis infection, blood should not be given if the patient is a hepatitis B carrier or was infected with hepatitis C.

4. Stress the need to follow precautions with blood and secretions until the patient is deemed free of HBsAg.

5. Explain to HBV carriers that their blood and secretions will remain infectious.

6. Emphasize that most hepatitis is self-limiting, but follow-up is needed for liver function tests.

H

Hernia, Abdominal

A *hernia* is a protrusion of an organ, tissue, or structure through the wall of the cavity in which it is normally contained. It is often called a "rupture." *Abdominal hernias* are likely to occur with congenital or acquired structural weakness or trauma to the abdominal wall, which yields to increased intraabdominal pressure from heavy lifting, obesity, pregnancy, straining, coughing, or proximity to a tumor. Many types of abdominal hernias occur, classified by site.

In an *inguinal hernia* (most common), viscera protrudes into the inguinal canal at the point where the spermatic cord emerges in the male, and the round ligament in the female. Through this opening, an indirect inguinal hernia extends down the inguinal canal and even into the scrotum or the labia. A direct inguinal hernia protrudes through the posterior inguinal wall.

A *femoral hernia* occurs where the femoral artery passes into the femoral canal, and appears below the inguinal ligament below the groin.

An *umbilical hernia* results from failure of the umbilical orifice to close. It occurs most often in obese women, in children, and in patients with increased intraabdominal pressure from cirrhosis and ascites.

A *ventral* or *incisional hernia* occurs through the abdominal wall because of weakness, possibly because of a poorly healed surgical incision.

A *parastomal hernia* may protrude through the fascial defect around a stoma and into the subcutaneous tissue.

Hernias may be reducible, where the protruding mass can be placed back into the abdominal cavity; irreducible, where the mass cannot be replaced; incarcerated, where intestinal flow is completely obstructed; or strangulated, where blood flow as well as intestinal flow are completely obstructed.

◆ Assessment

1. Hernia bulges when the patient stands or strains (Valsalva maneuver) and disappears when supine.
2. Discomfort or pulling sensation
3. Strangulation—severe pain, vomiting, swelling of hernial sac, rebound tenderness, fever

◆ Diagnostic Evaluation

1. Abdominal x-rays show abnormally high levels of gas in the bowel or bowel obstruction.
2. Complete blood count (CBC) and serum electrolytes may show hemoconcentration (increased hematocrit), increased white blood cells (WBC), and electrolyte imbalance.

◆ Collaborative Management

Therapeutic Interventions

1. If hernia is reducible and patient is poor surgical candidate, a truss (pad and belt) may be positioned snugly over the area to prevent viscera from entering the hernial sac. A similar appliance is available for a reducible parastomal hernia.

H

Surgical Interventions

1. Surgery is recommended to correct the defect and prevent strangulation. Procedures include:
   a. Herniorrhaphy—removal of hernial sac; contents replaced into the abdomen; layers of muscle and fascia sutured; may be done via laparoscopy as outpatient.
   b. Hernioplasty—involves reinforcement of suturing (often with mesh), for extensive hernia repair.
   c. Bowel resection for ischemic bowel along with hernia repair in strangulated hernia.

◆ Nursing Interventions

Monitoring

1. Monitor for signs of bowel obstruction, a common complication.
2. Monitor postoperative patient for signs and symptoms of infection: fever, chills, malaise, diaphoresis.

Supportive Care

1. If ordered, fit the patient with truss or belt when hernia is reduced. Advise the patient to wear truss under clothing, and to apply it before getting out of bed in the morning, when hernia is reduced.
2. Place the patient in Trendelenburg's position to reduce pressure on hernia, when appropriate.
3. Immediately report signs of hernial incarceration or strangulation. Keep patient NPO and insert nasogastric tube as directed to reduce intraabdominal pressure above the obstruction and relieve pressure on herniated sac.
4. Postoperatively, have the patient splint the incision site with hand or pillow when coughing to lessen pain and protect site from increased intraabdominal pressure.
5. Administer analgesics, as ordered.
6. Check scrotum or labia for swelling after inguinal hernia repair, and apply ice and other comfort measures.
7. Encourage ambulation as soon as permitted.
8. Advise patient that difficulty in urinating is common after surgery; encourage fluids to promote elimination. Catheterize, if necessary.

H

9. Check dressing for drainage and incision for redness and swelling; report signs of infection.
10. Administer antibiotics, if appropriate.

Patient Education and Health Maintenance

1. Teach using bed rest, intermittent ice packs, and scrotal elevation to reduce scrotal edema expected for 24 to 48 hours after repair of an inguinal hernia.
2. Teach the patient to monitor and report signs of infection: pain, drainage from incision, temperature elevation, continued difficulty in voiding.
3. Advise patient to avoid heavy lifting for 4 to 6 weeks. Athletics and extremes of exertion should be avoided for 8 to 12 weeks postoperatively, per provider instructions.

Hernia, Hiatal

A *hiatal hernia* is a protrusion of part of the stomach through the hiatus of the diaphragm and into the thoracic cavity. There are two types of hiatal hernias (Fig. 14). In a *sliding hernia*, the upper stomach and gastroesophageal junction move upward into the chest and slide in and out of the thorax (most common); in a *paraesophageal hernia* (rolling hernia), part of the greater curvature of the stomach rolls through the diaphragmatic defect next to the gastroesophageal junction. Hiatal hernia results from muscle weakening caused by aging or other conditions such as esophageal carcinoma, trauma, or after certain surgical procedures. Treatment can prevent incarceration of the involved portion of the stomach in the thorax, which constricts gastric blood supply.

◆ Assessment

1. May be asymptomatic
2. Patient may report feeling of fullness or chest pain resembling angina.
3. Sliding hernia may cause dysphagia, heartburn (with or without regurgitation of gastric contents into the

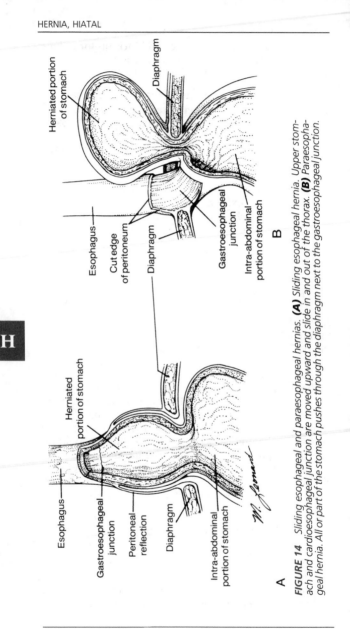

FIGURE 14 *Sliding esophageal and paraesophageal hernias. (**A**) Sliding esophageal hernia. Upper stomach and cardioesophageal junction are moved upward and slide in and out of the thorax. (**B**) Paraesophageal hernia. All or part of the stomach pushes through the diaphragm next to the gastroesophageal junction.*

H

mouth), or retrosternal or substernal chest pain from gastric reflux.
4. Severe pain or shock may result from incarceration of stomach in thoracic cavity with paraesophageal hernia.

◆ Diagnostic Evaluation

1. Upper GI series with barium contrast shows outline of hernia in esophagus.
2. Endoscopy visualizes defect and rules out other disorders, such as tumors or esophagitis.

◆ Collaborative Management

Therapeutic Interventions
1. Elevate head of bed 15 to 20 cm (6–8 in.) to reduce nighttime reflux.

Pharmacologic Interventions
1. Antacids neutralize gastric acid and reduce pain.
2. If patient has esophagitis, give histamine (H_2) receptor antagonist such as cimetidine or ranitidine.

Surgical Interventions
1. Gastropexy to fix the stomach in position is indicated if symptoms are severe. (See Gastrointestinal Surgery, p. 350.)

◆ Nursing Interventions

Supportive Care and Patient Education
1. Advise the patient on preventing reflux of gastric contents into esophagus by:
   a. Eating smaller meals to reduce stomach bulk
   b. Avoiding stimulation of gastric secretions by omitting caffeine and alcohol, which may intensify symptoms
   c. Refraining from smoking, which stimulates gastric acid secretion
   d. Avoiding fatty foods, which promote reflux and delay gastric emptying
   e. Refraining from lying down for at least 1 hour after meals

H

    f. Losing weight, if obese

    g. Avoiding bending from the waist or wearing tight-fitting clothes

2. Advise the patient to report to health care facility immediately at onset of acute chest pain—may indicate incarceration of paraesophageal hernia

---

Herniated Intervertebral Disk (Ruptured Disk)

A *herniated intervertebral disk* results from protrusion of the nucleus of the disk into the annulus (fibrous ring around the disk), with subsequent compression of nerve roots. Herniation may result from trauma, degeneration attributable to aging, and congenital malformations. It may take from months to years to develop, producing acute and chronic symptoms. Most herniations occur in the lumbar, lumbosacral, and cervical regions, but they can occur in any portion of the vertebral column (Fig. 15). If untreated, the disorder may cause permanent neurologic dysfunction (weakness, numbness).

◆ Assessment

1. Cervical herniation
   a. Pain and stiffness in the head, neck, top of shoulders, scapular region, and upper extremities
   b. Paresthesias, numbness, and weakness of upper extremities
2. Lumbar and lumbosacral herniation
   a. Low back pain with radiation into buttocks and down leg
   b. Positive straight leg raising test—radiation of pain below the knee when the leg is elevated at 45 degrees from supine position (indicates lumbosacral nerve root involvement). Pain at a lesser elevation may indicate a worsening condition.
   c. Varying degrees of sensory and motor dysfunction (weakness and asymmetric reflexes)

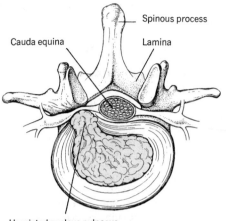

Cauda equina

Spinous process

Lamina

Herniated nucleus pulposus
compresses nerve root

FIGURE 15 *Ruptured vertebral disc.*

d. Postural deformity of the lumbar spine may also be evident.

H

❖ NURSING ALERT

Cauda equina syndrome is an emergency caused by compression of the cauda equina (a group of spinal nerves extending just below the end of the spinal cord proper). Symptoms include bowel, bladder, or sexual dysfunction, or saddle area numbness. It must be recognized early and compression relieved to prevent permanent loss of these functions.

Diagnostic Evaluation

1. Spinal x-rays to rule out bony abnormalities; and computed tomography or magnetic resonance imaging to identify herniated disk
2. Myelography, to determine the level of disk herniation

3. Electromyography, to localize spinal nerve involvement

◆ Collaborative Management

Therapeutic and Pharmacologic Interventions

1. Antiinflammatory drugs such as ibuprofen or prednisone
2. Narcotics may be necessary during acute phase.
3. Muscle relaxants to relieve associated spasm
4. Bed rest, initially, followed by physical therapy

Surgical Interventions

1. Surgery is indicated if there is progression of neurologic deficit or failure to improve with conservative management. Procedures include diskectomy, laminectomy, spinal fusion, microdiskectomy, or percutaneous diskectomy.
2. Chemonucleolysis for lumbar disk herniation, as a possible alternative to surgery. It involves injection of chymopapain to dissolve the nucleus pulposus and relieve pressure on the nerve root. This procedure is not very successful, however, and has fallen out of favor.

◆ Nursing Interventions

Monitoring

1. Assess the patient's response to conservative pain control regimen.
2. Inspect the skin several times a day (especially under a stabilizing device) for redness and evidence of pressure sore development.
3. Monitor for progression of motor, sensory, or reflex deficits.
4. If the patient has had surgery, monitor and report any sudden reappearance of radicular pain (may indicate nerve root compression from slipping of bone graft or collapsing of disk space) or burning back pain radiating to buttocks (may indicate arachnoiditis).
5. Monitor vital signs and surgical dressings frequently because hemorrhage is a possible complication.

Supportive Care

1. Be sure to administer or teach self-administration of antiinflammatory drugs with food or antacid to prevent GI upset.
2. Use bedboards under mattress and maintain bed rest except for short trips to bathroom; maintain the patient in supine or low Fowler's position or in side-lying position with slight knee flexion and a pillow between the knees.
3. Apply moist heat or ice massage to affected area of back as desired.
4. Encourage relaxation techniques such as imagery and progressive muscle relaxation.
5. Properly fit and use a cervical collar, back brace, or cervical skin traction (if appropriate) to maintain alignment.
6. Provide massage and good skin care to pressure-prone areas, especially around stabilizing devices.
7. Encourage range-of-motion exercises while in bed.
8. Encourage compliance with physical therapy treatments and activity restrictions as ordered, to prevent contractures and maintain rehabilitation potential.

H

COMMUNITY CARE CONSIDERATIONS

If cervical skin traction is ordered for home use, teach the patient how to apply the chin strap and head halter. The weight should hang freely over a the back of a chair or doorknob near the head of the bed. Make sure that the patient maintains proper neck alignment and removes traction before moving the head.

9. If the patient is undergoing surgery:
    a. Document baseline neurologic assessment to compare after surgery.
    b. Provide routine postoperative care, including frequent assessment of vital signs and neurologic function, frequent turning, coughing and deep breathing, pain control, and ambulation on the first postoperative day.
    c. Assess movement and sensation of extremities and report any new deficits.
    d. Administer analgesics and corticosteroid medica-

tions to control pain from surgical incision and resultant swelling around nerve roots and spinal cord.

e. Maintain cervical collar if ordered.

f. Position for comfort with small pillow under head (but avoid extreme neck flexion) and pillow under knees to take pressure off lower back.

g. If the patient has had cervical surgery, assess for hoarseness, indicating recurrent laryngeal nerve injury; may cause ineffective cough.

h. Provide fluids as soon as gag reflex and bowel sounds are noted.

i. Watch for dysphagia caused by edema of the esophagus, and provide blenderized diet.

j. Ensure that the patient voids after surgery; report urinary retention.

k. Encourage ambulation as soon possible by having the patient lie on side close to edge of bed and push up with arms while swinging legs toward floor in one motion; alternate walking with bed rest, discourage sitting.

Patient Education and Health Maintenance

1. Teach the patient the importance of complying with bed rest, use of cervical collar, and other conservative measures to reduce inflammation and heal disk herniation.

2. Tell the patient who has had a cervical disk herniation to avoid extreme flexion, extension, or rotation of the neck and to keep the head in a neutral position during sleep.

3. Encourage the patient with a lumbar disk herniation to remain on bed rest at home, with ambulation to the bathroom only, until inflammation and pain are sufficiently reduced; then ambulation can be increased, but lifting and sitting are discouraged for several weeks.

4. Encourage the patient to do stretching and strengthening exercises of extremities and abdomen after acute symptoms have subsided.

5. Teach the patient about proper body mechanics to prevent recurrence. Leg and abdominal muscles should always be used rather than the back. Knees should be bent on lifting and load carried close to midtrunk.

6. Encourage follow-up with physical therapy as indicated for reconditioning and work hardening.
7. Instruct the patient to report any changes in neurologic function or recurrence of radicular pain.
8. Encourage good nutrition, avoidance of obesity, and proper rest to reduce risk of recurrence.

Herpes Zoster

Herpes zoster (shingles) is an inflammatory skin condition in which the varicella zoster virus produces a painful vesicular eruption along the nerve tracks leading from one or more dorsal root ganglia. After a primary chickenpox infection, the virus persists in a dormant state in the dorsal ganglia. The virus may become active again in later years, either spontaneously or in association with immunosuppression, to cause the eruptions.

Herpes zoster may progress to chronic pain syndrome (postherpetic neuralgia), characterized by constant aching and burning pain or intermittent lancinating pain or hyperesthesia of affected skin after healing. Ophthalmic complications include involvement of the ophthalmic branch of the trigeminal nerve with keratitis, uveitis, corneal ulceration, and possibly blindness. Facial and auditory nerves may become involved, with hearing deficits, vertigo, and facial weakness. If the virus spreads to the viscera, it may cause pneumonitis, esophagitis, enterocolitis, myocarditis, or pancreatitis.

◆ Assessment

1. Inflammation is usually unilateral, involving the cranial, cervical, thoracic, lumbar, or sacral nerves in a bandlike configuration.
2. After 3 to 4 days, patches of grouped vesicles appear on erythematous, edematous skin.
3. Early vesicles contain serum; these later rupture and form crusts. Scarring usually does not occur unless the vesicles are deep and involve the dermis.
4. Patient may have a painful eye if ophthalmic branch of the facial nerve is involved.

H

5. Lesions usually resolve in 2 to 3 weeks.
6. Eruption may be accompanied or preceded by fever, malaise, headache, and pain. Pain may be burning, lancinating, stabbing, or aching.

❖

NURSING ALERT

A susceptible person can acquire chickenpox if he or she comes in contact with the infective vesicular fluid of a zoster patient. A person with a previous history of chickenpox is immune and thus is not at risk from infection after exposure to zoster patients. Varicella zoster virus may be a life-threatening condition to the patient who is immunosuppressed or is receiving cytotoxic chemotherapy or is a bone marrow transplant recipient.

◆ Diagnostic Evaluation

1. Culture of varicella zoster virus from lesions or detection by fluorescent antibody techniques, including monoclonal antibodies (MicroTrak).

◆ Collaborative Management

Pharmacologic Interventions

1. Antiviral drugs, particularly acyclovir, interfere with viral replication; may be used in all cases but especially for treatment of immunosuppressed or debilitated patients (IV route).
2. Corticosteroids *early* in illness for severe herpes zoster if symptomatic measures fail; given for antiinflammatory effect and relief of pain (controversial)
3. Aspirin, acetaminophen, nonsteroidal antiinflammatory drugs, or narcotics to manage pain during the acute stage. Not generally effective for postherpetic neuralgia.

◆ Nursing Interventions

Supportive Care

1. Assess the patient's level of discomfort and medicate as prescribed.
2. Teach the patient to apply wet dressings and calamine

lotion for soothing and cooling effect on inflamed tissue.

3. Encourage diversional activities.
4. Teach relaxation techniques, such as deep breathing, progressive muscle relaxation, and imagery to help control pain.
5. Apply antibacterial ointments (after acute stage) as prescribed to soften and separate adherent crusts and prevent secondary infection.

Patient Education and Health Maintenance

1. Teach the patient to use proper handwashing techniques to avoid spreading herpes zoster virus.
2. Advise the patient not to open the blisters to avoid secondary infection and scarring.
3. Reassure the patient that shingles is a viral infection of the nerves; "nervousness" does not cause shingles.
4. A caregiver may be required to assist with dressings and meals. In older persons, the pain is more pronounced and incapacitating. Dysesthesia and skin hypersensitivity are distressing.

High Blood Pressure
See Hypertension

Hip Arthroplasty
See Arthroplasty and Total Joint Replacement

Hip Dysplasia, Developmental

Developmental dysplasia of the hip (formerly known as congenital hip dysplasia or congenital dislocation of the hip) refers to conditions involving abnormal development of the proximal femur or the acetabulum. In this disorder, the acetabulum tends to be shallow and extremely oblique, and the head of the femur tends to be smaller than normal. Three forms are recognized: *unstable dyspla-*

sia, in which the acetabulum is shallow and the acetabular roof slants upward; *subluxation or incomplete dislocation,* in which the acetabular surface of the femoral head contacts the shallow dysplastic acetabular surface, but slides laterally and superiorly; and *complete dislocation,* in which the articular cartilage of the completely displaced femoral head does not contact acetabular articular cartilage.

The cause of hip dysplasia is unknown. Risk factors include twin births, firstborns, ligamentous laxity of fetal joints, breech presentation, in utero restrictions to fetal movement, and postnatal swaddling in which the hips are adducted and extended. Dysplasia may be unilateral or bilateral (20% of patients); unstable dysplasia occurs in 10 per 100 live births, whereas complete dislocation is rarer, occurring in 1 per 100 live births. Females are more commonly affected than males.

Unless treated early, hip dysplasia may lead to lost range of motion, early osteoarthritis, and recurrent dislocation or unstable hip. Avascular necrosis may occur after hip reduction.

◆ Assessment

1. Asymmetry of thigh folds or gluteal folds
2. Limitation in abduction of the hip
3. Leg length inequality
4. Ortolani's sign and positive Barlow's test
5. Abnormal gait pattern
6. Trendelenburg's sign—downward tilt of the pelvis on the affected side
7. Pain in the older child

◆ Diagnostic Evaluation

1. X-rays of the cartilaginous femoral head; it is difficult to visualize in the newborn. As the child ages, the ossification center can be better viewed, and the efficacy of this examination increases. It can be useful in ruling out other pelvic, spinal, and femoral anomalies.
2. Ultrasound examination by a skilled technician is highly accurate in diagnosing dysplasia.
3. Computed tomography is helpful in visualizing the femoral head after operative intervention such as re-

duction and casting (plain x-rays are obscured by the casting material).

4. Arthrograms can be useful to outline the cartilaginous portions of the acetabulum and femoral head.

5. Magnetic resonance imaging may be used to assess reduction, but it is costly, frequently requires the child to be sedated, and provides little in the way of additional information.

◆ Collaborative Management

Therapeutic Interventions

1. From birth to age 3 months, usually nonsurgical

2. Splinting or bracing the hips in flexion and abduction, using devices such as the Pavlik harness (treatment of choice), Frejka pillow, von Rosen splint, or Camp orthosis

3. The length of time varies with the stability of the hip at examination. If the hip remains unstable, a more aggressive management approach is considered.

Surgical Interventions

From age 3 months to 2 years:

1. Closed reduction under general anesthesia and placement of the child in a hip spica cast is the preferred treatment.
   a. There is usually a period of preoperative traction to increase the chances of reducing the hip as well as decreasing the chances of avascular necrosis after reduction.
   b. The cast is maintained for a period of 2 to 6 months based on clinical examination.

2. Open reduction of the hip with or without femoral shortening is decided on if the hip is not reducible in traction or at the time of attempted closed reduction.
   a. Followed by a period of immobilization, usually in a hip spica cast

3. Cast immobilization is usually followed by an abduction splint or orthosis, which is usually rigid.

After age 2 years:

1. Open reduction of the hip is usually accompanied by any combination of femoral or pelvic osteotomies de-

H

signed to restore the anatomic alignment of the hip and prevent the progression of joint destruction.

2. As the child ages, the risks of surgery increase. Risks may outweigh benefits, especially if the condition is bilateral.

◆ Nursing Interventions

Monitoring

1. Assess the skin around the edges of the cast or brace daily for signs of skin irritation.

2. Assess neurovascular status frequently after application of cast or brace, then daily to detect compromise. Watch for discoloration or cyanosis, impaired movement, loss of sensation, edema, absent pulses, and pain disproportionate to injury or not relieved by analgesics.

Supportive Care

1. Encourage parents to avoid swaddling the infant, and to hold the child with hips abducted.

2. Reassure parents that effective outcome depends on early intervention and compliance.

3. Prepare the child for casting or immobilization procedure by showing materials to be used and describing procedure in age-appropriate terms.

4. Assess the need for pain medication, sedation, distraction techniques, or restraint, and administer as ordered.

5. Assist with application of the immobilization device as indicated.

6. If a cast or plaster splint was applied, help facilitate drying in proper position.
   a. Keep the child or affected part still until thoroughly dry.
   b. Support the curves of the cast with pillows.
   c. Avoid excessive handling of the cast, and use palms of hands when handling it.

7. Try to prevent skin breakdown by padding edges of device and telling child to avoid placing anything inside the device.

8. If child is in hip spica cast, prevent skin breakdown from frequent soiling around perineum.

    a. Line cast edges around perineum with a plastic covering to prevent soiling of cast.

    b. Use a fracture bedpan or urinal to facilitate toileting.

    c. If child is not toilet trained, use a small diaper or perineal pad tucked under the edges of the cast, covered by a larger diaper, and change diapers as soon as soiled.

    d. Wash the perineum frequently and dry thoroughly.

    e. If the cast is synthetic and becomes soiled, clean it with a damp cloth and small amount of detergent.

9. Stimulate child with games and activities to exercise upper body and feet as able.

10. Turn the child frequently and encourage ambulation as able. Support the head and legs to reposition.

11. Encourage deep-breathing exercises at intervals to prevent atelectasis and hypostatic pneumonia. For example, children can blow whistles, party favors, soap bubbles, and cotton balls across the table as appropriate.

12. Encourage fluids and high-fiber diet to prevent constipation.

13. Prepare the child for cast removal by describing the sensation (warmth, vibration) and demonstrating the cast cutter by touching it lightly to your palm.

14. Provide and teach care of skin after cast, brace, or splint removal.

    a. Wash with warm, soapy water.

    b. Soak the area daily with warm water to facilitate removal of desquamated skin and secretions.

    c. Advise child to avoid scratching; instead apply lotion or oil to relieve itching.

    d. Encourage exercise as prescribed to regain strength and function.

Family Education and Health Maintenance

1. If the child is to be treated with an abduction splint, explain its purpose and demonstrate its application and removal to the parents.

    a. Instruct the parents as to if and when the device can be removed.

H

b. Instruct the parents to check fit of abduction splint at every diaper change.
c. Allow the parents to demonstrate their ability to properly place the device on the child.
d. Follow with written instructions whenever possible.

2. Teach child or parents to look for and report redness, skin breakdown, localized pain, or foul odor that may indicate open wounds under device.
3. Encourage regular follow-up evaluations and regular health maintenance visits.

Hirschsprung's Disease

Hirschsprung's disease (congenital aganglionic megacolon) is absence of or arrested development of parasympathetic ganglion cells in the colorectal wall, usually in the recto-sigmoid colon. The defect develops before the 12th week of gestation. Although the cause is unknown, a genetic component may be involved. Symptoms usually appear shortly after birth but may not be recognized until later in childhood, or (rarely) in adulthood.

In this disorder, the lack of colorectal innervation inhibits peristalsis, and the affected portion of intestine becomes spastic and contracted. The internal rectal sphincter fails to relax, which prevents evacuation of fecal material and gas and causes severe abdominal distention and constipation.

The disease occurs in 1 in 8,000 live births, mostly in Caucasians, and is three times more common in males than females. Complications of untreated disease include enterocolitis (a major cause of death); hydroureter or hydronephrosis; and cecal perforation.

◆ Assessment

1. In the newborn:
   a. No meconium passed
   b. Vomiting—bile-stained or fecal
   c. Abdominal distention
   d. Constipation—occurs in all patients

e. Overflow-type diarrhea
f. Anorexia, poor feeding
g. Temporary relief of symptoms with enema

PEDIATRIC ALERT
Suspect Hirschsprung's disease in any infant who fails to pass meconium within the first 24 hours and requires repeated rectal stimulation to induce bowel movements.

2. Older child (symptoms not prominent at birth):
   a. History of obstipation at birth
   b. Distention of abdomen—progressive enlarging
   c. Thin abdominal wall with observable peristaltic activity
   d. Constipation—no fecal soiling; relieved temporarily with enema
   e. Stool appears ribbonlike, fluidlike, or in pellet form
   f. Failure to grow—loss of subcutaneous fat; appears malnourished; perhaps has stunted growth
   g. Anemia

H

◆ Diagnostic Evaluation

1. Rectal examination demonstrates absence of fecal material.
2. Barium enema shows narrowed intestine proximal to anus and dilated intestine proximal to narrow segment.
3. Rectal biopsy may be done to demonstrate absent or reduced number of ganglion nerve cells, and confirm diagnosis.
4. Anorectal manometry may be done to record the reflex response of anal sphincter.
5. Ultrasonogram may be done to demonstrate dilated colon.

◆ Collaborative Management

Therapeutic Interventions
1. Enemas or colonic irrigation with physiologic saline solution

2. Older child whose symptoms are chronic but not severe may be treated with isotonic enemas, stool softeners, low-residue diet.

Pharmacologic Interventions
1. Antibiotics to control bowel flora

Surgical Interventions
1. Initially, a colostomy or ileostomy is performed to decompress intestine, divert fecal stream, and rest the normal bowel.
2. Definitive surgery is done to remove the nonfunctioning bowel segment with various pull-through procedures (abdominoperineal, endorectal, or rectorectal).
3. Surgery may be delayed until 9 to 12 months of age or until child is 6.8 to 9.0 kg (15–20 lb.).

◆ Nursing Interventions

Monitoring
Preoperative
1. Monitor for respiratory difficulty that may result from abdominal distention; watch for rapid shallow respirations, cyanosis, sternal retractions.
2. Monitor abdominal girths, for the presence of fluid waves, for increasing distension after enemas, and discrepancy in output from enemas, which may indicate intestinal obstruction.
3. Monitor hydration and nutritional status through intake and output, weights, and skin turgor.
4. Monitor characteristics of stool in older children being treated medically.
Postoperative
1. Monitor vital signs and respiratory status closely.

> **NURSING ALERT**
> To avoid injuring rectal mucosa, take axillary or external ear temperature.

2. Monitor for proper functioning of colostomy, if present.

a. Note drainage from colostomy—characteristics, frequency, fecal material, or liquid drainage.
b. Note abdominal distention.
c. Measure fluid loss from colostomy to help guide fluid replacement.

3. Monitor and report signs of obstruction (may be due to peritonitis, paralytic ileus, handling of bowel, or swelling): no output from colostomy, abdominal tenderness, irritability, vomiting, increased temperature.

4. Monitor for respiratory distress, infection, hemorrhage, and shock.

Supportive Care

Preoperative

1. Administer oxygen as ordered to support respiratory status.

2. Assist in emptying the bowel by giving repeated enemas and colonic irrigations.
   a. Procedure for enema in an infant is similar to that in an adult, except that less fluid and pressure are used.
   b. Warm physiologic saline solution should be used for irrigations. Tap water may result in water intoxication.
   c. Record all intake and output of irrigant and drainage. Report marked discrepancies in retention or loss of fluid.

3. Insert rectal tube to release accumulated fluid and gas, as ordered.

4. If abdominal distention is not relieved by enemas and discomfort is significant, insert a nasogastric tube, as ordered.
   a. Note drainage from nasogastric tube, and chart characteristics.
   b. Check for patency; saline irrigations may be requested. Carefully record input and output.
   c. Give frequent mouth care.
   d. Alternate nares when changing nasogastric tube every 24 hours, and use minimal amount of tape to prevent skin irritation.

5. Offer pacifier for infant to suck if on parenteral fluids.

6. Encourage parents to hold and rock infant.

7. Maintain position of comfort with head elevated.

H

Offer soothing stimulation (eg, music, touch, play therapy).

8. Offer small, frequent feedings. Low-residue diet will aid in keeping stools soft.

9. Administer parenteral nutrition if feeding causes additional discomfort because of distention and nausea.

10. For older child, provide demonstration and written and verbal instructions to family for saline enema administration and use of stool softeners.

Postoperative

1. Change wound dressing using sterile technique.

2. Prevent wound contamination from diaper.

3. Prevent perianal and anal excoriation by thorough cleansing and use of ointments after the infant soils.

4. Use careful handwashing technique.

5. Report any wound redness, swelling or drainage, evisceration, or dehiscence immediately.

6. Suction oral secretions frequently to prevent infection of the tracheobronchial tree and lungs.

7. In older child, encourage frequent coughing and deep breathing to maintain respiratory status.

8. Allow the infant to cry for short periods to prevent atelectasis.

9. Change position of infant frequently to increase circulation and allow for aeration of all lung areas.

10. Maintain patency of nasogastric tube immediately postoperatively.

    a. Watch for increasing abdominal distention; measure abdominal girth.

    b. Measure fluid loss because amount will affect fluid replacement.

11. Maintain NPO status until bowel sounds return and the bowel is ready for feedings as determined by health care provider.

12. Provide frequent oral hygiene while NPO.

13. Administer fluids to maintain hydration and replace lost electrolytes. Begin oral feedings as ordered.

14. Support the parents when teaching them to care for their child's colostomy. Reassure parents that colostomy will not cause delay in the child's normal development.

15. Initiate community nurse referral to help the parents

care for the child at home, and obtain necessary equipment.

Family Education and Health Maintenance

1. Involve the entire family in teaching colostomy care to enhance acceptance of body change of the child.
   a. An older child should become totally responsible for own colostomy care.
   b. Procedures need to be thoroughly understood and practiced, including preparation of skin, application of collecting appliance, care of appliance, and control of odor.
2. Teach parents to recognize and report signs of stomal complications: ribbonlike stool, diarrhea, failure of evacuation of stool or flatus, bleeding.
3. Prepare parents and older child for colostomy closure as appropriate.
4. Review gastrostomy feeding techniques as well as procedures for care and dilation of anus as indicated.
5. Allow the parents to learn and practice these procedures long before the infant is to be discharged.
6. Emphasize the importance of treating the child as normally as possible to prevent behavior problems later.
7. Teach about good nutrition—diet needs to be understood by parents before discharge. Involve the dietitian as necessary.
8. Encourage close medical follow-up for Hirschsprung's disease, as well as general growth and development and immunizations.
9. Refer parents to helping agencies such as:

> **American Pseudo-Obstruction and Hirschsprung's Disease Society**
> P.O. Box 772
> Medford, MA 02155
> 617-395-4255

HIV Disease and AIDS

Acquired immunodeficiency syndrome (AIDS) is defined as the most severe form of a continuum of illnesses associated with infection by the *human immunodeficiency virus* (HIV).

AIDS causes a slow degeneration of humoral and cell-mediated immune functions, eventually opening the way to the opportunistic infections and malignancies that characterize this disease.

HIV disease refers to the entire course of HIV infection from asymptomatic infection and early symptoms to fully developed AIDS.

HIV is transmitted by injection of blood or blood components, sexual contact (vaginal, anal, and oral intercourse), and perinatally from an infected mother to the child. High-risk groups for HIV transmission include homosexual or bisexual men, intravenous drug users, transfusion and blood product recipients (before 1985), heterosexual contacts of HIV-positive individuals, and newborns of HIV-positive mothers.

Most persons infected with HIV show no immediate signs of illness. However, some experience a brief flulike illness referred to as acute retroviral syndrome, in which the immune system is compromised by a sudden decrease in T4 lymphocytes for a brief period. Three to 6 months after initial infection, the body develops enough antibody to HIV to produce a positive serologic test (seroconversion). Staging of HIV disease is based on the medical findings and the CD4 count. Because HIV destroys CD4 molecules as it enters the T4 lymphocyte, the CD4 count diminishes over time (Fig. 16).

Because of declining immunity, frequent infections, severe opportunistic infections and malignancies develop years after the initial exposure to HIV, and death inevitably ensues.

◆ Assessment

1. Pulmonary manifestations:
   a. Persistent cough with and without sputum production, shortness of breath, chest pain, fever
   b. From *Pneumocystis carinii* pneumonia (most common), bacterial pneumonia, *Mycobacterium tuberculosis*, disseminated *Mycobacterium avium* complex, cytomegalovirus (CMV), *Histoplasma*, Kaposi's sarcoma, *Cryptococcus*, *Legionella*, and other pathogens
2. Gastrointestinal manifestations:

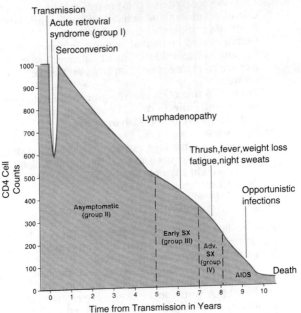

FIGURE 16 Natural history of HIV disease.

H

    a. Diarrhea, weight loss, anorexia, abdominal cramping, rectal urgency (tenesmus)

    b. From enteric pathogens including *Salmonella*, *Shigella*, *Campylobacter*, *Entamoeba histolytica*, cytomegalovirus (CMV), *M. avium* complex, and others

3. Oral manifestations:

    a. Appearance of oral lesions, white plaques on oral mucosa and angular cheilitis from *Candida albicans* of mouth and esophagus

    b. Vesicles with ulceration from herpes simplex virus

    c. White thickened lesions on lateral margins of tongue from hairy leukoplakia

    d. Oral warts attributable to human papilloma virus (HPV) and associated gingivitis

    e. Periodontitis progressing to gingival necrosis

4. Central nervous system (CNS) manifestations:
   a. Cognitive, motor, and behavioral symptoms (AIDS dementia complex/HIV encephalopathy)
   b. Demonstrated by mental slowing, impaired memory and concentration, loss of balance, lower extremity weakness, ataxia, apathy, and social withdrawal
   c. From CNS toxoplasmosis, cryptococcal meningitis, herpes virus infections, CMV (causing retinopathy and blindness), and CNS lymphoma
5. Malignancies:
   a. Kaposi's sarcoma (aggressive tumor involving skin, lymph nodes, gastrointestinal tract, and lungs)
   b. Non-Hodgkin's lymphoma (p. 552)
   c. Cervical carcinoma (p. 110)

◆ **Diagnostic Evaluation**

1. Enzyme-linked immunosorbent assay (ELISA) to detect antibody to HIV; Western blot test—used to confirm a positive result on ELISA test
   a. Once infected with HIV, it can take the body 3 to 6 months to develop enough antibody to HIV for the ELISA result to be positive (seroconversion). Risk of false-negative test if evaluated early.
   b. Occasionally, a sample that shows reactivity by ELISA may give an indeterminate result by Western blot. The cause of an indeterminate result may be early HIV seroconversion or error during interpretation of the test. The test should be repeated every 2 to 3 months until Western blot becomes positive or there is no longer suspicion of HIV disease.
2. Lymphocyte panel shows decreased CD4 count. Normal CD4 count is 800 to 1,000/mm^3.
3. A complete blood count (CBC) may show anemia and a low white blood cell count.
4. Presence of indicator disease (eg, *Pneumocystis carinii* pneumonia, candidiasis of esophagus, Kaposi's sarcoma, etc.)

◆ **Collaborative Management**

Therapeutic Interventions
1. Treatment of reversible illnesses
2. Nutritional support

H

3. Palliation of pain
4. Dental management
5. Evaluation and management of psychological and social aspects of AIDS
6. Treatment to relieve symptoms (cough, diarrhea)
7. Treatment of depression

Pharmacologic Interventions

1. Antiviral therapy; zidovudine (AZT), dideoxyinosine (DDI), zalcitabine (DDC)
   a. Therapy started at CD4 count of 500/mm^3 or less
   b. Decreases viral replication
   c. Prolongs quality of life; some studies show an extension of life by 1 to 2 years
   d. May not be tolerated well because of side effects.
2. Newer antivirals, such as lamivudine and stuvadine (reverse transcriptase inhibitors) and saquinavir and indinavir (protease inhibitors), have shown activity against HIV and are approved for combination therapy.

NURSING ALERT
If a patient on DDI develops abdominal pain or vomiting, discontinue the medication immediately and notify the health care provider. Mortality has been associated with DDI and acute pancreatitis.

H

3. *P. carinii* pneumonia prophylaxis: Trimethaprim-sulfamethoxazole, dapsone, aerosolized pentamidine
   a. Therapy is started at a CD4 cell count of 200/mm^3 or less.
   b. Decreases frequency, morbidity, and mortality of *P. carinii* infection

◆ Nursing Interventions

Monitoring

1. Monitor nutritional status by weighing, recording calorie count, taking anthropometric measurements, and evaluating serum albumin, blood urea nitrogen (BUN), protein, and transferrin levels.

2. Monitor CBC for severe anemia caused by acyclovir therapy.

3. Monitor for sore throat that progresses to dysphagia or odynaphagia (pain on swallowing) or persistent heartburn—suggestive of esophageal candidiasis.

4. Tell the patient to monitor stools for blood and try to determine if bleeding is before, with, or after bowel movement to help determine source of bleeding.

5. Monitor intake and output; assess skin and mucous membranes for poor turgor and dryness, indicating dehydration.

6. Assess for depressive or suicidal symptoms—AIDS represents a significant risk for suicide.

7. Assess mental status daily; monitor for changes in behavior, memory, concentration ability, and motor system dysfunction—the patient may become vegetative and unable to ambulate. Onset of dementia is usually insidious but may be abrupt, precipitated by acute infection.

8. Frequently assess for chills, fever, tachycardia, and tachypnea.

9. Watch for sudden change in respiratory function—the patient may be developing a secondary infection.

Supportive Care

1. Anticipate that the patient may pass through series of stages: initial crisis, transitional stage, acceptance state, and preparation for death.

   a. Allow the patient to use denial as a protective mechanism—gives some control over when and how the patient will confront mortality.

   b. Anticipate that drug abusers may exhibit antisocial behaviors, feelings of alienation and isolation.

NURSING ALERT

Never assume the family/loved ones know that the patient is HIV positive. Always ask the patient who knows of the HIV status. Confidentiality must be maintained. However, encourage the patient to share the diagnosis to decrease isolation. Offer to be with the patient when sharing the diagnosis; role playing before you meet with family/loved ones can be helpful.

2. Offer counseling services, especially when AIDS is initially diagnosed and as the patient enters terminal phase of illness.
3. Obtain social service referral for available resources and services such as housekeeping, food shopping, support groups, cancer counseling agencies, Social Security Administration.

COMMUNITY CARE CONSIDERATION

If the patient is home-bound, there are many agencies that are HIV specific and provide home visits for services such as legal counseling, hospice care, respite care, housekeeping, food preparation, care for pets, companionship. Assist the patient or significant other to locate these agencies in the community.

4. Encourage the patient to arrange personal business. Anticipate necessity of advance directives, guardianship, durable power of attorney for health care, informed consent, etc., because cognitive deterioration may make it impossible for the patient to act on own behalf at later date.
5. Assure the patient of palliative care, pain control, and help with anxiety and depression as disease progresses.
6. To help prevent infection and AIDS transmission, follow universal precautions for all patients. Use strict enteric precautions for diarrhea.
7. Administer and teach meticulous skin care, especially to the perianal area if having diarrhea.
8. Employ aseptic techniques when performing invasive procedures.
9. Consult with dietitian to develop strategies for nutritional therapy. Be aware that antiviral therapy and other drugs cause nausea and anorexia.
   a. Administer or teach the patient to administer prescribed antiemetic 30 minutes before meals.
   b. Encourage small, frequent meals because these may make best use of limited absorptive capacity.
10. For the patient with oral/esophageal pain from candida esophagitis, herpetic esophagitis, endotracheal Kaposi's sarcoma:

H

a. Avoid highly seasoned or acidic foods.
b. Offer fluids and blenderized foods to minimize chewing and ease swallowing.
c. Suggest nutrition-dense supplements such as instant breakfast drinks or protein-fortified juices for home care.

11. Discourage excessive alcohol intake—has immunosuppressive effect.

12. Prepare the patient for enteral or parenteral feedings when necessary.

13. Administer or teach the patient to administer prescribed antifungal mouth rinses or lozenges for oral candidiasis or acyclovir (oral or IV) for herpes simplex.

14. Perform or encourage oral care two to three times a day.

15. Advise the patient to eliminate caffeine, alcohol, dairy products, food high in fats, fresh juices, and acidic juices if diarrhea occurs. Drink liquids at room temperature.

16. Advise the patient to report increased weakness, dizziness, and continuing weight loss.

17. Reorient the patient to time and place frequently if dementia occurs; use structured plan of care.

18. Provide for patient safety: bed rails up; call signal available; things within the patient's reach.

19. Provide supplemental oxygen as indicated for pneumonia.

20. Encourage smoking cessation to enhance pulmonary ciliary defense.

21. Administer saline nebulization to induce sputum collection for culture and sensitivity.
a. Wear mask and gloves during sputum collection.
b. Instruct the patient to brush tongue, buccal surfaces, teeth, and palate with water before sputum induction—to decrease contamination of specimen.
c. Instruct the patient to gargle and rinse mouth with tap water.

Patient Education and Health Maintenance

1. Indicate that the patient is a source of infection to others and should take actions to prevent transmis-

sion (no exchange of blood or body fluids). Casual contact such as holding hands and hugging will not cause transmission, however.

2. Encourage the patient to disclose HIV status to sex and needle-sharing partners.

3. Emphasize to HIV-positive woman that children should be tested for HIV.

4. Discuss family planning with HIV-positive woman; the rate of transmission from mother to newborn is approximately 30%. If she does not want more children, discuss birth control options.

5. Establish a primary care provider for the patient and encourage the need for regular follow-up care. Should include yearly Pap smears for women, routine dental and eye examinations.

6. Teach the patient to recognize and report important symptoms:
   a. Change in pattern or magnitude of temperature elevation
   b. Development of a new focal complaint: skin spots, sore mouth, diarrhea

7. Emphasize to injection drug users that continued use may expose them to additional infection and such infections may activate viral replication.

8. Encourage the patient to modify sexual behaviors for safer sex:
   a. Use latex condoms (male or female) with spermicidal cream or jelly containing a viricidal agent if abstinence cannot be practiced.
   b. Refrain from oral and anal sex.
   c. Consult various AIDS action groups for additional safe-sex techniques.

9. If the patient is a substance abuser:
   a. Enroll in a treatment program.
   b. Do not share needles ("works").
   c. If no access to unused needles, clean needles before using with a bleach and water solution.

10. Teach the patient to optimize immune system function by sound dietary practices, exercise, and regular periods of sleep.

11. Refer the patient to resources such as:

National AIDS Hotline
800-342-AIDS

H

HIV Disease and AIDS in Children

An infant or child infected with human immunodeficiency virus (HIV) will, over time, show signs of impaired immune function, although the severity of the impairment can vary widely from mildly abnormal laboratory markers of immune function to full-blown acquired immunodeficiency syndrome (AIDS) defining illness. The causative agent is a retrovirus that damages the immune system by infecting and depleting the CD4 lymphocytes (T4 helper cells). HIV is transmitted by sexual contact, through exposure to blood and blood components, perinatally (in 90% of pediatric HIV cases), and through breast-feeding from an infected mother to her child. Perinatal transmission rate is 20% to 30%.

◆ Assessment

1. Generalized lymphadenopathy, especially in less common sites such as epitrochlear and axillary nodes
2. Persistent or recurrent oral candidiasis
3. Failure to thrive
4. Developmental delays or loss of previously acquired milestones
5. Hepatomegaly and splenomegaly
6. Persistent diarrhea
7. Parotitis (enlarged parotid glands)
8. Unexplained anemia, thrombocytopenia
9. Unexplained cardiac and kidney disease
10. Recurrent serious bacterial infections

◆ Diagnostic Evaluation

1. Enzyme-linked immunosorbent assay (ELISA) with confirmation by Western blot test is predictive of HIV disease after 15 months of age. Before that time, circulating maternal antibodies will be detected but not indicate the infant's infectious status.
2. Newer polymerase chain reaction and P24 antigen test are allowing earlier confirmation of infection (by 2–3 months of age).
3. CD4 lymphocyte counts should be done by 1 month

H

of age and then every 2 to 3 months until infant is known not to be infected, to determine pneumocystis pneumonia risk.

4. For the infected child, complete blood count, platelet count, CD4 count, and serum chemistry panel should be done every 3 to 6 months. Electrocardiogram and chest x-ray should be done yearly.

◆ Collaborative Management

Therapeutic Interventions

1. Nutritional support
2. Evaluation and treatment of developmental delays
3. Support for child and family in the areas of disclosure issues, parental guilt, and long-term care (including caretakers for child in the event of maternal death)

Pharmacologic Interventions

1. Initiation of PCP prophylaxis when indicated by low CD4 counts based on age (Table 10) with trimethoprim-sulfamethoxazole (first choice), pentamidine, or dapsone.
2. Initiation of antiretroviral therapy in known infected children when symptomatic or CD4 counts 250 cells/mm^3 above the threshold for initiation of PCP prophylaxis. Zidovudine (AZT), didanosine, and other agents (through clinical trials) are currently in use.
3. Use of intravenous immune globulin (IVIG) in infected children who have had two or more serious bacterial

H

TABLE 10 Guidelines for *Pneumocystis carinii* Pneumonia Prophylaxis

Age	Percent CS4 Cells	Absolute Number CS4 Cells
1–12 mo	≤20%	≤1,500/mm^3
12–24 mo	≤20%	≤750/mm^3
24–72 mo	≤20%	≤500/mm^3
>6 y	≤20%	≤200/mm^3

Any age: Prior episode of *Pneumocystic carinii* pneumonia

infections within 1 year or for the treatment of HIV-related thrombocytopenia

4. Antifungal drugs such as nystatin or fluconazole for oral candidiasis

5. Prompt treatment of additional infections

◆ Nursing Interventions

Monitoring

1. Monitor absolute neutrophil counts, which may drop with antiretroviral therapy and predispose to infection.
2. Monitor hydration status if diarrhea is present through intake and output, skin turgor, and skin and mucous membrane dryness.
3. Monitor for fever and report any core temperature over 101°F (38.4°C).
4. Monitor growth parameters and developmental milestones.

Supportive Care

1. Prevent secondary infections by maintaining a clean environment, employing aseptic technique for invasive procedures, providing good skin care, and encouraging proper food preparation.
2. Encourage high-calorie, nutritious diet in small frequent feedings.
3. Provide fluids and blenderized foods and avoid highly seasoned or acidic foods if oral candidiasis is present.
4. If diarrhea is present, avoid foods that increase intestinal motility and provide careful skin care of anal area, including application of barrier cream. Use strict enteric precautions.
5. While child is febrile, institute comfort measures such as sponge baths, dry linens, and antipyretics, as ordered.
6. Assess the family's coping skills and provide emotional and situational support. Refer to social services and community resources.
7. Allow the family to use denial as a protective mechanism, if needed, but help them move toward setting realistic goals and expectations for the child.
8. Accept that some families may not be able to disclose the nature of the disease with their child, even after

H

much support and guidance. Answer the child's questions as honestly as possible within parental constraints.

9. Assess the child for pain and administer analgesics as indicated. Allay fear by explaining all procedures in age-appropriate terms and providing distraction techniques.

Family Education and Health Maintenance

1. Teach universal precautions. Gloves are recommended when handling any potentially contaminated body fluids but are not considered necessary for routine diaper changes unless bloody diarrhea or hematuria exists.

2. Offer guidance as to how to initiate discussion of the child's HIV status with school and day care settings. It is not currently required that schools and day care settings be advised, but it is advantageous in that this alerts the school to notify parents in the event of a breakout of infectious disease (such as varicella) that could pose a threat to the HIV-infected child.

3. Advise reporting fever over 101°F (38.4°C) and other signs of illness.

4. Encourage all recommended immunizations according to pediatric schedule with the addition of pneumococcal vaccine (after age 2) and yearly influenza (after age 6 months).

COMMUNITY CARE CONSIDERATIONS
HIV-infected children, and those noninfected children living with HIV-infected parents and siblings, should not receive the oral polio vaccine, but rather the inactivated polio vaccine (IPV), which is injectable. This is because of the prolonged shedding of the virus from the live oral vaccine, which may prove to be hazardous for immune-compromised individuals.

Hodgkin's Disease

Hodgkin's disease is a malignant lymphoma of the reticuloendothelial system that results in an accumulation of dysfunctional, immature lymphoid-derived cells. The disease generally spreads by lymphatic channels, involving lymph nodes, spleen, and ultimately (through the bloodstream) to extralymphatic sites such as GI tract, bone marrow, skin, upper air passages, and other organs. Hodgkin's disease is most common in patients aged 20 to 40 years and in those older than age 60. Its cause is unknown.

Hodgkin's disease is more readily cured than other lymphomas. More than one treatment strategy is available, and combinations of radiation and chemotherapy are commonly used. Depending on location and extent of malignancy, complications may include splenomegaly, hepatomegaly, thromboembolism, and spinal cord compression.

◆ Assessment

1. Fatigue, fever, chills, night sweats, painless swelling of lymph nodes (generally unilateral), pruritis, weight loss
2. Wide variety of symptoms may occur if there is pulmonary involvement, superior vena cava obstruction, hepatic or bone involvement, and involvement of other structures.

◆ Diagnostic Evaluation

Tests are used to determine extent of disease involvement before treatment and repeated periodically to assess response to treatment.

1. Lymph node biopsy to detect characteristic Reed-Sternberg giant cell, helping to confirm diagnosis
2. Complete blood count, bone marrow aspiration and biopsy to determine whether there is bone marrow involvement
3. X-rays, computed tomography, and magnetic resonance imaging to detect deep nodal involvement
4. Lymphangiogram to detect size and location of deep nodes involved, including abdominal nodes, which may not be readily seen by CT
5. Liver function tests and liver biopsy to determine hepatic involvement
6. Surgical staging (laparotomy with splenectomy, liver

biopsy, multiple lymph node biopsies) may be done in selected patients.

◆ Collaborative Management

Therapeutic Interventions

1. Radiation therapy is treatment of choice for localized disease.
   a. Areas of body where lymph node chains are located can generally tolerate high radiation doses.
   b. Vital organs are protected during radiation treatments with lead shielding.

Pharmacologic Interventions

1. Chemotherapy may be used in combination with radiation.
   a. Initial treatment often begins with a specific four-drug regimen.
   b. Three or four drugs may be given in intermittent or cyclical courses, with periods of treatment to allow recovery from toxicities.

Surgical Interventions

1. Autologous or allogenic bone marrow transplantation has been tried.

◆ Nursing Interventions

Supportive Care

1. To protect the skin receiving radiation, avoid rubbing, powders, deodorants, lotions, or ointments (unless prescribed) or application of heat or cold.
2. Encourage patient to keep clean and dry, and to bathe the area affected by radiation gently with tepid water and mild soap.
3. Encourage wearing loose-fitting clothes and to protect skin from exposure to sun, chlorine, temperature extremes.
4. To protect oral and GI tract mucous membranes, encourage frequent small meals, using bland and soft diet at mild temperatures.
5. Teach patient to avoid irritants such as alcohol, tobacco, spices, extremely hot or cold foods.

H

6. Administer or teach self-administration of pain medication or antiemetic before eating or drinking, if needed.
7. Encourage mouth care at least twice a day and after meals using soft toothbrush or toothette and mild mouth rinse.
8. Assess for ulcers, plaques, or discharge that may be indicative of superimposed infection.
9. For diarrhea, switch to low-residue diet and administer antidiarrheals as ordered.

Patient Education and Health Maintenance

1. Teach patient about risk of infection; advise to monitor temperature and report any fever or other sign of infection promptly; avoid crowds; use condoms and other safe sex practices.
2. Teach patient how to take medications as ordered; advise about possible side effects and their management.
3. Explain to patients that radiation therapy may cause sterility; male patients should be given opportunity for sperm banking before treatment; female patients may develop ovarian failure and require hormone replacement therapy.
4. Refer patient to support group if appropriate.
5. Reassure the patient that fatigue will decrease after treatment is completed; encourage frequent naps and rest periods.

Human Immunodeficiency Virus
See HIV Disease and AIDS

Hydrocephalus

Hydrocephalus is characterized by an abnormal increase in cerebrospinal fluid volume within the intracranial cavity and by enlargement of the head in infancy. Pressure from increased fluid volume can damage brain tissue.

Hydrocephalus results from two major causes: obstruction of CSF flow (noncommunicating hydrocephalus) or faulty CSF absorption (communicating hydrocephalus). In the noncommunicating type, obstruction may result from congenital defects, infections, trauma, spontaneous intracranial bleeding, and neoplasms. In the communicating type, faulty CSF absorption may result from meningeal adhesions or excessive production of cerebrospinal fluid caused by a tumor or from unknown causes. Complications include seizures, spontaneous arrest due to natural compensatory mechanisms, persistent increased intracranial pressure (IICP), brain herniation, and developmental delays.

Hydrocephalus occurs in approximately 3 to 4 births per 1,000, including those associated with spina bifida. Approximately two thirds of children with hydrocephalus die at an early age if they do not receive surgical treatment.

◆ Assessment

Infants
1. Excessive head growth (may be seen up to 3 years of age)
2. Forehead becomes prominent ("bossing")
3. Scalp appears shiny, with prominent scalp veins
4. Infant has difficulty holding head up
5. Delayed closure of the anterior fontanel
6. Fontanel tense and elevated above the surface of the skull
7. Signs of IICP—vomiting, restlessness and irritability, high-pitched and shrill cry, alteration in vital signs (increased systolic blood pressure, decreased pulse), pupillary changes, lethargy, seizures
8. Eyebrows and eyelids may be drawn upward, exposing the sclera above the iris.
9. Infant cannot gaze upward, causing "sunset eyes"
10. Strabismus, nystagmus, and optic atrophy may occur.
11. Alteration of muscle tone of the extremities

Older Children—present with signs of IICP
1. Headache, especially on awakening
2. Vomiting
3. Lethargy, fatigue apathy
4. Personality changes
5. Separation of cranial sutures (may be seen up to 10 years old)

H

6. Double vision, constricted peripheral vision, sudden appearance of internal strabismus, pupillary changes
7. Alteration in vital signs similar to those seen in infants
8. Difficulty with gait
9. Stupor, coma
10. Papilledema

◆ Diagnostic Evaluation

1. Transillumination of the infant's skull indicates abnormal fluid collection.
2. Percussion of the skull may produce a typical "cracked pot" sound (MacEwen's sign).
3. Computed tomography (CT) scan is the diagnostic tool of choice; helps differentiate between hydrocephalus and other intracranial lesions.
4. Skull x-rays show widening of the fontanelle and sutures and erosion of intracranial bone.
5. Ventriculography (rarely used) visualizes abnormalities in the ventricular system or the subarachnoid space.

H

◆ Collaborative Management

Surgical Interventions

1. Surgical procedures include
   a. Extracranial shunt (most common), diverts fluid from the ventricular system to an extracranial compartment, frequently the peritoneum or right atrium.
   b. Intracranial shunt may be used in selected cases of noncommunicating hydrocephalus, to divert fluid from the obstructed segment of the ventricular system to the subarachnoid space.
   c. Direct operation on the lesion causing the obstruction, such as a tumor
2. Most shunts have the following components:
   a. Ventricular tubing
   b. A one-way or unidirectional pressure-sensitive flow valve
   c. A pumping chamber
   d. Distal tubing

3. Shunt complications
   a. Need for shunt revision frequently occurs because of occlusion, infection, or malfunction.
   b. Shunt revision may be necessary because of growth of the child. Newer models, however, include coiled tubing to allow the shunt to grow with the child.
   c. Shunt dependency frequently occurs. The child rapidly manifests symptoms of IICP if the shunt does not function optimally.
   d. Children with ventriculoatrial shunts may experience endocardial contusions and clotting, leading to bacterial endocarditis, bacteremia, and ventriculitis, or thromboembolism and cor pulmonale.

◆ **Nursing Interventions**

Monitoring

1. Observe for evidence of IICP and report immediately.

PEDIATRIC ALERT
Brain stem herniation can occur with increased intracranial pressure and is manifested by opisthotonic positioning (flexion of head and feet backward). This is a grave sign and may be followed by respiratory arrest. Obtain help and prepare ventricular tap. Have emergency equipment on hand for resuscitation.

H

2. After surgery, monitor the child's temperature, pulse, respiration, blood pressure, and pupillary size and reaction every 15 minutes until stable; then monitor every 1 to 2 hours.
3. Monitor postoperatively for excessive drainage of cerebrospinal fluid.
   a. Sunken fontanel, agitation, restlessness (infant)
   b. Decreased level of consciousness (older child)
4. Monitor postoperatively for IICP, indicating shunt malfunction.
   a. Note especially change in level of consciousness, change in vital signs, vomiting, pupillary changes.
   b. Report these changes immediately to prevent cerebral hypoxia and possible brain herniation.

5. Accurately measure and record total fluid intake and output.

6. When oral feeding is begun after surgery, observe for and report any decrease in urine output, increased urine specific gravity, diminished skin turgor, dryness of mucous membranes, or lethargy, indicating dehydration.

7. After surgery, assess for fever (temperature normally fluctuates during the first 24 hours after surgery), purulent drainage from the incision, or swelling, redness, and tenderness along the shunt tract.

Supportive Care

1. If ventriculography is done, administer prescribed sedatives 30 minutes before the procedure to ensure its effectiveness.

> **NURSING ALERT**
> Sedatives are contraindicated in many cases because IICP predisposes the child to hypoventilation or respiratory arrest. If sedatives are administered, observe the child very closely for evidence of respiratory depression.

a. Observe the child closely for leaking of cerebrospinal fluid from the sites of subdural or ventricular taps. These tap holes should be covered with a small piece of gauze or cotton saturated with collodion.

b. Observe for changes in vital signs indicative of shock.

c. Observe for signs of IICP, which may occur if air has been injected into the ventricles.

2. Offer small, frequent feedings.

a. Be aware that feeding is often a problem because the child may be listless, anorectic, and prone to vomiting.

b. Complete nursing care and treatments before feeding so that the child will not be disturbed after feeding.

c. Hold the infant in a semi-sitting position with head well supported during feeding. Allow ample time for bubbling.

H

   d. Place the child on side with head elevated after feeding to prevent aspiration.

3. Because pressure sores of the head are a frequent problem, prevent sores by placing the child on a sponge rubber or lamb's-wool pad or an alternating-pressure or egg-crate mattress to keep weight evenly distributed. Keep the scalp clean and dry.

4. Provide meticulous skin care to all parts of the body and observe skin for the effects of pressure.

5. Turn the child's head frequently; change position at least every 2 hours.
   a. When turning the child, rotate head and body together to avoid straining the neck.
   b. A firm pillow may be placed under the head and shoulders for further support when lifting the child.

6. Perform passive range-of-motion exercises with the extremities, especially the legs.

7. Keep the eyes moistened with artificial tears if the child is unable to close eyelids normally. This prevents corneal ulcerations and infections.

8. Prepare the parents for their child's surgery by answering questions, describing what nursing care will take place postoperatively, and explaining how the shunt will work.

9. Prepare the child for surgery by using dolls or other form of play to describe what interventions will occur.

10. After surgery, take precautions to prevent hypothermia or hyperthermia.

11. Aspirate mucus from the nose and throat as necessary to prevent respiratory difficulty.

12. Turn the child frequently.

13. Promote optimal drainage of cerebrospinal fluid through a surgical shunt by pumping the shunt and positioning the child as directed.
   a. Report any difficulties in pumping the shunt.
   b. Gradually elevate the head of child's bed to 30 to 45 degrees as ordered. (Initially the child is positioned flat to prevent excessive cerebrospinal fluid drainage.)

14. Avoid placing excessive pressure of skin overlying shunt.

H

15. Administer intravenous fluids as prescribed; carefully monitor infusion rate to prevent fluid overload.
16. Use a nasogastric tube if necessary for abdominal distention.
    a. Most frequently used when a ventriculoperitoneal shunt has been performed
    b. Measure the drainage and record the amount and color.
    c. Monitor for return of bowel sounds after nasogastric suction has been disconnected for at least 30 minutes.
17. Give frequent mouth care while the child is NPO.
18. Begin oral feedings once the child is fully recovered from the anesthetic and displays interest.
19. Encourage the parents to treat the child as normally as possible, providing appropriate toys and love.
20. Help the parents to assist siblings to understand hydrocephalus and the child's special needs. Encourage parents to spend individual time with siblings and not neglect their needs as well. Suggest family counseling if needed.
21. Assist parents in locating additional resources, such as a social worker, discharge planner, visiting or home health nurse or aide, parent group or community agencies, and special programs at school.

Family Education and Health Maintenance

1. Stress the importance of recognizing symptoms of IICP and reporting them immediately.
2. Advise parents to report shunt malfunction or infection immediately to prevent IICP.
3. Teach parents that illnesses that cause vomiting and diarrhea or that prevent an adequate fluid intake are a great threat to the child who has had a shunt procedure. Advise parents to consult with the child's health care provider about immediate treatment of fever, control of vomiting and diarrhea, and replacement of fluids.
4. Tell the parents that few restrictions are required for children with shunts and to consult with the health care provider about specific concerns.

Hyperglycemic Hyperosmolar Nonketotic Syndrome

Hyperglycemic hyperosmolar nonketotic syndrome (HHNKS), also called hyperosomolar coma, is an acute complication of diabetes mellitus (particularly type II) characterized by hyperglycemia, dehydration, and hyperosmolarity, but little or no ketosis. The disorder is caused by inadequate levels of endogenous or exogenous insulin to control hyperglycemia. Precipitating factors include cardiac failure, burns, or chronic illness that increases need for insulin; use of agents such as corticosteroids or immunosuppressants that increase blood glucose levels; and procedures that cause stress and increase blood glucose levels such as hyperosmolar hyperalimentation or peritoneal dialysis.

HHNKS is a medical emergency which can cause coma and death if not treated properly.

◆ Assessment

1. Early symptoms include fatigue, malaise, polyuria, signs of dehydration, nausea, and vomiting.
2. Later signs are muscle weakness, hypothermia, seizures, stupor, and coma.

◆ Diagnostic Evaluation

1. Serum glucose and osmolality greatly elevated
2. Serum and urine ketone bodies minimal to absent
3. Serum sodium and potassium may be elevated, depending on degree of dehydration, despite total body losses.
4. Serum BUN and creatinine may be elevated because of dehydration.
5. Urine specific gravity elevated because of dehydration.

◆ Collaborative Management

Therapeutic Interventions

1. Correct fluid and electrolyte imbalances with IV fluids.
2. Evaluate complications such as stupor, seizures, shock, and treat appropriately.

H

3. Identification and treatment of underlying illnesses or events that precipitated HHNKS

Pharmacologic Interventions

1. IV regular insulin drip to counteract hyperglycemia

◆ Nursing Interventions

Monitoring

1. Assess for signs of dehydration such as poor turgor, flushing, dry mucous membranes.
2. Monitor glucose and electrolyte levels during IV therapy.
3. Monitor hourly intake and output and urine specific gravity for hydration status.
4. Monitor for shock: rapid, thready pulse, cool extremities, hypotension.
5. Monitor respiratory rate and breath sounds for signs of aspiration pneumonia.

Supportive Care

1. Institute fluid replacement therapy as ordered (usually normal or half-strength saline initially), maintaining patent IV line.
2. Assess patient for signs and symptoms of fluid overload and cerebral edema as IV therapy progresses.

NURSING ALERT
Too-rapid infusion of IV fluids can cause cerebral edema and death.

3. Administer regular insulin IV as ordered, and add dextrose to IV infusion as blood glucose falls below 300, to prevent hypoglycemia.
4. Be aware that patient is at risk for aspiration; assess patient's level of consciousness and ability to handle oral secretions (cough and gag reflex, ability to swallow).
5. Properly position patient to reduce possibility of aspiration.
   a. Elevate head of bed unless contraindicated.
   b. If nausea present, use side lying position.

6. Suction as often as needed to maintain patent airway.
7. Withhold oral intake until patient is no longer in danger of aspiration.
8. If patient is comatose, insert nasogastric tube to prevent aspiration.
9. Provide mouth care to maintain adequate mucosal hydration.

Patient Education and Health Maintenance

1. Advise the patient and family that it may take 3 to 5 days for symptoms to resolve.
2. Instruct patient and family about signs and symptoms of hyperglycemia and use of sick day guidelines (see p. 263).
3. Explain possible causes of HHNKS.
4. Review any changes in medication, activity, meal plan, or glucose monitoring for home care. It may not be necessary to continue insulin therapy after HHNKS; many patients can be treated with diet and oral agents alone.

Hyperparathyroidism

H

Hyperparathyroidism results from hypersecretion of parathyroid hormone (PTH), which causes calcium resorption by bone and increased calcium absorption by the kidneys and gut, among other effects. The disorder occurs in primary and secondary forms. Primary hyperparathyroidism most commonly results from a single parathyroid adenoma (approximately 80% of cases), and primarily affects women older than age 50. Secondary hyperparathyroidism is usually caused by kidney failure, which stimulates excessive compensatory production of PTH.

Early diagnosis is difficult. Complications include renal stones and kidney disease, gastrointestinal ulceration, demineralization of bones causing fractures, and hypoparathyroidism following surgery.

◆ Assessment

1. Depression of neuromuscular function: The patient may trip, drop objects, show general fatigue, loss of

memory for recent events, emotional instability, changes in level of consciousness with stupor and coma.
2. Cardiac dysrhythmias, hypertension, possible cardiac standstill.
3. Skeletal pain, backache, pain on weight bearing, muscular weakness, and possible vertebrae and ribs fractures.

◆ Diagnostic Evaluation

1. Persistently elevated serum calcium (11 mg/100 mL); test is performed on at least two occasions to determine consistency of results. Other causes of hypercalcemia must be ruled out: malignancy (usually bone or breast cancer), vitamin D excess, multiple myeloma, sarcoidosis, milk–alkali syndrome, Cushing's disease, hyperthyroidism, or effects of drugs such as thiazides.
2. PTH levels are increased.
3. Alkaline phosphatase levels are elevated, and serum phosphorus levels are decreased.
4. X-rays show skeletal changes such as deformities and bony cysts.
5. Cine CT will disclose parathyroid tumors more readily than x-ray.

◆ Collaborative Management

Therapeutic Interventions

1. Restrict dietary calcium, and discontinue all drugs that might cause hypercalcemia (thiazides, vitamin D) as directed.
2. Dialysis may be necessary in patients with resistant hypercalcemia or who have renal failure.

Pharmacologic Interventions

1. Hydration with IV saline solution and diuretics to increase urinary excretion of calcium in patients *not* in renal failure
2. Reduce digitalis dosage, as patient with hypercalcemia is more sensitive to drug's toxic effects.
3. Oral phosphate may be used as an antihypercalcemic agent.

4. Plicamycin, calcitonin, and etidronate disodium inhibit bone resorption of calcium.

Surgical Interventions

1. Primary hyperparathyroidism is treated surgically to remove parathyroid lesion.
2. Treatment risks hypoparathyroidism if too much of the gland tissue is removed.

◆ Nursing Interventions

Monitoring

1. Closely monitor the patient's fluid input and output and dietary calcium intake.
2. Monitor serum BUN, creatinine, and calcium.
3. Observe for signs of urinary tract infection, hematuria, and renal colic. Strain all urine.
4. Monitor ECG to detect changes secondary to hypocalcemia: shortened Q-T interval; with extreme hypercalcemia, widening of the T wave is seen.
5. After surgery, monitor serum calcium level and evaluate for signs and symptoms of hypocalcemia and onset of tetany.

Supportive Care

1. Prevent or promptly treat dehydration by reporting vomiting or other sources of fluid loss promptly.
2. Increase fluid intake to 3,000 mL/day to maintain hydration and prevent precipitation of calcium and formation of stones.
3. Assist the patient in hygiene and activities if bone pain is severe or if the patient experiences musculoskeletal weakness.
4. Protect the patient from falls or injury.
5. Turn the patient cautiously, and handle extremities gently to avoid fractures.
6. Encourage the patient to participate in mild exercise gradually as symptoms subside.
7. Instruct and demonstrate correct body mechanics to reduce strain, backache, and injury.
8. Administer analgesia as prescribed; assess level of pain and the patient's response to analgesia.
9. Reassure the patient about skeletal recovery: bone pain

H

diminishes fairly quickly, and fractures can be treated by orthopedic procedures.

Patient Education and Health Promotion

1. Instruct the patient about administration and side effects of calcium-reducing medications.
   a. Teach subcutaneous administration of calcitonin.
   b. Avoid calcium-containing foods within 2 hours of etidronate.
   c. Plicamycin is an antineoplastic drug that may cause nausea and vomiting, stomatitis.
2. Instruct the patient to avoid dietary sources of calcium, such as dairy products, broccoli, calcium-containing antacids.
3. Teach the patient to recognize and report signs and symptoms of hypocalcemic tetany (apprehensiveness, numbness and tingling in extremities or around the mouth).

H

Hypertension

Hypertension (high blood pressure) is a disease of vascular regulation resulting from malfunction of arterial pressure control mechanisms (CNS, renin-angiotensin-aldosterone system, extracellular fluid volume). The cause is unknown, and there is no cure. The basic explanation is that blood pressure is elevated when there is increased cardiac output plus increased peripheral vascular resistance.

The two major types of hypertension are *primary (essential) hypertension*, in which diastolic pressure is 90 mm Hg or higher in absence of other causes of hypertension (approximately 90% of patients); and *secondary hypertension*, which results primarily from renal disease, endocrine disorders, and coarctation of the aorta (approximately 5%–10% of patients). Either of these conditions may give rise to *accelerated hypertension*—a medical emergency—in which blood pressure elevates very rapidly to threaten one or more of the target organs: the brain, kidney, and heart (Box 2).

Hypertension is one of the most prevalent chronic diseases for which treatment is available; however, most patients with hypertension are untreated. Because hypertension presents no overt symptoms, it is termed the "silent killer." The untreated disease may progress to retinopathy, renal failure, coronary artery disease, left ventricular hypertrophy and congestive heart failure, and stroke.

◆ Assessment

1. History for associated risk factors:
   a. Age—between 30 and 70 years
   b. Race—black
   c. Use of medications that could elevate blood pressure— oral contraceptives, corticosteroids, nonsteroidal antiinflammatory agents, nasal decongestants, appetite suppressants, or tricyclic antidepressants
   d. Overweight
   e. Family history of high blood pressure, or previous episodes of high blood pressure
   f. Cigarette smoking
   g. Excessive salt intake
   h. Lipid abnormalities
   i. Sedentary lifestyle
   j. Stress
   k. Diabetes mellitus
2. Elevated blood pressure above 140/90 mm Hg on two occasions
   a. Measure blood pressure under the same conditions each time, and avoid taking blood pressure readings immediately after stressful or taxing situations.
   b. Use correct size blood pressure cuff; width should be 20% greater than width of measured extremity, and length should be sufficient to encircle measured extremity.
   c. Be aware that falsely elevated blood pressures may be obtained with a cuff that is too narrow; falsely

H

■ BOX 2 ACCELERATED HYPERTENSION

Accelerated hypertension (malignant hypertension) is severely elevated and sustained diastolic blood pressure that puts strain on the arterial walls, possibly leading to cerebral, myocardial, and renal ischemia. The blood pressure must be reduced promptly but not too rapidly because the patient's usual range may not be tolerated. The patient may manifest headaches, vision problems, confusion, disorientation, irritability, lethargy, and nausea and vomiting. Be alert for signs of seizure activity and pulmonary edema. If diastolic blood pressure exceeds 115 to 130 mm Hg, hospitalization in an ICU is recommended. Antihypertensive treatment includes vasodilators, adrenergic inhibitors, and possibly a calcium antagonist, all given IV. Diuretics also may be administered. Vasopressor agents should be available if the blood pressure responds too vigorously to antihypertensive agents.

Nursing responsibilities include continuous monitoring of blood pressure; monitoring urine output; monitoring for side effects of medications such as tachycardia and orthostatic hypotension; maintaining seizure precautions; providing a restful, quiet environment; maintaining cardiac monitoring; and reporting signs of central nervous system or cardiac complications.

low readings may be obtained with a cuff that is too wide.
   d. Auscultate and record precisely the systolic and diastolic pressures based on Korotkoff sounds.
3. Associated findings:
   a. Shift of the point of maximal impulse (PMI) to the left, which occurs in heart enlargement caused by chronic strain.

b. Bruits over peripheral arteries indicating the presence of atherosclerosis, which may be manifested as obstructed blood flow.
c. Possible vascular changes on funduscopic examination of the eyes: edema, spasm, and hemorrhage of the eye vessels
4. Headache, dizziness, and blurred vision, which indicate greatly elevated BP, and possibly development of accelerated hypertension

NURSING ALERT
The finding of an isolated elevated blood pressure does not necessarily indicate hypertension. However, the patient should be regarded as at risk for high blood pressure until further assessment through history taking and diagnostic testing either confirms or denies the diagnosis.

◆ Diagnostic Evaluation

1. 12-lead ECG, to evaluate effects of hypertension on the heart (left ventricular hypertrophy, ischemia) and to detect underlying heart disease
2. Chest radiographs to detect possible cardiomegaly
3. Blood samples for chemistry evaluation:
   a. Elevated serum BUN and creatinine indicate kidney disease as a cause or effect of hypertension.
   b. Decreased serum potassium indicates primary hyperaldosteronism; increased potassium indicates Cushing's syndrome—both conditions cause secondary hypertension.
4. 24-hour urine samples to evaluate extent of renal disease or to detect increased catecholamines indicating pheochromocytoma
5. Renal scan, computed tomography, and other special tests to detect causes of secondary hypertension

◆ Collaborative Management

Therapeutic Interventions

1. Lifestyle modifications as initial therapy:
   a. Lose weight, if more than 10% above ideal weight.

b. Limit alcohol (no more than 1 oz of ethanol per day).
c. Get regular aerobic exercise three times per week.
d. Cut sodium intake to less than 2 g/day.
e. Include recommended daily allowances of potassium, calcium, and magnesium in diet.
f. Stop smoking.
g. Reduce dietary saturated fat and cholesterol.

Pharmacologic Interventions

1. Antihypertensive medications, if, despite lifestyle changes, the blood pressure remains at or above 140/90 mm Hg over 3 to 6 months. Depending on the patient's condition, possible drugs include diuretics, beta-adrenergic blockers, alpha-receptor blockers, angiotensin-converting enzyme (ACE) inhibitors, and calcium antagonists (calcium channel blockers).
2. If hypertension is not controlled with the first drug within 1 to 3 months, three options can be considered:
   a. If the patient has faithfully taken the drug and not developed any side effects, the dose of the drug may be increased.
   b. If the patient has had adverse effects, another class of drugs can be substituted.
   c. A second drug from another class could be added. If adding the second drug lowers the pressure, the first drug may be slowly withdrawn.
3. A third drug or a diuretic if the desired blood pressure is still not achieved after adding a second drug. Medications may include centrally-acting alpha-agonists, peripheral adrenergic antagonists, or direct vasodilators.

◆ Nursing Interventions

Monitoring

1. Monitor the patient's blood pressure at regular intervals.
2. Monitor patient's response to drug therapy. Check for orthostatic changes caused by medication.
3. Monitor patient's weight and diet.
4. Monitor urinalysis for proteinuria, a sign of renal involvement.
5. Monitor for signs of target organ disease.

Supportive Care and Patient Education

1. Educate the patient about the disease, its treatment, and control. The goals of treatment are to control blood pressure, reduce risk of complications, and use minimum number of drugs with lowest dosage necessary to accomplish control.

2. Warn that unless BP is greatly elevated, the patient cannot tell by the way he or she feels whether blood pressure is normal or elevated.

3. Stress that hypertension is chronic and requires persistent therapy and mandatory follow-up health care visits.

4. Explain the pharmacologic control of hypertension. Discuss possible side effects of drugs.

GERONTOLOGIC ALERT
The multiple drugs required to control blood pressure may be difficult for the elderly patient to comprehend. The names of drugs are frequently difficult for the patient to pronounce. Color coding of medication bottles with an accompanying color-coded time of administration chart is one way to help the patient remember when to take medications. Elderly patients are also more sensitive to therapeutic levels of drugs and may demonstrate side effects while on an otherwise average dosage. They may be more sensitive to postural hypotension and should be cautioned to change positions with great care.

5. Educate the patient to be aware of toxic manifestations and report them so that pharmacotherapy can be adjusted.
    a. Remember that certain circumstances produce vasodilation—a hot bath, hot weather, febrile illness, consumption of alcohol.
    b. Be aware that blood pressure is decreased when circulating blood volume is reduced—dehydration, diarrhea, hemorrhage. '
    c. Consider the presence of edema as a reportable symptom, particularly when guanethidine is taken; medications are less effective in the presence of edema.

6. Teach a low-sodium diet and enlist the patient's cooperation in redirecting lifestyle in keeping with therapy guidelines.

◆

COMMUNITY CARE CONSIDERATIONS
Teach the patient how to take blood pressure at home and at work if the health care provider so desires. Tell the patient which readings should be reported. Have patient bring home blood pressure monitor to health care facility to check accuracy against sphygmomanometer.

Hyperthyroidism

Hyperthyroidism is overproduction of thyroid hormone, which creates far-reaching metabolic effects. The condition is more common in women than in men and occurs in several forms.

Graves' disease, the most prevalent form in adults and children, has been linked to an autoimmune reaction. It may also occur after an emotional shock, stress, or infection. The disorder can be mild, characterized by remissions and exacerbations, or it may progress to emaciation, extreme nervousness, delirium, disorientation, thyroid storm, and death.

In toxic nodular goiter, one or more thyroid nodules becomes hyperproductive. It is more common in older women with preexisting goiter.

Autoimmune thyroiditis (Hashimoto's disease) may cause initial hyperthyroidism before developing into hypothyroidism.

Factitious hyperthyroidism results from ingestion of excessive amounts of thyroid hormone medication.

Thyroid storm (thyrotoxicosis, thyroid crisis), can be precipitated by stress (surgery, infection, etc.) or inadequate surgical preparation of a patient with known hyperthyroidism. It requires emergency treatment. Other complications include infiltrative ophthalmopathy in 50% of patients with Graves' disease, development of goiter (hy-

H

perplasia of thyroid) from overstimulation, and hypothyroidism caused by overtreatment.

◆ Assessment

1. Nervousness, emotional lability, irritability, apprehension, insomnia
2. Fine tremor of hands
3. Profuse perspiration; flushed skin (eg, hands may be warm, soft, moist); heat intolerance
4. Increased appetite but progressive weight loss
5. Change in bowel habits; constipation or diarrhea; frequent stools
6. Muscle fatigability and weakness
7. Amenorrhea
8. Children may be tall and underweight for age.
9. Rapid pulse at rest as well as on exertion (ranges between 90 and 160 beats/min)
10. Palpitations, possible atrial fibrillation
11. Infiltrative ophthalmopathy
    a. Exophthalmos (bulging eyes) creates a startled expression.
    b. Weakness of extraocular muscles, lid edema, lid lag
12. Possible enlarged thyroid gland (goiter); a bruit may be auscultated over gland

H

NURSING ALERT
Thyroid storm is characterized by hyperpyrexia, diarrhea, dehydration, tachycardia, dysrhythmias, extreme irritation, and delirium. Coma, shock, and death result if not adequately treated.

◆ Diagnostic Evaluation

1. Elevated T_3 and T_4, elevated serum T_3 resin uptake; possibly suppressed thyroid-stimulating hormone (TSH)
2. Microsomal antibodies elevated in initial stage of autoimmune thyroiditis
3. Thyroid scan to show increased uptake of radioactive iodine ^{131}I. (Results may also be below normal, de-

pending on the underlying cause of the disorder.) Also needed to rule out cold nodules that may indicate thyroid cancer.

◆ Collaborative Management

Therapeutic Interventions

1. Treatment aims to restore the patient's basal metabolic rate to normal as soon as possible, and then to maintain it. The specific approach depends on the cause, age of the patient, severity of disease, and complications.
2. Radioactive iodine therapy limits thyroid hormone secretion by destroying thyroid tissue. Dosage is controlled to avoid provoking hypothyroidism.
   a. Chief advantage over thionamides is that a lasting remission can be achieved; chief disadvantage is that permanent hypothyroidism can be caused by overmedication.
   b. Radiation thyroiditis (a transient exacerbation of hyperthyroidism) may result from leakage of thyroid hormone into the circulation from damaged follicles.
3. Emergency management of thyroid storm includes treatment of hyperthermia with cooling blanket and acetaminophen; reversal of dehydration with IV fluids and electrolytes. The precipitating event must also be identified and treated, if possible.

Pharmacologic Interventions

1. Thyroid hormone antagonists—thionamide drugs such as propylthiouracil and methimazole—inhibit thyroid hormone formation. Often used for Graves' disease; remissions occur spontaneously within 1 to 2 years; however, 50% of patients suffer a relapse.
   a. Duration of treatment depends on reduction of thyroid gland, and normalization of T_4 and T_3 uptake. Treatment continues until patient becomes clinically euthyroid (from 3 months to 1–2 years).
   b. Drug is withdrawn gradually to prevent exacerbation.
   c. If euthyroidism cannot be maintained without therapy, then radiation or surgery is recommended.

❖

NURSING ALERT
Observe the patient for evidence of iodine toxicity when taking thionamides: swelling of buccal mucosa, excessive salivation, coryza, skin eruptions. Discontinue thionamides if these occur.

2. Beta-adrenergic blocking agent propranolol may be given to abolish tachycardia, tremor, excess sweating, nervousness until antithyroid drugs or radioiodine can take effect.
3. Glucocorticoids may be given to suppress peripheral conversion of thyroxine to triiodothyronine, a more potent thyroid hormone.
4. Lugol's iodine solution may be used to inhibit hormone release in thyroid storm.

Surgical Interventions

1. Used for patients with very large goiters, or for those who cannot be treated with thionamides or radioiodine. Surgery or radioiodine are preferred for nodular toxic goiter and thyroid carcinoma.
2. Subtotal thyroidectomy involves removal of most of the thyroid gland (see p. 840). Entire thyroid gland is not removed to spare parathyroid function.

◆ Nursing Interventions

Monitoring

1. Monitor for signs of thionamide toxicity (acute agranulocytosis)—fever, sore throat, upper respiratory infection or rash, fever, urticaria, or enlarged salivary glands.
2. Monitor temperature for impending thyroid storm.
3. Monitor the patient's fluid and nutritional status: weigh the patient daily, accurately record daily intake and output.
4. Monitor vital signs and assess skin turgor, mucous membranes, and neck veins for signs of increased or decreased fluid volume.

Supportive Care

1. To provide adequate nutrition, give high-calorie foods and fluids consistent with the patient's requirements.

H

2. Provide a quiet, calm environment.
3. Restrict stimulants (tea, coffee, chocolate) and alcohol; explain rationale of requirements and restrictions to patient.
4. Assess for fatigue and prevent overactivity.
5. To avoid upsetting the patient, limit visitors; avoid stimulating conversations or television.
6. Reduce environmental stressors; reduce noise and lights.
7. Promote sleep and relaxation through use of prescribed medications, massage, relaxation exercises, and clustering nursing care activities.
8. Employ safety measures to reduce risk of trauma or falls if patient is agitated.
9. Bathe the patient frequently with cool water (avoid soap to prevent drying skin) to counteract diaphoresis; change linens when damp. Use lubricant skin lotions to protect pressure points.
10. Clear up treatment misconceptions, especially about radioactive iodine.
    a. Radioactive iodine pill will cause destruction of thyroid tissue only.
    b. Small levels of radiation will be eliminated through urine and feces, which should be disposed of promptly.

Family Education and Health Maintenance

1. Emphasize to the patient and family the importance of following the prescribed medication regimen.
2. Advise the patient to have periodic blood evaluations to monitor thyroid hormone levels.
3. Teach about signs of hypothyroidism due to overtreatment, which need to be reported.
4. Teach the patient and family to recognize and immediately report signs and symptoms of thyroid storm (tachycardia, hyperpyrexia, extreme irritation) and alert them to predisposing factors (infection, surgery, stress, abrupt withdrawal of antithyroid medications and adrenergic blocking agents).
5. Encourage well-child visits for evaluation of growth and development.

Hypoparathyroidism

Hypoparathyroidism results from a deficiency of parathyroid hormone (PTH) caused by accidental surgical removal or destruction, malignancy, idiopathic (may be familial or autoimmune), or resistance to parathyroid hormone (PTH) action. With inadequate PTH secretion, less calcium is resorbed by the kidneys and bones, and less calcium is absorbed by the GI tract, causing serum calcium levels to fall.

Acute complications related to hypocalcemia include seizures, tetany, and mental disorders, all of which can be reversed with calcium therapy.

Long-term complications include subcapsular cataracts, calcification of the basal ganglia, and papilledema, caused by precipitation of calcium out of serum and deposition in tissues; shortening of the fingers and toes, and bowing of the long bones, caused by inadequate PTH and additional genetic abnormalities. Of these complications, only papilledema is reversible.

H

◆ Assessment

1. Tetany—general muscular hypertonia; severe anxiety and apprehension; attempts at voluntary movement result in tremors and spasmodic or uncoordinated movements
   a. Positive Chvostek and Trousseau's signs (see p. 843)
   b. If onset is acute, may cause laryngeal spasm.
2. Renal colic is often present if the patient has history of stones; preexisting stones loosen and migrate into the ureter—also cause hematuria, and signs of infection.

◆ Diagnostic Evaluation

1. Serum phosphorus is elevated; serum calcium is decreased to low level (7.5 mg/100 mL or less).
2. PTH is decreased in most cases; may be normal or elevated in pseudohypoparathyroidism.

◆ Collaborative Management

Therapeutic and Pharmacologic Interventions

1. IV calcium solution is used to treat hypocalcemic tetany.
   a. Ensure that a syringe and ampule of a calcium solution (calcium chloride, calcium gluceptate, calcium gluconate) is kept at the bedside at all times.
   b. Most rapidly effective calcium solution is ionized calcium chloride (10% solution).
   c. For rapid relief of severe tetany, infuse prescribed calcium solution every 10 minutes.

NURSING ALERT

Administer all IV calcium preparations slowly, at rates of approximately 0.5 to 1 mL/min, to avoid severe irritation, thrombosis, flushing, and possible cardiac arrest.

---

   d. When tetany is controlled, give IM or oral calcium as prescribed.
   e. Later, add vitamin D to calcium intake to increase calcium absorption and raise serum calcium levels.
   f. Thiazide diuretic may also be added because of its calcium-retaining effect on the kidney; doses of calcium and vitamin D may then be lowered.
2. Treat kidney stones and possible hypercalciuria.

◆ Nursing Interventions

Monitoring

1. Monitor respiratory and neuromuscular status closely for impending tetany and laryngeal spasm.
2. Closely monitor patient's intake and output and serum calcium and phosphorous levels.
3. During treatment for tetany, monitor for hypercalciuria. Periodic 24-hour urinary calcium determinations are recommended.

Supportive Care

1. Promote high-calcium diet if prescribed—dairy products, green leafy vegetables.

2. Instruct the patient about signs and symptoms of hypo-calcemia and hypercalcemia that should be reported.
3. Use caution in administering other drugs to the patient with hypocalcemia.
   a. The hypocalcemic patient is sensitive to digoxin; as hypocalcemia is reversed, the patient may rapidly develop digitalis toxicity.
   b. Cimetidine interferes with normal parathyroid function, especially in the patient with renal failure, which increases the risk of hypocalcemia.

Patient Education and Health Maintenance

1. Explain to the patient and family the function of PTH and the role of vitamin D and calcium in maintaining good health.
2. Discuss the importance of complying with the medica-tion regimen. Warn the patient not to substitute any over-the-counter drugs without prior advice and con-sent of the health care provider.
3. Teach the patient to recognize and report symptoms of hypercalcemia or hypocalcemia.
4. Advise the patient to wear a medical alert tag.
5. Stress the rationale and importance of lifelong periodic follow-up examinations.

H

Hypospadias

Hypospadias is a congenital malposition of the urethral opening. It is the most common congenital anomaly in-volving the penis, and may result partly from decreased testosterone production in early gestation. In males, the urethra opens on the ventral aspect of the penis. In severe cases, the urethra may open on the shaft of the penis and deflect the penis downward. Hypospadias is rare in females, in which the urethra opens into the vagina. The disorder is frequently associated with other urogenital tract anomalies, as well as with undescended testicles and inguinal hernia. Subsequent male siblings are at increased risk of hypospadias. Severe forms may interfere with the ability to procreate.

◆ Assessment

1. Inspection of the genitalia shows abnormal placement of urethra.
2. The male infant or child cannot void with the penis in the normal elevated position.

◆ Diagnostic Evaluation

1. Usually not difficult to diagnose because of visual anomaly
2. Severe cases require genotypic or phenotypic sex determination, chromosomal, and hormonal studies.
3. Renal ultrasound, intravenous pyelography, or voiding cystourethrography may be done to determine associated defects.

◆ Collaborative Management

Surgical Interventions

1. Surgical reconstruction may be required beginning before 1 year of age
2. Two-stage procedure is needed for extensive defects.

◆ Nursing Interventions

Monitoring

1. Postoperatively, monitor daily weights and intake and output.
2. Monitor vital signs for hypotension or tachycardia.
3. Assess patient's skin turgor and mucous membranes for signs of dehydration.
4. Observe and record characteristics of urinary drainage, occurrence of bladder spasms, appearance of dressing and the incision. Report urine or bloody drainage from the incision promptly.

Supportive Care

1. Explain all diagnostic tests before their occurrence and prepare the parents and child for surgery.
2. Emphasize that the parents or child are in no way to blame for the illness.
3. Postoperatively, maintain patency of suprapubic cath-

H

eter and perineal dressing. Restrain child as necessary to prevent inadvertent removal.

4. Maintain child in bed in the supine position for 2 to 3 days and with limited activity in bed for several more days to prevent disruption of surgical site. Use bed cradle as necessary to prevent pressure of bedclothes on surgical site.

5. Administer analgesics as needed and anticholinergics for sharp painful bladder spasms.

6. Encourage fluids and high-fiber diet to prevent constipation associated with bed rest.

7. Provide diversional activity and reassurance while on bed rest.

Family Education and Health Management

1. Teach prompt diaper changes and cleaning of skin after bowel movements to prevent irritation of skin and contamination of healing wound.

2. Encourage long-term follow-up to ensure healing and acceptable cosmetic appearance.

3. Advise parents to report curvature of the penis, decreased force of urinary stream, or any change in voiding that may indicate complication requiring dilation or other surgical intervention.

H

Hypothermia

Hypothermia is a condition in which the core temperature of the body falls below 95°F (35°C) as a result of exposure to cold. In response to a decreased core temperature, the body will attempt to produce or conserve more heat through three mechanisms: by shivering, which produces heat through muscular activity; by peripheral vasoconstriction, which decreases heat loss; and by raising the basal metabolic rate. Treatment of this life-threatening condition requires immediate resuscitation, careful monitoring, and gradual rewarming of the body without precipitating cardiac dysrhythmias.

◆ Assessment

1. Initial tachypnea followed by slow and shallow respirations; possibly 2 or 3 breaths/min in severe hypothermia

2. Breath may have fruity or acetone odor, indicating metabolism of fat because of decreased insulin levels.

3. If the body temperature falls below 30°C (86°F) (severe hypothermia), heart sounds may not be audible even if the heart is still beating. Tissues conduct sound poorly at low temperatures.

4. Blood pressure readings may be extremely difficult to hear because cold tissue conducts sound waves poorly.

5. Pupil reflexes may be blocked by a decrease in cerebral blood flow, so the pupils may appear fixed and dilated.

NURSING ALERT
A patient with a weak heartbeat may present like a patient in cardiac arrest, with fixed dilated pupils, no pulse, and no blood pressure.

H

6. A variety of cardiac dysrhythmias may be seen. A hypothermic heart is extremely susceptible to ventricular fibrillation. Very cold hearts do not respond to drugs or defibrillation.

7. Progressive neurologic deterioration marked by apathy, poor judgment, ataxia, dysarthria, drowsiness, and eventually coma.

8. Speech is slow and may be slurred.

9. Shivering may be suppressed below a temperature of 32.2°C (90°F).

◆ Diagnostic Evaluation

1. Electrocardiogram and continuous cardiac monitoring to determine rate and rhythm

2. Arterial blood gases (ABGs) to detect acidosis

3. Serum electrolytes and kidney function tests to monitor condition

Therapeutic Interventions

1. Assist breathing and oxygenation with supplemental O_2 at 100%, or bag-valve-mask device.

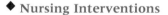

NURSING ALERT
If intubation is necessary, extreme caution should be used, because ventricular fibrillation may be precipitated.

2. If pulse and respirations are absent, provide CPR until the patient is adequately rewarmed and further evaluation through ECG and hemodynamic monitoring can be done.
3. Start IV therapy with normal saline. Ringer's lactate is not recommended, because a cold liver may not be able to metabolize the lactate.
4. Initiate rewarming. The type of rewarming (passive or active external rewarming; active core rewarming) depends on the degree of hypothermia. Rewarming should continue until the core body temperature is 34°C (93.2°F). If the patient is in cardiac arrest, rewarming should continue until a temperature of 32°C (89.6°F) has been reached. Death in hypothermia is defined as a failure to revive after rewarming.

◆ **Nursing Interventions**

Monitoring

1. Continuously monitor core temperatures with a low-reading rectal thermometer.
2. Continuously monitor ECG. Because pulse may be unobtainable because of hypothermia, rely on the cardiac monitor to determine the need for CPR.
3. Monitor the patient's condition through vital signs, central venous pressure, urinary output, ABGs, and other hemodynamics methods.
   a. Maintain an arterial line for recording blood pressure and to facilitate blood sampling. This allows rapid detection of acid–base disturbances and assessment of adequacy of ventilation and oxygenation.

H

b. Urine output may show increase in response to peripheral vasoconstriction, "cold diuresis."

Supportive Care

1. Handle the patient *carefully and gently*—to avoid triggering ventricular fibrillation.

> **NURSING ALERT**
> Extreme caution should be used in moving or transporting patients because the heart is near fibrillation threshold in hypothermia.

2. Provide passive external rewarming for patients with temperature above 28°C (82.4°F).
   a. Remove all the wet or cold clothing and replace with warm clothing.
   b. Provide insulation by wrapping the patient in several blankets.
   c. Provide warmed fluids to drink.
3. Provide active external rewarming for patients with temperature above 28°C (82.4°F), as directed.
   a. Apply external heat, for example, warm hot water bottles to the armpits, neck, or groin (do not apply hot water bottles directly to the skin), or warm water immersion.
   b. May cause peripheral vasodilation, returning cool blood to the core, causing an initial lowering of the core temperature
   c. May cause acidosis because of the "washing out" of lactic acid from the peripheral tissues
   d. May cause an increase in the metabolic demands before the heart is warmed to meet these needs
4. Active core rewarming for patient with temperature less than 28°C (82.4°F), as directed
   a. Inhalation of warmed, humidified oxygen by mask or ventilator
   b. Warmed intravenous fluids
   c. Warmed gastric lavage
   d. Peritoneal dialysis with warmed standard dialysis solution
   e. Mediastinal irrigation through open thoracotomy

H

has been used successfully but has serious complications.

f. Cardiopulmonary bypass

Family Education and Health Maintenance

1. Ensure adequate follow-up to ensure full recovery.
2. Review safety measures to prevent hypothermia such as wearing adequate warm, dry clothing when exposed to cool, wet, windy weather conditions.
3. Discourage the use of alcohol while engaging in sports and recreation outdoors in cool weather, because alcohol increases the risk of hypothermia.

Hypothyroidism

Hypothyroidism (also known as myxedema if symptomatic) refers to a low level of thyroid hormone in the bloodstream. This condition is caused by thyroid dysfunction, which may result from surgery (thyroidectomy), therapy with radioactive iodine, or overtreatment with antithyroid drugs.

Hypothyroidism may also be congenital (1 in 4,000 live births) or result from chronic immunologic dysfunction, as in Hashimoto's thyroiditis.

Hypothyroidism in the newborn results in abnormal development of the central nervous system. As the disorder progresses, there is a general depression of most cellular enzyme systems and oxidative processes. The signs and symptoms of the disorder range from vague, nonspecific complaints that make diagnosis difficult, to severe symptoms that may be life threatening if unrecognized and untreated. Complications include mental retardation in the young child who is untreated from birth; short stature and delayed physical development in the older child; and myxedema coma, which has a high mortality rate.

◆ Assessment

1. The newborn may have very subtle signs, if any: markedly open posterior fontanel, prolonged physiologic

H

jaundice, feeding difficulties, cool and mottled skin, hypotonia, umbilical hernia.

2. After 6 months of age, signs may include: growth failure, large and protruding tongue, coarse facial features, poor feeding, and constipation.

3. Older children with acquired hypothyroidism may exhibit: slow growth rate, lethargy, obedient and nonaggressive behavior, cold intolerance, and poor school performance.

4. Signs and symptoms in adults include:
   a. Fatigue and lethargy
   b. Weight gain
   c. Complaints of cold hands and feet
   d. Decreased libido
   e. Menorrhagia or amenorrhea; difficulty conceiving or spontaneous abortion
   f. Subnormal temperature and pulse rates
   g. Thick, puffy skin; subcutaneous swelling in hands, feet, and eyelids (myxedema); thinning hair, with loss of the lateral one-third of each eyebrow
   h. Polyneuropathy, ataxia, muscle aches or weakness, clumsiness, prolonged deep tendon reflexes (especially ankle jerk)
   i. Constipation, decreased peristalsis

5. Severe hypothyroidism is evidenced by hypotension, bradycardia, hyponatremia, (possibly) convulsions, hypothermia, cerebral hypoxia, and myxedema coma

◆ Diagnostic Evaluation

1. Thyroid function tests show low T_3 and T_4 levels and elevated TSH level.
2. Thyroid microsomal antibodies may be elevated in autoimmune thyroiditis.
3. Elevated cholesterol
4. Possible enlarged heart on chest x-ray
5. Children may have delayed bone age on x-ray
6. ECG may show sinus bradycardia, low voltage of QRS complexes, and flat or inverted T waves.

◆ Collaborative Management

Therapeutic Interventions

1. In severe hypothyroidism with myxedema coma, vital functions are supported.

2. IV fluids are given cautiously if hyponatremia is present to prevent water intoxication.
3. Rapid rewarming techniques are avoided to prevent increased oxygen requirements and possible cardiovascular collapse.

Pharmacologic Interventions

1. To restore normal metabolic state (euthyroid) in severe hypothyroidism:
   a. Because triiodothyronine (T_3) acts more quickly than thyroxine (T_4), this is given by nasogastric tube if patient is unconscious.
   b. Levothyroxine can be administered parenterally until consciousness is restored to restore thyroxine level.
   c. Later, the patient is continued on oral thyroid hormone therapy.
   d. With rapid administration of thyroid hormone, plasma thyroxine levels may initiate adrenal insufficiency; hence, steroid therapy may be initiated.
2. Mild symptoms in the alert patient or asymptomatic cases (with abnormal laboratory work only) require only low-dose thyroid hormones, such as levothyroxine, to be given orally.

H

GERONTOLOGIC ALERT
Care must be taken with elderly patients and those with coronary artery disease when starting thyroid hormone replacement, to avoid coronary ischemia caused by increased oxygen demands of heart. It is preferable to start with low doses and increase very gradually, taking 1 to 2 months to reach full replacement doses.

◆ Nursing Interventions

Monitoring

1. Monitor the effects of sedatives, narcotics, and anesthetics closely because patient is more sensitive to these agents.
2. Monitor the patient to anticipate successful response to treatments:

a. Diuresis, decreased puffiness
b. Improved reflexes and muscle tone
c. Accelerated pulse rate
d. A slightly higher T_4 level and decreased TSH
e. All signs of hypothyroidism should disappear over a 3- to 12-week period.
3. As thyroid hormone levels gradually return to normal, monitor for dysrythmias, chest pain, and signs of heart failure.
4. Monitor a child's behavior, including sleep, eating pattern, bowel habits, level of alertness, and school performance.
5. Assess a child's growth pattern, weight gain, and head circumference.

Supportive Care

1. Prevent chilling to avoid increasing metabolic rate, which, in turn, places strain on the heart. Provide bed socks, bed jacket, warm environment.
2. Administer all prescribed drugs with caution before and after thyroid replacement begins. After thyroid replacement is initiated, the thyroid hormones may increase the effects of digitalis (monitor pulse) and anticoagulants (watch for signs of bleeding).
3. Report occurrence of angina.
4. Teach energy conservation techniques and need to increase activity gradually.

Family Education and Health Maintenance

1. Stress that thyroid hormone replacement therapy is a life-long treatment.
2. Teach patients to take medications every day.

PEDIATRIC ALERT
Advise parents not to mix thyroid medication in a bottle because feeding may not be finished; instead mix with small amount of fluid and give with dropper or syringe. If thyroid hormone pill is being chewed rather than swallowed, have child avoid brushing teeth immediately after to avoid washing away some of dose.

---

3. Teach about signs and symptoms of insufficient and excessive medication.
4. Reinforce the necessity of having blood evaluations periodically to determine thyroid levels.
5. Encourage adequate fluid intake and use of fiber to prevent constipation.
6. Advise controlling dietary intake to limit calories and reduce weight.

Hysterectomy

Hysterectomy is the surgical removal of the uterus, primarily to treat cancer, benign tumors, bleeding disorders of the uterus, and endometriosis. Sixty-five percent of these procedures occur during the reproductive years. Hysterectomy is classified as subtotal, total, or radical. In subtotal hysterectomy, the corpus of the uterus is removed, but a cervical stump remains. In total hysterectomy, the entire uterus, including cervix, is removed, but tubes and ovaries remain. In radical hysterectomy with bilateral salpingo-oophorectomy (BSO), all of the reproductive organs are removed. Sometimes the uterus is removed through a vaginal rather than an abdominal approach.

◆ Potential Complications

1. Incisional or pelvic infection
2. Hemorrhage
3. Urinary tract injury

◆ Collaborative Management

Preoperative Care

1. Determine if the patient knows reason for hysterectomy, what the procedure involves, and what to expect postoperatively.
2. Keep the patient NPO from midnight the night before surgery and have the patient void before surgery.
3. Administer an enema before surgery to evacuate the bowel and prevent contamination and trauma during surgery.

H

4. Perform vaginal irrigation before surgery to cleanse the area and ensure that a skin preparation is done if ordered.
5. Administer preoperative medication to help the patient relax.

Postoperative Care

1. Provide adequate pain control.
2. Encourage the patient to splint incision when moving.
3. Encourage the patient to ambulate as soon as possible to decrease flatus and abdominal distention.
4. Institute sitz baths or ice packs as prescribed to alleviate perineal discomfort.
5. Monitor intake and output, bladder distention, signs and symptoms of bladder infection.
6. Ensure that patient voids after surgery. Catheterize the patient intermittently if uncomfortable or has not voided in 8 hours. Maintain patency of indwelling catheter if one is in place.
7. Catheterize for residual urine after the patient voids, if ordered; should be less than 100 mL. Continue to check if more than 100 mL to prevent bladder infection.
8. Encourage the patient to empty bladder around the clock, not only when feeling the urge, because of loss of sensation of bladder fullness.
9. Ensure adequate hydration to decrease risk of urinary infection.
10. Assess vaginal drainage for amount, color, and odor. Assess incision site and vital signs for signs of infection.
11. Administer antibiotics as prescribed.
12. Assist with use of incentive spirometer, coughing and deep breathing, and ambulation to decrease risk of pulmonary infection.
13. Discuss changes regarding sexual functioning such as shortened vagina and possible dyspareunia due to dryness.
14. Offer suggestions to improve sexual functioning.
    a. Use of water-soluble lubricants
    b. Change position—female dominant offers more control of depth of penetration.

H

◆ Patient Education and Health Maintenance

1. Advise the patient that a total hysterectomy with BSO produces a surgical menopause. The patient may experience hot flashes, vaginal dryness, and mood swings unless hormonal replacement therapy is instituted.
2. Advise the patient not to sit too long at one time, as in driving long distances, because of risk of pooling of blood in the lower extremities or pelvis, causing thromboembolism.
3. Suggest that the patient delay driving a car until the third postoperative week, because even pressing the brake pedal puts stress on the lower abdomen.
4. Tell the patient to expect a tired feeling for the first few days at home and, therefore, not to plan too many activities for the first week. She will be able to perform most of her usual daily activities within 1 month, and feel herself again within 2 months.
5. Tell the patient not to feel discouraged if at times during convalescence she experiences depression, feels like crying, and seems unusually nervous. This is common but will not last.
6. Remind the patient to ask her surgeon about any strenuous or lifting activities, which are usually delayed for 4 to 6 weeks.
7. Reinforce instructions given by the surgeon on intercourse, douching, and use of tampons, which are usually discouraged for 4 to 6 weeks. Sexual intercourse should be resumed cautiously to prevent injury and discomfort.
8. Showers are permitted, but tub baths are deferred until healing is complete.
9. Instruct the patient to report fever over 37.8°C (100°F), heavy vaginal bleeding, drainage, and foul odor of discharge.
10. Emphasize the importance of follow-up and routine physical and gynecologic examinations.

H

Imperforate Anus

Imperforate anus refers to all congenital abnormalities of the anorectal canal or in the vicinity of the anus within the perineum. These conditions include anal stenosis (abnormally small anal opening); imperforate anal membrane; and anal or rectal agenesis, with or without perineal, urethral, or vaginal fistulas. These conditions result from arrested embryologic development of the anus, lower rectum, and urogenital tract at the eighth week of gestation. Although the cause is unknown, imperforate anus is linked to other congenital abnormalities, including (in descending order of importance) genitourinary anomalies, spinal malformations, esophageal atresia with tracheoesophageal fistula, low birth weight/CNS anomalies, and congenital heart disease. Imperforate anus occurs in 1 of every 5,000 births and is more likely to affect infants with Down syndrome.

◆ Assessment

1. Anal stenosis—anal opening is very small; defecation is difficult; stools may be ribbonlike
2. Imperforate anal membrane—infant fails to pass meconium; greenish, bulging membrane is seen
3. Anal agenesis—anal dimple is present; stimulation of perianal area leads to puckering; signs of intestinal obstruction develop if no fistula; fistula may be visible in perineal or vulvar area in girl, perineal or urethral area in boy; meconium-stained urine or vaginal drainage
4. Rectal agenesis—no anal opening; fistulas not externally visible (posterior urethra in boys, high in vagina in girls)

PEDIATRIC ALERT
A newborn who does not pass a stool in the first 24 hours of birth requires further assessment.

◆ Diagnostic Evaluation

1. Urine examination may show meconium and epithelial debris, indicating fistula.
2. Voiding cystourethrogram shows abnormality.
3. Wangensteen-Rice x-ray (upside-down position) is useful only after infant is 24 hours of age; has limited accuracy in locating rectal pouch.
4. Sonogram may be done to locate rectal pouch.

◆ Collaborative Management

Surgical Interventions

Surgical procedure depends on the location, type of imperforate anus, and sex of child.

1. Low—female
   a. Decompression of bowel with catheter irrigations
   b. Dilatation of fistula for 8 to 12 months thereafter
   c. Definitive repair
2. Low—male
   a. Rectal cutback anoplasty or Y-V plasty
   b. Local dilatation of fistula
3. High—male
   a. Colostomy for decompression
   b. Definitive pull-through surgery; deferred until about 1 year of age or when child attains 6.75 to 9 kg (15–20 lb.)
4. High—female
   a. Colostomy
   b. Definitive repair done when infant is 1 year of age or 6.75 to 9 kg (15–20 lb.)

◆ Nursing Interventions

Monitoring

1. Observe the patient carefully for any signs of distress, abdominal distension, vomiting. Monitor abdominal girth and intake and output.
2. Check vital signs frequently.
3. Monitor nasogastric decompression before and after surgery for amount and character of drainage.
4. Observe postoperatively for abdominal distention,

I

bleeding from perineum, and respiratory difficulty. Especially note any vomiting or stooling.

5. Monitor for return of peristalsis through auscultation after clamping of nasogastric tube.

6. Monitor parenteral fluids and discontinue when oral intake is sustained.

Supportive Care

Preoperative care

1. Withhold feedings. Note color and amount of any vomiting.

2. Maintain nasogastric tube passed to decompress the stomach.

3. Use an Isolette or radiant warmer to maintain stable temperature.

4. Keep fistula area clean.

Postoperative care

1. Prevent infection of suture line.
   a. Do not put anything in rectum after anoplasty.
   b. Expose perineum to air.
   c. Position the infant for easy access to perineum for cleansing and minimal irritation of site.

2. Observe for redness, drainage, poor healing.

3. Prevent skin breakdown around colostomy site with appropriate appliances and skin barrier. Consult an enterostomal therapist.

4. Start oral feedings as ordered (usually within hours after an anoplasty, longer with colostomy or pull-through).

5. Reassure the parents that colostomy is temporary.

6. Encourage parents to participate in care and provide emotional security for the child.

7. Initiate referral to community nurse, especially if the parents are particularly anxious about caring for the child at home.

Family Education and Health Maintenance

1. Review special care and procedures to be continued at home (colostomy, anal dilation). Involve parents and other caregivers in teaching.

2. Explain problems that may be encountered as the child grows:
   a. Fecal impaction because of lack of sensation to defecate

    b. Future surgery if primary repair was not done
    c. Toilet training may be delayed, especially after a pull-through procedure.
    d. Inability to control fecal seepage from rectum
3. Provide some practical guidelines to help parents cope:
    a. Fecal control may not be achieved until age 10.
    b. Encourage bowel habit training or patterning of defecation (eg, after breakfast) early.
    c. Promote diet modifications; teach foods that produce laxative effect (plums, prunes, chocolate, nuts, corn) and foods that have binding effect (peanut butter, hot cereal, cheese).
    d. Stool softeners or antidiarrheal medications may be effective.
    e. Rectal inertia may cause fecal impaction in rectosigmoid colon with soiling from fluid overflow. Bisacodyl suppository or cleansing enema provide assistance in management.
4. Encourage mutual support form other families who have a child with an anorectal malformation.

Infective Endocarditis
See Endocarditis, Infective

I

Intestinal Obstruction

Intestinal obstruction is an interruption in the normal flow of intestinal contents along the intestinal tract. The block may occur in the small or large intestine, may be complete or incomplete, may be mechanical or paralytic, and may or may not compromise the vascular supply. Obstruction most frequently occurs in the very young and the very old.

Mechanical obstruction does not restrict the bowel's blood supply, and can result from postsurgical adhesions (90% of mechanical obstructions), hernia (most common nonsurgical cause), volvulus, hematoma, tumor, intussusception (telescoping of intestinal wall into itself), stricture, stenosis, foreign body, fecal or barium impaction, or polyp.

Paralytic obstruction (paralytic ileus), in contrast, involves no physical obstruction. Peristalsis is ineffective, blood supply is not interrupted, and the condition disappears spontaneously after 2 to 3 days. Causes include spinal cord injuries, vertebral fractures, peritonitis, pneumonia, gastrointestinal or abdominal surgery, and wound dehiscence (breakdown).

Strangulated obstruction compromises the blood supply, leading to gangrene of the intestinal wall. It is caused by prolonged mechanical obstruction.

Untreated, intestinal obstruction leads to ischemia, necrosis, shock, and death.

◆ Assessment

1. *Simple mechanical—high small bowel:* Colic (cramps) mid-to-upper abdomen, some distention, early bilious vomiting, increased bowel sounds (high-pitched tinkling heard at brief intervals), minimal diffuse tenderness.
2. *Simple mechanical—low small bowel:* Significant colic (cramps) midabdominal, considerable distention, vomiting—slight or absent—later feculent, increased bowel sounds and "hush" sounds, minimal diffuse tenderness.
3. *Simple mechanical—colon:* Cramps (mid-to-lower abdomen), later-appearing distention, then vomiting may develop (feculent), increase in bowel sounds, minimal diffuse tenderness.
4. *Partial chronic mechanical obstruction:* May occur with granulomatous bowel in Crohn's disease. Symptoms are cramping abdominal pain, mild distention, and diarrhea.
5. *Strangulation:* Symptoms progress rapidly; pain is severe, continuous, and localized; moderate distention; persistent vomiting; usually decreased bowel sounds and marked localized tenderness. Stools or vomitus become melenous or bloody or contain occult blood.

GERIATRIC ALERT
Watch for air–fluid lock syndrome in elderly patients, who often remain in the recumbent position for extended periods. In this syndrome, fluid collects in dependent bowel loops and peristalsis is too weak to push fluid "uphill." The obstruction primarily occurs in the large bowel. Turn the patient every 10 minutes until enough flatus is passed to decompress the abdomen. A rectal tube may help.

◆ Diagnostic Evaluation

1. Abdominal x-rays show intestinal gas or fluid.
2. Barium enema shows a distended, air-filled colon or a closed sigmoid loop.
3. Decreased serum sodium, potassium, and chloride levels because of vomiting; elevated WBC counts with necrosis, strangulation, or peritonitis; and increased serum amylase levels from irritation of the pancreas by the bowel loop
4. Arterial blood gases may indicate metabolic acidosis or alkalosis.

◆ Collaborative Management

Therapeutic Interventions
1. Correct fluid and electrolyte imbalances:
   a. Na^+, K^+, blood component therapy
   b. Ringer's lactate to correct interstitial fluid deficit
   c. Dextrose and water to correct intracellular fluid deficit
2. Nasoenteral long-tube decompression of intestine proximal to the blockage site; the tube can be passed more effectively with the patient lying on right side.
3. Implement treatment for shock and peritonitis.
4. Hyperalimentation to correct protein deficiency from chronic obstruction, paralytic ileus, or infection

Surgical Interventions
1. Bowel resection with end-to-end anastomosis
2. Double-barrel ostomy if end-to-end anastomosis too risky

I

3. Loop colostomy to divert fecal stream and decompress bowel, with bowel resection to be done as second procedure

◆ Nursing Interventions

Monitoring

1. Frequently check the patient's level of responsiveness; decreasing responsiveness may point to impending shock or increasing electrolyte imbalance.
2. Observe for signs of shock—pallor, tachycardia, hypotension.
3. Watch for signs of metabolic alkalosis—slow, shallow respirations, changes in sensorium, tetany.
4. Watch for signs of metabolic acidosis—disorientation, deep rapid breathing, weakness, and shortness of breath on exertion.
5. Monitor urinary output; urinary retention may occur from bladder compression by distended intestine.

Supportive Care

1. Recognize the patient's concerns and provide care confidently and calmly to ensure cooperation and allay fears.
2. Evaluate effectiveness of pain relief regimen.
3. Maintain nasoenteral suction and monitor drainage.
4. Record intake and output, taking into account IV fluids, hyperalimentation, and blood products.
5. Minimize factors that would enhance gastric secretions to prevent fluid loss (via nasoenteral suction); avoid conversations about food and prevent meals from being served within patient's range of seeing or smelling.
6. After enterostomy, connect tube to drainage bottle at side of bed; expect considerable amount of fecal drainage during the first 12 to 15 hours (500–1,000 mL).
   a. Observe drainage equipment frequently for patency.
   b. If there is difficulty with drainage, it may be necessary to inject 15 mL warm saline solution into the enterostomy tube every 2 to 4 hours, with approval of health care provider.
   c. Protect skin around enterostomy tube with a skin barrier such as a karaya preparation.

I

7. Record amount and consistency of stools, and save all stools to test for occult blood.
8. Keep the patient in Fowler's position to promote ventilation and relief from abdominal distention.
9. Avoid use of enemas to prevent distortion of x-ray (by introducing gas into the tract distal to the obstruction) and to prevent worsening of a partial obstruction.

Patient Education and Health Maintenance

1. Teach care following bowel resection or temporary colostomy (see p. 350).
2. Teach proper diet, fluid intake, and activity to prevent prevent constipation and recurrence of partial obstruction.
3. Advise prompt recognition and reporting of recurrent symptoms.

Intracranial Aneurysm

See Aneurysm, Intracranial

Intussusception

Intussusception is the invagination or telescoping of a portion of the intestine into an adjacent, more distal section of the intestine (most commonly, the ileum invaginates into ascending colon). The cause of intussusception is unknown, but it may be initiated by increased intestinal motility and lymphoid hyperplasia. Possible contributing factors in older children include Meckel's diverticulum, bowel polyps or cysts, intestinal malrotation, acute enteritis, abdominal injury or surgery, cystic fibrosis, or celiac disease.

Intussusception is the most common cause of bowel obstruction in the first year of life. It is twice as common in male infants as in females, and is most likely to occur when the infant is aged 6 to 18 months. Without prompt treatment, intussusception progresses to hemorrhage, necrosis of the involved segment, shock, perforation, and peritonitis.

◆ Assessment

1. Paroxysmal abdominal pain
2. "Currant jelly" stools containing blood and mucus; positive Hemoccult test
3. Vomiting
4. Increasing absence of stools
5. Abdominal distention and tenderness
6. Sausagelike mass palpable in abdomen
7. Unusual-looking anus; may look like rectal prolapse
8. Dehydration and fever
9. Shocklike state with rapid pulse, pallor, marked sweating

PEDIATRIC ALERT
Episodic and severe, colicky abdominal pain combined with vomiting suggests intussusception.

◆ Diagnostic Evaluation

1. Flat plate of abdomen shows staircase pattern (invagination appears like stair steps).
2. Barium enema under fluoroscopy shows "coiled spring" appearance of bowel.
3. Ultrasonogram may be done to locate area of telescoped bowel.

◆ Collaborative Management

Therapeutic Interventions

1. Hydrostatic reduction of telescoped bowel with barium enema used during first 48 hours after onset may reduce intussusception in 75% of patients.

Surgical Interventions

1. Intussusception can be surgically reduced; resection may be necessary if bowel is gangrenous.

◆ Nursing Interventions

Monitoring

1. Monitor IV fluids, intake and output.
2. Be alert for respiratory distress because of abdominal

distention. Watch for grunting or shallow and rapid respirations if in shocklike state.

3. Monitor vital signs and general condition postoperatively.

Supportive Care

Preoperative care

1. Observe infant's behavior as indicator of pain; may be irritable and very sensitive to handling or lethargic or unresponsive. Handle very gently.
2. Explain cause of pain and reassure parents as to purpose of diagnostic tests and treatments.
3. Administer analgesics as prescribed.
4. Maintain NPO status as ordered.
   a. Wet lips and give mouth care.
   b. Give infant pacifier to suck.
5. Restrain infant as necessary for intravenous therapy.
6. Insert nasogastric tube if ordered to decompress stomach.
   a. Irrigate at frequent intervals.
   b. Note drainage and return from irrigation.
7. Continually reassess condition because increased pain and bloody stools may indicate perforation.

❖❖

NURSING ALERT

Passage of one normal brown stool may occur, clearing the colon distal to the intussusception. Passage of more than one normal brown stool may indicate that the intussusception has reduced itself. Report any stools immediately to the health care provider.

8. Prepare the patient for surgery if shocklike or febrile.
   a. Administer blood or plasma to restore circulating blood volume, and observe for transfusion reactions.
   b. Monitor pulse rate carefully, and know appropriate pulse range for age of child. Report tachycardia, indicating shock.
   c. Reduce temperature because fever increases metabolism and makes oxygenation during anesthesia more complicated.

Postoperative care

1. After reduction by hydrostatic barium enema:
   a. Monitor vital signs and general condition, especially

abdominal tenderness, bowel sounds, lethargy, and tolerance to fluids.
2. After surgical reduction or resection:
   a. Similar to general postabdominal surgical care (p. 350)
   b. Administer antipyretics and cooling measures to reduce fever. Fever is usually present from absorption of bacteria through the damaged intestinal wall.

Family Education and Health Maintenance

1. Explain that recurrence is rare and usually occurs within 36 hours after reduction. Review signs and symptoms with parents.
2. Review activity restrictions with parents (eg, positioning on back or side, quiet play, and avoidance of water sports until wound heals).
3. Encourage follow-up care.
4. Provide anticipatory guidance for developmental age of child.

Iron Deficiency Anemia
See Anemia, Iron Deficiency

Kawasaki Disease

Kawasaki disease (mucocutaneous lymph node syndrome) is a form of vasculitis identified by a febrile illness and involvement of vital body systems. It is the leading cause of acquired heart disease in children in the United States, especially in those younger than age 5. The cause is unknown, but autoimmunity, infection, and genetic predisposition are believed to be involved.

Although Kawasaki disease is a multisystem disease, the cardiovascular system appears to be the primary site. Vascular damage proceeds in stages. Initially, arterioles, venules, and capillaries are involved, progressing to panvasculitis and perivasculitis of coronary arteries. Aneurysm formation, pericarditis, myocarditis, endocarditis, and phlebitis may result. In late disease, coronary arterial scarring, stenosis, and calcification may occur, possibly with myocardial fibrosis and endocardial fibroelastosis. Approximately 15% to 20% of patients develop cardiac complications (coronary arteritis, aneurysmal thrombosis or rupture, myocardial infarction, congestive heart failure, coronary insufficiency, and ischemia). However, the mortality rate is less than 0.3%.

◆ Assessment

Stage I—Acute febrile phase (days 1–11):
1. The child appears severely ill and irritable.
2. Major diagnostic criteria established by Centers for Disease Control and Prevention (CDC) are as follows:
   a. High, spiking fever for 5 or more days
   b. Bilateral conjunctival injection
   c. Oropharyngeal erythema, "strawberry" tongue, red and dry lips
   d. Indurative edema of hands and feet; or erythema of palms and soles; or general edema; or periungual desquamation
   e. Erythematous rash
   f. Cervical lymphadenopathy greater than 1.5 cm (0.6 in.)
3. Carditis, such as pericarditis, myocarditis, cardiomegaly, congestive heart failure, coronary thrombosis
4. Iridocyclitis and aseptic meningitis

Stage II—Subacute phase (days 11–21):
1. Acute symptoms of stage I subside as temperature returns to normal. The child remains irritable and anorectic.
2. Dry, cracked lips with fissures

K

3. Desquamation of toes and fingers
4. Arthralgia, arthritis (temporary)
5. Coronary thrombosis, aneurysms

Stage III—Convalescent phase (days 21–60):
1. The child appears well.
2. Transverse grooves of fingers and toenails (Beau's lines)
3. Coronary thrombosis, aneurysms may occur.

◆ Diagnostic Evaluation

1. The CDC requires that the patient demonstrate fever and four of the six stage I criteria listed above.
2. Electrocardiogram, echocardiograms, cardiac catheterization, and angiocardiography may be required to diagnose abnormalities.
3. Although there are no specific laboratory tests, the following may help support diagnosis or rule out other diseases:
   a. CBC shows leukocytosis during stage I.
   b. ESR is elevated during stage I.
   c. Erythrocytes and hemoglobin are slightly decreased.
   d. C-reactive protein is positive.
   e. Platelet count is increased during second to fourth weeks of illness.
   f. IgM, IgA, IgG, and IgF are transiently elevated.
   g. Urinalysis detects proteinuria and leukocytes.

◆ Collaborative Management

Therapeutic Interventions

1. Treatment aims to ameliorate symptoms and prevent coronary thrombosis, coronary aneurysm, and death.
2. Supportive measures:
   a. Maintain fluid and electrolyte balance; give nutritional support.
   b. Provide comfort.
3. Cardiac follow-up by pediatric cardiologist with serial two-dimensional echocardiograms, angiography, and cardiac isoenzyme studies

K

Pharmacologic Interventions

1. Immune globulin (gamma globulin) IV therapy—
   IVGG (2 g/kg per day) is initiated during stage I in
   one 10- to 12-hour infusion to reduce the incidence
   of coronary artery abnormalities.

NURSING ALERT
Infusion of IVGG sometimes causes blood pressure to drop
sharply, which may mimic anaphylaxis. This effect may be related
to the infusion rate. Monitor blood pressure and heart rate at
the start of infusion, after 30 minutes, 1 hour, and then every
2 hours until infusion is complete. Slow the infusion and have
the patient evaluated for any drop in blood pressure. Have epinephrine available to treat any anaphylactic reaction.

2. Aspirin therapy
   a. Antiinflammatory dose (80–100 mg/kg/day) dur-
      ing stage I
   b. Antiplatelet dose (3–5 mg/kg/day) given after fever
      is controlled, then continued for 2 to 3 months post-
      illness (when the echocardiogram is normal), or
      until ESR and platelet count are normal, to reduce
      risk of spontaneous coronary thrombosis. Aspirin
      may be continued indefinitely if there are coronary
      abnormalities.
3. Thrombolytic therapy may be required during stages
   I, II, or III. Dipyridamole may be given as a platelet
   aggregation inhibitor if aneurysms are present.

◆ **Nursing Interventions**

Monitoring
1. Monitor pain level and child's response to analgesics.
2. Institute continual cardiac monitoring and assessment
   for complications.
   a. Take vital signs and blood pressure every 2 hours;
      report abnormalities.
   b. Ensure proper functioning of cardiac monitor; ob-
      serve for and report any arrhythmia.
   c. Assess the child for signs of myocarditis (tachycar-
      dia, gallop rhythm, chest pain).

K

    d. Monitor the child for congestive heart failure (dyspnea, nasal flaring, grunting, retractions, cyanosis, orthopnea, crackles, moist respirations, distended neck veins, edema).

3. Closely monitor intake and output and administer oral and IV fluids as ordered.
4. Monitor hydration status by checking skin turgor, weight, urinary output, specific gravity, and presence of tears.
5. Monitor temperature every 4 to 8 hours, every 2 hours if elevated. Give tub or sponge baths for temperature over 101°F (38.3°C), or use a cooling blanket for higher temperatures not responsive to antipyretics.
6. Observe mouth and skin frequently for signs of infection.

Supportive Care

1. Allow the child periods of uninterrupted rest. Offer pain medication routinely rather than PRN during stage I.
2. Perform comfort measures related to the eyes:
   a. Conjunctivitis can cause photosensitivity, so darken the room, offer sunglasses.
   b. Apply cool compresses.
   c. Discourage rubbing eyes.
   d. Instill artificial tears to soothe conjunctiva.
3. Perform comfort measures related to joint pain and tender lymph nodes.
   a. Use passive range-of-motion exercises every 4 hours while the child is awake, because movement may be restricted.
   b. Encourage the child to move about freely under supervision; provide soft toys and quiet play and encourage use of hands and fingers.
4. Provide quiet, peaceful environment with diversional activities.
5. Provide care measures for oral mucous membranes.
   a. Offer cool liquids (ice chips and popsicles); progress to soft, bland foods.
   b. Give mouth care every 1 to 4 hours with special mouth swabs; use soft tooth brush only after healing has occurred.
   c. Apply petroleum to dried, cracked lips.

K

6. Provide care measures to improve skin integrity.
   a. Avoid use of soap because it tends to dry skin and make it more likely to break down.
   b. Elevate edematous extremities.
   c. Use sheepskin, egg-crate mattress, and smooth sheets.
   d. If clothes are used, encourage use of soft flannel or terry cloth that fit loosely.
   e. Apply emollients to skin, as ordered.
   f. Protect peeling skin; observe for signs of infection.
7. Offer clear liquids every hour when child is awake.
8. Encourage the child to eat meals and snacks to prevent nutritional deficit.
9. Infuse IV fluids through a volume control device if dehydration is present, and check the site and amount hourly.
10. Explain all procedures to the child and family.
11. Provide respite for parents during irritable stage of illness when child may be inconsolable.
12. Encourage the parents and child to verbalize their concerns, fears, and questions.
13. Practice relaxation techniques with child such as relaxation breathing, guided imagery, and distraction.
14. Prepare the child for cardiac surgery or thrombolytic therapy if complications develop.
15. Keep the family informed of progress and reinforce stages and prognosis.

Family Education and Health Maintenance

1. Ensure that the family understands the medications, follow-up tests, and physical activity levels that have been prescribed for the child based on specific categories. For long-term follow-up care children can be categorized into one of three groups: those with no cardiac involvement, those with small coronary aneurysms, and those with aneurysms greater than 8 mm (0.31 in.).
2. Teach parents that long-term care after discharge is critical because of risk of complications.
3. Provide written instructions about cardiac complications and stress the need to report the development of symptoms.
4. Teach family members cardiopulmonary resuscitation.

5. Teach parents to recognize and report signs of possible salicylate toxicity—tinnitus, nausea and vomiting, gastrointestinal distress, blood in stool, increased respirations.

6. Encourage parents not to overprotect the child. Discuss with parents the grief and mourning process of denial, anger, bargaining, depression, and acceptance that they may be going through because of the chronic illness.

7. Advise parents to allow child to be as active as desired unless coronary ischemia is present or the child is on anticoagulants. Try to protect the child from injury if on anticoagulants (no sharp toys, no contact sports).

8. Discuss regression that might occur as a result of hospitalization or the disease process and suggest ways to deal with these changes.

9. Refer for additional information to agencies such as:

    American Heart Association
    7272 Greenville Ave.
    Dallas, TX 75231-4596
    214-373-6300

Kidney Surgery and Urinary Diversion

Kidney surgery may include nephrectomy, kidney transplantation, procedures to remove obstruction such as stones or tumors, and procedures to insert drainage tubes for nephrostomy or ureterostomy. Incisional approaches vary, but may involve the flank, thoracic, and abdominal regions. Nephrectomy is most often performed for malignant tumors of the kidney, but also may be indicated for trauma and kidneys that no longer function because of obstructive disorders and other renal disease. Loss of one kidney does not impair renal function when the remaining kidney is normal. Kidney transplantion is done for end-stage renal failure, as an alternative to hemodialysis. *Urinary diversion* refers to providing an alternate pathway for urinary excretion other than through the bladder and urethra. Urinary diversion is most commonly done in cystectomy, and may also be done in GU cancer, congenital malformation, or in severe urinary tract infections that threaten the kidneys. A number of operative procedures are performed to achieve this (Box 3).

◆ Potential Complications

1. Hemorrhage and shock
2. Pulmonary complications (atelectasis, pneumonia, pneumothorax)
3. Thromboembolism (thrombophlebitis and pulmonary embolism)
4. Paralytic ileus
5. Infection
6. Obstruction of urinary drainage
7. Rejection of transplant
8. Postinfarction syndrome (if renal artery embolization was done)

◆ Collaborative Management

Preoperative Care

1. Prepare the patient for surgery with information about operating room routine and postoperative care; administer preoperative antibiotics and bowel-cleansing regimen.
2. Assess for risk factors for thromboembolism (smoking, oral contraceptive use, varicosities of lower extremities) and apply anti-embolism stockings if ordered. Review leg exercises with the patient and describe pneumatic/sequential compression stockings that will be used postoperatively.
3. Assess pulmonary status (presence of dyspnea, productive cough, other related cardiac symptoms) and teach deep-breathing exercises, effective coughing, and use of an incentive spirometer.
4. If embolization of the renal artery is being done preoperatively for patients with renal cell carcinoma, monitor for and treat symptoms of postinfarction syndrome (flank pain, fever, leukocytosis, and hypertension), which may last for up to 3 days.

Postoperative Care

1. Closely monitor intake and output, especially after kidney transplantation.

(text continues on p. 519)

K

■ **BOX 3 METHODS OF URINARY DIVERSION**

■ **Ileal Conduit**

Most common; ureters are transplanted into an isolated section of the terminal ileum; one end is brought through the abdominal wall to create a stoma. Urine flows from the kidney through the ileal conduit and exits through the stoma. The ureters also may be transplanted into the transverse colon (colon conduit).

■ **Continent Urinary Reservoir (Kock pouch, Indiana pouch, Mainz pouch, and others)**

Transplants the ureters into a pouch created from small bowel or large and small bowel. The existing ileocecal valve or a surgically created intussuscepted nipple valve provide the continence mechanism. The patient does not have to war an external appliance, but the procedure does require intermittent self-catheterization of the pouch.

■ **Orthotopic Bladder Replacement (Hemi–Kock pouch, Mainz pouch, and others)**

Pouch created from small or large and small bowel is anastomosed to urethral stump in men; voiding is through the urethra. The patient usually has nocturnal incontinence. Not all patients are candidates for this procedure.

■ **Nursing Considerations**

1. Advise patient that enterostomal therapist or surgeon will mark stoma site preoperatively in good anatomic location where patient can see it. Site may also be marked for orthotopic bladder replacement in case intraoperative findings prevent such a procedure.

continued

K

■ BOX 3 *(Continued)*

2. Postoperatively monitor drains—Sudden increase in drainage suggests a urine leak; send specimen of drainage for BUN and creatinine, if ordered. (Presence of measureable BUN and creatinine in drainage indicates urine in drainage, confirming a urine leak.)

3. Maintain protection of ureteral stents used to protect ureterointestinal anastomoses (with ileal or colon conduit); stents will emerge from stoma or through separate wound and are removed in approximately 3 weeks.

4. Maintain transparent urostomy pouch over stoma postoperatively to allow easy assessment. Observe for normal urine (but not fecal) drainage at all times.

5. Inspect stoma for color; size; whether it is flush, nippled, or retraced; and the condition of peristomal skin; document baseline information.

6. With continent urinary diversions, maintain patency of drainage catheters placed into internal urinary pouch during surgery; irrigate with 30 mL saline every 2 to 4 hours to prevent obstruction from mucus accumulation.

7. Teach patient how to change pouch. Emphasize that peristomal skin must be clean and dry or appliance will not ahdere.

   a. Tell patient that frequency of pouch changes depends on type of pouch used—generally, pouches should be changed every 3 days (for one-piece pouches) to every 4 to 7 days (for two-piece pouches).

   b. Advise emptying the pouch when it is one-third to one-half full to prevent weight of urine from loosening adhesive seal—open drain valve (spigot) for periodic emptying.

K

continued

■ **BOX 3** *(Continued)*

COMMUNITY CARE CONSIDERATIONS
Advise changing pouch in morning before fluids are taken or before bedtime when urine output is lowest. Suggest inserting a tampon partially into stoma to soak up urine during changing of pouch, if necessary

    c. Advise using a belt to keep the pouch in place during the day and using a bedside urinary drainage bag at night if desired.

8. Teach patient with continent urinary reservoir how to catheterize stoma every 2 hours at first and gradually lengthen time until reservoir is holding 400 to 500 mL urine and catheterizing 4 to 5 times a day.

9. For patients with orthotopic bladder replacement, after removal of catheter, teach patient to void by straining abdominal muscles. Initially voiding must be done every 2 hours during day and 3 hours at night, and gradually intervals are lengthened.

    a. Teach pelvic floor–strengthening exercises to minimize incontinence.

    b. Patience with exercise and voiding schedule will optimize results.

10. Advise reporting problems with peristomal skin or with leakage from pouch or development of fever, chills, pain, change in color of urine (cloudy, bloody), diminishing urine output.

11. For additional information and support refer to:

    United Ostomy Association, Inc.
    36 Executive Park, Suite 120
    Irvine, CA 92714
    714-660-8624

K

a. Expect normal urine output to be 30 to 100 mL/hr.

b. Report oliguria with less than 30 mL/hr, or polyuria of 100 to 500 mL/hr.

2. Monitor serum electrolyte results and ECG for changes caused by electrolyte imbalance. Report dysrhythmias or other cardiac symptoms immediately.

3. Monitor blood pressure and heart rate, CVP, and pulmonary artery pressure (if indicated) to anticipate adjustment of fluid replacement.

NURSING ALERT

Frequently monitor blood pressure, pulse, and respirations to recognize signs of hemorrhage (and shock), the chief dangers after renal surgery. Watch for pain, blood in wound drainage, or an expanding flank mass. Prepare for rapid blood and fluid replacement and reoperation.

4. Avoid using the same extremity being used for dialysis access when inserting IV or intraarterial lines. Prepare for hemodialysis in postoperative period if kidney transplant was done, until transplanted kidney is functioning well. Monitor patency of vascular access.

5. Assess pain location, intensity, and characteristics.
   a. Transient renal colic-like pain may be caused by passage of blood clots down the ureter; report increased, persistent pain that may indicate hemorrhage or obstruction of urinary drainage.
   b. Assess bowel sounds, abdominal distention and pain that may indicate paralytic ileus and need for nasogastric decompression.

6. Administer pain medications; evaluate effectiveness of patient-controlled analgesia.

7. Assist the patient with use of incentive spirometer, coughing and deep breathing, and ambulation to decrease risk of pulmonary infection. Provide meticulous chest tube care. Encourage splinting of incision when turning or coughing.

8. Maintain patency of urinary drainage tubes or catheters as indicated. Prevent kinking or pulling.

K

9. Use frequent handwashing and asepsis when providing care and handling of urinary drainage system (especially important for the patient on immunosuppressants).
10. Make sure indwelling catheter is dependent and draining.
    a. Report any decrease in output or excessive clots.
    b. Be alert for signs of urinary infection such as cloudy urine, fever, aching pain in bladder or flank.
11. Administer antibiotics as prescribed.
12. Change dressings promptly if drainage is present.
13. Provide regular skin care and assist with hygiene.
14. Obtain specimens for bacteriologic testing of urine, wound drainage, sputum, and discontinued catheters, drains, and IV lines as indicated.
15. For kidney transplant patients, administer immunosuppressant drugs, and monitor for early signs of rejection:
    a. Temperature greater than 100.4°F (38.5°C)
    b. Decreased urine output
    c. Weight gain of 3 or more pounds overnight
    d. Pain or tenderness over the graft site
    e. Hypertension
    f. Increased serum creatinine
16. For kidney transplant patients, give oral antifungal agent to prevent mucosal candidiasis, which often occurs because of immunosuppression.

K

◆ Family Education and Health Maintenance

1. Provide information about postoperative recovery measures: regular exercise, refraining from heavy lifting or strenuous activities, resuming normal dietary intake.
2. Advise wearing a medical alert bracelet and informing all health care providers of single-kidney status.
3. Reinforce the need for close follow-up and urge the patient to to seek immediate medical attention for any signs of urinary infection or urinary tract disease involving the remaining kidney.
4. After kidney transplant:
    a. Explain and reinforce symptoms of rejection—fe-

ver, chills, sweating, lassitude, hypertension, weight gain, peripheral edema, decrease in urine output. Reassure the patient that acute rejection, while common, is usually reversible. It often occurs in first 2 months after transplant.

b. Prepare the patient for possible need for maintenance dialysis when rejection occurs. If the transplanted kidney is rejected, it may be removed in the initial postoperative period. In chronic rejection, the kidney is not usually removed.

c. Explain need for continued protection of vascular access graft, which may still be enlarged and tender, which is associated with edema of overlying tissue.

d. Encourage compliance with laboratory tests (serum and urine chemistry, hematology, bacteriology) to monitor immune status and detect early signs of rejection.

e. Instruct the patient and family about prescribed immunosuppressants and possible complications of therapy (infection or incomplete control of rejection). Review other medications, such as antacids to prevent stress ulcers, vitamins, and iron replacement.

f. Review in detail postoperative self-care regimen (may be inpatient or outpatient), including adequate fluid intake, daily weight, measurement of urine, stool test for occult blood, prevention of infection, exercise.

g. Advise the patient to avoid contact sports for life to prevent trauma to the transplanted kidney.

h. Stress that follow-up care after transplantation is a lifelong necessity.

5. For additional support and information, refer to:

American Association of Kidney Patients
100 South Ashley Dr., Suite 280
Tampa, FL 33602
800-749-AAKP

K

Knee Arthroplasty
See Arthroplasty and Total Joint Replacement

Knee Injuries

Knee injuries result from rapid position changes involving flexing and twisting of the joint. Severe stresses are applied to knee ligaments and cartilage during many sport activities. The knee ligaments provide stability to the knee joint. These ligaments promote rotational stability (anterior and posterior cruciate ligaments) and prevent varus and valgus instability (medial and lateral collateral ligaments). Pieces of cartilage that stabilize the knee internally are known as the medial and lateral menisci. Anterior cruciate ligament (ACL) injuries and medial meniscus tears are common because of sports injuries.

◆ Assessment

1. Torn cartilage (meniscus)
   a. Pain, tenderness, joint effusion
   b. Clicking sensations
   c. Decreased range of motion
2. Torn ligaments
   a. Pain on ambulation, swelling
   b. Joint instability
   c. Possible rupture of patellar tendon

◆ Diagnostic Evaluation

1. Special assessment techniques are done to detect injury to the anterior cruciate ligament (ACL):
   a. Anterior drawer test: Patient placed supine with knee in 90 degrees of flexion with foot flat on table. Proximal tibia is pulled forward by examiner using two hands. Forward subluxation of tibia on femur indicates ACL injury.
   b. Lachman test: Patient placed supine with knee in 15 to 20 degrees of flexion. Distal femur is grasped by examiner with one hand while other hand grasps proximal tibia and applies forward pressure. Forward subluxation of tibia on femur indicates ACL injury.
   c. Pivot shift test: Evaluates anterolateral rotational stability. Patient is placed supine with knee slightly

K

flexed. Examiner grasps patient's ankle in one hand and places palm of other hand over lateral aspect of knee distal to the joint. Lower leg is extended and internally rotated, applying a valgus (lateral) stress to knee. Tibia subluxes and reduces itself ("pivots and shifts"), indicating ACL injury.

2. Magnetic resonance imaging shows extent of soft tissue injury.

◆ Collaborative Management

Therapeutic Interventions

1. Some injuries may be immobilized (splint, brace, or cast) and treated with physical therapy.

Surgical Interventions

1. Anterior cruciate ligament reconstruction frequently indicated.
   a. Arthroscopic surgery preferred using synthetic ligaments where ligaments failed. Graft rejection is a complication.
   b. Postoperative continuous passive motion used.
   c. Postoperative anterior cruciate ligament rehabilitation program includes progressive range of motion, bracing (not done with synthetic ligaments).
   d. Long-term bracing during sports controversial
2. Meniscal injury—damaged cartilage removed
   a. Arthroscopic or open meniscectomy
   b. Rehabilitation includes progressive range of motion and quadriceps strengthening.

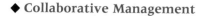

◆ Nursing Interventions

Supportive Care

1. After arthroscopic surgery, ensure proper use of crutches and encourage pain control through medications as prescribed and rest, ice, compression, and elevation.
2. For open joint surgery, evaluate incision for drainage and signs of infection. Maintain immobility as ordered.
3. Encourage exercises prescribed by physical therapy.

Patient Education and Health Maintenance

1. Teach the patient strengthening exercises for affected extremity.
2. Teach the patient to prevent fatigue through rest periods, conservation of energy.
3. Advise on prevention of injuries, using proper equipment and footwear for sports.

Laryngeal Cancer
See Cancer, Laryngeal

Lead Poisoning

Lead poisoning is a chronic disorder resulting from consumption of lead in some form. Lead poisoning is the best-known cause of environmental illness in children, who commonly ingest the element from nonfood substances such as paints and coating on toys, furniture, window sills, household fixtures, and plaster painted with lead-containing paint. Other sources include water dispensed from lead pipes, dirt containing lead fallout from automobile exhaust, or accidental ingestion of lead-containing objects (fish sinkers, pie weights).

Lead is absorbed from the gastrointestinal (GI) tract and primarily affects the central nervous system (CNS), bone marrow, and kidneys. CNS effects include learning disabilities, mental retardation, encephalopathy, paralysis, blindness, and seizures. Lead in bone marrow impairs production of hemoglobin and red blood cells, resulting in anemia and respiratory distress. In the kidneys, lead damages proximal tubules, causing increased excretion of amino acids, protein, glucose, and phosphate.

Incidence of lead poisoning is highest in children aged 1 to 3 years, especially if they live in older, deteriorated housing. Symptomatic lead poisoning occurs most frequently in the summer months. The recurrence rate is high, especially if lead is not removed from the home environment. A small number of affected children may die, and many survivors are left with irreversible mental, emotional, and physical deficits.

Adults may acquire the disorder because of exposure to leaded gas fumes or occupational- or hobby-related exposure to lead compounds.

◆ Assessment

1. Gastrointestinal: anorexia, sporadic vomiting, intermittent abdominal pain (colic), constipation
2. CNS: hyperirritability; decreased activity; personality changes; loss of recently acquired developmental skills; falling, clumsiness, loss of coordination (ataxia); local paralysis; peripheral nerve palsies
3. Hematologic: anemia, pallor
4. Cardiovascular: hypertension, bradycardia
5. Encephalopathy may occur 4 to 6 weeks after first symptoms:
   a. Sudden onset of persistent vomiting
   b. Severe ataxia
   c. Altered state of consciousness
   d. Coma
   e. Seizures
   f. Massive cerebral edema in younger children

L

COMMUNITY CARE CONSIDERATIONS
Assess for pica (appetite for nonfood substances such as paint chips or dirt) in the child suspected of lead poisoning. Also assess other children in the home for lead poisoning.

◆ Diagnostic Evaluation

1. Elevated serum lead levels
2. Complete blood count indicates iron deficiency anemia.
3. Erythrocyte protoporphyrin (EP) level: not sensitive enough to identify lead levels below approximately 25 mg/dL. Can be used to follow blood lead levels after medical and environmental interventions for poisoned children. A progressive decline in EP levels indicates that management is successful.
4. 24-hour urine specimen is more accurate than a single voided specimen in determining elevated urine components that correspond with elevated blood lead levels.
5. Edetate calcium disodium (CaEDTA) provocation chelation test: used only in selected medical centers treating large numbers of lead-poisoned children, demonstrates increased lead levels in urine over an 8-hour period after injection of CaEDTA
6. Flat plate of abdomen: may show radiopaque material if lead has been ingested during the preceding 24 to 36 hours
7. Radiologic examination of long bones: unreliable for diagnosis of acute lead poisoning; may provide some indication of past lead poisoning or length of time poisoning has occurred

◆ Collaborative Management

Therapeutic Interventions

1. Removal of leaded paint/paint chips or lead-containing objects from the child's environment. Child should be away from environment during paint-stripping process.
2. Low-fat, high-iron diet and iron supplements to treat associated anemia
3. For the child with encephalopathy, corticosteroids are given, and intensive care management is maintained until acute stage is resolved.

Pharmacologic Interventions

1. Edetate calcium disodium (CaEDTA), British anti-Lewisite (BAL), and succimer (Chemet) bind with

L

lead in the blood to form nontoxic compounds that are excreted by bowel and kidney.

2. Effectiveness of therapy is dependent on degree and duration of lead poisoning.
3. BAL is given first to decrease the chance of seizures.
   a. Used alone in patients with encephalopathy
   b. Do not give with iron supplements and avoid in patients with plant allergies.
   c. Avoid in patients with glucose-6-phosphate dehydrogenase deficiency caused by hemolysis.
   d. Administered deep intramuscularly, results in pain and tissue necrosis at the injection site
4. CaEDTA may be toxic to the kidneys.
   a. Monitor urinary output as well as kidney and liver function studies.
   b. Administer IV.
5. Succimer: approved for use in 1991
   a. Not given to patients with encephalopathy
   b. Administer orally.
6. Dosage: depends on individual drug, the child's weight, severity of poisoning, history, and whether other chelating agents are being used simultaneously
7. Chelating drugs are usually given every 4 hours for 5 days. A second course of therapy may be needed if there is a rebound in the blood lead level.
8. Increased oral and IV fluids are given to enhance excretion, except if increased intracranial pressure is present.
9. D-penicillamine, another drug that chelates heavy metals, may be given for long-term chelation only if current exposure to lead is definitely excluded. If this drug is used, it should be given on an empty stomach, 2 hours before breakfast.
10. Supplemental calcium, phosphorus, and vitamin D are given to help lead move from the blood (where it is toxic) to the bones (where it is nontoxic).

◆ Nursing Interventions

Monitoring

1. In a child with encephalopathy, observe for signs of increased intracranial pressure:
   a. Rising blood pressure

L

  b. Papilledema
  c. Slow pulse
  d. Seizures
  e. Unconsciousness
2. In chelation therapy, monitor intake and output and blood studies such as electrolytes, and liver and kidney function tests as directed.

Supportive Care

1. Maintain seizure precautions for a child with encephalopathy.
   a. Crib or bed rails elevated and padded
   b. Have tongue blade and suction equipment at bedside.
2. Provide supportive care to maintain vital functions. Care is similar to that of child with Reye's syndrome (see p. 744).
3. In chelation therapy, plan appropriate play activities to prepare the child for injections and as an outlet for pain and anger child feels.
4. Implement measures to decrease pain at injection site.
   a. Rotate sites of injection.
   b. Apply warm packs to site to decrease pain.
   c. Move painful areas slowly.
5. Provide diversional activities, fluids, and meals between injections.
6. Provide and encourage activities that will help the child to learn and progress from current developmental state to meet next appropriate milestone.
7. Initiate appropriate referrals in cases of obvious developmental delays or learning difficulties.
8. Share the results of developmental testing with the parent(s) and discuss ways to provide stimulation for the child at home.
9. Use sensitivity in interviewing and teaching to avoid causing or increasing guilt feelings about the poisoning and to establish a positive, trusting relationship between the family and the health care facility.

Family Education and Health Maintenance

1. Teach the parents why long-term follow-up is important. Explain that residual lead is liberated gradually

L

after treatment and may result in renewal of symptoms, increase serum lead to a dangerous level, and cause additional CNS damage, which may not become apparent for several months.

2. Stress that acute infections must be recognized and treated promptly because these may reactivate the disease.
3. Inform that iron supplementation may be continued to treat anemia. Advise on administration and side effects and periodic CBC monitoring.
4. Advise parents that the single most important factor in managing childhood lead poisoning is reducing the child's re-exposure to lead.

PEDIATRIC ALERT
Children should not be discharged from the hospital until their home environment is lead free.

5. Initiate referrals to community outreach workers so that environmental case management is conducted. Lead abatement must be conducted by experts, not untrained parents, property owners, or contractors.
6. Suggest periodic, focused household cleaning to remove the lead dust; use a wet mop.
7. Encourage handwashing before meals and at bedtime to eliminate lead consumption from normal hand-to-mouth activity.
8. Make certain that the family can closely supervise the child, or assist them to make necessary arrangements.

L

COMMUNITY CARE CONSIDERATIONS
Initiate and support educational campaigns through schools, day-care centers, and news media to alert parents and children to hazards and symptoms of lead poisoning.

Learning Disabilities
See Attention Deficit Disorder and Learning Disabilities

Legg-Calvé-Perthes Disease

Legg-Calvé-Perthes disease is a self-limiting condition of the proximal femur, in which avascular necrosis of the femoral head leads to its eventual deformation. Four stages are recognized. In stage I (avascularity), the blood supply to the upper femoral epiphysis is halted spontaneously and bone growth is halted. In stage II (revascularization), new blood vessels arise to supply the necrotic area, and bone resorption and deposition take place. However, the new bone lacks strength and pathologic fractures may occur; the weakened epiphysis may be progressively deformed. In stage III (reossification), the head of the femur gradually reforms as dead bone is replaced with new bone, which gradually spreads to heal the lesion. Finally, in stage IV (postrecovery), the femoral head becomes permanently distorted, with resultant joint misalignment.

Legg-Calvé-Perthes disease occurs primarily in boys aged 4 to 8 years for unknown reasons, and is bilateral in 12% to 20% of cases. Without treatment, early degenerative joint disease and loss of hip function may result in later life. With timely treatment, the femoral head can be reformed to preserve joint function and mobility.

◆ Assessment

1. Synovitis causing limp and pain in the hip (may be intermittent initially)
2. Referred pain to knee, inner thigh, and groin
3. Limited abduction and internal rotation of the hip
4. Mild to moderate muscle spasm

◆ Diagnostic Evaluation

1. Hip x-ray findings are related to the stage of the disease process. Early x-rays may be normal.
2. Magnetic resonance imaging has been useful in demonstrating the pathologic process.

530

3. Bone scans can detect avascular stage early.
4. Arthrograms may be useful to evaluate sphericity of femoral head.

◆ Collaborative Management

Therapeutic Interventions
1. Limitation of activities, bed rest with or without skin traction
2. To prevent deformity of the femoral head, it is contained within the acetabulum by means of a non–weight-bearing abduction cast or brace (Petrie casts), or a weight-bearing abduction brace (Scottish Rite orthosis).

Pharmacologic Interventions
1. Salicylates or antiinflammatory agents are given to relieve synovitis, muscle spasm, and pain in the joint and help restore motion.

Surgical Interventions
1. Osteotomy of the proximal femur, acetabulum (Salter innominate), or a combination of these may be required.

◆ Nursing Interventions

Monitoring
1. If child is in cast or brace:
   a. Assess the skin around the edges of the device daily for signs of skin irritation.
   b. Assess neurovascular status frequently after application of the device, then daily to detect compromise.

Supportive Care and Family Education
1. Instruct child and parents as to which activities can be continued and which to avoid (eg, collision sports, high-impact running).
2. Encourage activities to maintain range of motion (eg, swimming, bicycle riding).
3. Encourage parents to allow activities that involve unaffected body parts within restriction guidelines.

L

4. Provide equipment to assist with mobility (eg, wheel-chair, walker).
5. Assess parents' ability to care for child at home. Provide community-based referral to assist if indicated.
6. Teach parents and siblings to assist only as needed.
7. Allow child to care and participate for self as able.
8. Reinforce to child that he or she is only temporarily restricted. Stress positive aspects of activity.
9. Provide opportunities for child to express fears and emotions. Offer support when needed.
10. Prepare the child for casting or immobilization procedure by showing materials to be used and describing procedure in age-appropriate terms.
11. Assess the need for pain medication, sedation, distraction techniques, or restraint and administer as ordered.
12. Try to prevent skin breakdown by padding edges of device and telling child to avoid placing anything inside the device.

Leukemia, Acute Lymphocytic and Acute Myelogenous

Leukemias are malignant disorders of the blood and bone marrow that result in an accumulation of dysfunctional immature white blood cells (blasts) in bone marrow, peripheral blood, and body tissues. Acute leukemias are characterized by rapid progression of symptoms. High numbers (greater than 50,000/mm^3) of circulating blasts weaken blood vessel walls, with high risk for rupture and bleeding, including intracranial hemorrhage.

When lymphocytes are the predominant malignant cell, the disorder is called acute lymphocytic leukemia (ALL); when monocytes or granulocytes are predominant, it is called acute myelogenous leukemia (AML). Approximately half of new leukemias are acute. Approximately 85% of acute leukemias in adults are AML. ALL is the most common cancer in children, with peak incidence between ages 2 and 9 years.

Although the cause of leukemias is unknown, predis-

L

posing factors include genetic susceptibility, exposure to ionizing radiation or certain chemicals and toxins, some genetic disorders (Down syndrome, Fanconi's anemia), and human T cell leukemia-lymphoma virus (HTLV-1). Complications include infection and hemorrhage.

◆ Assessment

1. Weight loss, fever, frequent infections (with ALL), weakness, progressively increasing fatigability, abnormal bleeding and bruising, and lymphadenopathy (ALL)
2. Bone and joint pain, headache, splenomegaly, hepatomegaly, and neurologic dysfunction

◆ Diagnostic Evaluation

1. White blood cell count varies widely from 1,000/mm^3 to 100,000/mm^3. Peripheral smear shows large number of lymphoblasts and lymphocytes in 90% of cases.
2. Anemia may be profound (decreased hemoglobin and hematocrit); platelet count may be low, and coagulopathies (abnormal prothrombin time and partial thromboplastin time) may exist.
3. Bone marrow aspiration and biopsy to classify leukemia and to check for chromosomal abnormalities and immunologic markers
4. Lymph node biopsy to detect disease spread
5. Lumbar puncture to detect leukemic cells (especially in ALL) with central nervous system spread

◆ Collaborative Management

Therapeutic Interventions

1. Radiation therapy, particularly of CNS in ALL or for testicular involvement
2. Autologous or allogenic bone marrow transplant for failure to respond to conventional therapy

Pharmacologic Interventions

1. High-dose chemotherapy given as an induction course to obtain a remission (elimination of abnormal cells from bone marrow and blood) and then in cycles as

L

consolidation or maintenance therapy to prevent disease recurrence
2. Granulocyte colony-stimulating factor to stimulate neutrophil production and prevent serious infection while undergoing chemotherapy
3. Antibiotics to treat infection
4. Analgesics and antiemetics

◆ Nursing Interventions

Monitoring
1. Monitor vital signs every 4 hours.
2. Monitor for fever and signs of infection.

NURSING ALERT
Fever may not develop with infection if patient is immunosuppressed because of chemotherapy. A fever of 101°F (38.4°C) may indicate overwhelming infection and impending septic shock.

3. Assess respiratory function every 4 hours while symptoms are present; otherwise, every 8 hours.
4. Assess for changes in mental status every 8 hours.
5. Monitor platelet counts daily.
6. Monitor granulocyte counts. Concentrations under 500 μL indicate serious risk of infection.
7. Monitor for signs of minor bleeding such as petechiae, ecchymosis, conjunctival injection, epistaxis, bleeding gums, oozing at puncture sites, vaginal spotting, heavy menses.

NURSING ALERT
Be alert for and report signs of serious bleeding such as headache with change in responsiveness, blurred vision, hemoptysis, hematemesis, melena, hypotension, tachycardia, and dizziness.

8. Monitor urine, stool, and emesis for gross and occult blood.

L

Supportive Care

1. Use meticulous handwashing; observe reverse isolation precautions or use laminar airflow room, as directed.
2. Avoid invasive procedures and trauma to skin or mucous membrane to prevent entry of microorganisms.
3. Use the following rectal precautions to prevent infection:
   a. Avoid diarrhea and constipation, which can irritate the rectal mucosa.
   b. Avoid rectal thermometers.
   c. Avoid foods that increase bacterial colonization of the GI tract, such as fresh fruits, vegetables, undercooked meat or eggs, or buttermilk.
   d. Keep perianal area clean.
4. Encourage and assist the patient with personal hygiene, bathing, and oral care.
5. Keep the patient on bed rest during bleeding episodes.

Family Education and Health Maintenance

1. Teach the use of good handwashing and avoidance of sources of infection such as crowds, unnecessary hospital visits, etc.
2. Teach recognition and reporting of signs and symptoms of infection.
3. Advise reporting any exposure to chicken pox if child has not had them or the vaccine.

PEDIATRIC ALERT

Immunosuppressed children are at risk for developing disseminated varicella if they are exposed to chicken pox, and they may be treated prophylactically with varicella immune globulin.

---

4. Encourage adequate nutrition to prevent emaciation from chemotherapy.
5. Encourage regular dental visits to detect and treat dental infections and disease.
6. Teach avoidance of constipation with increased fluid and fiber, and good perianal care.
7. Teach bleeding precautions such as use of electric

razor, avoidance of aspirin or nonsteroidal antiinflammatory drugs (NSAIDs), avoidance of sharp objects, avoidance of straining at stool or forceful nose-blowing.

Leukemia, Chronic Lymphocytic

Chronic lymphocytic leukemia (CLL) involves more mature cells than acute leukemia and is characterized by proliferation of lymphocytes. Five forms are recognized according to cell origin: B cell, T cell, lymphosarcoma, prolymphocytic leukemia, and hairy cell leukemia. B cell lymphocytic leukemia is the most common type (95% of cases) and is also the most common leukemia in the United States and Europe. It occurs in twice as many men as women; most patients are older than age 50 years.

Usually insidious in onset, CLL may be discovered during a routine physical examination. The specific cause is unknown, although hereditary and hormonal factors may play a role. As the disease progresses, thrombophlebitis may develop because of venous or lymphatic obstruction, and opportunistic bacterial, fungal, and viral infections may occur. Survival time varies from 2 to 7 years.

◆ Assessment

1. Early signs include frequent skin or respiratory infections, symmetric lymphadenopathy, and mild splenomegaly
2. Advanced symptoms include pallor, fatigue, activity intolerance, easy bruising and bleeding, skin lesions, bone tenderness, and abdominal discomfort

◆ Diagnostic Evaluation

1. Increased lymphocytes (10,000–150,000/mm^3); decreased hemoglobin and hematocrit; decreased platelets on complete blood count (CBC)
2. Decreased serum immunoglobulins also may be evident.

3. Bone marrow aspiration and biopsy to detect lymphocytic infiltration
4. Lymph node biopsy to detect spread of disease

◆ Collaborative Management

Therapeutic Interventions

1. Splenic irradiation or splenectomy for painful splenomegaly, platelet sequestration, or hemolytic anemia
2. Irradiation of painful enlarged lymph nodes
3. Supportive treatment includes transfusion therapy to replace platelets and red cells.

Pharmacologic Interventions

1. Chemotherapy (chlorambucil, cyclophosphamide, prednisone) to decrease lymphadenopathy and splenomegaly
2. IV immunoglobulins or gamma globulin to treat hypogammaglobulinemia.

◆ Nursing Interventions

Monitoring

1. Monitor for signs of infection, especially pneumonia.
2. Monitor for signs of thrombophlebitis—swollen, painful extremity with tenderness and red streaking.
3. Monitor platelet count and for signs of bleeding.

Supportive Care

1. Administer or teach the patient to administer analgesics on regular schedule, as prescribed.
2. Teach the use of relaxation techniques such as relaxation breathing, progressive muscle relaxation, distraction, and imagery to control pain.
3. Encourage frequent rest periods alternating with ambulation and light activity as tolerated.
4. Assist with hygiene and physical care as necessary.
5. Encourage balanced diet or nutritional supplements as tolerated.
6. Teach the patient to use energy conservation techniques while performing activities of daily living, such as sitting while bathing.

L

Patient Education and Health Maintenance

1. Teach the patient to minimize risk of infection: immediately cleanse any abrasion or wound of mucous membranes or skin; monitor temperature and report any fever or other sign of infection promptly; use condoms and other safe sex practices.
2. Teach use of medications as ordered, and possible side effects and their management; also to avoid aspirin and nonsteroidal antiinflammatory drugs, which may interfere with platelet function.
3. For information and support, refer to agencies such as:

   Leukemia Society of America
   600 Third Ave.
   New York, NY 10016
   212-573-8484

Leukemia, Chronic Myelogenous

Chronic myelogenous leukemia (CML), also known as chronic granulocytic or chronic myelocytic leukemia, results from malignant transformation of pluripotent hematopoietic stem cells, which leads to proliferation of granulocytes, monocytes, platelets, and occasionally red cells. The specific cause is unknown. This disorder accounts for 25% of adult leukemias, generally in ages 25 to 60 years, with peak incidence in the mid-40s. It causes fewer than 5% of childhood leukemias.

In its terminal phase, CML resembles an acute leukemia, with an accelerated phase and possibly a blast crisis. With the exception of possible cures using bone marrow transplant, CML is usually fatal, with an average survival time of 3 years. Complications include leukostasis from overproduction of cell types, infection, bleeding, and organ damage.

◆ Assessment

1. Insidious onset, may be discovered on routine physical examination by laboratory changes or splenomegaly
2. Common symptoms include fatigue, pallor, weight loss, night sweats, activity intolerance.

◆ Diagnostic Evaluation

1. Complete blood count shows increased granulocytes (often more than $100,000/mm^3$) and platelets initially; later thrombocytopenia.
2. Bone marrow aspiration and biopsy shows hypercellular marrow and usually demonstrates presence of Ph (Philadelphia) chromosome.

Therapeutic and Pharmacologic Interventions

1. Treatment during chronic phase is usually palliative to control symptoms. May include chemotherapy (busulfan, hydroxyurea), irradiation, splenectomy, or biotherapy (interferon).
2. Allogenic bone marrow transplant (related or unrelated donor) is potentially curative.
3. Treatment during accelerated phase or blast crisis aims to restore chronic phase through use of high-dose chemotherapy, leukopheresis.
4. Supportive care—generally terminal

◆ Nursing Interventions

Monitoring

Also see Acute Leukemia, p. 532.
1. Monitor for signs of infection.
2. Monitor for signs of bleeding.
3. Monitor for signs of thrombophlebitis caused by leukostasis.

Supportive Care

1. Encourage the patient to verbalize feelings and concerns.
2. Prevent infection by using good handwashing technique, encouraging good hygiene, and preventing exposure to pathogens.
3. Provide good skin care, handle the patient gently, and prevent falls that may lead to bleeding.
4. Encourage fluids and ambulation to counteract leukostasis.
5. Assist the patient in identifying resources and support (eg, family and friends, spiritual support, community or national organizations, support groups).

L

Patient Education and Health Maintenance

1. Teach the patient to take medications as prescribed and monitor for side effects.
2. For information and support, refer to agency listed on p. 538.

Liver Cancer

See Cancer, Liver

Liver Failure, Fulminant

Fulminant liver failure (FLF), also called fulminant hepatitis, is acute, massive necrosis of liver tissue in the absence of preexisting chronic liver disease, resulting in collapse of liver function. This rare syndrome is usually a complication of hepatitis B or D, or of drug toxicity. It progresses rapidly to hepatic encephalopathy within 8 weeks of onset. Acute respiratory failure, infections and sepsis, cardiac dysfunction, kidney failure, and hemorrhage also may occur. Mortality is high (60%–85%) despite intensive treatment.

Drugs such as acetaminophen, tetracycline, isoniazid, halogenated anesthetics, monoamine oxidase inhibitors, valproate, amiodarone, and methyldopa have been implicated. Other nondisease causes include various poisons and ingestion of *Amanita* mushrooms. Fulminant liver failure may also result from ischemia and hypoxia caused by hepatic vascular occlusion, hypovolemic shock, acute circulatory failure, septic shock, heat stroke, Budd-Chiari syndrome, acute fatty liver of pregnancy, partial hepatectomy, and liver transplantation.

◆ Assessment

1. Malaise, anorexia, nausea, vomiting, fatigue
2. Jaundice of skin and sclera; tea-colored, frothy urine; pruritus
3. Steatorrhea and diarrhea caused by decreased fat absorption
4. Ascites and edema caused by hypoproteinemia
5. Easy bruising, petechiae, overt bleeding caused by clotting deficiency

6. Fetor hepaticus: breath odor of acetone
7. Altered levels of consciousness, ranging from irritability and confusion to stupor, somnolence, and coma
8. Asterixis; change in deep tendon reflexes—initially hyperactive, become flaccid

◆ Diagnostic Evaluation

1. Prolonged prothrombin time, decreased platelet count
2. Elevated ammonia, amino acid, and mercaptan levels
3. Hypoglycemia or hyperglycemia
4. Dilutional hyponatremia or hypernatremia, hypokalemia, hypocalcemia, and hypomagnesemia

◆ Collaborative Management

Therapeutic Interventions

1. Restrict dietary protein and sodium while maintaining adequate caloric intake with prescribed diet or hypertonic dextrose solutions.
2. Hemodialysis, hemofiltration, hemoperfusion, or plasmapheresis may be indicated.

Pharmacologic Interventions

1. Administer lactulose orally or rectally to minimize formation of ammonia and other nitrogenous by-products in the bowel.
2. Administer neomycin rectally to suppress urea-splitting enteric bacteria in the bowel and decrease ammonia formation.
3. Administer low-molecular-weight dextran or albumin followed by a potassium-sparing diuretic (spironolactone) to enhance fluid shift from interstitial back to intravascular spaces.
4. Administer pancreatic enzymes, if diarrhea and steatorrhea are present, to permit better tolerance of diet.
5. Administer supplemental vitamins (A, B complex, C, and K) and folate.
6. If indicated, administer mannitol IV to manage cerebral edema.
7. Administer cholestyramine to promote fecal excretion of bile salts and reduce itching.
8. Administer antacids and H_2 antagonists to reduce the risk of bleeding from stress ulcers.

L

9. Administer infusion of fresh frozen plasma to maintain prothrombin time; give cryoprecipitate as needed for bleeding.

Surgical Interventions

1. Liver transplantation is the treatment of choice.

◆ Nursing Interventions

Monitoring

1. Monitor vital signs frequently.
2. Weigh patient daily and keep an accurate intake and output record; record frequency and characteristics of stool.
3. Measure and record abdominal girth daily.
4. Monitor respiratory rate, depth, use of accessory muscles, nasal flaring, and breath sounds.
5. Evaluate results of arterial blood gases and hemoglobin and hematocrit evaluations.
6. Be alert for signs of infection such as fever, cloudy urine, abnormal breath sounds.
7. Observe for subtle changes in behavior, worsening of sample of handwriting, and change in sleeping pattern to detect worsening hepatic encephalopathy.

Supportive Care

1. Elevate the head of the bed to lower diaphragm and decrease respiratory effort.
2. Turn the patient frequently to prevent pressure sores and pooling of respiratory secretions.
3. Administer oxygen therapy as needed.
4. Provide small, frequent meals or dietary supplements to conserve the patient's energy.
5. Encourage the patient to eat in a sitting position to decrease abdominal tenderness and feeling of fullness.
6. Provide frequent mouth care if the patient has bleeding gums or fetor hepaticus.
7. Provide enteral and parenteral feedings as needed.
8. Bathe the patient without soap and apply soothing lotions.
9. Keep the patient's fingernails short to prevent scratching from pruritus. Administer antipruritics as prescribed.
10. Assess for signs of bleeding from broken areas on the skin.

L

11. Use good handwashing and aseptic technique when caring for any break in the skin or mucous membranes.

12. Restrict visits with anyone who may have an infection.

13. Maintain close observation, side rails, and nurse call system.

14. Assist with ambulation as needed and avoid obstructions, to prevent falls.

15. Have well-lit room and reorient the patient frequently.

Patient Education and Health Maintenance

1. Teach the patient and family to notify health care provider of increased abdominal discomfort, bleeding, increased edema or ascites, hallucinations, or lapses in consciousness.

2. Instruct the patient to avoid activities that increase the risk of bleeding: scratching, falling, forceful nose blowing, aggressive tooth brushing, use of straight-edged razor.

3. Advise the patient to limit activities when fatigued and to rest frequently.

4. Maintain close follow-up for laboratory testing and evaluation.

Lou Gehrig's Disease
See Amyotrophic Lateral Sclerosis

Low Back Pain
See Back Pain, Low

L

Lung Cancer
See Cancer, Lung

Lupus Erythematosus, Systemic

Systemic lupus erythematosus (SLE) is a chronic, multisystem disease involving connective tissue that appears to result from production of inappropriate autoantibodies. Immune complexes and other immune system constituents combine to form complement that is deposited in organs, causing inflammation and tissue necrosis. The disease can resemble rheumatoid arthritis and may be mistaken for it, especially early in the course of the disease. Course of the disease is highly variable, but complications of SLE include infection, renal failure, permanent neurologic impairment, and death. The disease is more common in women than men, usually of childbearing age, but can affect children 5 to 15 years of age.

PEDIATRIC ALERT
The neonatal variant of SLE involves transient skin lesions, heart block, and hematologic abnormalities.

◆ Assessment

1. Skin-related manifestations:
   a. "Butterfly" rash characterized by erythema and edema
   b. Ringed-shaped lesions involving the shoulders, arms, and upper back
   c. Discoid lesions resulting in erythematous, scaly plaques on the face, scalp, external ear, and neck; alopecia is common
2. Arthritis:
   a. Generally bilateral and symmetric, involving the hands and wrists as well as other joints
   b. May resemble rheumatoid arthritis, but is nonerosive (no joint destruction is seen on x-ray)
   c. Tendon involvement is common and may lead to deformities or tendon rupture.
3. Cardiac manifestations:
   a. Pericarditis
   b. Pleural effusion
   c. Myocarditis
   d. Endocarditis
   e. Coronary arteritis—less common
4. Pulmonary manifestations:
   a. Pleuritis

L

    b. Pleural effusion
    c. Lupus pneumonitis
    d. Pulmonary hemorrhage
    e. Pulmonary embolism
5. Gastrointestinal manifestations:
    a. Oral ulcers
    b. Acute or subacute abdominal pain
    c. Pancreatitis
    d. Spontaneous bacterial peritonitis
    e. Bowel infarction
6. Renal manifestations: occur in 50% of patients, with up to 15% developing renal failure
    a. Nephritis (several forms)
    b. Renal vein thrombosis (rare)
7. Central nervous system manifestations:
    a. Neuropsychiatric disorders: depression, psychosis
    b. Transient ischemic attacks and stroke
    c. Epilepsy
    d. Migraine headache
    e. Myelopathy
    f. Guillain-Barré syndrome
    g. Chorea and other movement disorders
8. Hematologic manifestations:
    a. Hemolytic anemia
    b. Leukopenia
    c. Thrombocytopenia
9. Systemic manifestations:
    a. Fever
    b. Weight loss
    c. Fatigue
    d. Lymphadenopathy
    e. Hepatomegaly and splenomegaly

L

◆ Diagnostic Evaluation

1. Complete blood count: Leukopenia, anemia (may be hemolytic), thrombocytopenia
2. Antinuclear antibodies: positive in more than 90% of patients with SLE. Predominant pattern is homogeneous. Additional antibodies such as anti-dsDNA, anti-ssDNA, anti-nRNP, anti-Ro, and anti-La may be done if diagnosis is unclear.
3. Erythrocyte sedimentation rate: generally elevated

4. Complement levels: generally decreased in active disease
5. Hematuria, proteinuria, and "active sediment" (red cell casts) on urinalysis
6. 24-hour urine for protein may be elevated, and creatinine clearance may be decreased in kidney disease.
7. Hand and wrist x-rays may show nondestructive arthritis.
8. CT scan or MRI of the brain, to define any neurologic manifestations; of the abdomen, to rule out other abdominal processes in a patient with abdominal pain
9. Cerebral arteriography may be done to detect cerebral vasculitis.

◆ Collaborative Management

Therapeutic Interventions

1. Avoid direct exposure to sunlight to reduce the chance of exacerbation.
   a. Sunscreens: SPF 15 or higher on all sun-exposed areas
   b. Protective clothing: hats, long-sleeved shirts, lightweight
2. Joint protection and energy conservation
3. Application of heat or cold to affected areas

Pharmacologic Interventions

1. Antiinflammatories such as nonsteroidal antiinflammatory drugs (NSAIDS) and corticosteroids to control pain, fever, and inflammation
2. Antimalarials such as hydroxychloroquine to relieve joint symptoms and rash
3. Immunosuppressants such as azathioprine or cyclophosphamide for severe disease, especially nephritis
4. Topical corticosteroids may suppress skin lesions.

◆ Nursing Interventions

Monitoring

1. Monitor degree of renal involvement:
   a. Intake and output, urine specific gravity
   b. Measure urine protein, microalbumin, or obtain 24-hour creatinine clearance, as ordered.

L

   c. Check serum blood urea nitrogen (BUN) and creatinine.

2. Monitor control of joint pain.
3. Monitor temperature every 4 hours, and provide analgesics and comfort measures.
4. Monitor for signs of dehydration such as decreased urine output, dry mucous membranes, poor skin turgor, and thirst.
5. Monitor for side effects of medication such as hyperglycemia caused by corticosteroids.

Supportive Care

1. Suggest the use of hot or cold applications, relaxation techniques, and nonstrenuous exercise to enhance pain relief.
2. Instruct the patient in avoidance of factors that may exacerbate disease.
   a. Avoid prolonged exposure to sunlight and ultraviolet light. Use sunscreen SPF 15 or greater; wear protective clothing, hats, lightweight long-sleeved shirts.
   b. Avoid exposure to drugs or chemicals such as hairspray or hair coloring agents.
   c. Obtain health care provider's advice before taking medications.
3. Encourage good nutrition, sleep habits, exercise, rest, and relaxation to improve general health and help prevent infection.
4. Suggest alternate hairstyles, wearing scarves, wigs to cover significant areas of alopecia.
5. Encourage good oral hygiene and inspect mouth for oral ulcers.
6. Advise the patient that fatigue level will fluctuate with disease activity. Encourage the patient to modify schedule to include several rest periods during the day; use energy conservation techniques in daily activities.
7. Teach relaxation techniques such as deep breathing, progressive muscle relaxation, and imagery to reduce emotional stress that causes fatigue.

Patient Education and Health Maintenance

1. Stress that close follow-up is mandatory, even in times of remission, to detect early progression of organ in-

L

volvement and to alter drug therapy. Laboratory tests may be needed to monitor medication effects.

2. Advise frequent ophthalmologic examinations with hydroxychloroquine therapy to detect corneal and retinal changes to prevent blindness.
3. Advise using special cosmetics to cover skin lesions.
4. Advise about reproduction:
   a. Avoid pregnancy during time of severe disease activity.
   b. Immunomodulators may have teratogenic effects.
   c. Use of some drugs for treatment of SLE can cause sterility.
5. Advise on need for all regular childhood immunizations as well as pneumococcal vaccine and yearly influenza vaccine.
6. For additional information and support, refer to agencies such as:

   American Lupus Society
   260 Maple Court, Suite 123
   Ventura, CA 93003
   805-339-0443

Lyme Disease

Lyme disease is a chronic, inflammatory, multisystemic disorder caused by a spirochete, *Borrelia burgdorferi.* This organism is transmitted by small ticks, which inject the organism into the bloodstream as they feed. Originally found in Lyme, Connecticut, in 1975, the disease is endemic to the northeast (Massachusetts to Maryland), midwest (Minnesota, Wisconsin), and the west (California, Oregon). Lyme disease has also been reported from 43 other states as well as several foreign countries.

Onset is commonly in the summer, among persons visiting in heavily wooded areas. Three to 32 days after initial infection, *Borrelia* spreads through the skin to form a characteristic circular rash, erythema chronicum migrans (ECM). It then migrates through the blood and lymphatics to large joints and meningeal sites, where it may eventually cause meningitis, arthritis, various neuropathies (chorea), or cardiac abnormalities (AV block).

◆ Assessment

1. Erythema chronicum migrans (ECM) is the initial manifestation of acute infection.
   a. Annular lesion appears at site of tick bite, expands over days or weeks to up to 15 cm in diameter, bright red with central clearing.
   b. Lesion is warm to touch but not painful.
   c. Frequently appear on axilla, thighs, and groin.
   d. Occurs in 80% of patients.
2. Flulike symptoms develop along with ECM (or alone if no rash)—malaise, fever, headache, myalgia, lymphadenopathy. Some patients have no rash or flulike symptoms.
3. Migratory arthritis, debilitating fatigue, severe headache, and stiff neck develop within several weeks, indicating disseminated infection.
   a. Cardiac involvement may occur in 5% to 10% of patients within several weeks, with heart block lasting 3 to 6 weeks.
   b. Neurologic involvement occurs in 15% to 20% of patients with meningitis and cranial and peripheral neuropathies occurring several weeks to months after infection.
   c. Frank arthritis develops in 60% of untreated patients up to 6 months after acute infection.
4. Chronic infection may develop after several months of latency with continued neurologic impairment, arthritis, and skin changes.

◆ Diagnostic Evaluation

1. Erythrocyte sedimentation rate: high in early disease
2. Enzyme-linked immunosorbent assay (ELISA) testing for immunoglobulin (Ig) M and IgG antibodies—detectable several weeks after infection and remaining elevated indefinitely. Test is nonspecific and has high false-positive rate.

◆ Collaborative Management

Pharmacologic Interventions

1. Oral antibiotics over 10- to 21-day course for early Lyme disease: doxycycline, amoxicillin, or erythromycin

L

2. For meningitis or cranial/peripheral neuropathies, 14 to 21 days: IV penicillin-G, IM or IV ceftriaxone, IV chloramphenicol, or oral or IV doxycycline
3. For Lyme arthritis:
   a. IV penicillin-G or ceftriaxone for 14 to 21 days.
   b. Oral doxycyline or amoxicillin for 30 days

◆ Nursing Interventions

Supportive Care

1. Reassure the patient and family that Lyme disease cannot be transmitted person to person, and although treatment may be long, prognosis is good for most patients.
2. Administer pain relief medications as ordered.
3. Ask about drug allergies before giving prescribed antibiotics.
4. Monitor cardiac rhythm if heart block develops.

Family Education and Health Maintenance

1. Teach avoidance of tick-infested areas.
2. Advise use of insect repellent while outdoors.
3. Advise checking body and clothing every 3 or 4 hours while working or playing in infested area.
4. Emphasize that ticks should be removed from skin with tweezers or forceps to avoid leaving mouthparts in skin.

Lymphedema and Lymphangitis

Lymphedema is a swelling of the lymphatic tissues in the extremities (particularly in the dependent position), produced by obstructed lymph flow of the lymph nodes and lymphatic vessels. Lymphedema may be associated with radical mastectomy, varicose veins, chronic phlebitis, or a congenital condition.

Lymphangitis is an acute inflammation of lymphatic channels, which most commonly arises from a focus of infection in an extremity. Recurrent lymphangitis is often associated with lymphedema.

Complications include abscess formation, lymphedema

praecox (firm, nonpitting lymphedema unresponsive to treatment), septicemia, or elephantiasis (chronic fibrosis of subcutaneous tissue).

◆ Assessment

1. Edema may be massive and is often firm in lymphedema.
2. Red streaks extend up the extremity in lymphadenitis, with local pain, tenderness, and swelling along involved lymph vessels. Lymph nodes may be enlarged, red, tender.
3. Areas of necrotic, pus-producing abscesses indicate suppurative lymphadenitis (rare).
4. Fever and chills accompany lymphangitis.

◆ Diagnostic Evaluation

1. Lymphangiography to outline the lymphatic system.
2. Lymphoscintigraphy, a reliable alternative to lymphangiography using a radioactive contrast medium to help detect obstruction and inflammation.

◆ Collaborative Management

Therapeutic Interventions
1. External compression devices to treat lymphedema

Pharmacologic Interventions
1. Diuretics in lymphedema to control excess fluid (controversial)
2. Antibiotics in lymphangitis because causative organisms usually are streptococci and staphylococci

Surgical Interventions
1. For lymphedema not responsive to other approaches, procedures include replacement of affected subcutaneous tissue and fascia with skin grafts; or transfer of superficial lymphatics to the deep lymphatic system by means of a buried dermal flap.
2. In lymphangitis, incision and drainage may be necessary if necrosis and abscess formation take place.

L

◆ Nursing Interventions

Monitoring

1. Assess extremity for response to therapy or worsening inflammation and edema.
2. Observe for signs of postoperative infection.
3. Watch for postoperative complications such as flap necrosis, hematoma, abscess under flap, cellulitis.

Supportive Care

1. Advise the patient to rest frequently with the affected part elevated, each joint higher than the preceding one. In lymphangitis, apply hot, moist dressings.
2. Apply elastic bandages or stocking (in lymphedema or after acute attack with lymphangitis).
3. To relieve postoperative pain:
   a. Encourage comfortable positioning and immobilization of affected area.
   b. Use a bed cradle to relieve pressure from bed covers.
   c. Administer, or teach patient to administer, analgesics as prescribed; monitor for side effects.
4. Recommend isometric exercises with extremity elevated.
5. Advise the patient to restrict dietary sodium.

Patient Education and Health Maintenance

1. Encourage use of elastic bandage or stocking when ambulatory. May need for several months to prevent long-term edema.
2. Advise the patient to avoid trauma to extremity.
3. Advise the patient to practice good hygiene to avoid superimposed infections.

Lymphoma, Non-Hodgkin's

Non-Hodgkin's lymphomas are a group of malignancies of lymphoid tissue arising from T or B lymphocytes or their precursors. Although the cause is unknown, the disorder may be associated with defective or altered immune function. Incidence is higher in patients receiving immunosuppression for organ transplantation, in human immunodeficiency virus (HIV)-positive individuals, and in the presence of some viruses. Incidence rises steadily from approximately age 40 years. Unlike Hodgkin's disease, this disorder is more likely to be in an advanced stage at presentation. Complications of non-Hodgkin's lymphomas depend on the location and extent of malignancy and may include splenomegaly, hepatomegaly, thromboembolism, and spinal cord compression.

◆ Assessment

1. Common symptoms include fatigue, fever, chills, night sweats, painless enlargement of lymph nodes (generally unilateral), and weight loss.
2. Examination findings include splenomegaly, hepatomegaly, and generalized lymphadenopathy.
3. Wide variety of manifestations may occur if there is pulmonary involvement, superior vena cava obstruction, hepatic or bone involvement, etc.

◆ Diagnostic Evaluation

1. Lymph node biopsy to determine the type of lymphoma
2. Complete blood count and bone marrow aspiration and biopsy to determine whether there is bone marrow involvement
3. X-rays, CT, MRI to detect deep nodal involvement
4. Lymphangiogram to detect size and location of deep nodes involved, including abdominal nodes, which may not be readily seen by CT
5. Liver function tests and liver scan to detect liver involvement
6. Surgical staging (laparotomy with splenectomy, liver biopsy, multiple lymph node biopsies) may be done in selected patients.

◆ Collaborative Management

Therapeutic Interventions

1. Radiation therapy is palliative, not curative treatment.
2. Autologous or allogenic bone marrow transplantation has been tried.

L

Pharmacologic Interventions

1. Chemotherapy regimens, including CHOP regimen of cyclophosphamide, doxorubicin, vincristine, and prednisone, or BACOP regimen of bleomycin, doxorubicin, cyclophosphamide, vincristine, and prednisone

◆ Nursing Interventions

Monitoring

1. Monitor vital signs, breath sounds, level of consciousness, and skin and mucous membranes frequently for signs of infection.
2. Monitor for complications of radiation therapy and chemotherapy, such as leukopenia.

Supportive Care

1. To minimize the risk of infection in a patient with altered immune response, provide care in protected environment with strict handwashing technique.
2. If possible, avoid invasive procedures such as urinary catheterization.
3. Assess frequently for signs of infection, and notify health care provider if fever exceeds 101°F (38.3°C) or the patient's condition changes.
4. If infection is suspected, obtain cultures of suspected infected sites or body fluids.

Patient Education and Health Maintenance

1. Teach the patient infection precautions: Avoid crowds and infected individuals; avoid raw or undercooked food; wash hands frequently; use condoms and other safe sex practices.
2. Encourage frequent follow-up for monitoring of complete blood count (CBC) and condition.

Malabsorption Syndrome

Malabsorption syndrome is a group of symptoms and physical signs resulting from poor nutrient absorption in the small intestine, especially of fats and fat-soluble vitamins A, D, E, and K. Poor absorption of other nutrients, including carbohydrates, mineral, and proteins, also may occur. Malabsorption has multiple causes, including gallbladder or pancreatic disease, lymphatic obstruction, vascular impairment, or bowel resection (Table 11). Two common causes are lactase deficiency and celiac disease. In lactase deficiency, the lack of this enzyme prevents the digestion of lactose found in milk, causing osmosis of water into the lumen of the intestine when milk products are ingested.

Celiac disease, also called celiac sprue, is a disease of the small intestine (primarily duodenum and jejunum), marked by atrophy of the villi and microvilli caused by an intolerance to gluten, a protein found in common grains such as wheat, rye, oats, and barley. Cause is unknown, but genetic, environmental, and immunologic elements may be involved. Celiac disease affects more females than males, primarily persons of northwestern European ancestry; it is most common in young children 6 to 24 months of age but can occur at any age. Complications include impaired growth, inability to fight infection, electrolyte imbalance, clotting disturbance, and possible predisposition to malignant lymphoma of the small intestine. Celiac disease will be highlighted in this entry, but other malabsorption syndromes present similar manifestations.

M

◆ Assessment

3 to 9 Months of Age
1. Acutely ill; severe diarrhea and vomiting
2. Possible failure to thrive

TABLE 11 Malabsorption Syndromes

Reduced Digestion

Pancreatic exocrine deficiency	Cystic fibrosis, pancreatitis, Schwachman syndrome
Bile salt deficiency	Cholestasis, biliary atresia, hepatitis, cirrhosis, bacterial deconjugation
Enzyme defects	Lactase, sucrase, enterokinase, lipase deficiencies

Reduced Absorption

Primary absorption defects	Glucose–galactose malabsorption, abetalipoproteinemia, cystinuria, Hartnup disease
Decreased mucosal surface area	Crohn's disease, malnutrition, short bowel syndrome, antimetabolite chemotherapy, familial villous atrophy
Small intestinal disease	Celiac disease, tropical sprue, giardiasis, immune/allergic enteritis, Crohn's disease, lymphoma, acquired immunodeficiency syndrome

Lymphatic Obstruction

	Lymphagiectasia, Whipple disease, lymphoma, chylous ascites

Other

Drugs	Antibiotics, antimetabolites, neomycin, laxatives
Collagen vascular	Scleroderma
Infestations	Hookworms, tapeworm, giardiasis, immune defects

M

9 to 18 Months of Age
1. Slackening of weight followed by weight loss
2. Abnormal stools
   a. Pale, soft, bulky
   b. Offensive odor
   c. Greasy (steatorrhea)
   d. May increase in number
3. Abdominal distension
4. Anorexia
5. Muscle wasting: most obvious in buttocks and proximal parts of extremities
6. Hypotonia
7. Mood changes: ill humor, irritability, temper tantrums, shyness
8. Mild clubbing of fingers
9. Vomiting: often occurs in evening

Older Child and Adult
1. Signs and symptoms are often related to nutritional or secondary deficiencies resulting from disease.
   a. Anemia, vitamin deficiency (A, D, E, K)
   b. Hypoproteinemia with edema
   c. Hypocalcemia, hypokalemia, hypomagnesemia
   d. Hypoprothrombinemia from vitamin K deficiency
   e. Disaccharide (sugar) intolerance
2. Anorexia, fatigue, and weight loss
3. May have colicky abdominal pain, distension, flatulence, constipation, and large, pale stools

Celiac Crisis (This is rare and most often seen in very young children and toddlers.)
1. Profound anorexia
2. Severe vomiting and diarrhea
3. Weight loss
4. Marked dehydration and acidosis (secondary to intractable diarrhea and vomiting)
5. Decreased activity
6. Grossly distended abdomen
   a. Fluid rattle is present
   b. Abdomen flattens with passage of large, liquid stool
7. Appears shocklike and profoundly depressed

◆ Diagnostic Evaluation

1. Small bowel biopsy, which demonstrates characteristic abnormal mucosa

M

    a. Severely damaged or flat, villous lesions
    b. Histologic recovery after gluten elimination
    c. Histologic recurrence of villous injury within 2 years of gluten reintroduction
2. Hemoglobin levels—may be reduced
3. Prothrombin time—may be prolonged
4. Immunoglobulins—IgA may be increased in acute stage of disease.
5. Total protein and albumin may be decreased.
6. 72-hour stool collection for fecal fat is increased.
7. D-xylose absorption test—decreased blood and urine levels
8. Sweat test and pancreatic function studies may be done to rule out cystic fibrosis in child.

◆ Collaborative Management

Therapeutic Interventions

1. Dietary modifications include a lifelong gluten-free diet, avoiding all foods containing wheat or rye (and possibly barley and oats).
    a. Biopsy reverts to normal with appropriate diet.
    b. Clinical signs of improvement should be seen 1 to 4 weeks after proper diet is initiated.
2. In some cases, fats may be reduced.
3. Lactose may be eliminated from diet for 6 to 8 weeks, based on reduced disaccharidase activity.

Pharmacologic Interventions

1. Supplemental vitamins and minerals:
    a. Folic acid for 1 to 2 months
    b. Vitamins A and D because of decreased absorption
    c. Iron for 1 to 2 months if anemic
    d. Vitamin K if there is evidence of hypoprothrombinemia and bleeding
    e. Calcium lactate if milk is restricted
2. Treatment of celiac crisis:
    a. IV fluids and electrolytes
    b. Corticosteroids
    c. Parenteral hyperalimentation with amino acids, medium-chain triglycerides, and glucose for short course

M

d. Initial oral feedings are disaccharide free or completely sugar free.

◆ Nursing Interventions

Monitoring

1. Note child's reaction to food, to determine effectiveness of therapy and detect other possible intolerances.
   a. Foods taken and those refused
   b. Appetite
   c. Change in behavior after eating
   d. Characteristics and frequency of stools
   e. General disposition—behavior improvement often seen within 2 to 3 days after diet control is initiated
2. Monitor blood pressure and pulse for shock; changes in activity level and consciousness; and respirations for increased rate and depth, indicating acidosis, all signs of celiac crisis.

Supportive Care

1. Ensure that initial diet is high in protein, relatively low in fat, and starch free. Consult with dietitian.
   a. Add individual foods one at a time at several-day intervals, such as lean meat, cottage cheese, egg white, and raw ground apple.
   b. Add starchy foods to diet last.
2. Maintain NPO (nothing by mouth) status during initial treatment of celiac crisis or during diagnostic testing; take special precautions to ensure proper restriction if the child is ambulatory.
3. Encourage small frequent meals, but do not force eating if child has anorexia.
4. Be prepared to temporarily eliminate food items if symptoms increase.
5. Avoid exposing the child to sources of infection and use good handwashing technique.
6. Teach parents that child usually perspires freely and has a subnormal temperature with cold extremities; prevent dampness and chilling and dress child appropriately.
7. Assess for fever, cough, irritability, or other signs of infection.
8. Teach the parents to develop an awareness of the

M

child's condition and behavior; recognize changes and care for child accordingly.

a. Explain that diet and eating have a direct effect on behavior, and that behavior may indicate how the child is feeling.

b. Avoid conflict or emotional upset in child's presence; these may precipitate diarrhea, vomiting, and celiac crisis.

9. Explain that the toddler may cling to infantile habits for security. Allow this behavior; it may disappear as physical condition improves.

10. Help the parents to understand that after initial rapid weight gain, further improvement may be slow.

Family Education and Health Maintenance

1. Teach dietary therapy guidelines.

   a. Provide a specific list of restricted and acceptable foods.

   b. Teach how to read labels on foods to rule out those containing wheat and rye glutens.

   c. Provide information on substitutes for wheat, rye, barley, and oats, such as corn, rice, soybean flour, and gluten-free starch.

   d. Warn that advancing diet too rapidly may result in a setback.

2. Encourage regular medical follow-up and prompt attention to signs of upper respiratory infections that might trigger celiac crisis if untreated.

3. Advise that prolonged fasting and use of anticholinergic drugs may precipitate celiac crisis.

4. Encourage good hygiene to prevent infection.

5. Explain that the emotional climate in the home and around the patient is vitally important in maintaining the patient's medical and physical stability.

6. Stress that the disorder is lifelong; however, changes in the mucosal lining of the intestine and in general clinical condition are reversible when dietary gluten is avoided.

7. For additional information and support, refer to:

> **Celiac Sprue Association**
> P.O. Box 31700
> Omaha, NE 68131-0700
> (402) 558-0600

M

Manic Depression
See Bipolar Disorders

Mastectomy and Other Breast Cancer Surgery

Surgery for breast cancer may involve breast and lymph node removal (mastectomy) or a breast-preserving procedure (lumpectomy and axillary dissection). Breast-preserving procedures aim to achieve a cosmetically acceptable breast while completely excising the tumor.

Simple mastectomy (removal of the breast with some nearby axillary nodes) is indicated for carefully selected patients who are at high risk for developing breast cancer. Modified radical mastectomy (removal of the entire breast with all axillary nodes) is indicated in advanced disease involving large or multifocal tumors, or in women with very small breasts that preclude local tumor excision, or who are ineligible for radiation therapy. Radical mastectomy itself (removal of the entire breast, pectoral muscles, and axillary nodes) is rarely performed except in advanced disease. If appropriate, breast reconstructive surgery may be performed after mastectomy (Box 4).

Research studies comparing breast conservation (lumpectomy) with mastectomy have demonstrated equivalent patient survival. The following discussion covers mastectomy and axillary node dissection.

◆ Potential Complications

1. Infection
2. Hematoma, seroma
3. Lymphedema
4. Paresthesias, pain of axilla and arm
5. Impaired mobility of arm

◆ Collaborative Management

Preoperative Care
1. Explain the nature of the procedure and expected postoperative care, including care of surgical drains, location of the incision, and mobility of the involved arm.

M

■ BOX 4   BREAST RECONSTRUCTION AFTER
            MASTECTOMY

B reast reconstruction (mammoplasty) may be
   performed immediately or as long after surgery
as desired. Benefits include improved psychological
coping because of improved body image and self-
esteem.

Implants are indicated for patients with
inadequate breast tissue and skin of good quality.
Prosthetic implants made of saline (and in the past,
silicone) are placed in pocket under skin or
pectoralis muscle. TIssue expansion with saline may
be necessary before inserting implants. If opposite
breast is ptotic (protruding downward), mastopexy
may be necessary for symmetry. Complications
include capsular contracture resulting in firmness,
pain, and infection.

Nursing considerations for implants include:
1. Teach signs and symptoms of infection,
   hematoma, migration, and deflation.
2. Teach patient to massage breast to decrease
   capsule formation around implant.
3. Teach patient she may feel discomfort with the
   expansions, if used.

Flap grafts involve transfer of skin, muscle, and
subcutaneous tissue from another part of the body to
the mastectomy site. Latissimus dorsi flap graft
tunnels skin, fat, and muscles of the back between
shoulder blades under skin to front of chest.
Transverse rectus abdominis myocutaneous (TRAM)
flap tunnels muscle, fat, skin, and blood supply from
abdomen to breast area. There is increased cost,
hospitalization, time, and morbidity associated with
this procedure. Complications include flap loss,
hematoma, infection, seroma, and abdominal hernia.

continued

M

■ BOX 4 *(Continued)*

Nursing considerations for TRAM flap grafts include:
1. Assess flap and donor site for color, temperature, and wound drainage.
2. Control pain.
3. Provide support with bra or abdominal binder to maintain position of prosthesis.
4. Teach patient to perform BSE monthly and that she may have some asymmetry.

Nipple–areolar reconstruction is usually done at a separate time from breast reconstruction. This procedure uses skin and fat from the reconstructed breast for the nipple, and upper thigh for the areola. Tanning or tatooing is done to obtain appropriate color.

---

2. Reinforce the health care provider's information about diagnosis and possibility of further therapy.
3. Recognize the extreme anxiety and fear that the patient, family, and significant others are experiencing.
   a. Discuss patient's concerns and usual coping mechanisms.
   b. Explore support systems with patient.
   c. Discuss concerns regarding body image changes.

GERONTOLOGIC ALERT
Assessing the preoperative mental status of the older patient will help determine if cognitive changes occur postoperatively.

M

Postoperative Care
1. Assess dressing and wound after dressing is removed to note erythema, edema, tenderness, odor, and drainage.

    a. Initial dressing may consist of gauze held in place by elastic wrap; usually removed within 24 hours.

    b. Wound may be left open to the air or elastic wrap may be replaced if desired.

    c. Elastic wrap bandage should fit snugly but not so tightly that it hinders respiration. It should fit comfortably and support unaffected breast.

2. Assess drainage via suction drain for amount, color, and odor. Record amounts.

    a. May have 100 to 200 mL serous to serosanguinous drainage in the first 24 hours.

    b. Report grossly bloody or excessive drainage.

3. Assess the involved arm for edema, erythema, and pain.

    a. Do not take blood pressure, draw blood, inject medications, or start IVs in affected arm. Post sign over bed.

    b. Elevate affected arm on pillows, above level of heart, and position hand above elbow to promote gravity drainage of fluid.

    c. Teach the patient to massage the arm if prescribed, to increase circulation and decrease edema.

    d. Provide the patient with information on arm and hand care.

NURSING ALERT

At particular risk for lymphedema are patients who undergo axillary node dissection in combination with radiation therapy to axilla.

4. Assess mobility of affected arm and the patient's ability to perform self-care.

    a. Initially encourage wrist and elbow flexion and extension. Encourage use of arm for washing face, combing hair, applying lipstick, and brushing teeth. Encourage the patient to gradually increase use of the arm.

    b. Encourage the patient to avoid abduction initially to help prevent seroma formation. If prescribed, support arm in sling to prevent abduction of the arm.

M

   c. Instruct and provide patient with prescribed exercises to do when permitted.
5. Inspect wound and instruct patient to recognize and report signs of infection, hematoma, or seroma formation. Teach drain care, if appropriate.

GERONTOLOGIC ALERT
Signs and symptoms of infection may not be obvious in older patients. Assess patients for mental status changes or urinary incontinence.

6. Teach patient to bathe the incision gently and blot carefully to dry, and later, with approval, massage the healed incision gently with cocoa butter to encourage circulation and increase skin elasticity.
7. Assess the mastectomy patient's knowledge of prosthesis and reconstruction options, and provide information as needed.
   a. Suggest clothing adjustments to camouflage loss of breast.
   b. Help the patient obtain a temporary prosthesis (may be provided by Reach to Recovery, an American Cancer Society program). Initial prosthesis should be light and soft to allow incision to heal. The patient may wear a heavier type, usually after 4 to 8 weeks, with the surgeon's approval.
8. Encourage the patient to allow herself to experience the grief process over the loss of her breast and to learn to cope with these feelings.
9. Discuss with the patient the effects of diagnosis and surgery on her view of herself as a woman.
   a. Encourage the patient to discuss these concerns with her partner.
   b. Assist the patient and partner to look at the incision when ready.

M

◆ Patient Education and Health Maintenance

1. Explain to the patient how the wound will gradually change and that the newly healed wound may have less sensation because of severed nerves.

TABLE 12 Hand and Arm Care to Help Prevent Lymphedema and Infection

After a mastectomy or axillary dissection, the arm may swell because of the excision of lymph nodes and their connecting vessels. Circulation of lymph fluid is slowed, making it more difficult for the body to combat infection. Special precautions should be taken to prevent lymphedema and infection.

Avoid burns while cooking or smoking.

Avoid sunburns.

Have all injections, vaccinations, blood samples, and blood pressure tests done on the other arm whenever possible.

Use an electric razor with a narrow head for underarm shaving to reduce the risk of nicks and scratches.

Carry heavy packages or handbags on the other arm.

Never cut cuticles; use hand cream or lotion instead.

Wear protective gloves when gardening and when using strong detergents, etc.

Use a thimble when sewing.

Avoid harsh chemicals and abrasive compounds.

Use insect repellent to avoid bites and stings.

Avoid elastic cuffs on blouses and nightgowns.

From *Mastectomy: A Treatment for Breast Cancer*. NIH Pub No. 91-658.

2. Teach the patient how to care for arm to prevent lymphedema and infection after axillary node dissection (Table 12).
3. Teach importance of breast self-examination (BSE), mammograms, and regular follow-up visits.
4. Encourage discussion with health care provider about pregnancy after breast cancer, if indicated. Advise patient of premature menopause as side effect of chemotherapy.
5. Refer the patient to a postmastectomy support group as needed and desired. Community resources may be accessed through the telephone directory, the hospital information system, or the American Cancer Society (1-800-ACS-2345).
6. Remind patient that stress related to breast cancer and mastectomy may persist for 1 year or more and to seek counseling as needed.

7. Encourage female relatives, especially sisters, daughters, and mother, to seek breast cancer surveillance.

Mastitis, Acute

Acute mastitis is inflammation of the breast caused by infection. The infection may be from hands of patient, personnel caring for patient, baby's nose or throat, or blood borne. Most common causative agents are *Staphylococcus aureus, Escherichia coli,* and *Streptococcus.*

The disorder usually occurs in first-time breast-feeding mothers. It may also occur later in chronic lactation mastitis and central duct abscesses. Milk stasis may lead to obstruction, followed by noninfectious inflammation, then infectious mastitis. If untreated, the disorder can progress to a breast abscess.

◆ Assessment

1. Fever of 101°F (38.3°C) or higher
2. Redness, warmth, edema; breast may feel doughy and tough
3. Patient may complain of dull pain in affected area and may have nipple discharge.
4. No diagnostic tests are necessary.

◆ Collaborative Management

Therapeutic and Pharmacologic Interventions

1. Apply heat to resolve tissue reaction; however, may cause increased milk production and worsen symptoms
2. May apply cold to decrease tissue metabolism and milk production

Pharmacologic Interventions

1. Antibiotics for infection
2. Antipyretics and nonnarcotic analgesics as needed
3. If abscess develops, may need incision and drainage

M

◆ Nursing Interventions

Monitoring

1. Monitor or teach the patient to monitor temperature and response to fever and pain control measures.
2. Inspect the breasts daily to note skin changes.
3. Observe for mammary abscess: increased fever, chills, malaise, purulent nipple discharge, and a palpable mass

Supportive Care and Patient Education

1. Have the patient wear firm breast support.
2. Encourage the breast-feeding patient to practice meticulous personal hygiene to prevent mastitis.
3. Discuss the issue of stopping or continuing breast-feeding with patient and health care provider; support the patient in her decision.

Meniere's Disease

Meniere's disease (endolymphatic hydrops) is a chronic disease of unknown cause that involves the inner ear. In this disorder, fluid distension of the endolymphatic spaces of the labyrinth destroy cochlear hair cells, which causes a triad of symptoms: vertigo, hearing loss, and tinnitus. If untreated, irreversible hearing loss results, with concomitant disability and social isolation. Meniere's disease occurs most frequently in patients aged 30 to 60 years.

◆ Assessment

1. Sudden attacks of dizziness occur in which the patient feels the sensation of spinning (vertigo); attacks may last 10 minutes to several hours.
2. Tinnitus and reduced hearing occur on the involved side.
3. The patient reports headache, nausea, vomiting, and incoordination. Sudden head motion may precipitate vomiting.

568

◆ Diagnostic Evaluation

1. Electronystagmography (ENG) testing to help differentiate Meniere's disease from an intracranial lesion. This test battery evaluates the vestibuloocular reflex. One test (water/caloric) involves introducing water into the ear canal so that it hits the eardrum. Normal response is dizziness; lack of response may indicate an acoustic neuroma; and a severe attack of vertigo indicates Meniere's disease.
2. Audiometric tests to evaluate sensorineural hearing loss
3. CT scan, MRI may be used to rule out tumor.

◆ Collaborative Management

Therapeutic Interventions

1. Have the patient keep a diary noting presence of aural symptoms (eg, tinnitus, distorted hearing) when episodes of vertigo occur, to help determine which ear is involved and if surgery will be needed.
2. Lifestyle changes to decrease attacks: smoking cessation; avoidance of coffee, tea, alcohol, and stimulating drugs

Pharmacologic Interventions

1. Acetazolamide, a vestibular suppressant and diuretic, may reduce symptoms when attacks are infrequent.
2. Antihistamines, diazepam, and antiemetics also may be used to control symptoms.
3. Corticosteroids may be used to try to preserve hearing, and streptomycin may be used in severe bilateral disease to reduce symptoms.

Surgical Interventions

1. If drug therapy is ineffective, a conservative approach involves decompressing the endolymphatic sac or implanting an endolymphatic subarachnoid or mastoid shunt to relieve symptoms without destroying vestibular function.
2. Destructive procedures (labyrinthectomy or vestibular nerve neurectomy) may be required to provide relief. These cause total deafness of the affected ear.

M

◆ Nursing Interventions

Supportive Care

1. Help the patient recognize aura symptoms to allow time to prepare for an attack. Also help the patient to identify specific trigger factors to control attacks.
   a. Move slowly because jerking or sudden movements may precipitate an attack.
   b. Avoid noises and glaring, bright lights, which may initiate an attack. Have patient close eyes if this lessens symptoms.
   c. Eliminate smoking and the intake of coffee, tea, alcohol, and stimulating drugs, because of vasoconstriction effects.
   d. Control environmental factors and personal habits that may cause stress or fatigue.
   e. If there is a tendency to allergic reactions to foods, eliminate those foods from the diet.
2. Encourage the patient to lie still in a safe place during the attack. Put side rails up on bed if in hospital.
3. Inform the patient that the dizziness may last for varying lengths of time. Maintain safety precautions until attack is complete.

Patient Education and Health Maintenance

1. Teach the patient about medication regimen, including side effects of antihistamines, such as drowsiness, dry mouth.
2. Advise sodium restriction as adjunct to diuretic (acetazolamide) therapy.
3. Advise the patient to maintain a diary of attacks, triggers, and severity of symptoms.
4. Encourage follow-up hearing evaluations.
5. Teach patient to be aware of other sensory cues from the environment (visual, olfactory, tactile) if hearing is affected.

M

Meningitis

Meningitis is an inflammation of the brain and spinal cord meninges. This disorder is usually a complication of other bacterial infections such as sinusitis, otitis media, pneumonia, endocarditis, or osteomyelitis. Common causative organisms include *Neisseria meningitides* (meningococcal meningitis), *Haemophilus influenzae,* and *Streptococcus pneumoniae. Escherichia coli* and *Listeria monocytogenes* may also affect infants from birth to 3 months of age. Onset is either insidious or fulminant, depending on causative organism.

If meningitis is caused by a virus, it is called aseptic meningitis. This type of meningitis may result also from a noninfectious cause such as blood in the subarachnoid space. Infants, children, and the elderly are at highest risk for meningitis. Complications include seizures, increased intracranial pressure (IICP), syndrome of inappropriate antidiuretic hormone secretion (SIADH), hearing loss, hydrocephalus, blindness, developmental delays, and learning disabilities.

◆ Assessment

1. History of recent infection (upper respiratory, ear, sinus) or procedure or trauma that may have penetrated the central nervous system
2. Headache, backache, neck stiffness, and photophobia
3. Fever and vomiting are more likely to occur in children than in adults.
4. Altered mental status
5. Characteristic signs of meningeal irritation: nuchal rigidity, positive Brudzinski's and Kernig's signs (Fig. 17).
6. Petechial or purpuric rash, which may indicate meningococcal meningitis
7. In children, the following may occur:
   a. Infants younger than 2 months—irritability, lethargy, vomiting, poor feeding, seizures, high-pitched cry, fever, or hypothermia
   b. Infants 2 months to 2 years—above signs plus altered sleep pattern, tenseness of fontanel, fever, signs of menigeal irritation
   c. Children older than 2 years—signs and symptoms similar to those of adult with progressive decline in responsiveness

M

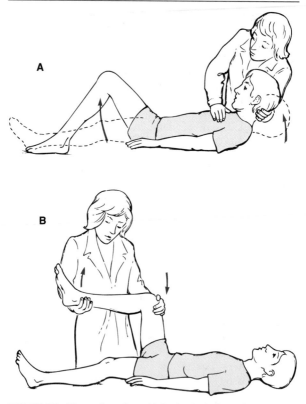

FIGURE 17 *Signs of meningeal irritation include nuchal rigidity, a positive Brudzinski's and Kernig's signs.* **(A)** *To elicit Brudzinski's sign, place the patient supine and flex the head upward. Resulting flexion of both hips, knees, and ankles with neck flexion indicate meningeal irritation.* **(B)** *To test for the Kernig's sign, once again place the patient supine. Keeping one leg straight, flex the other hip and knee to a bent knee to form a 90-degree angle. Slowly extend the lower leg. This places a stretch on the meninges, resulting in pain and spasm of the hamstring muscle. Resistance to further extension can be felt.*

M

◆ Diagnostic Evaluation

1. Complete blood count (CBC) with differential shows elevated white blood cells (WBCs) and neutrophils.
2. Blood, urine, and nasopharyngeal cultures to help identify the causative organism
3. Lumbar puncture to obtain cerebrospinal fluid (CSF) cultures, to show elevated cell counts and possibly isolate causative organism
4. CT or MRI with and without contrast, to rule out other neurologic disorders

◆ Collaborative Management

Pharmacologic Interventions

1. Antibiotics in large doses IV to allow adequate amount to cross blood–brain barrier: penicillins, cephalosporins, vancomycin
2. Corticosteroids and osmotic diuretic to reduce cerebral edema
3. Supportive care to critically ill or comatose child or adult

◆ Nursing Interventions

Monitoring

1. Monitor level of consciousness, vital signs, and neurologic parameters frequently. Notify the health care provider of increasing temperature, decreasing alertness, onset of seizures, or periods of apnea, which signal deterioration.
2. Monitor for IICP (see p. 372) or SIADH. SIADH causes inappropriate fluid retention and dilutional hyponatremia with signs and symptoms of anorexia, nausea, vomiting, edema, decreased urine output, lethargy, seizures, sluggish deep tendon reflexes, tachycardia, hyponatremia, and decreased serum osmolality.
3. Monitor central venous pressure and infusion of IV fluids to avoid fluid overload, which may worsen cerebral edema.
4. Monitor peak and trough blood levels of antibiotics to ensure adequate therapy.

M

Supportive Care

1. To reduce fever, administer antipyretics as ordered, and institute other cooling measures (eg, hypothermia blanket) as indicated. Administer IV fluids as ordered to avoid dehydration.
2. Administer analgesics as ordered; monitor for response and adverse reactions. Narcotics should be avoided to prevent interference in assessment of level of consciousness.
3. Maintain infection precautions for at least 24 hours after starting appropriate antibiotic therapy. Good handwashing and careful disposal of respiratory secretions is essential. Gowns and gloves may be considered.
4. Maintain quiet, calm environment to prevent agitation, which may cause IICP.
5. Darken the room if photophobia is present.
6. Assist with positioning the patient for neck stiffness; be sure to turn the patient slowly and carefully with head and neck in alignment.
7. Be prepared to treat seizures in the child.

Family Education and Health Maintenance

1. Advise the patient's close contacts that prophylactic treatment with rifampin may be indicated to protect against meningococcal meningitis; check with their health care providers or the local public health department.
2. Encourage following medication regimen as directed because infectious agent must be fully eradicated from body.
3. Advise on reporting recurrent fever, tense fontanel in infant, or neurologic impairments after meningitis.
4. Encourage routine health evaluations for children to identify any developmental delays or other long-term complications.

M

Menopause

Menopause is described as the physiologic cessation of menses. It is caused by failing ovarian function and decreased estrogen production by the ovary. Climacteric is the transition period (perimenopausal) during which the woman's reproductive function gradually diminishes and disappears. It usually occurs at approximately age 50 years. Artificial or surgical menopause may occur secondary to surgery or radiation involving the ovaries.

◆ Assessment

1. Genitalia: atrophy of vulva, vagina, urethra results in dryness, bleeding, itching, burning, dysuria, thinning of pubic hair, loss of labia minora, decreased lubrication
2. Sexual function: dyspareunia, decreased intensity and duration of sexual response, but can still have active function
3. Vasomotor: 60% to 70% of women experience "hot flashes," which may be preceded by an anxious feeling and accompanied by sweating.
4. Osteoporosis: decreased bone mass results in increased hip fractures, spinal compression fractures.
5. Cardiovascular: increased coronary artery disease, cholesterol level, and palpitations
6. Psychological: insomnia, irritability, anxiety, memory loss, fear, and depression may be experienced.

◆ Diagnostic Evaluation

1. Hormonal levels of luteinizing hormone (LH) and follicle-stimulating hormone (FSH) (increased), and estradiol (decreased) may be measured to confirm menopause.

◆ Collaborative Management

Pharmacologic Interventions

1. Estrogen replacement therapy
   a. Indicated to reduce symptoms and to prevent osteoporosis and coronary artery disease
   b. Topical preparations may be used for atrophic vaginitis.
   c. Progesterone preparation also given if uterus is intact to prevent endometrial hyperplasia and possible cancer

M

2. Vaginal lubricants such as Replens to decrease vaginal dryness and dyspareunia
3. Vitamin E and B supplements—to decrease hot flashes
4. Calcium supplements to prevent bone loss

◆ Nursing Interventions

Supportive Care

1. Provide patient with information related to estrogen replacement therapy, including dosage schedule, route, side effects, and what to expect of menstrual bleeding. Women who still have a uterus can expect a period at the end of every month if they are taking hormones cyclically. A newer method of hormone replacement, giving estrogen and lower-dose progesterone daily, may cause some irregular spotting for 3 months to up to 1 year, then most women experience no bleeding.
2. Explore with patient her feelings about menopause, clear up misconceptions about sexual functioning, and encourage her to discuss her feelings with her partner.
3. Instruct patient how to use water-based lubricant for intercourse to decrease dryness.

Patient Teaching and Health Maintenance

1. Teach patient that sexual functioning does not decrease during menopause but may even increase because of loss of fear of pregnancy and increased time if children are grown.
2. Teach patient about foods that are high in calcium—dairy products, broccoli, and some fortified cereals—and to maintain weight-bearing activities to prevent osteoporosis.

3. Counsel patient on reducing risk factors for coronary artery disease.
4. Encourage patient to keep regular medical and gynecologic follow-up visits.
5. Advise patient that vulvovaginal infection and trauma are possible because of the dryness of the tissue, and to seek prompt evaluation if pain and discharge occur.

Multiple Myeloma

Multiple myeloma is a malignant disorder of plasma cells. Neoplastic plasma cells produce a homogeneous immunoglobulin (M protein or Bence-Jones protein) without any apparent antigenic stimulation. Bence-Jones protein affects renal function and platelet function, lowers resistance to infection, and may cause hyperviscosity of blood. The abnormal plasma cells also produce osteoclast-activating factor (OAF), which causes extensive bone loss, severe pain, pathologic fractures, and, in some cases, spinal cord compression.

Multiple myeloma has no known cause. It generally affects the elderly (median age at diagnosis is 68 years) and is more common among African Americans. Multiple myeloma has a median survival of 3 to 4 years. Complications include bacterial infections, renal failure or pyelonephritis, bleeding, and thromboembolism.

◆ Assessment

1. Constant, often severe bone pain caused by bone lesions and pathologic fractures. Sites commonly affected include thoracic and lumbar vertebrae, ribs, skull, pelvis, and proximal long bones.
2. Fatigue and weakness related to anemia caused by crowding of marrow by plasma cells
3. Bone deformities

◆ Diagnostic Evaluation

1. Bone marrow aspiration and biopsy to demonstrate increased number and abnormal form of plasma cells

M

2. Decreased hemoglobin and hematocrit related to anemia
3. Bence-Jones protein found in urine and serum
4. Hypercalcemia (from bone destruction)
5. Skeletal x-rays to detect osteolytic bone lesions

◆ Collaborative Management

Therapeutic Interventions

1. Plasmapheresis to treat hyperviscosity or bleeding
2. Radiation therapy for painful bone lesions
3. Hemodialysis to manage renal failure
4. Stabilization and fixation of fractures

Pharmacologic Interventions

1. Oral melphalan or cyclophosphamide
2. Corticosteroids alone or in combination with chemotherapy
3. Allopurinol and fluids to treat hyperuricemia

◆ Nursing Interventions

Monitoring

1. Report any sudden, severe pain, especially of back, which could indicate pathologic fracture.
2. Watch for nausea, drowsiness, confusion, polyuria, which could indicate hypercalcemia caused by bony destruction and immobilization.
3. Monitor serum calcium levels.
4. Monitor serum blood urea nitrogen (BUN) and creatinine to detect renal insufficiency.
5. Monitor intake and output, and weigh the patient daily.

Supportive Care

1. Administer analgesics as needed to control pain. Use adequate doses, regularly scheduled around the clock.
2. Encourage the patient to wear back brace for lumbar lesion.
3. Recommend physical/occupational therapy consultation.
4. Discourage bed rest to prevent hypercalcemia, but ensure safety of environment to prevent fractures.
5. Assist the patient with measures to prevent injury and

M

decrease risk of fractures. Avoid lifting and straining; use walker and other assistive devices as appropriate.

6. Reassure the patient that you are available for support, to provide comfort measures, and to answer questions.

7. Encourage the patient to use own support network, such as church and community services and national agencies.

Patient Education and Health Maintenance

1. Teach the patient about risk of infection caused by impaired antibody production; instruct to monitor temperature and report any fever or other sign of infection promptly; also use condoms and other safe sex practices.

2. Teach the patient to take medications as prescribed and monitor for possible side effects; avoid aspirin and nonsteroidal antiinflammatory drugs unless prescribed, because these drugs may interfere with platelet function.

3. Teach the patient to minimize risk of fractures: Use proper body mechanics and assistive devices as appropriate; avoid bed rest, remain ambulatory.

4. Advise the patient to report new onset of pain, new location, or sudden increase in pain intensity immediately. Report new onset or worsening of neurologic symptoms (eg, changes in sensation) immediately.

5. Encourage the patient to maintain high fluid intake (2–3 L/day) to avoid dehydration and prevent renal insufficiency; also not to fast before diagnostic tests.

Multiple Sclerosis

Multiple sclerosis (MS) is a chronic central nervous system disorder marked by demyelination of small areas of the white matter of the optic nerve, brain, and spinal cord. Demyelination results in disordered transmission of nerve impulses; concurrent inflammatory changes lead to scarring of the affected nerve fibers. The cause of MS is unknown but may be related to autoimmune dysfunction, genetic factors, or an infectious process. Although classed as a chronic disease, MS may flare up in acute exacerbations, after which the patient may go into remission. Com-

M

plications include respiratory dysfunction, infection or sepsis, and complications of immobility.

◆ Assessment

1. Muscle weakness, fatigue, tremor, uncoordinated movements
2. Cranial nerve dysfunction, including visual disturbances (impaired and double vision, nystagmus) and impaired speech (slurring, dysarthria)
3. Absent or exaggerated deep tendon reflexes
4. Paresthesias, impaired deep sensation, impaired vibratory and position sense
5. Urinary dysfunction (hesitancy, frequency, urgency, retention, incontinence)

◆ Diagnostic Evaluation

1. Visual, auditory and somatosensory evoked potential testing: slowed conduction is evidence of demyelination
2. Lumbar puncture: Electrophoresis shows abnormal immunoglobulin (Ig) G antibody in cerebrospinal fluid.
3. MRI: visualizes small plaques of demyelination scattered throughout white matter of CNS

◆ Collaborative Management

Therapeutic Interventions
1. Physical and occupational therapy to facilitate rehabilitation and maintenance of functional capacity.
2. Nerve block for severe spasticity

Pharmacologic Interventions
1. Corticosteroids or adrenocorticotropic hormone (ACTH) to decrease inflammation and shorten duration of exacerbation of MS
2. Immunosuppressive agents to help stabilize the course of the disease
3. Beta-interferon is being used for treatment of rapidly progressing disease in some individuals.
4. Centrally acting muscle relaxants to control spasticity
5. Amantadine for fatigue
6. Antidepressants and counseling for depression

M

7. Anticholinergics for bladder control
8. Stool softeners, bulk laxative, suppositories to control bowel function
9. Carbamazepine to control dystonia and chronic pain

◆ Nursing Interventions

Monitoring

1. Observe for adverse reactions to drug therapy.
2. Monitor vital signs to detect changes.
3. Monitor for signs of respiratory or urinary infection, sepsis.
4. Monitor for signs of complications of immobility, such as pressure ulcers, contractures, constipation, pneumonia, deep vein thrombosis.

Supportive Care

1. Perform muscle stretching and strengthening exercises daily or teach patient or family to perform, using stretch–hold–relax routine to minimize spasticity and prevent contractures.
2. Encourage ambulation and activities.
   a. Teach use of braces, canes, walker, etc. when necessary.
   b. Advise the patient to avoid sudden changes in position and to use a wide-based gait, to avoid injury from falls.
3. Encourage frequent position changes while immobilized to prevent contractures; advise that sleeping prone will minimize flexor spasm of hips and knees.
4. Explore ways to minimize fatigue.
   a. Advise the patient to plan ahead and prioritize activities, and to take brief rest periods throughout the day.
   b. Teach energy conservation techniques, and avoidance of overheating or overexertion.
5. Advise the patient to avoid exposure to infectious agents.
6. Optimize sensory function.
   a. Suggest use of an eye patch or frosted lens (alternate eyes) for patients with double vision.
   b. If necessary, advise ophthalmologic consultation to maximize vision.
   c. Provide a safe environment for a patient with any

M

sensory alteration. Orient patient and make sure floors are free of obstacles or slippery areas.

7. Maintain urinary function.
   a. Ensure adequate fluid intake to help prevent infection and stone formation.
   b. Assess for urinary retention, catheterize for residual urine as indicated.
   c. Initiate bladder training program to reduce incontinence.

8. Promote the patient's sense of independence and well-being.
   a. Encourage verbal communication between patient and family members related to the disease and treatment.
   b. Explore adaptation of some roles so that patient can still function in family unit; suggest dividing up household duties, child care responsibilities to prevent strain on one individual.
   c. Encourage counseling and use of church or community resources.
   d. If appropriate, encourage open communication between sexual partners; suggest consultation with sexual therapist to help promote sexual function.

Patient Education and Health Maintenance

1. Encourage the patient to maintain previous activities although at a lowered level of intensity.
2. Teach the patient to respect fatigue and avoid physical overexertion and emotional stress; remind patient that activity tolerance may vary from day to day.
3. Encourage nutritious diet that is high in fiber to promote health and good bowel elimination.
4. Advise the patient that some medications may accentuate weakness, such as some antibiotics, muscle relaxants, antiarrhythmics and antihypertensives, antipsychotics, oral contraceptives, and antihistamines; urge the patient to check with health care provider before taking any new medications.
5. Teach the patient receiving beta-interferon to expect side effects of flulike symptoms, fever, asthenia, chills, myalgias, sweating, and local reaction at the injection site. Liver function test elevation and neutropenia may also occur. Side effects may persist for up to 6 months of treatment before subsiding.

M

6. Instruct patient in self-injection technique for beta-interferon.
7. Refer the patient and family to agencies such as:

> **National Multiple Sclerosis Society**
> 733 3rd Ave.
> New York, NY 10017
> 212-986-3240

Muscular Dystrophy

Muscular dystrophy is a group of hereditary disorders marked by progressive, symmetric weakness and wasting of skeletal muscles. Despite wasting, muscle groups tend to physically enlarge because of excessive adipose and connective tissue deposition. Common types include: *Duchenne's (pseudohypertrophic) muscular dystrophy, Becker's (benign pseudohypertrophic) muscular dystrophy, facioscapulohumeral dystrophy, and limb-girdle dystrophy.* These disorders typically strike in childhood. Complications include infections and sepsis, cardiac dysrhythmias, respiratory insufficiency, and depression.

◆ Assessment

1. Progressive weakening and atrophy of muscles
   a. *Duchenne's, Becker's:* involvement of iliopsoas, gluteal, and quadriceps muscles, pseudohypertrophy of calves, waddling gait, difficulty walking and climbing stairs; later, weakening of pretibial, pectoral girdle, and upper limbs
   b. *Facioscapulohumeral:* inability to raise arms over head; scapular winging, "Popeye" effect of arms (large forearms, slim upper arms); atrophy of facial, shoulder and arm muscles; lordosis
   c. *Limb-girdle:* involvement of upper arm and pelvis, scapular winging (but absence of pseudohypertrophy of calves, sparing of facial muscles); lordosis; waddling gait
2. Inability to close eyes or purse lips, with *facioscapulohumeral MD*

M

◆ Diagnostic Evaluation

1. Muscle biopsy shows deposits of fat and connective tissue (definitive diagnosis).
2. Nerve conduction test and electromyogram show weak bursts of electrical activity in affected muscles.
3. Serum creatinine kinase (CK) level is usually elevated.

◆ Collaborative Management

Therapeutic Interventions

1. Physical and occupational therapy to preserve mobility and independence
2. Immobilization devices and possibly surgical tendon release to treat contractures and preserve mobility

Pharmacologic Interventions

1. Antiarrhythmics, anticonvulsants, and corticosteroids are given to control manifestations.
2. Analgesics and antidepressants may be given to facilitate participation in activities.

◆ Nursing Interventions

Monitoring

1. Monitor vital signs, cardiac rhythm, and signs of congestive heart failure such as edema, adventitious breath sounds, and weight gain.
2. Monitor for signs of infections (pulmonary, urinary, systemic).
3. Monitor patient's mental status; be alert for signs of depression.

Supportive Care

1. When respiratory involvement occurs, encourage upright positioning to provide for maximum chest excursion.
2. Encourage coughing and deep breathing or perform chest physiotherapy as indicated, to strengthen respiratory muscles.
3. Suggest energy conservation techniques and avoidance of exertion.
4. Perform range-of-motion exercises to preserve mobility and prevent atrophy and encourage stretching and

M

strengthening exercises as taught by physical therapist.

5. Schedule activity with consideration of energy highs throughout the day.

6. Consult with occupational therapist for assistive devices to maintain independence.

7. Apply braces and splints, as directed to prevent contractures.

8. Evaluate swallowing (gag reflex) and chewing.

9. Provide a diet that the patient can handle; blenderizing food may be necessary.

10. Encourage eating in upright position without talking and in small, frequent meals.

11. Administer alternate enteral feeding if gag reflex is diminished.

12. Monitor intake and output and maintain IV or oral fluid intake as ordered.

13. Encourage diversional activities that prevent overexertion and frustration, but discourage long periods of bed rest and inactivity, such as TV watching.
    a. If upper extremities are mostly affected, suggest walking or riding a stationary bike.
    b. If lower extremities are mostly affected, encourage use of a wheel chair to promote mobility, and performing simple crafts.

14. Help the patient investigate various methods of stress management to deal with frustration.

Family Education and Health Maintenance

1. Instruct the patient and family in range-of-motion exercises, pulmonary care, and methods of transfer and locomotion.

2. Stress the importance of maintaining fluid intake to decrease risk of urinary and pulmonary infections.

3. Advise the patient or family to report signs of respiratory infection immediately to obtain treatment and prevent congestive heart failure.

4. Encourage genetic counseling if indicated to determine options of family planning.

5. Refer the patient and family to agencies such as:

   The Muscular Dystrophy Association
   3300 East Sunrise Dr.
   Tucson, AZ 85718
   602-529-2000

M

Myasthenia Gravis

Myasthenia gravis is a neuromuscular disorder affecting impulse transmission in the voluntary muscles of the body. The cause is unknown, but it is thought to result from impairment or destruction of acetylcholine receptors at neuromuscular junctions by an autoimmune reaction. Muscle contraction is impaired, leading to muscle weakness.

Complications include *myasthenic crisis,* severe weakness and respiratory distress caused by deterioration of condition, emotional stress, upper respiratory infection, surgery, trauma, or as a result of adrenocorticotropic hormone (ACTH). A related emergency, *cholinergic crisis,* can result from overmedication with anticholinergic drugs, which release too much acetylcholine (ACh) at the neuromuscular junction. Presentation is similar to myasthenic crisis. *Brittle crisis* occurs when receptors at the neuromuscular junction become insensitive to anticholinergic medication.

◆ Assessment

1. Cranial nerve dysfunction:
   a. Visual disturbances: diplopia and ptosis from ocular weakness
   b. Masklike facial expression from involvement of facial muscles
   c. Dysarthria and dysphagia from weakness of laryngeal and pharyngeal muscles
2. Extreme muscular weakness and easy fatigability with repetitive activity and speech
3. Possible respiratory involvement with decreased vital capacity

◆ Diagnostic Evaluation

1. Serum test for ACh receptor antibodies, which is positive in up to 90% of patients
2. Tensilon test: IV injection temporarily improves motor response and relieves symptoms in myasthenic crisis; temporarily worsens symptoms in cholinergic crisis.

3. Electrophysiologic testing to show decremental response to repetitive nerve stimulation.
4. Computed tomography may show thymus hyperplasia, which is thought to initiate the autoimmune response.

◆ Collaborative Management

Therapeutic Interventions
1. In myasthenic or cholinergic crisis, maintain a patent airway and give oxygen and mechanical ventilation as indicated.
2. Plasmapheresis may be used to temporarily remove circulating ACh-receptor antibodies from the blood.

Pharmacologic Interventions
1. Anticholinergics such as neostigmine and pyridostigmine to enhance neuromuscular transmission. Neostigmine is given IV in myasthenic crisis.
2. Prednisone or azathioprine to suppress immune response.
3. Atropine is given IV in cholinergic crisis to reduce excessive ACh secretions.

Surgical Interventions
1. Thymectomy when thymoma or hyperplasia exist; may provide remission in some patients

◆ Nursing Interventions

Monitoring
1. Monitor the patient's respiratory status to watch for possible respiratory failure and myasthenic or cholinergic crisis.
2. Be alert for signs of an impending crisis:
   a. Sudden respiratory distress
   b. Signs of dysphagia, dysarthria, ptosis, and diplopia
   c. Tachycardia, anxiety
   d. Rapidly increasing weakness of extremities and trunk
3. Monitor the patient's response to drug therapy.

M

◆◆

NURSING ALERT

Many medications can accentuate the weakness experienced by the patient with myasthenia—including some antibiotics, antiarrhythmics, local and general anesthetics, muscle relaxants, and analgesics. Assess neurologic function after administering any new drug and report any changes in the patient's condition.

Supportive Care

1. Administer medications so that their peak effect coincides with meals or essential activities.
2. Help the patient develop a realistic activity schedule.
3. Allow for rest periods throughout the day to minimize fatigue.
4. Provide assistive devices to help patient perform activities of daily living (ADLs) despite weakness.
5. If the patient has diplopia, provide an eye patch to use on alternate eye to minimize risk of tripping and falling.
6. To avoid aspiration:
   a. Teach the patient to position the head in a slightly flexed position to protect the airway during eating.
   b. Have suction available that the patient can operate.
   c. If the patient is in crisis or has impaired swallowing, administer fluids IV and foods through nasogastric (NG) tube; elevate the head of bed after feeding.
   d. If the patient is on a mechanical ventilator, provide frequent suction, assess breath sounds, and check chest x-ray reports.
7. Show the patient how to cup chin in hands to support lower jaw to assist with speech.
8. If speech is severely affected, encourage the patient to use an alternate communication method such as flash cards or a letter board.

Patient Education and Health Maintenance

1. Instruct the patient and family regarding the symptoms of myasthenic crisis.
2. Teach the patient ways to prevent crisis and aggravation of symptoms.
   a. Avoid exposure to colds and other infections.
   b. Avoid excessive heat and cold.

M

  c. Tell the patient to inform the dentist of condition, because use of procaine (Novocaine) is not well tolerated and may provoke crisis.
  d. Avoid emotional upset.
3. Teach the patient and family regarding the use of home suction.
4. Review the peak times of medications and how to schedule activity for best results.
5. Stress the importance of scheduled rest periods, to avoid fatigue.
6. Encourage the patient to wear a medical alert bracelet.
7. Refer the patient and family to agencies such as:

The Myasthenia Gravis Foundation, Inc.
61 Grammercy Park North, Room 605
New York, NY 10010
212-533-7005

Myocardial Infarction

Myocardial infarction (MI) refers to a dynamic process by which one or more regions of the heart muscle experience a severe and prolonged decrease in oxygen supply because of insufficient coronary blood flow. The affected muscle tissue subsequently becomes necrotic. Onset of an MI may be sudden or gradual, and the process takes 3 to 6 hours to run its course.

Approximately 90% of MIs are precipitated by acute coronary thrombosis (partial or total) secondary to severe coronary artery disease (greater than 70% narrowing of the artery). Other causative factors include coronary artery spasm, coronary artery embolism, infectious diseases causing arterial inflammation, hypoxia, anemia, and severe exertion or stress on the heart in the presence of significant coronary artery disease (ie, surgical procedures or shoveling snow).

In MI, the heart muscle experiences different degrees of damage, for example, necrosis, injury, and ischemia. In the *zone of necrosis*, death of the heart muscle has occurred; in the *zone of injury*, the muscle is inflamed and injured but can still be kept viable; and in the *zone of ischemia*, the tissue is at risk if the infarction spreads.

M

589

MIs are classified according to the layers of the heart muscle involved. In a transmural (Q wave) infarction, necrosis occurs throughout the entire thickness of the heart muscle. In a subendocardial (nontransmural/non–Q wave) infarction, the necrotic area is confined to the innermost layer of the myocardium lining the chambers.

> **NURSING ALERT**
> Patients with subendocardial infarctions should be considered as having an uncompleted MI; monitor carefully for signs and symptoms of spreading heart muscle damage.

MIs are also classified by the location of damaged heart muscle within the left ventricle (most common): anterior, inferior, lateral, and posterior wall. When an MI occurs in the right ventricle, it is commonly associated with damage to the inferior or posterior wall of the left ventricle. The region of the heart muscle that sustains damage is determined by the specific coronary artery that becomes obstructed (Fig. 18).

◆ Assessment

1. Chest pain:
   a. *Character:* variable, but often diffuse, steady substernal chest pain. Other sensations include a crushing and squeezing feeling in the chest.
   b. *Severity:* pain may be severe; not relieved by rest or sublingual vasodilator therapy, requires narcotics
   c. *Location:* variable, but often pain resides behind upper or middle third of sternum
   d. *Radiation:* Pain may radiate to the arms (commonly the left), and to the shoulders, neck, back, or jaw.
   e. *Duration:* Pain continues for more than 15 minutes.
2. Associated manifestations include anxiety, diaphoresis, cool clammy skin, facial pallor, hypertension or hypotension, bradycardia or tachycardia, premature ventricular or atrial beats, palpitations, dyspnea, disorientation, confusion, restlessness, fainting, marked weakness, nausea, vomiting, hiccoughs.
3. Atypical symptoms of MI include epigastric or abdominal distress, dull aching or tingling sensations, shortness of breath, and extreme fatigue.

M

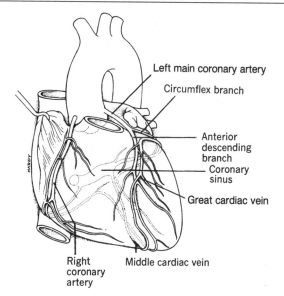

FIGURE 18 *Diagram of the coronary arteries arising from the aorta and encircling the heart. Some of the coronary veins also are shown.*

NURSING ALERT
Some patients are asymptomatic, particularly diabetics; these "silent myocardial infarctions" still cause damage to the heart.

GERONTOLOGIC ALERT
Elderly patients are more likely to experience silent MIs or have atypical symptoms: hypotension, low body temperature, vague complaints of discomfort, mild perspiration, strokelike symptoms, dizziness, change in sensorium.

M

4. Risk factors for MI: smoking, high blood cholesterol levels, and hypertension (these three increase chances

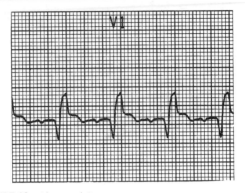

FIGURE 19 *Abnormal Q wave.*

of having another MI); family history of myocardial infarction, diabetes, obesity, stress, and lack of exercise

◆ Diagnostic Evaluation

1. Serial 12-lead electrocardiograms (ECGs) detect changes that usually occur within 2 to 12 hours, but may take 72 to 96 hours.
   a. ST segment depression and T wave inversion indicate a pattern of ischemia; ST elevation indicates an injury pattern.
   b. Q waves indicate tissue necrosis and are permanent (Fig. 19).

NURSING ALERT
A normal ECG does not rule out the possibility of infarction, because ECG changes can be subtle and obscured by underlying conditions (bundle branch blocks, electrolyte disturbances).

M

2. Serum cardiac enzymes including creatine kinase (CK), lactic dehydrogenase (LDH), and aspartate transaminase (AST) are taken every 6 to 24 hours. Isoenzymes CK-MB and LDH1 and LDH2 show characteristic elevation after MI.

3. White blood cell count and sedimentation rate may be elevated.
4. Radionuclide imaging, chest x-ray, and positron emission tomography may be done to evaluate heart muscle.

◆ Collaborative Management

Therapeutic Interventions

1. Oxygen via nasal cannula to improve oxygenation of ischemic heart muscle
2. Bed rest to reduce myocardial oxygen demands

Pharmacologic Interventions

1. Pain control drugs to reduce catecholamine-induced oxygen demand to injured heart muscle
   a. Opiate analgesics: morphine (to relieve pain, improve cardiac hemodynamics, and provide anxiety relief); meperidine (if allergic to morphine or sensitive to respiratory depression)
   b. Vasodilators: nitroglycerin (sublingual, IV, paste) (to promote venous [low-dose] and arterial [high-dose] relaxation as well as to relax coronary vessels and prevent coronary spasm; also to reduce myocardial oxygen demand with subsequent pain relief). Persistent chest pain requires IV nitroglycerin.
   c. Anxiolytics: benzodiazepines (used with analgesics when anxiety complicates chest pain and its relief).
2. Thrombolytic therapy by IV or intracoronary route, to dissolve thrombus formation and reduce the size of the infarction.
   a. Must be administered within 6 hours of the onset of chest pain to be effective, and they carry a risk of allergic reaction and bleeding
   b. Reperfusion dysrhythmias may follow successful therapy.
3. Anticoagulants, as adjunct to thrombolytic therapy
4. Beta-adrenergic blocking agents, to improve oxygen supply and demand, decrease sympathetic stimulation to the heart, promote blood flow in the small vessels of the heart, and provide antidysrhythmic effects
5. Antidysrhythmics such as lidocaine decrease ventricular irritability commonly occurring post-MI.
6. Calcium channel–blockers, to improve oxygen supply and demand.

M

Surgical Interventions

1. Percutaneous transluminal coronary angioplasty (PTCA) or coronary artery bypass graft (CABG) surgery (see p. 163) if revascularization of an evolving MI is deemed desirable.

◆ Nursing Interventions

Monitoring

1. Monitor continuous ECG to watch for life-threatening dysrhythmias (common within 24 hours after infarctions) and evolution of the MI (changes in ST segments and T waves). Be alert for any type of premature ventricular beats—these may herald ventricular fibrillation or ventricular tachycardia.
2. Monitor baseline vital signs before and 10 to 15 minutes after administering drugs; also monitor blood pressure continuously when giving nitroglycerin IV.
3. Observe for signs of anxiety.
4. Monitor blood pressure every 2 hours or as indicated.
5. Monitor respirations and auscultate lung fields every 2 to 4 hours or as indicated for crackles associated with left ventricular failure or pulmonary edema.

NURSING ALERT
Dyspnea, tachypnea, frothy pink sputum, and orthopnea may indicate left ventricular failure, or pulmonary edema. Auscultation of clear lungs in the presence of cool, clammy skin, jugular vein distension, and hypotension may indicate right ventricular infarction.

6. Evaluate heart rate and heart sounds every 2 to 4 hours or as directed. Auscultate heart for the presence of a third heart sound (failing ventricle), fourth heart sound (stiffening ventricular muscle due to MI), friction rub (pericarditis), murmurs (valvular and papillary muscle dysfunction), or intraventricular septal rupture.
7. Evaluate major arterial pulses (weak pulse or presence of pulsus alternans indicates decreased cardiac output; irregularity results from dysrhythmias).

8. Monitor body temperature every 4 hours or as directed (most patients with MI develop increased temperature within 24–48 hours because of tissue necrosis).
9. Monitor skin color and temperature (cool, clammy skin and pallor—associated with vasoconstriction secondary to decreased cardiac output).
10. Observe for changes in mental status such as confusion, restlessness, disorientation.
11. Evaluate urine output (30 mL/h)—decrease in volume reflects a decrease in renal blood flow.
12. Employ hemodynamic monitoring as indicated, including central venous pressure (CVP) monitoring, pulmonary artery (PA) and pulmonary capillary-wedge pressure (PCWP) monitoring, and arterial blood pressure monitoring.

Supportive Care

1. Handle the patient carefully while providing initial care, starting IV infusion, obtaining baseline vital signs, and attaching electrodes for continuous ECG monitoring.
2. Reassure the patient that pain relief is a priority and administer analgesics promptly. Place the patient in supine position during administration to minimize hypotension.

GERONTOLOGIC ALERT
Elderly patients are extremely susceptible to respiratory depression in response to narcotics. Substitute analgesic agents with less profound effects on the respiratory center. Anxiolytic agents also should be used with caution.

NURSING ALERT
Intravenous administration is the preferred route for analgesic medication, because intramuscular injections can cause elevations in serum enzymes, resulting in an incorrect diagnosis of myocardial infarction.

M

3. Emphasize importance of reporting any chest pain, discomfort, or epigastric distress without delay.

4. Explain equipment, procedures, and need for frequent assessment to the patient and significant others to reduce anxiety associated with hospital environment.

5. Offer back massage to promote relaxation, decrease muscle tension, and improve skin integrity.

6. Promote rest with early gradual increase in mobilization to prevent deconditioning, which occurs with bed rest.

    a. Minimize environmental noise, provide a comfortable environmental temperature, and avoid unnecessary interruptions and procedures.

    b. Promote restful diversional activities for the patient (reading, listening to music, drawing, crossword puzzles, crafts).

    c. Encourage frequent position changes while in bed.

    d. Assist the patient to rise slowly from a supine position to minimize orthostatic hypotension caused by some drugs.

    e. Encourage passive and active range-of-motion exercises as directed while on bed rest.

    f. Elevate the patient's feet on chair when out of bed to promote venous return.

7. Take measures to prevent bleeding if patient is receiving thrombolytic therapy.

    a. Take vital signs every 15 minutes during infusion of thrombolytic agent and then hourly.

    b. Observe for presence of hematomas or skin breakdown, especially in potential pressure areas such as the sacrum, back, elbows, ankles.

    c. Be alert to the patient's complaints of back pain, which may indicate retroperitoneal bleeding.

    d. Observe all puncture sites every 15 minutes during infusion of thrombolytic therapy and then hourly for bleeding.

    e. Apply manual pressure to venous or arterial sites if bleeding occurs. Use pressure dressings to cover all access sites.

    f. Observe for blood in stool, emesis, urine, and sputum.

    g. Minimize venipunctures and arterial punctures; use heparin lock for blood sampling and medication administration.

M

   h. Avoid intramuscular injections.

   i. Avoid use of automatic BP device above puncture sites or hematoma. Use care in taking BP; use arm not used for thrombolytic therapy.

   j. Caution the patient about vigorous tooth brushing, hair combing, or shaving.

   k. Monitor laboratory work: prothrombin time (PT), partial thromboplastin time (PTT), hematocrit (Hct), hemoglobin (Hgb), and check for current blood type and crossmatch.

   l. Administer antacids as directed to prevent stress ulcers.

8. Observe for persistence or recurrence of signs and symptoms of ischemia—chest pain, diaphoresis, hypotension—may indicate extension of MI or reocclusion of coronary vessel. Report these manifestations immediately.

9. Be alert to signs/symptoms of sleep deprivation—irritability, disorientation, hallucinations, diminished pain tolerance, aggressiveness.

10. Minimize possible adverse emotional response to transfer from the intensive care unit to the intermediate care unit. Introduce the admitting nurse from the intermediate care unit to the patient before transfer and inform the patient what to expect relative to physical layout of unit, nursing routines, and visiting hours.

Patient Education and Health Maintenance

1. Explain basic cardiac anatomy and physiology; identify the difference between angina and MI; and describe how the heart heals and that healing is not complete for 6 to 8 weeks after attack.

2. Emphasize the importance of rest and relaxation alternating with activity.

   a. Instruct the patient how to take pulse before and after starting activity, and to slow activity pace if sudden increase in heart rate occurs.

   b. Review signs/symptoms indicating a poor response to increased activity levels: chest pain, extreme fatigue, shortness of breath.

3. Reinforce cardiac rehabilitation program with guidelines such as 1) walk daily, gradually increasing dis-

M

tance and time as prescribed; 2) avoid activities that tense muscles, such as weight lifting, lifting heavy objects, isometric exercises, pushing or pulling heavy loads; 3) avoid working with arms overhead; 4) gradually return to work; 5) avoid extremes in temperature; 6) Do not rush; avoid tension.

4. Tell the patient that sexual relations may be resumed on advice of health care provider, usually after exercise tolerance is assessed. If the patient can walk briskly or climb two flights of stairs, sexual activity can usually be resumed with familiar partner. Advise the patient that sexual activity should be avoided after eating a heavy meal, after drinking alcohol, or when tired.

5. Advise the patient to get at least 7 hours of sleep each night and take 20- to 30-minute rest periods twice a day.

6. Advise eating three to four small meals per day rather than large heavy meals. Rest 1 hour after meals.

7. Advise limiting caffeine and alcohol intake.

8. Advise that driving a car must be cleared with health care provider at follow-up.

9. Teach the patient about medication regimen and side effects.

10. Instruct the patient to report the following symptoms: chest pressure or pain not relieved in 15 minutes by nitroglycerin or rest, shortness of breath, unusual fatigue, swelling of feet and ankles, fainting, dizziness, very slow or rapid heart beat.

11. Assist the patient to reduce risk of another MI by modifying risk factors (see CAD, p. 220).

12. For additional information and support, refer to:

> **American Heart Association**
> 7272 Greenville Ave.
> Dallas, TX 75231
> 214-373-6300

M

Myocarditis

Myocarditis is a focal or diffuse inflammation of the myocardium. It may be acute or chronic and can occur at any age. Myocarditis may be caused by viral infections (particularly Coxsackie group B viruses, as well as influenza A or B, and herpes simplex); infections by bacteria, fungi, parasites, protozoans, rickettsiae, and spirochetes; sarcoidosis and collagen vascular disorders; and chemotherapy (especially doxorubicin [Adriamycin]), or immunosuppressive therapy. Myocarditis may be self-limiting or progress to congestive heart failure or cardiomyopathy.

◆ Assessment

1. Fatigue, fever, dyspnea, palpitations, and occasional chest pains. Be aware that disease severity depends on the type of infection, degree of myocardial damage, recuperative capacity of the myocardium, and host resistance. In some cases, symptoms may be minor and go unnoticed.
2. History of recent episodes of infection, chronic disease, and drugs that are myocardial toxins such as doxorubicin
3. Third heart sound, a systolic murmur in the apical area, and possibly a pericardial friction rub, if pericarditis is also present
4. Signs of congestive heart failure such as pulsus alternans, dyspnea, and crackles

NURSING ALERT
Have equipment ready for resuscitation, cardiac defibrillation, and cardiac pacing if a life-threatening dysrhythmia occurs.

◆ Diagnostic Evaluation

1. 12-lead electrocardiogram (ECG) may show transient ECG changes including flattened ST segment, T wave inversion, conduction defects, extrasystoles, and supraventricular and ventricular ectopic beats.
2. Chest x-ray to evaluate for cardiomegaly of inflamed heart
3. White blood cell (WBC) count and sedimentation rate—elevated

M

4. Throat or stool cultures to isolate the offending bacteria or virus

◆ Collaborative Management

Pharmacologic Interventions

1. Antipyretics to reduce fever
2. Antidysrhythmic therapy (usually quinidine or procainamide)
3. Antimicrobial therapy if causative bacteria is isolated
4. Diuretics and digoxin to treat symptoms of CHF

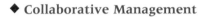

NURSING ALERT
Patients with myocarditis may be sensitive to digitalis—assess for toxic signs and symptoms such as anorexia, nausea, fatigue, weakness, yellow-green halos around visual images, prolonged PR interval.

◆ Nursing Interventions

Monitoring

1. Monitor body temperature every 4 hours.
2. Record daily intake and output, daily weights, and check for edema to monitor for congestive heart failure (CHF).
3. Maintain continuous ECG monitoring if dysrhythmia develops.
4. Evaluate for clinical evidence that disease is subsiding by monitoring pulse, auscultating heart for improvement in murmur, auscultating lung fields, and monitoring respirations.

Supportive Care

1. Ensure strict bed rest to reduce heart rate, stroke volume, blood pressure, and heart contractility; bed rest also helps to decrease residual damage and complications of myocarditis, and promotes healing. Advise patient that bed rest may be prolonged until heart size is reduced and cardiac function improves.
2. Elevate the head of the bed, if necessary, to enhance respiration.

3. Allow the patient to use a bedside commode rather than a bedpan, to reduce cardiovascular workload.
4. Provide diversional activities for the patient.

Family Education/Health Maintenance

1. Because some residual heart enlargement is usually present, advise the patient that physical activity may be *slowly* increased. Discuss with the patient activities that can be continued after discharge to avoid fatigue. The patient should begin with chair rest for increasing periods, followed by walking in the room, then outdoors for longer periods.
2. Tell the patient to immediately report any symptom in which the heart starts beating rapidly.
3. Advise the patient to avoid competitive sports, alcohol, and other myocardial toxins (such as doxorubicin).
4. Inform a female patient to avoid pregnancy if she has a cardiomyopathy.
5. Advise the patient to get appropriate immunizations to avoid infectious diseases.

Myxedema
See Hypothyroidism

Neck Dissection, Radical

Radical neck dissection involves surgical removal of all subcutaneous tissue from the ramus of the jaw down to the clavicle; from midline back to the angle of the jaw. In modified (functional) radical neck dissection, only the lymph nodes are removed. In some cases, part or all of the larynx may also be removed. The procedure is commonly followed by radiation therapy. Surgical reconstruction may be performed with a rotational flap, skin graft, or free flap to promote healing and improve aesthetics.

This surgery is indicated for head and neck cancers (mostly squamous cell carcinomas), including tumors of the upper respiratory and digestive tracts. Specific sites include the ear, nasopharynx, nose and paranasal sinuses, palate, oral cavity, larynx, hypopharynx, and thyroid gland. Local extension to adjacent muscle, bone, and vital structures often occurs before detection, and metastasis to cervical lymph nodes is common.

◆ Potential Complications

1. Salivary incontinence
2. Malocclusion
3. Unintelligible speech
4. Difficulty eating or swallowing
5. Unacceptable deformity

◆ Collaborative Management

Preoperative Care

1. Improve nutritional status preoperatively through the use of nutritional supplements, hyperalimentation, alcohol withdrawal, and counseling.
2. Assist with general health status evaluation and detection and treatment of underlying conditions such as cirrhosis or obstructive pulmonary or cardiovascular disease.
3. Assess level of understanding of disease process, treatment regimen, and follow-up care.
4. Provide intensive teaching and emotional preparation for major surgery, long rehabilitation, and change in body image.

Postoperative Care

1. Protect the airway and support respiration.
   a. After the patient has fully recovered from anesthesia, the endotracheal tube is removed (unless respiratory compromise occurs).

b. Place the patient in Fowler's position.

c. Observe for signs of respiratory difficulty such as dyspnea, cyanosis, stridor, hoarseness, or dysphagia.

d. Provide supplemental oxygen by face mask if necessary; if tracheostomy is present, provide oxygen by collar or T-piece to provide adequate humidification.

e. Auscultate for decreased breath sounds, crackles, wheezes; auscultate over the trachea in the immediate postoperative period to assess for stridor indicative of laryngeal edema.

f. Encourage deep breathing and coughing.

g. Assist the patient in assuming a sitting position to bring up secretions (support the patient's neck with the nurse's hands).

h. Suction secretions orally or aseptically by tracheostomy if patient is unable to cough them up.

2. Administer prophylactic antibiotics as directed to prevent infection because of extensive incision, lymph node resection, and close proximity to oral secretions.

3. Assess vital signs for indication of infection (increased heart rate, elevation of temperature).

4. Closely monitor wound for hemorrhage, drainage, or tracheal constriction; reinforce dressings as needed.

5. Inspect incision for signs of infection (redness, warmth, swelling, and drainage). Assure the incision site remains clean and dry; cleanse away secretions immediately.

6. If portable suction is used, expect approximately 80 to 120 mL serosanguineous secretions to be drawn off during the first postoperative day; this diminishes with each day. Aseptically cleanse skin area around drain exit, using saline or prescribed solution.

7. Provide IV fluids and hyperalimentation, tube feedings by nasogastric tube or gastrostomy tube, or oral feedings of pureed food as soon as swallowing is established. Continue until oral intake is adequate and nutritional status is improved.

8. Provide mouth care before and after meals.

9. Watch for excessive or decreased salivation.

10. Assure that emergency suctioning and airway equip-

N

ment is available at the bedside during meals in the event of choking or aspiration.

11. Position patient in an upright position for feeding, supporting shoulders and neck with pillows if necessary.

12. If tracheostomy or laryngectomy has been performed, provide alternative methods of communication (letter board, chalk and slate, paper and pencil). Difficulty writing may result from denervation of the trapezius muscle.

13. Allow adequate time for patient to communicate. Recognize that patient may have difficulty nodding "yes" or "no" because of neck dissection.

14. Observe for lower facial paralysis, because this may indicate facial nerve injury.

15. Watch for shoulder dysfunction, which may follow resection of spinal accessory nerves. Muscle exercises can improve range of motion.

16. Encourage the patient to verbalize concerns and feelings about body image and lifestyle changes in the areas of alcohol consumption and cigarette smoking.

◆ Patient Education and Health Maintenance

1. Advise the patient and family regarding exercises to prevent limited range of motion and discomfort.
   a. Instruct the patient to perform exercises morning and evening. At first exercises are done only once; then the number is increased by one each day until each exercise is done 10 times. The patient must relax after each exercise.
   b. For neck, gently rotate head to each side as far as possible; tilt head to the right side as far as possible, then the left; drop chin to chest and then raise chin as high as possible.
   c. For shoulder, place hand from unoperated side on chair for support and gradually swing arm on operated side up and back as far as tolerated. Each day, work toward finishing a complete circle.

2. Emphasize the need for frequent follow-up visits and completion of radiation therapy if prescribed.

N

3. If patient has a permanent tracheostomy or laryngectomy, instruct the patient and family regarding:
   a. Need for humidification
   b. Protection measures
   c. Activities to avoid that may cause aspiration
   d. Referral for speech–language pathologist, social worker to meet ongoing communication needs

Nephrolithiasis and Urolithiasis

Nephrolithiasis refers to the presence of stones, or calculi, in the renal pelvis, and *urolithiasis* refers to their presence in the urinary system. Stones are formed by crystallization of urinary solutes (calcium oxalate, uric acid, calcium phosphate, struvite, and cystine). They vary in size from granular ("sand or gravel") deposits to orange-sized bladder stones. In 80% of patients with urolithiasis, gravel stones pass spontaneously. Men are affected more frequently than women, and recurrences are possible.

Causes and predisposing factors include hypercalcemia and hypercalciuria caused by hyperparathyroidism; renal tubular acidosis; multiple myeloma; excessive intake of vitamin D, milk, and alkali; chronic dehydration, poor fluid intake, and prolonged immobility; abnormal purine metabolism (hyperuricemia and gout); genetic disorders (cystinuria); chronic infection with urea-splitting bacteria *(Proteus vulgaris)*; chronic obstruction by foreign bodies in the urinary tract; and excessive oxalate absorption in inflammatory bowel disease, bowel resection, or ileostomy. Complications include obstruction, infection, and impaired renal function.

◆ Assessment

1. Pain pattern (referred to as colic) depends on site of obstruction (Fig. 20).
2. Chills, fever, dysuria, frequency, and hematuria may occur if infection is present.
3. Nausea, vomiting, diarrhea, and general abdominal discomfort may occur.

N

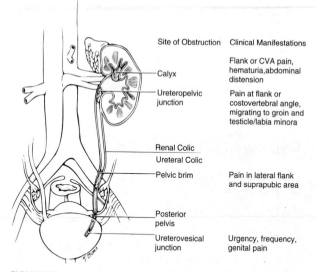

Site of Obstruction	Clinical Manifestations
Calyx	Flank or CVA pain, hematuria, abdominal distension
Ureteropelvic junction	Pain at flank or costovertebral angle, migrating to groin and testicle/labia minora
Renal Colic	
Ureteral Colic	
Pelvic brim	Pain in lateral flank and suprapubic area
Posterior pelvis	
Ureterovesical junction	Urgency, frequency, genital pain

FIGURE 20. *Areas where calculi may obstruct the urinary system. The ensuing clinical manifestations depend on the site of obstruction. Stones that have broken loose may obstruct the flow of urine, cause severe pain, and injure the kidney.*

◆ Diagnostic Evaluation

1. Intravenous pyelography (IVP), to locate stone(s) and evaluate degree of obstruction
2. Retrograde or antegrade pyelography may be necessary when stones are radiolucent.
3. Laboratory analyses of passed or retrieved stone material to identify type of stone
4. Urinalysis may show hematuria and pyuria; culture and sensitivity studies to identify infective organisms

◆ Collaborative Management

Therapeutic and Pharmacologic Interventions

1. Because most stones are passed spontaneously, conservative therapy aims to facilitate this process.

a. Hydration to maintain high urinary volume
b. Straining of urine and observation
c. Dietary measures designed to reduce urinary solutes
d. Pain management

2. *Extracorporeal shock wave lithotripsy (ESWL)*, in which high-energy shock waves are directed at the kidney stone, disintegrating it into minute particles that pass in the urine
   a. Treatment of choice for stones smaller than 2 cm ($\frac{3}{4}$ inch) in diameter (80% of stones fall into this category)
   b. Eliminates need for surgery in most patients and can be repeated for recurrent stones with no apparent risk to kidney structure or function

Surgical Interventions

1. *Percutaneous nephrolithotomy (PCNL)*, in which stones are broken apart with hydraulic shock waves or a laser beam administered by nephroscope; fragments are removed using forceps, graspers, or basket
   a. May be combined with ESWL
   b. Used for stones larger than 2.5 cm in diameter

2. *Percutaneous stone dissolution (chemolysis)*, in which a solvent is infused into the stone through a nephrostomy tube placed in the kidney. Used to dissolve struvite, uric acid, and cystine stones

3. *Ureteroscopy*, in which stones are either removed by ureteroscope with basket or grasper, or are fragmented with electrohydraulic, ultrasonic, or laser equipment
   a. Used for distal ureteral calculi; may be used for mid-ureteral calculi
   b. Stent may be inserted to maintain patency of ureter.

4. Open surgical procedures are indicated for only 1% to 2% of all stones. Procedures include *pyelolithotomy, nephrolithotomy, nephrectomy, ureterolithotomy,* and *cystolithotomy*. See p. 514.

◆ Nursing Interventions

Monitoring

1. Monitor for complications of procedures for stone removal, including renal infection, hemorrhage, extrav-

N

asation of urine, obstruction from remaining stone fragments.

2. Monitor response to analgesics; large doses of narcotics are often necessary so monitor for respiratory depression and decrease in blood pressure.

3. Monitor urine output and patterns of voiding. Report oliguria or anuria.

4. Monitor for fever and foul-smelling urine, indicating infection.

Supportive Care

1. Encourage the patient to assume position of comfort.

2. Administer antiemetics (via intramuscular [IM] or rectal suppository) as indicated for nausea.

3. Encourage oral fluid intake if able, or give IV (if vomiting) to ensure adequate urine output.

4. Strain all urine through strainer or gauze to harvest the stone; uric acid stones may crumble. Crush clots and inspect sides of urinal/bedpan for clinging stones or fragments.

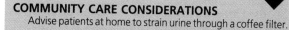

COMMUNITY CARE CONSIDERATIONS
Advise patients at home to strain urine through a coffee filter.

5. Assist the patient to walk, if possible, because ambulation may help move the stone through the urinary tract.

Patient Education and Heath Maintenance

To aid postoperative or postprocedure recovery:

1. Encourage fluids to accelerate passing of stone particles.

2. Teach about analgesics, which still may be necessary for colicky pain that may accompany passage of stone debris.

3. Warn that some blood may appear in urine for up to several weeks.

4. Encourage frequent walking to assist in passage of stone fragments.

To prevent recurrent stone formation:

1. Instruct on dietary requirements related to specific stone type: avoid excessive calcium and phosphorus

for calcium oxalate stones; reduced purines (red meat, fish, and fowl) for uric acid stones

2. Encourage compliance with prescribed drug therapy such as thiazide diuretics to reduce urine calcium excretion, allopurinol to reduce uric acid formation, d-penicillamine to lower cystine concentration, and sodium bicarbonate to alkalinize urine.

3. Teach patients with uric acid or cystine stones how to monitor urine pH with a test strip for alkalinity.

4. Teach patients with struvite stones to recognize and report signs and symptoms of urinary infection and seek prompt treatment.

5. Encourage weight-bearing activity and avoidance of prolonged bed rest, which alters calcium metabolism.

6. Advise all patients with stone disease to drink enough fluids to achieve a urinary volume of 2,000 mL to 3,000 mL or more every 24 hours.

Nephrotic Syndrome

Nephrotic syndrome is a clinical disorder of unknown cause characterized by proteinuria, hypoalbuminemia, edema, and hyperlipidemia. These conditions result from excessive leakage of plasma proteins into the urine because of impairment of the glomerular capillary membrane. Nephrotic syndrome is seen in chronic glomerulonephritis, diabetes mellitus with intercapillary glomerulosclerosis, renal amyloidosis, systemic lupus erythematosus, renal vein thrombosis, and is secondary to malignancy in older adults. Precipitating events in children may be upper respiratory infection or immunization. Nephrotic syndrome is mild in 80% of children affected. The loss of proteins, particularly immunoglobulins, predisposes young patients to infection. Other complications include thromboembolism, altered drug metabolism caused by decreased plasma proteins, and progression to end-stage renal disease.

N

◆ Assessment

1. Insidious onset of pitting edema and weight gain
2. Decreased urine output

3. Irritability, fatigue, anorexia, nausea and vomiting
4. Wasting of skeletal muscles

◆ Diagnostic Evaluation

1. Urinalysis:
   a. Protein: 2+ or greater
   b. Casts: numerous
   c. Blood: absent or transient
   d. Note "foamy" appearance of urine.
2. Elevated 24-hour urine for protein; may be normal creatinine clearance
3. Serum chemistry:
   a. Total protein and albumin reduced
   b. Cholesterol and triglycerides elevated
4. Needle biopsy of kidney may be necessary to confirm diagnosis.

◆ Collaborative Management

Therapeutic Interventions
1. Treat causative glomerular disease
2. Restrict sodium and fluids to control edema
3. Give dietary protein supplements
4. Paracentesis for severe ascites

Pharmacologic Interventions
1. Corticosteroids or immunosuppressant agents to decrease proteinuria
2. Diuretics to control edema if renal insufficiency is not severe
3. Infusion of salt-poor albumin to raise oncotic pressure and shift fluid from interstitial to intravascular space

◆ Nursing Interventions

Monitoring

1. Monitor edema, daily weights, urine specific gravity, and intake and output to gauge severity of condition.
2. Monitor central venous pressure (if indicated), vital signs, and orthostatic blood pressure and heart rate measurements to detect hypovolemia.
3. Monitor serum blood urea nitrogen (BUN) and creatinine to assess renal function.

4. Monitor for signs and symptoms of infection secondary to loss of immunoglobulins and therapy with immunosuppressants.

NURSING ALERT

No immunizations should be given during active nephrosis or while child is receiving immunosuppressant therapy because response will be muted.

5. Monitor temperature and laboratory values for neutropenia.
6. Monitor the patient's response to drug therapy; drug metabolism may be altered because of reduced plasma proteins.

Supportive Care

1. Encourage bed rest for a few days to help mobilize edema; however, some ambulation is necessary to reduce risk of thromboembolic complications.
2. Enforce mild to moderate sodium and fluid restriction if edema is severe; offer small amounts of fluid in appropriate-size cup at regular intervals.
3. Use aseptic technique for all invasive procedures and strict handwashing by the patient and all contacts; prevent patient contact with persons who may transmit infection.
4. Handle edematous extremities carefully, encourage change of position frequently, and inspect skin for breakdown caused by pressure of the edema.
5. Encourage high-protein, high-carbohydrate diet according to patient's interest.
6. Suggest quiet diversion activities during periods of bed rest.

Family Education and Health Maintenance

1. Teach the patient signs and symptoms of nephrotic syndrome; also review causes, purpose of prescribed treatments, and importance of long-term therapy to prevent end-stage renal disease.
2. Instruct patient and family in side effects of prescribed medications and methods of preventing infection if on immunosuppressant.

N

3. Carefully review with patient and family dietary and fluid restrictions; consult dietitian for assistance in meal planning.
4. Discuss the importance of maintaining exercise, decreasing cholesterol and fat intake, and changing other risk factors such as smoking, obesity, and stress to reduce risk of atherosclerosis and severe thromboembolic complications.
5. Encourage extended follow-up to ensure resolution of proteinuria.

Neuroblastoma

Neuroblastoma is a malignant tumor that arises from embryonic cells along the craniospinal axis of the sympathetic nervous system. Neuroblastoma is the most common extracranial solid tumor of childhood, occurring in approximately 1 per 100,000 children, mostly infants and young children. The tumor may spread to the liver, soft tissue, bones, and bone marrow. The overall survival rate is approximately 30% to 35%, with almost all recurrences or deaths occurring within the first 2 years after diagnosis. In some cases, neuroblastoma may undergo spontaneous remission.

◆ Assessment

1. Symptoms depend on the location of the tumor and the stage of the disease.
2. Most tumors are located within the abdomen and present as firm, nontender, irregular masses that cross the midline.
3. Other common signs include:
   a. Bowel or bladder dysfunction resulting from compression by a paraspinal or pelvic tumor
   b. Neurologic symptoms caused by compression by the tumor on nerve roots or because of tumor extension
   c. Supraorbital ecchymoses, periorbital edema, and exophthalmos resulting from metastases to the skull bones and retrobulbar soft tissue

N

    d. Lymphadenopathy, especially in the cervical area
    e. Bone pain and joint swelling with skeletal involvement
    f. Swelling of the neck or face, and cough with thoracic masses
    g. Pallor, anorexia, weight loss, and weakness with widespread metastasis

◆ Diagnostic Evaluation

1. Workup done to document the extent of the disease throughout the body includes: chest and skeletal x-rays, bone scan, bone marrow aspiration and possible biopsy, complete blood count, platelet count, ferritin level, 24-hour urine collection to detect elevated excretion of homovanillic acid and vanillylmandelic acid, liver and kidney function tests.
2. Additional studies may include:
    a. Computed tomography scan of primary site and chest
    b. Ultrasound examination
    c. Liver/spleen scan
3. N-*myc* oncogene blood screening—multiple copies associated with a poor prognosis
4. Tumors are staged primarily on the basis of the extent of disease.
    a. Evans staging system: stage I (tumor is confined to the organ or structure of origin) to stage IV (there is remote disease involving the skeleton, parenchymal organs, soft tissue, distant lymph nodes, or bone marrow)
    b. Pediatric oncology group staging: stages A to D; examine regional lymph nodes for presence of disease

◆ Collaborative Management

Pharmacologic Interventions

1. Chemotherapy drugs of choice include vincristine, dacarbazine, cyclophosphamide, doxorubicin, cisplatin, carboplatinum, and ifosphamide.
2. Neuroblastoma is one of few childhood tumors that has not responded dramatically to modern antitumor therapy. The use of newer chemotherapy drugs and

N

other techniques, such as immunotherapy and bone marrow transplantation, may improve survival rates for these children.

Surgical Interventions

1. Surgery is both diagnostic and therapeutic. Either primary (before chemotherapy or radiation) or delayed/secondary (after therapy).
2. When complete surgical resection of a stage I tumor is possible, this may be the only treatment required.
3. Children with other than stage I disease generally receive a combination of surgery, radiation therapy, and chemotherapy.

◆ Nursing Interventions

Monitoring

1. Observe the surgical incision for erythema, drainage, or separation of the incision. Report any of these changes.
2. Monitor and report any elevated temperature or sign of infection.
3. If the child is receiving chemotherapy or radiation, monitor for side effects, hydration status, and nutritional status.

Supportive Care

1. Encourage the parents to ask questions and to understand fully the risks and benefits of surgery.
2. Prepare the child for surgery; explain procedures at the appropriate developmental level.
3. Continue supporting the parents during the postoperative period. They may be frightened and upset by the appearance of their child.
4. Explain why fatigue and shortness of breath may occur.
5. Plan frequent rest periods between daily activities.
6. Caution the child about physical overexertion; encourage rest frequently and warn child to expect a tired feeling.
7. Assess normal elimination patterns the child had before the illness began.
8. Keep careful intake and output records.

N

9. Assess for urinary overflow incontinence and loss of bowel function, depending on the age of the child.
10. Administer pain control medications as ordered in the immediate postoperative period.
11. Encourage the child to express feelings regarding the threat to body image resulting from chemotherapy.
12. Reassure the child that he or she will be able to wear a wig or a hat after recovery; hair will grow back from chemotherapy.

Family Education and Health Maintenance

1. Teach parents about the laboratory tests and x-rays needed at diagnosis and periodically throughout therapy.
2. Instruct parents about chemotherapy medications used and their potential side effects.
3. Inform parents about potential treatment methods, such as radiation therapy and bone marrow transplantation.
4. Advise parents to use good handwashing and preventing exposure to children with communicable diseases.

Obesity

Obesity is an overabundance of body fat resulting in body weight 20% more than the average weight for the person's age, height, sex, and body frame. The root cause is unknown, but a wide variety of predisposing factors have been identified. These include heredity, environment (eg, socioeconomic status), psychological factors (eg, depression, anxiety), age (puberty, old age), and, rarely, endocrine abnormalities (eg, Cushing's syndrome, hypothyroidism, hypogonadism, or hypothalamic lesions). Obes-

O

ity may progress to serious complications such as diabetes mellitus or cardiovascular disease, and it is a risk factor in gallbladder disease, osteoarthritis, and high blood pressure.

◆ Assessment and Diagnostic Evaluation

1. Nutritional assessment to evaluate dietary habits and calorie intake
2. Anthropometric assessment, including height, weight, triceps skinfold measurement, and mid–upper arm circumference, to evaluate body mass and fat
3. Complete physical examination to determine effect of obesity on body
4. Selected hormonal studies (thyroid, adrenal) to look for underlying cause

◆ Collaborative Management

Therapeutic Interventions

1. Diet therapy is instituted to eliminate 1,000 calories per day to lose 1 kg (2.2 lbs) of body weight per week.
   a. A 1,200-calorie diet for women and a 1,500-calorie diet for men (adjusted to the patient's size and activity level) are basic to diet management.
   b. Fats should compose no more than 30% of all calories, proteins approximately 20% to 25%, with carbohydrates constituting the remainder. Nutrient supplements may be necessary (iron, vitamin B6, zinc, and folate).
   c. Vitamin and mineral deficiencies may result from a severely restricted diet. A very-low-calorie diet (800–1,000 calories per day) requires careful monitoring and use of vitamin and mineral supplements.
2. Daily exercise, such as walking or other aerobic activity for approximately 30 minutes a day
3. Behavior modification to reinforce diet program
   a. Use food diary to identify and eliminate situations or cues leading to overeating or high-calorie foods.
   b. Provide positive reinforcement of proper diet habits.
   c. Stress reduction techniques such as visual imagery

O

or progressive relaxation and peer support may be helpful.

Pharmacologic Interventions

1. Appetite suppressants are being used for some patients unable to achieve satisfactory weight loss with diet and exercise. Serotonin modulators are proving successful.
2. Controversy exists on length of therapy. Most anorectants are recommended for short-term use to avoid tolerance and abuse potential; however, weight is usually regained after discontinuation.

Surgical Interventions

1. Generally reserved for morbidly obese patients unable to lose weight through nonsurgical therapies
   a. Gastroplasty (gastric stapling) is the current procedure of choice. Most common procedure is vertical banding involving creation of a 30-mL pouch along the lesser gastric curvature with a small outlet.
   b. Gastric (jejunoileal) bypass creates distal and proximal stomach pouches with horizontal stapling; distal jejunum is attached to proximal pouch, bypassing distal stomach pouch. This procedure creates vitamin and mineral deficiency (malabsorption syndrome).

◆ Nursing Interventions

Monitoring

1. Monitor dietary intake for calorie count and essential nutrients.
2. Postoperatively, monitor vital signs and surgical wound for signs of wound infection and dehiscence.

Supportive Care

1. Assist the patient in assessing current dietary habits and identifying poor dietary habits.
2. Assist the patient in developing appropriate diet plan based on likes and dislikes, activity level, and lifestyle.
3. Suggest behavior modification strategies such as shortening lunch break, preventing access to quick snacks, and eating only at mealtimes at the table.
4. Provide emotional support to the patient during weight

O

reduction efforts through positive reinforcement and creative problem solving.

5. Provide the patient with alternative coping mechanisms, including stress reduction techniques such as progressive relaxation and guided imagery.

6. Assess the patient's ability to tolerate exercise through measurement of vital signs before, during, and after exercise and asking about symptoms of shortness of breath and chest pain.

7. Provide postoperative care.
   a. Observe for and report increased pain and distension, which may indicate leakage at staple sites or obstruction.
   b. When bowel sounds return, give oral fluids to prevent dehydration.
   c. If fluids are tolerated, begin six small feedings for a total of 600 to 800 calories per day.
   d. Watch for and report signs of dehydration (thirst, oliguria, dry mucous membranes) and hypokalemia (muscle weakness, anorexia, nausea, decreased bowel sounds, and dysrhythmias).
   e. Warn patients that overeating will cause vomiting and painful esophageal distension.

Patient Education and Health Maintenance

1. Explain the purpose of a balanced diet based on the food pyramid (Fig. 21) and the need for vitamins and minerals.

2. Review the health hazards of obesity and the danger of regaining weight if good diet and exercise habits are not maintained.

3. Advise the patient of plateau period without weight loss for some time that may occur, but not to get discouraged.

4. Tell the patient to keep a food diary to show to nutritionist and to weigh self no more than once a week.

5. Refer to agencies such as:

> **TOPS (Take Off Pounds Sensibly)**
> P.O. Box 07360
> 4575 South Fifth St.
> Milwaukee, WI 53207
> 414-482-4620

O

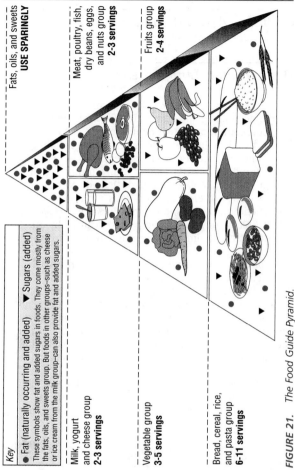

Key

● Fat (naturally occurring and added)   ▼ Sugars (added)

These symbols show fat and added sugars in foods. They come mostly from the fats, oils, and sweets group. But foods in other groups—such as cheese or ice cream from the milk group—can also provide fat and added sugars.

Fats, oils, and sweets
USE SPARINGLY

Meat, poultry, fish,
dry beans, eggs,
and nuts group
2-3 servings

Fruits group
2-4 servings

Milk, yogurt
and cheese group
2-3 servings

Vegetable group
3-5 servings

Bread, cereal, rice,
and pasta group
6-11 servings

FIGURE 21.   The Food Guide Pyramid.

O

Occlusive Arterial Disease
See Arterial Occlusive Disease

Occupational Lung Diseases

Occupational lung diseases result from long-term exposure to organic or inorganic (mineral) dusts and noxious gases. The most common occupational lung diseases include *silicosis,* a chronic pulmonary fibrosis caused by inhaling silica dusts encountered in mining, ceramic, abrasive, and foundry industries; *asbestosis,* a diffuse interstitial fibrosis caused by inhaling asbestos dust and particles from products encountered in numerous manufacturing and construction industries; and *coal worker's pneumoconiosis* (CWP, "black lung"), a tissue reaction caused by inhaling coal dust (also kaolin, mica, or silica) from mining industries.

In silicosis, fibrotic nodular lesions cause restrictive and obstructive lung disease. In asbestosis, the alveoli are gradually obliterated by fibrous tissue and fibrous pleural thickening, and plaque formation occurs, which leads to restrictive lung disease and eventual pulmonary heart disease (cor pulmonale). In CWP, the bronchioles and alveoli become clogged by coal macules (coal dust, macrophages, and fibroblasts), which leads to focal or centrilobular emphysema.

Occupational lung diseases usually develop slowly (over 20–30 years) and are asymptomatic in the early stages. Complications include respiratory failure and lung cancer.

NURSING ALERT
Asbestosis is strongly associated with bronchogenic cancer and with mesotheliomas of the pleura and peritoneal surfaces. Smoking increases the risk of lung cancer 50 to 100 times.

◆ Assessment

1. Characteristic symptoms include cough (chronic in asbestosis, productive in silicosis and CWP); dyspnea on

O

exertion (progressive and irreversible in asbestosis and CWP); and expectoration of varying amounts of black fluid in CWP.

2. Auscultation of breath sounds shows bibasilar crackles with asbestosis.

◆ Diagnostic Evaluation

1. Chest x-ray may show nodules of upper lobes in silicosis and CWP and diffuse parenchymal fibrosis, especially of lower lobes, in asbestosis.
2. Pulmonary function tests primarily show a pattern of restrictive lung disease with possibly some obstructive component.
3. Bronchoscopy (with lavage) helps identify the specific exposure.
4. CT, sputum examination, lung biopsy, and tuberculin testing may be done to rule out other disorders.

Therapeutic Interventions

1. Be aware that there is no specific treatment; the exposure agent is eliminated, and the patient is treated symptomatically.
2. Home oxygen therapy may be required.

Pharmacologic Interventions

1. Isoniazid (INH) is given prophylactically to a patient with positive tuberculin test, because silicosis is associated with high risk of tuberculosis.
2. Bronchodilators are given if any degree of airway obstruction is present.

◆ Nursing Interventions

Monitoring

1. Monitor for changes in baseline respiratory function.
2. Monitor changes in sputum quantity and quality.
3. If the patient has asbestosis, watch for signs and symptoms of lung cancer, such as changing cough, hemoptysis, weight loss.

Supportive Care

1. Encourage smoking cessation, especially in patients who have been exposed to asbestos fibers, to decrease risk of lung cancer.

O

2. Encourage hydration and breathing and coughing exercises to mobilize secretions.
3. Advise the patient to pace activities to prevent exertion.

Patient Education and Health Maintenance

1. Teach patient how to use bronchodilating inhalers or nebulizers.
2. Instruct the patient in methods of health maintenance, such as adequate nutrition and exercise, to avoid additional medical problems.
3. Advise the patient that compensation may be obtained for impairment related to occupational lung disease through the Workman's Compensation Act.
4. Provide information to healthy workers on preventing occupational lung disease, such as enclosing toxic substances to minimize their release into the air; using engineering controls to reduce exposure; monitoring air samples; ensuring adequate ventilation to reduce dust levels in the work atmosphere; and using protective devices such as face masks, respirators, fume hoods, etc.

Oral Cancer
See Cancer, Oral

Orthopedic Surgery

Orthopedic surgery includes a wide variety of procedures performed on bones, joints, and surrounding structures for trauma, musculoskeletal, and systemic disorders. Procedures include:

1. Open reduction: reduction and alignment of the fracture through surgical incision
2. Internal fixation: stabilization of the reduced fracture by use of metal screw, plates, nails, or pins
3. Bone graft: placement of autologous or homologous bone tissue to replace, promote healing of, or stabilize diseased bone

4. Arthroplasty: repair of a joint; may be done through arthroscope (arthroscopy) or open joint repair
5. Joint replacement: type of arthroplasty that involves replacement of joint surface(s) with metal or plastic materials
6. Total joint replacement: replacement of both articulatory surfaces within a joint
7. Meniscectomy: excision of damaged meniscus (fibrocartilage) of the knee
8. Tendon transfer: movement of tendon insertion point to improve function
9. Fasciotomy: cutting muscle fascia to relieve constriction or contracture
10. Amputation: removal of a body part

◆ Potential Complications

1. Compartment syndrome
2. Shock
3. Atelectasis and pneumonia
4. Osteomyelitis, wound infections
5. Thromboembolism
6. Fat embolus

◆ Collaborative Management

Preoperative Care

1. Assess nutritional status; hydration, protein and caloric intake. Maximize healing and reduce risk of complications by providing IV fluids, vitamins, and nutritional supplements as indicated.

GERONTOLOGIC ALERT
Many elderly are at risk for poor healing because of undernutrition.

2. Determine if person has had previous corticosteroid therapy—could contribute to current orthopedic condition (aseptic necrosis of the femoral head; osteopo-

O

rosis), as well as affect the patient's response to anesthesia and the stress of surgery. May need adrenocorticotropic hormone (ACTH) postoperatively.

3. Determine if the person has an infection (cold, dental, skin, urinary tract infection); could contribute to development of osteomyelitis after surgery. Administer preoperative antibiotics as ordered.

4. Prepare patient for postoperative routines: coughing and deep breathing, frequent vital sign and wound checks, repositioning.

5. Have the patient practice voiding in bedpan or urinal in recumbent position before surgery. This helps reduce the need for postoperative catheterization.

6. Acquaint the patient with traction apparatus and the need for splint, cast, as indicated by type of surgery.

Postoperative Care

1. Monitor for hemorrhage and shock, which may result from significant bleeding and poor hemostasis of muscles that occurs with orthopedic surgery.
   a. Evaluate the blood pressure and pulse rates frequently—report rising pulse rate or slowly decreasing blood pressure.
   b. Watch for increased oozing of wounds.
   c. Measure suction drainage if used. Anticipate up to 200 to 500 mL drainage in the first 24 hours, decreasing to less than 30 mL per 8 hours within 48 hours, depending on surgical procedure.
   d. Report increased wound drainage or steady increase in pain of operative area.

2. Administer IV fluids or blood products as ordered.

3. Monitor neurovascular status.
   a. Watch circulation distal to the part where cast, bandage, or splint has been applied.
   b. Prevent constriction leading to interference with blood or nerve supply.
   c. Watch toes and fingers for healthy color and good capillary refill.
   d. Check pulses of affected extremity; compare with unaffected extremity.
   e. Note skin temperature.

O

NURSING ALERT

If neurovascular problems are identified, notify surgeon and loosen cast or dressing at once.

4. Elevate affected extremity and apply ice packs as directed to reduce swelling and bleeding into tissues.
5. Immobilize the affected area and limit activity to protect the operative site and stabilize musculoskeletal structures.
6. Avoid or give respiratory depressant drugs in minimal doses. Monitor respiration depth and rate frequently. Narcotic analgesic effects may be cumulative.
7. Change position and encourage use of incentive spirometer and coughing and deep-breathing exercises every 2 hours to mobilize secretions and prevent atelectasis. Auscultate lungs frequently.
8. Monitor vital signs for fever, tachycardia, or increased respiratory rate, which may indicate infection.
   a. Examine incision for redness, increased temperature, swelling, and induration.
   b. Note character of drainage.
9. Maintain aseptic technique for dressing changes and wound care.
10. Encourage the patient to move joints that are not fixed by traction or appliance through their range of motion as fully as possible. Suggest muscle-setting exercises (quadriceps setting) if active motion is contraindicated.
11. Apply antiembolism stockings and give prophylactic anticoagulants, if prescribed, to prevent thromboembolism.
12. Encourage early resumption of activity.
13. Monitor for anemia, especially after fracture of long bones.
14. Avoid giving large amounts of milk to orthopedic patients on bed rest and encourage other fluids to prevent urinary calculi.

O

◆ **Family Education and Health Maintenance**

1. Instruct the patient in dietary considerations to facilitate healing and minimize development of constipation and renal calculi.
   a. Encourage high-iron diet.
   b. Ensure adequate protein and vitamin C.
   c. Ensure balanced diet with increase fluids and fiber.
2. Inform the patient of techniques that facilitate moving while minimizing associated discomforts (eg, supporting injured area and practicing smooth, gentle position changes).
3. Encourage long-term follow-up and physical therapy exercises as prescribed to regain maximum functional potential.

Osteoarthritis

Osteoarthritis (OA), or degenerative joint disease (DJD), is a chronic, noninflammatory, progressive disorder that causes deterioration of articular cartilage, ulceration and inflammation of joints, and formation of abnormal bone spurs caused by hypertrophy of subchondral bone. Osteoarthritis affects weight-bearing joints (hips and knees) as well as joints of the distal and proximal interphalangeal joints of the fingers. The cause is unknown, but aging and obesity are contributing factors; the disease generally affects adults aged 50 to 90 years, occurring equally in both sexes. Untreated disease leads to limited mobility and, in some cases, neurologic deficits associated with spinal involvement.

◆ **Assessment**

1. Deep, aching joint pain; pronounced after weight bearing or exercise, usually relieved at rest
2. Joint swelling or deformity
3. Joint stiffness on awakening, usually lasting less than 30 minutes
4. Hard nodes on distal or proximal interphalangeal joints

O

of the fingers; known as Heberden's nodes when present on distal interphalangeal (DIP) joints and Bouchard's nodes when present on proximal interphalangeal (PIP) joints

◆ Diagnostic Evaluation

1. X-rays of affected joints show joint space narrowing, osteophytes (bone spurs), and sclerosis.
2. Radionuclide imaging (bone scan) may show increased uptake in affected bones.
3. Synovial fluid analysis will differentiate osteoarthritis from rheumatoid arthritis.

◆ Collaborative Management

Therapeutic Interventions

1. Conservative management includes physical therapy, isometric exercises, and graded exercises; diet to control weight if indicated; application of heat; use of splints, traction, other means of support as needed.
2. Patient education on joint conservation techniques to stop the progression of degeneration

Pharmacologic Interventions

1. Analgesics, including acetaminophen, nonsteroidal antiinflammatory drugs (NSAIDs), and narcotics, as indicated

Surgical Interventions

1. Surgical intervention is considered when the pain becomes intolerable to the patient, and mobility is severely compromised. Options include osteotomy, debridement, joint fusion, arthroscopy, and arthroplasty.

◆ Nursing Interventions

Monitoring

1. Monitor mobility and functional capacity to perform activities of daily living.
2. Monitor the patient's response to pain medications.
3. Monitor for adverse effects to NSAIDs such as renal impairment and GI bleeding.

GERONTOLOGIC ALERT

Elderly patients are at greater risk for GI bleeding associated with NSAID use. Encourage administration with meals and monitor stool for occult blood.

Supportive Care

1. Provide rest for involved joints. Excessive use aggravates the symptoms and accelerates degeneration.
   a. Use splints, braces, cervical collars, traction, lumbosacral corsets as necessary.
   b. Have prescribed rest periods in recumbent position.
2. Advise the patient to avoid activities that precipitate pain.
3. Apply heat as prescribed to relieve muscle spasm and stiffness; avoid prolonged application of heat, which may cause increased swelling and flare symptoms.
4. Teach correct posture and body mechanics. Postural alterations lead to chronic muscle tension and pain.
5. Advise sleeping with a rolled terrycloth towel under the neck, to relieve cervical pain.
6. Provide crutches, braces, or cane when indicated to reduce weight-bearing stress on hips and knees. Teach use of cane in hand on side opposite involved hip or knee.
7. Encourage wearing corrective shoes and metatarsal supports for foot disorders; also to help in treating arthritis of the knee.
8. Encourage weight loss to decrease stress on weight-bearing joints.
9. Support the patient undergoing orthopedic surgery for unremitting pain and disabling arthritis of joints. See p. 622.
10. Teach range-of-motion exercises to maintain joint mobility and muscle tone for joint support, to prevent capsular and tendon tightening, and to prevent deformities. Avoid flexion and adduction deformities by prolonged sitting.
11. Refer to physical and occupational therapy.

O

Patient Education and Health Maintenance

1. Teach isometric exercises and graded exercises to improve muscle strength around the involved joint.
2. Advise putting joints through range of motion after periods of inactivity (eg, automobile ride).
3. Suggest performing important activities in morning, after stiffness has been abated and before fatigue and pain become a problem.
4. Advise on modifications, such as wearing looser clothing without buttons, placing bench in tub or shower for bathing, sitting at table or counter in kitchen to prepare meals.
5. Help with obtaining assistive devices, such as padded handles for utensils and grooming aids, to promote independence.
6. Suggest swimming or water aerobics (eg, offered by the YMCA) as a form of nonstressful exercise to preserve mobility.
7. Encourage adequate diet and sleep to enhance general health.
8. Refer for additional information and support to local chapter of The Arthritis Foundation.

Osteomyelitis

Osteomyelitis is an infection of the bone. It results from hematogenous spread (through the bloodstream) of infection to an area of bone with lowered resistance, or by direct extension from a soft tissue infection or open wound. It may occur at any age. The most common causative organisms include *Staphylococcus aureus* (70%–80%), *Escherichia coli, Pseudomonas, Klebsiella, Salmonella,* and *Proteus.* In acute osteomyelitis, the organisms grow and form pus within the bone, accompanied by edema, vascular congestion, thrombosis, and necrosis. The infection spreads into the medullary cavity and into adjacent soft tissue and joints. If an abscess forms, the area must be completely drained and excised for complete healing to take place. If treatment is unsuccessful, recurrent abscesses develop in chronic osteomyelitis. Other complications include pathologic fracture, joint destruction, skeletal deformities, and unequal limb length. Osteomyelitis may be life threatening if unrecognized and untreated.

◆ Assessment

1. Localized pain
2. Swelling, erythema
3. Elevated temperature
   (Note: Above signs may be masked in early disease)
4. Malaise, irritability
5. Generalized signs of sepsis

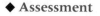

NURSING ALERT
Those at risk for osteomyelitis include the elderly, obese, poorly nourished, diabetics, those with rheumatoid arthritis, and those on long-term corticosteroid therapy.

◆ Diagnostic Evaluation

1. Blood cultures obtained before initiation of antibiotic therapy to identify causative agent
2. Needle aspiration of bone may be done if necessary to help identify causative agent. (Negative aspirate does not always rule out infection.)
3. CBC shows marked leukocytosis, low hemoglobin.
4. Erythrocyte sedimentation rate (ESR) is elevated.
5. X-ray may be negative in early stages.
   a. Rules out fracture
   b. Will eventually show periosteal elevation
6. Bone scan to rule out multiple lesions
7. MRI to differentiate soft tissue from bone marrow involvement

◆ Collaborative Management

Therapeutic Interventions
1. Immobilization of affected bone by traction or plaster cast

Pharmacologic Interventions
1. Broad-spectrum antibiotics until organism sensitivity obtained

O

2. IV antibiotics for 4 to 8 weeks
3. Additional 4 to 8 weeks of oral antibiotics at completion of IV therapy is recommended.

Surgical Interventions

1. Surgical incision and drainage if infection site is abscessed.
2. Chronic disease requires surgical removal of sequestra (dead bone).

◆ Nursing Interventions

Supportive Care

1. Maintain rest and immobilization of affected part.
2. Administer analgesics as indicated.
3. Increase fluid intake to prevent dehydration.
4. Monitor temperature and administer antipyretics as indicated.
5. Inspect and cleanse surgical wounds every 4 to 8 hours. Use strict aseptic technique.
6. Instruct patient and family in proper care of surgical wounds.
7. Teach proper IV catheter and site care.
8. Instruct on allowable activities: generally no weight bearing on affected limb and bed rest during acute phase.
9. Encourage use or exercise of unaffected limbs and joints.
10. Initiate appropriate home care referrals for reinforcement and monitoring of IV therapy.

Family Education and Health Maintenance

1. Teach the patient and family to recognize and report signs and symptoms of recurrent or chronic infection.
2. Stress the importance of compliance with treatment. Reinforce the need for maintaining serum levels of antibiotics after discharge even after signs and symptoms improve.
3. Encourage long-term follow-up to prevent recurrent abscesses.
4. Encourage early medical intervention of subsequent infections.

O

Osteoporosis

Osteoporosis is a condition in which the rate of bone resorption increases over the rate of bone formation, causing loss of calcium and phosphate salts and bone mass. Loss of bone mass and structure weakens the bones and makes them more susceptible to fractures. The disease occurs frequently in postmenopausal women, especially whites and Asians. Other risk factors include prolonged inactivity, chronic illness, medications such as corticosteroids, calcium and vitamin D deficiency, smoking, caffeine intake, and genetic predisposition.

◆ Assessment

1. Asymptomatic until later stages
2. Fracture after minor trauma may be first indication.
3. Most frequent fractures associated with osteoporosis include fractures of the distal radius, vertebral bodies, proximal humerus, pelvis, and proximal femur (hip).
4. May have vague complaints related to aging process (stiffness, pain, weakness)

◆ Diagnostic Evaluation

1. X-rays show changes only after 30% to 60% bone loss.
2. Studies that show decreased density of bone include CT, dual-photon absorptiometry, and dual-energy x-ray absorptiometry (DEXA).
3. Serum bone gla-protein (a marker for bone turnover) is elevated.
4. Bone biopsy shows thin, porous bone structure.

◆ Collaborative Management

Therapeutic Interventions

1. Management is primarily preventive.
2. Prevention of falls in the elderly to prevent fractures
3. Weight-bearing exercise (walking) throughout life
4. Adequate intake of vitamin D through milk, exposure to sunlight, and dietary supplements to enhance absorption of calcium
5. Intake of calcium (1–1.5 g/day) may be preventive.

O

Pharmacologic Interventions

1. Calcium supplements
2. Use of estrogen replacement therapy for postmenopausal women, which is viewed as more effective than calcium supplements. Ideally start within 5 years of menopause before osteoporosis is established, but may be of benefit in late stages as well.
3. Other agents such as 25-hydroxyvitamin D, calcitonin, flouride, biphosphonates, and thiazide diuretics may have some benefit.
   a. Calcitonin-salmon is available as a nasal spray or IM or subcutaneous injection.
   b. Alendronate sodium, a biphosphonate, has recently been shown to increase bone density and reduce fracture risk.

◆ Nursing Interventions

Supportive Care

1. Administer analgesics as indicated for acute exacerbations of pain.

GERONTOLOGIC ALERT
Prolonged use of narcotics in the elderly is especially dangerous because of impairment of mental status and may contribute to falls and other accidents.

---

2. Assist with putting on back brace and ensure proper fit. Encourage use as much as possible, especially while ambulatory.
3. Encourage compliance with physical therapy and practicing of exercises to increase muscle strength surrounding bones and to relieve pain.
4. Ensure safety measures to prevent falls.

Patient Education and Health Maintenance

1. Encourage exercise for all patients. Teach the value of walking daily throughout life to provide stress required for strong bone remodeling.
2. Explain that calcium can be obtained through milk and dairy products, vegetables, and supplements. Advise

O

that anyone with a history of urinary tract stones should consult with health care provider before increasing calcium intake.

3. Encourage young women at risk to maximize bone mass through nutrition and exercise.

4. Suggest that perimenopausal women confer with the doctor concerning need for calcium supplements and estrogen therapy.

5. Teach strategies to prevent falls. Assess home for hazards (eg, scatter rugs, slippery floors, extension cords, inadequate lighting). Encourage use of walking aids when balance is poor and muscle strength weakens.

COMMUNITY CARE CONSIDERATIONS

Identify women at high risk for osteoporotic fractures in the community—frail, elderly white or Asian women with poor dietary intake of dairy products and little exposure to sun—and provide education and safety measures to prevent falls and fractures.

Otitis Externa

Otitis externa (swimmer's ear) is an inflammation of the external ear canal that may occur 2 to 3 days after swimming and diving, especially in contaminated water. Infection may be caused by bacteria, usually *Pseudomonas, Proteus vulgaris,* streptococci, and *Staphylococcus aureus,* or fungi, such as *Aspergillus niger* or *Candida albicans.* Predisposing factors include seborrhea, psoriasis, stagnant water in the ear canal, and trauma to the canal from cleaning ears with blunt objects.

◆ Assessment

1. Pain may be mild to severe, increased by jaw movement or manipulation of auricle or tragus or may be pulsating ache.

2. Ear canal may be red and swollen and have foul-smelling, white, or purulent discharge. Fungal infection may produce blackish deposits.

3. Fever and periauricular lymphadenopathy may be present.

O

◆ Diagnostic Evaluation

1. Otoscopic evaluation may be difficult because of pain and swelling but shows characteristic swelling and exudate.
2. Culture and sensitivity tests may be done but are usually not necessary.

◆ Collaborative Management

Therapeutic and Pharmacologic Interventions

1. Apply warm compresses and give analgesics for pain.
2. Topical antibiotics or acetic acid (modifies pH) solution are used to treat infection.
3. Topical corticosteroids may be used to decrease inflammation and swelling.
4. If acute inflammation and closure of the ear canal prevent drops from saturating canal, a wick may need to be inserted so that drops will penetrate to walls of entire ear canal. Irrigation may be necessary to clear drainage when acute swelling subsides.
5. Burow's solution (aluminum acetate solution) reduces drainage caused by eczema.
6. Alcohol may be used as a drying agent to prevent recurrences.

◆ Nursing Interventions

Supportive Care

1. Provide comfort measures such as warm compresses and frequent cleansing of drainage from around ear canal to relieve irritation.
2. Demonstrate proper application of eardrops:
    a. Lie or sit with head tilted to side and affected ear up.
    b. Pull auricle upward and outward (for adults) or downward and backward (for children) and instill four drops or amount prescribed.
    c. Maintain position for 5 minutes to ensure proper saturation.
    d. Do not put cotton in ear, because cotton will soak up drops and impair contact with canal.

3. Advise the patient that external otitis can be prevented or minimized by thoroughly drying the ear canal after coming into contact with water or moist environment.

Family Education and Health Maintenance

1. Tell the patient and family to use eardrops after swimming to help prevent swimmer's ear.
2. Advise the use of properly fitting ear plugs for recurrent cases.
3. Teach proper ear hygiene: clean auricle and outer canal with washcloth only, do not insert anything smaller than finger wrapped in washcloth in ear canal.

COMMUNITY CARE CONSIDERATIONS

Use of cotton-tipped applicators to dry the canal or remove earwax should be avoided because:
a. Cerumen may be forced against the tympanic membrane.
b. The canal lining may be abraded, making it more susceptible to infection.
c. Cerumen that coats and protects the canal may be removed.

Otitis Media, Acute and Chronic

Otitis media is an inflammation and infection of the middle ear caused by a dysfunctional eustachian tube. In suppurative otitis media, infection usually results from bacterial infection by *Streptococcus pneumoniae, Haemophilus influenzae, Branhamella catarrhalis,* and *Staphylococcus aureus.* In serous (secretory) otitis media, no purulent infection occurs, but blockage of the eustachian tube causes negative pressure and transudation of fluid from blood vessels and development of effusion in the middle ear. Chronic secretory disease may lead to conductive hearing loss.

Acute otitis media, with its rapid onset of signs and symptoms, is a major problem in children but may occur at any age. If not treated successfully, or if the causative organism is resistant to drugs, it can progress to chronic otitis media and possibly mastoiditis, in which the accumulation of pus under pressure in the middle ear cavity

O

causes tissue necrosis and extension of infection into the mastoid cells.

If advanced chronic ear disease is left untreated, inner ear and life-threatening CNS complications may develop because of erosion of surrounding structures.

◆ Assessment

1. In acute disease, pain is usually the first symptom; in chronic disease, may be painless or dull ache and tenderness of mastoid.
2. Fever may reach 40° to 40.6°C (104°–105°F).
3. Postauricular erythema and edema in chronic disease
4. Purulent drainage (otorrhea) is present if tympanic membrane is perforated; may be odorless or foul-smelling.
5. Pain and tenderness of mastoid process occurs in mastoiditis.

PEDIATRIC ALERT
In infants and young children, look for irritability, difficult feeding or anorexia, nausea, and vomiting, indicating otitis media.

◆ Diagnostic Evaluation

1. Pneumatic otoscopic examination shows a tympanic membrane that is full, bulging, and opaque with impaired mobility (or retracted with impaired mobility).
2. Specimens of ear discharge (from ruptured tympanic membrane) for cultures to help identify causative organism
3. Audiometry may be ordered to evaluate conductive hearing loss in chronic disease.
4. X-ray of mastoid area may show mastoid pathologic condition, for example, cholesteatoma (soft ball of dead skin cells that erodes surrounding vital structures) or haziness of mastoid cells.

O

◆ Collaborative Management

Pharmacologic Interventions

1. In acute disease, oral antibiotics are given, including broad-spectrum penicillins, cephalosporins, and sulfa preparations.
2. In chronic disease, antibiotic and corticosteroid eardrops may control infection and inflammation, but once mastoiditis develops, parenteral antibiotic therapy is necessary.
3. Nasal decongestants and antihistamines help promote eustachian tube drainage.
4. Frequent removal of epithelial debris and purulent drainage in chronic disease may protect tissue from damage.

Surgical Interventions

1. In acute otitis media, myringotomy (incision in tympanic membrane to relieve pressure and drain pus from middle ear) may be done for antimicrobial failure, for severe, persistent pain, or for persistent conductive hearing loss.
2. In children with middle ear effusions lasting 3 months or longer, myringotomy with ventilating tube placement may be done.
3. In chronic otitis media, mastoidectomy may be done for cholesteatoma, or serious signs that may signal progression to meningitis or brain abscess (pain, profound deafness, dizziness, sudden facial paralysis, or stiff neck).
   a. Simple mastoidectomy: removal of diseased bone and insertion of a drain
   b. Radical mastoidectomy: remnants of the tympanic membrane, and malleus and incus are also removed
   c. Posteroanterior mastoidectomy: simple mastoidectomy combined with tympanoplasty (reconstruction of middle ear structures)

◆ Nursing Interventions

Monitoring

1. Monitor for headache, increasing irritability, fever, stiff neck, nausea, and vomiting, which indicate meningeal involvement.

2. After mastoidectomy, monitor for facial nerve paralysis, bleeding, and local infection.
3. Monitor hearing status regularly.
4. Check for speech and language delays in young children at regular intervals, caused by hearing impairment.

Supportive Care

1. Administer or teach self-administration of aspirin and other analgesics as prescribed. Sedation is usually avoided because it may interfere with early detection of CNS complications.
2. Encourage use of warm compresses to promote comfort and help resolve infectious process.
3. Perform and teach postoperative dressing changes because area is packed with gauze for drainage—this may be done daily or every other day; packing is removed on third or fourth day.
4. Warn the patient that transient vertigo and nausea may be present after radical mastoidectomy. Ensure safety measures.

Family Education and Health Maintenance

1. Instruct the patient on activities that are to be avoided after tympanic membrane rupture or surgery until healing takes place (swimming, shampooing hair, showering).
2. Advise the patient of hygienic practices that will prevent tympanic membrane injury (avoid ear-picking, inserting objects into ear).
3. Advise reporting of symptoms that indicate recurrence (discomfort, pain, fever, dizziness).
4. Teach patients with serous otitis to take decongestants as directed and to perform Valsalva maneuver several times per day to help open the eustachian tube.
5. Advise elevation of head at night to promote drainage of middle ear into pharynx.
6. Postoperatively, teach dressing changes and compliance with antibiotic therapy as ordered.
7. Stress the importance of follow-up hearing evaluations.
   a. If stapes has been removed or dislodged, then hearing is lost.

  b. If stapes or cochlea has not been removed or disturbed, then hearing will probably be regained; a hearing aid may be required.
8. Advise parents that episodes of otitis may be minimized by breast-feeding, bottle-feeding in upright position, using specially designed bottles to allow upright feeding, and eliminating identified allergens such as milk products, mold, and dust.
9. Advise parents of children with ventilating tubes that water should not enter ear canal, ear drops should not be instilled into that ear, and tubes will come out spontaneously in 6 to 12 months.

Ovarian Cancer
See Cancer, Ovarian

Ovarian Cysts

Ovarian cysts are benign growths that arise from various ovarian tissues. They often arise from functional changes in the ovary, as from the graafian follicle or from persistent corpus luteum; dermoid ovarian cysts may develop from abnormal embryonic epithelium. Incidence is highest during childbearing years. Masses found in women older than age 50 years are more likely to become malignant. Ruptured cysts may cause peritoneal inflammation.

◆ Assessment

1. Cysts may be asymptomatic or cause minor pelvic pain.
2. Menstrual irregularity may be noted.
3. Tender, palpable mass may be palpated.
4. Rupture causes acute pain and tenderness and may mimic appendicitis or ectopic pregnancy.

◆ Diagnostic Evaluation

1. Pelvic sonogram to determine cyst size and characteristics

2. Pregnancy test as directed to rule out ectopic pregnancy
3. Suspicious cysts may be examined through biopsy at time of surgery.

◆ Collaborative Management

Pharmacologic Interventions

1. Oral contraceptives for 1 to 3 months to suppress functional cysts smaller than 5 cm in diameter.

Surgical Interventions

1. Laparoscopy or laparotomy to remove large or leaking cysts.

◆ Nursing Interventions

Monitoring

1. Postoperatively, monitor vital signs frequently.
2. Assess frequently for abdominal distension caused by fluid and gas pooling in abdominal cavity.
3. Assess for effectiveness of pain management and return of bowel sounds.

Supportive Care

1. Encourage the use of analgesics as prescribed.
2. Teach the patient the proper use of oral contraceptives if prescribed, along with side effects; encourage monthly follow-up to determine if cyst is resolving.
3. Tell the patient that heavy lifting, strenuous exercise, and sexual intercourse may increase pain.
4. Encourage deep breathing and coughing postoperatively
5. Administer antiemetics and insert a nasogastric tube as ordered to prevent vomiting.
6. Place the patient in semi-Fowler's position for greatest comfort and encourage early ambulation after surgery to reduce distension. Help the patient arise slowly to prevent orthostatic hypotension.
7. As distension resolves and bowel sounds return, advance oral intake slowly.

Patient Education and Health Maintenance

1. Reassure the patient that, in most cases, ovarian function and fertility are preserved.

O

P

2. Reassure the patient about low malignancy rate of cysts.
3. Encourage the patient to report recurrent symptoms or worsening of pain if cyst is being treated medically.

Pancreatic Cancer
See Cancer, Pancreatic

Pancreatitis

Acute *pancreatitis* refers to inflammation of the pancreas, which is most commonly caused by alcoholism and biliary tract diseases such as cholelithiasis and cholecystitis. Other causes include infections, trauma, pancreatic tumors, and use of certain drugs (corticosteroids, thiazide diuretics, and oral contraceptives). Attacks may resolve with complete recovery, may recur without permanent damage, or may progress to chronic pancreatitis. Mortality is high (10%) because of shock, anoxia, hypotension, or fluid and electrolyte imbalances.

Chronic pancreatitis (Box 5) results in destruction of the secreting cells of the pancreas, causing maldigestion and malabsorption of protein and fat, and possibly diabetes mellitus if islet cells have been affected. As cells are replaced by fibrous tissue, the pancreatic and common bile ducts may be obstructed.

◆ Assessment

1. Abdominal pain, usually constant in nature, midepigastric or periumbilical, radiating to the back or flank

■ BOX 5 CHRONIC PANCREATITIS

In chronic pancreatitis, pain is similar to that of acute pancreatitis, but it is more constant and occurs at unpredictable intervals. As the disease progresses, recurring attacks of pain are more severe, more frequent, and of longer duration. As pancreatic cells are destroyed, malabsorption and steatorrhea occur, along with diabetes mellitus.

Treatment involves chronic pain management, pancreatic enzyme replacement, and insulin treatment for hyperglycemia. Surgery may be necessary to reduce pain, restore drainage of pancreatic secretions, correct structural abnormalities, and manage complications. Pancreaticojejunostomy is the side-to-side anastomosis of pancreatic duct to jejunum to drain pancreatic secretions into jejunum. Other procedures include revision of sphincter of ampulla of Vater, drainage of pancreatic cyst into stomach, resection or removal of pancreas (pancreatectomy), and autotransplantation of islet cells.

Nursing interventions involve assessing and assisting in pain management; assessing and assisting in nutritional management; teaching low concentrated carbohydrate diet and insulin therapy; and assessment of gastrointestinal symptoms and characteristics of stool to guide pancreatic enzyme replacement. After surgery, provide meticulous care to prevent infection, promote wound healing, and prevent routine complications of surgery. Support total abstinence from alcohol to control symptoms and prevent progression.

❖

NURSING ALERT
Warn the patient that a dangerous hypoglycemic reaction may result from use of insulin while still drinking and skipping meals.

2. Nausea and vomiting, diarrhea, and passage of stools containing fat
3. Low-grade fever
4. Involuntary abdominal guarding, epigastric tenderness to deep palpation, and reduced or absent bowel sounds
5. Dry mucous membranes, hypotension, cold, clammy skin, cyanosis, and tachycardia, which may reflect mild to moderate dehydration from vomiting or capillary leak syndrome (third space loss)
6. Shock may be the presenting manifestation in severe episodes, along with respiratory distress and acute renal failure.
7. Purplish discoloration of the flanks (Turner-Grey sign) or of the periumbilical area (Cullen's sign) occurs in extensive hemorrhagic necrosis

◆ Diagnostic Evaluation

1. Serum amylase, lipase, glucose, bilirubin, alkaline phosphatase, serum transaminases, potassium, and cholesterol—may be elevated
2. Serum albumin, calcium, sodium, magnesium, and possibly potassium—low because of dehydration, vomiting, and the binding of calcium in areas of fat necrosis
3. Abdominal x-rays—to show pancreatic calcification, or peripancreatic gas pattern of a pancreatic abscess
4. Chest x-ray—to detect infiltrate or pleural effusion as a complication
5. Ultrasonography and CT to identify pancreatic structural changes such as calcifications, masses, ductal irregularities, enlargement, and cysts

◆ Collaborative Management

Therapeutic Interventions

1. Oxygen therapy to maintain adequate oxygenation, which is reduced by pain, anxiety, acidosis, abdominal pressure, or pleural effusions
2. Withhold oral feedings to decrease pancreatic secretions.
3. Nasogastric intubation and suction to relieve gastric stasis, distention, and ileus

4. IV crystalloid or colloid solutions or blood products to restore circulating blood volume
5. Parenteral nutrition to treat malnutrition

Pharmacologic Interventions

1. Narcotic analgesics to alleviate pain and anxiety, which increases pancreatic secretions
2. Histamine 2 (H_2) antagonists and antacids to suppress acid drive of pancreatic secretions and prevent stress ulcer complications of acute disease.
3. Sodium bicarbonate to reverse metabolic acidosis
4. Regular insulin to treat hyperglycemia
5. Antibiotics to treat infection or sepsis

Surgical Interventions

1. Surgery is indicated if complications occur. Care is similar to that for the patient undergoing abdominal surgery (see p. 350).
2. Incision and drainage of infection and pseudocysts
3. Debridement or pancreatectomy to remove necrotic pancreatic tissue
4. Cholecystectomy for gallstone pancreatitis

◆ Nursing Interventions

Monitoring

1. When giving narcotic analgesics, monitor for hypotension and respiratory depression.
2. Monitor and record vital signs, skin color and temperature, and intake and output, including nasogastric drainage.
3. Assess respiratory rate and rhythm, effort, oxygen saturation, and breath sounds frequently.

GERONTOLOGIC ALERT
The incidence of severe, systemic complications of pancreatitis increases with age. Monitor kidney function and respiratory status closely in elderly patients.

Supportive Care

1. Keep the patient NPO (nothing by mouth) to decrease pancreatic enzyme secretion; administer adequate replacement IV fluids.

P

2. Provide frequent oral care.
3. Administer antacids followed by clamping of nasogastric tube. Check pH of gastric aspirate periodically.
4. Report any increase in severity of pain, which may indicate pancreatic hemorrhage, rupture of a pseudocyst, or inadequate analgesic dosage.
5. Evaluate laboratory results for hemoglobin, hematocrit, albumin, calcium, potassium, sodium, and magnesium levels and administer replacements as prescribed.
6. Position the patient in upright or semi-Fowler's position to enhance diaphragmatic excursion.
7. Administer oxygen supplementation as prescribed to maintain adequate oxygen levels.
8. Instruct the patient in coughing and deep breathing to improve respiratory function.

Patient Education and Health Maintenance
1. Instruct the patient to gradually resume a low-fat diet.
2. Instruct the patient to increase activity gradually, providing for daily rest periods.
3. Reinforce information about the disease process and precipitating factors. Stress that subsequent bouts of acute pancreatitis destroy more and more of the pancreas and cause additional complications.
4. If the pancreatitis results from alcohol abuse, remind the patient of the importance of eliminating all alcohol; advise joining Alcoholics Anonymous or obtaining other substance abuse counseling.

Parkinson's Disease

Parkinson's disease is a progressive neurologic disease affecting the brain centers responsible for control and regulation of movement. A deficiency of dopamine in the substantia nigra produces the symptoms of parkinsonism. The cause is not known. Complications include dementia, aspiration, and injury from falls.

◆ Assessment

1. Characteristic resting tremor
2. Masklike facies, bradykinesia (slowness of movement), and muscle rigidity in performing all movements

3. Voice may be high-pitched, monotonal
4. Signs of autonomic dysfunction (sleeplessness, salivation, sweating, orthostatic hypotension)
5. Depression and dementia

◆ Diagnostic Evaluation

1. Diagnosis is based on observation of clinical symptoms and consideration of patient's age and history.
2. Computed tomography and magnetic resonance imaging may be performed to rule out other disorders.

◆ Collaborative Management

Pharmacologic Interventions

1. Anticholinergics to reduce activation of cholinergic pathways, which are thought to be overactive in dopamine deficiency
2. Amantadine, which may improve dopamine release in the brain
3. Levodopa–carbidopa to inhibit destruction of L-dopa in the bloodstream, making more available to the brain.
4. Bromocriptine, a dopaminergic agonist that activates dopamine receptors in the brain
5. Monoamine oxidase inhibitors (deprenyl, selegiline) as an adjunct to levodopa therapy

GERONTOLOGIC ALERT
Elderly patients may have reduced tolerance to antiparkinsonian drugs and may require smaller doses. Watch for and report psychiatric reactions such as anxiety and confusion; cardiac effects such as orthostatic hypotension and pulse irregularity; and blepharospasm (twitching of the eyelids), an early sign of toxicity.

◆ Nursing Interventions

Monitoring

1. Monitor drug treatment to note adverse reactions and allow for dosage adjustments. Monitor for diabetes, glaucoma, hepatotoxicity, and anemia during drug therapy.

P

2. Monitor the patient's nutritional intake and check weight regularly.
3. Monitor ability to perform activities of daily living.

Supportive Care

1. To improve mobility, encourage the patient in daily exercise such as walking, riding a stationary bike, swimming, or gardening.
2. Advise the patient to perform stretching and postural exercises as outlined by physical therapist.
3. Teach walking techniques to offset parkinsonian shuffling gait and tendency to lean forward.
4. Encourage the patient to take warm baths and massage muscles to help relax muscles.
5. Instruct the patient to rest often to avoid fatigue and frustration.

COMMUNITY CARE CONSIDERATIONS

Suggest a variety of aids around the house to promote the patient's mobility and to help avoid injury from falls, such as grab rails on the tub or shower, raised toilet seat, handrails on both sides of stairway, a rope secured to the foot of the bed to help pull up to sitting position, straight-backed wooden chair with armrests.

---

6. To improve the patient's nutritional status, teach the patient to think through the sequence of swallowing:
   a. Close lips with teeth together; lift tongue up with food on it; then back and swallow while tilting head forward.
   b. Chew deliberately and slowly, using both sides of mouth.
7. Urge the patient to make a conscious effort to control accumulation of saliva (drooling) by holding head upright and swallowing periodically. Be alert for aspiration hazard.
8. Have the patient use secure, stabilized dishes and eating utensils.
9. Suggest taking smaller meals and additional snacks.
10. To prevent constipation, encourage foods with mod-

erate fiber content (whole grains, fruits, and vegetables), and have the patient increase water intake.

11. Obtain a raised toilet seat to help the patient sit and stand.
12. Encourage the patient to follow regular bowel routine.
13. Maintain the patient's communication ability.
    a. Encourage compliance with medication regimen to help preserve speech function.
    b. Suggest referral to a speech therapist.
    c. Teach the patient facial exercises and breathing methods to obtain appropriate pronunciation, volume, and intonation.
14. Strengthen the patient's coping ability.
    a. Help the patient establish realistic goals and outline ways to achieve goals.
    b. Provide emotional support and encouragement.
    c. Encourage use of outside resources such as therapists, primary care provider, social worker, social support network.
    d. Encourage open communication, discussion of feelings, and exchange of information about Parkinson's disease.
    e. Have the patient take an active role in activity planning and evaluating the treatment plan.

Patient Education and Health Maintenance

1. Teach the patient about the medication regimen and about adverse reactions such as orthostatic hypotension, dry mouth, dystonia, muscle twitching, urinary retention, impaired glucose tolerance, anemia, and elevated liver function tests.
2. Instruct the patient to avoid sedatives, unless specifically prescribed, which have additive effects with other medications.
3. Instruct the patient to avoid vitamin B preparations and vitamin-fortified foods that can reverse effects of medication.
4. Encourage follow-up visits and monitoring for diabetes, glaucoma, hepatotoxicity, and anemia while on drug therapy.
5. Teach the patient ambulation cues to avoid "freezing" in place:

   a. Raise head, raise toes, then rock from one foot to another while bending knees slightly
   b. Or raise arms in a sudden short motion
   c. Or take a small step backward, then start forward
   d. Or step sideways, then start forward
6. Instruct the family not to pull the patient during such "freezing" episodes, which may cause falling.
7. Refer the patient to agencies such as:

United Parkinson's Foundation
866 West Washington Blvd.
Chicago, IL 60607
312-733-1893

Pelvic Inflammatory Disease

Pelvic inflammatory disease (PID) may involve the fallopian tubes, ovaries, uterus, or peritoneum. It is caused by infection with *Neisseria gonorrhoeae, Chlamydia trachomatis,* or *Mycoplasma hominis.* Predisposing factors include multiple sexual partners, early onset of sexual activity, use of intrauterine devices, and procedures such as therapeutic abortion, cesarean sections, and hysterosalpingograms. The disease has a high recurrence rate because of reinfections. Complications may include abscess rupture and sepsis; infertility caused by adhesions of fallopian tubes and ovaries; and ectopic pregnancy.

◆ Assessment

1. Pelvic pain is the most common presenting symptom; it is usually dull and bilateral.
2. Fever (especially with gonococcal infection), vaginal discharge, irregular bleeding, and urinary symptoms may be present.
3. On pelvic examination, mucopurulent cervical discharge and cervical motion tenderness may be present (especially with gonococcal infection).
4. Nausea and vomiting, abdominal tenderness, rebound, guarding, or presence of a mass may indicate abscess.

NURSING ALERT

Localized right or left lower quadrant tenderness with guarding, rebound, or palpable mass signifies tubo-ovarian abscess with peritoneal inflammation. Immediate evaluation and surgery are necessary to prevent rupture and widespread peritonitis.

5. Presentation with chlamydia may be mild.

◆ Diagnostic Evaluation

1. Smears for endocervical culture or immunodiagnostic testing to identify causative organisms
2. CBC—may show elevated leukocytes
3. Laparoscopy may be done to visualize the fallopian tubes.

◆ Collaborative Management

Pharmacologic Interventions

1. Oral or parenteral antibiotics: combinations of tetracyclines, penicillins, quinolones, and cephalosporins

COMMUNITY CARE CONSIDERATIONS

If patient with PID is to be treated at home, stress the importance of follow-up, usually within 48 hours, to determine if oral antibiotic treatment is effective. Advise the patient to report worsening symptoms immediately.

2. Inpatient treatment is required in uncertain diagnosis, abscess, pregnancy, severe infection, inability to take oral fluids, if the patient is prepubertal, or if more aggressive antibiotic therapy is required to preserve fertility.

Surgical Interventions

1. Surgery may be needed to drain an abscess, or later to treat adhesions or tubal damage.

P

◆ Nursing Interventions

Monitoring

1. Monitor vital signs and intake and output closely.
2. Monitor for abdominal rigidity and bowel sounds to detect development of peritoneal inflammation.
3. Monitor pain control.

Supportive Care

1. Administer or teach self-administration of analgesics as prescribed. Alert the patient to side effects or drowsiness.
2. Assist the patient to a position of pelvic dependence, with head and feet elevated slightly.
3. Encourage the patient to apply a heating pad to lower abdomen or lower back.
4. Advise the patient to rest in bed for first 1 to 3 days.
5. Administer or teach self-administration of antibiotics as prescribed. Advise the patient to keep strict dosage schedule and notify health care provider if a dose is lost through vomiting.
6. Administer antiemetics as indicated.
7. Maintain IV infusion of fluids until oral intake is adequate.
8. Restart oral intake with ice chips and sips of water after vomiting has ceased for 2 hours.
9. Provide clear fluids followed by soft bland diet as tolerated.

Patient Education and Health Maintenance

1. Encourage compliance with antibiotic therapy for full length of prescription.
2. Stress the need for sexual abstinence until repeat cultures prove cure at follow-up, approximately 2 weeks after treatment.
3. Tell the patient to advise partner(s) to seek treatment.
4. Teach the patient methods of preventing sexually transmitted diseases (STDs): abstinence, monogamy, proper condom use.

Peptic Ulcer Disease

A *peptic ulcer* is a lesion in the mucosa of the lower esophagus, stomach, pylorus, or duodenum (Fig. 22). This disor-

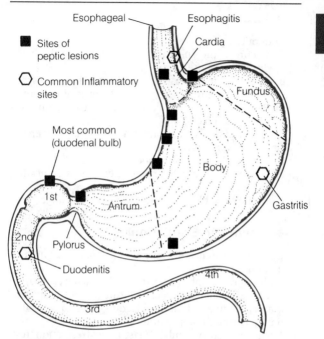

FIGURE 22 *The stomach is divided on the basis of its physiologic functions into two main portions. The proximal two thirds, the fundic gland area, acts as a receptacle for ingested food and secretes acid and pepsin. The distal third, the pyloric gland area, mixes and propels food into the duodenum and produces the hormone gastrin. "Peptic" lesions may occur in the esophagus (esophagitis), stomach (gastritis), or duodenum (duodenitis). Note peptic ulcer sites and common inflammatory sites.*

der is caused by mucosal infection by the bacterium *Helicobacter pylori* (mechanism unclear); use of nonsteroidal antiinflammatory drugs (NSAIDs), especially aspirin; hypersecretion of acid related to methylxanthines (tea, coffee, cola, and chocolate); Zollinger–Ellison syndrome (excessive secretion of gastrin); and genetic factors. Complications include gastrointestinal (GI) hemorrhage, perforation, and gastric outlet obstruction.

P

◆ Assessment

1. Abdominal pain
   a. Occurs in the epigastric area radiating to the back; described as dull, aching, gnawing
   b. Pain may increase when the stomach is empty, at night or approximately $\frac{1}{2}$ to 2 hours after eating. Pain is relieved by taking antacids (common with duodenal ulcers).
2. Nausea and anorexia (common with gastric ulcers)
3. Gastrointestinal bleeding
   a. Positive fecal occult blood
   b. Decreased hemoglobin and hematocrit indicating anemia
   c. Orthostatic blood pressure and pulse changes

◆ Diagnostic Evaluation

1. Upper GI series usually outlines ulcer or area of inflammation.
2. Endoscopy (esophago-gastroduodenoscopy, EGD) to visualize duodenal mucosa and help identify inflammatory changes, lesions, bleeding sites, and malignancy (through biopsy and cytology).
3. Gastric secretory studies (gastric acid secretion test, serum gastrin level test)—elevated in Zollinger–Ellison syndrome.
4. *H. pylori* antibody titer may be positive, especially in recurrent ulcers; however, there is a high rate of false positive results.

◆ Collaborative Management

Therapeutic Interventions

1. Diet therapy includes well-balanced diet high in fiber content; meals given at regular intervals; avoid caffeine, colas, and alcohol.
2. Avoid smoking, which decreases rate of healing and increases rate of recurrence.

Pharmacologic Interventions

1. Histamine (H_2)-receptor antagonists such as ranitidine to reduce gastric acid secretion

2. Antisecretory or proton-pump inhibitor such as ome-prazole to help ulcer heal quickly in 4 to 8 weeks
3. Cytoprotective drug sucralfate, which protects ulcer surface against acid, bile, and pepsin
4. Antacids to reduce acid concentration and help reduce symptoms
5. Antibiotics such as tetracycline and metronidazole may be given with bismuth subsalicylate as "triple therapy" to eradicate *H. pylori.*
6. For NSAID ulcers—discontinue NSAIDs and treat as mentioned above. If NSAID is restarted, administer with misoprostol, a prostaglandin analogue, antisecretory, and cytoprotective drug.

Surgical Interventions

1. Surgery is indicated in emergency situations for un-controlled bleeding or bleeding that developed in spite of chronic drug maintenance therapy Procedures in-clude:
   a. Gastrojejunostomy and vagotomy
   b. Antrectomy and vagotomy
   c. Subtotal gastrectomy
   d. Vagotomy and pyloroplasty
2. Vagotomy (severed vagus nerve) reduces acid secre-tion and movement of stomach.

◆ Nursing Interventions

Monitoring

1. Monitor for signs of bleeding through fecal occult blood, vomiting, persistent diarrhea, change in vital signs.
2. Monitor intake and output.
3. Monitor hemoglobin and hematocrit and electrolytes.

Supportive Care

1. Administer prescribed intravenous fluids and blood re-placement, if acute bleeding is present.
2. Maintain nasogastric tube for acute bleeding, perfora-tion, and postoperatively, and monitor tube drainage for amount and color.
3. Perform saline lavage if ordered for acute bleeding.
4. Encourage bed rest to reduce stimulation that may en-hance gastric secretion.

P

5. Provide small frequent meals to prevent gastric distension if not actively bleeding.
   a. Decreases distension and release of gastrin.
   b. Neutralizes gastric secretions and dilutes stomach contents. However, small frequent meals or snacks can lead to acid rebound, which occurs 2 to 4 hours after eating.
6. Watch for diarrhea caused by antacids and other medications. Restrict foods and fluids that promote diarrhea and encourage good perianal care.
7. Advise the patient to avoid extremely hot or cold food or fluids, to chew thoroughly, and to eat in a leisurely fashion to reduce pain.

Patient Education and Health Maintenance

1. Advise the patient to modify lifestyle to include health practices that will prevent recurrences of ulcer pain and bleeding.
   a. Plan for rest periods and avoid or learn to cope with stressful situations; avoid fatigue.
   b. Avoid specific foods known to cause gastric distress and pain.
   c. Avoid aspirin and NSAIDs, alcohol, smoking.
2. Instruct patient to immediately report evidence of bleeding, tarry stools, or dizziness; may indicate an acute bleeding episode
3. Instruct about medications:
   a. Take antacids 1 hour after meals, at bedtime, and when needed. Be aware that antacids may cause changes in bowel habits.
   b. Do not take H_2-receptor antagonists at the same time as sucralfate. This reduces the therapeutic effect of H_2 blockers.
   c. Take medications for as long as prescribed (usually 8 weeks), even if symptoms subside.
4. Encourage follow-up to determine adequate healing.

Pericarditis

Pericarditis is an inflammation of the pericardium, the membranous sac enveloping the heart. It is often a manifestation of a more generalized disease. A *pericardial effusion* may occur in pericarditis, in which excess fluid accumulates in the pericardial cavity. In *constrictive pericarditis*, chronic inflammatory thickening of the pericardium compresses the heart so that it is unable to fill normally during diastole. Acute idiopathic pericarditis is the most common form; its cause is unknown.

Other causes of pericarditis include infection by viruses (influenza and Coxsackie virus), bacteria (staphylococcus, meningococcus, streptococcus, pneumococcus, gonococcus, and *Mycobacterium tuberculosis*), fungi, and parasites; connective tissue disorders such as systemic lupus erythematosus and periarteritis nodosa; myocardial infarction (early, 24–72 hours; or late, 1 week to 2 years, known as Dressler's syndrome); uremia; malignant disease such as lung or breast cancer; thoracic irradiation; chest trauma; heart surgery (including pacemaker implantation); or drug-induced reaction (as with procainamide or phenytoin).

Complications of pericarditis include cardiac tamponade, congestive heart failure, and hemopericardium (especially in patients post–myocardial infarction [MI] receiving anticoagulants).

◆ Assessment

1. Pain in anterior chest, which is aggravated by thoracic motion and relieved by sitting up and leaning forward
   a. May vary from mild to sharp and severe
   b. Located in the precordial area (may be felt beneath clavicle, neck, scapular region)
   c. In post-MI patients, a dull, crushing pain may radiate to the neck, arm, and shoulders, mimicking an extension of infarction.
2. Associated symptoms of dyspnea (from compression of the heart and surrounding thoracic structures) and fever, sweating, and chills caused by inflammation of the pericardium
3. Pericardial friction rub—a scratchy, grating, or creaking sound occurring in the presence of pericardial inflammation

P

◆ Diagnostic Evaluation

1. Chest x-ray to detect cardiac enlargement
2. Echocardiogram if pericardial effusion is suspected
3. 12-lead electrocardiogram (ECG) to rule out acute MI
4. White blood cell count and differential to determine if infection is the cause; blood urea nitrogen (BUN) to rule out uremia; antinuclear antibodies (ANA) to rule out systemic lupus erythematosus (SLE); and antistreptolysin-O (ASO) titers to rule out rheumatic fever.
5. Tuberculin testing
6. Pericardiocentesis to evaluate pericardial fluid and determine cause
   a. Position patient with head elevated 45 degrees and apply limb leads of ECG for cardiac monitoring.
   b. Have defibrillator and temporary pacemaker available.
   c. After pericardiocentesis, monitor for signs of cardiac tamponade.

NURSING ALERT
Because pericardiocentesis carries some risk of fatal complications, such as laceration of the myocardium or of a coronary artery, have emergency equipment ready at bedside.

◆ Collaborative Management

Therapeutic Interventions
1. Dialysis and biochemical control of end-stage renal disease in uremic pericarditis
2. Radiation therapy for neoplastic pericarditis
3. Emergency pericardiocentesis if cardiac tamponade develops

Pharmacologic Interventions
1. Antimicrobial agents such as a penicillin for bacterial pericarditis or amphotericin B for fungal pericarditis
2. Corticosteroids to treat rheumatic fever or SLE
3. Antituberculosis chemotherapy to treat tuberculosis
4. Intrapericardial chemotherapy to treat neoplastic pericarditis

5. Aspirin, NSAIDs, or corticosteroids in postmyocardial infarction syndrome, as well as other types of pericarditis to provide symptomatic relief of inflammation and pain

Surgical Interventions

1. Partial pericardiectomy (pericardial "window") or total pericardiectomy for recurrent constrictive pericarditis

◆ Nursing Interventions

Monitoring

1. Monitor heart rate, rhythm, blood pressure, and respirations at least hourly in the acute phase.
2. Assess for signs of cardiac tamponade (increased heart rate, decreased BP, presence of paradoxical pulse, distended neck veins, restlessness, muffled heart sounds).

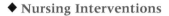

NURSING ALERT
The normal pericardial sac contains less than 25 mL to 30 mL fluid; pericardial fluid may accumulate slowly without noticeable symptoms. However, a rapidly developing effusion can produce serious hemodynamic alterations.

3. Assess for signs of congestive heart failure (see p. 393).
4. Institute continuous cardiac monitoring and monitor closely for the development of dysrhythmias caused by compression of the heart.

Supportive Care

1. Give prescribed drug regimen on timely basis for pain and symptomatic relief.
2. Encourage the patient to remain on bed rest when chest pain, fever, and friction rub occur.
3. Help the patient to a position of comfort, usually sitting upright.
4. Help relieve anxiety by explaining to the patient and family the difference between pain of pericarditis and pain of recurrent myocardial infarction. (Patients may fear extension of myocardial tissue damage.) Explain

P

that pericarditis does not indicate further heart damage.

Patient Education/Health Maintenance

1. Instruct the patient about signs and symptoms of pericarditis and stress the need for long-term medication therapy to help relieve symptoms.
2. Review all medications with the patient—purpose, side effects, dosages, and special precautions.

Peritonitis

Peritonitis is a generalized or localized inflammation of the peritoneum, the membrane that lines the abdominal cavity and covers visceral organs. This condition most often results from contamination by gastrointestinal secretions and is a complication of appendicitis, diverticulitis, peptic ulceration, biliary tract disease, colitis, volvulus, strangulated obstruction, or abdominal neoplasms. It may also occur after abdominal trauma (gunshot or stab wounds, blunt trauma from motor vehicle accident) or gastrointestinal surgery.

Primary peritonitis is relatively rare, occurring in patients with nephrosis or cirrhosis by *Escherichia coli;* or in young women because of infection introduced through fallopian tubes or through hematogenous spread.

Complications include intraabdominal abscess, septicemia, and death.

◆ Assessment

1. Localized abdominal pain becomes more diffuse, constant, and intense.
2. Fever and tachycardia develop.
3. Anorexia, nausea, and vomiting develop as peristalsis decreases.
4. Abdominal distention and tenderness become prominent. Abdomen becomes rigid with rebound tenderness and absent bowel sounds. Note that patient lies very still, usually with legs drawn up.

5. Percussion shows resonance and tympany indicating paralytic ileus; loss of liver dullness may indicate free air in abdomen.
6. Shock may develop.

◆ Diagnostic Evaluation

1. CBC shows leukocytosis (increased white blood cells) or leukopenia if severe.
2. Abdominal x-ray detects gas and fluid accumulation in small and large intestines, generalized dilation.
3. CT of abdomen may show abscess formation.
4. Paracentesis may be done to demonstrate blood, pus, bile, bacteria, and amylase in the peritoneal cavity. Gram stain and culture can be done.
5. Arterial blood gases may show metabolic acidosis with respiratory compensation.
6. Laparotomy may be necessary to identify the underlying cause.

◆ Collaborative Management

Therapeutic and Pharmacologic Interventions

1. Treatment of inflammatory conditions preoperatively and postoperatively with antibiotics aims to prevent peritonitis.
   a. Initially, broad-spectrum antibiotics to cover aerobic and anaerobic organisms
   b. Specific antibiotic therapy follows culture and sensitivity results.
2. Give parenteral replacements of fluid and electrolytes.
3. Give analgesics for pain; antiemetics for nausea and vomiting.
4. Nasogastric intubation to decompress the bowel; possibly rectal tube to facilitate passage of flatus

Surgical Interventions

1. May be necessary to close perforations of abdominal organs, remove infection source (ie, inflamed organ, necrotic tissue), drain abscesses, and lavage peritoneal cavity

◆ Nursing Interventions

Monitoring

1. Monitor fluid status because large volumes of fluid can be shifted into peritoneal space.
   a. Weakness, pallor, diaphoresis, and cold skin result from loss of fluid, electrolytes, and protein into the abdomen.
   b. Observe for signs of hypovolemia: dry mucous membranes, oliguria, postural hypotension, tachycardia, diminished skin turgor.
   c. Hypotension and hypokalemia may occur.
2. Monitor blood pressure continuously in shock.
3. Monitor central venous pressure to guide fluid replacement.
4. Monitor intake and output, including amount of nasogastric (NG) tube drainage and paracentesis fluid.

Supportive Care

1. Place the patient on bed rest in semi-Fowler's position to enable less painful breathing.
2. Maintain NPO status to reduce peristalsis.
3. Infuse IV fluids, for initial fluid replacement and fluid maintenance needs; administer hyperalimentation, as ordered, to maintain positive nitrogen balance until patient can resume oral diet.
4. Reduce parenteral fluids and give oral food and fluids as directed, when the following occur:
   a. Temperature and pulse return to normal.
   b. Abdomen becomes soft.
   c. Bowel sounds return.
   d. Flatus is passed, and patient has bowel movement.

Family Education and Health Maintenance

1. Teach the patient and family how to care for open wounds and drain sites, if appropriate.
2. Assess the need for home care nursing to assist with wound care and assess healing; refer as necessary.
3. Teach signs to report for recurrence of infection—fever, increasing abdominal pain, anorexia, nausea, vomiting, abdominal distention.

Pheochromocytoma

P

Pheochromocytoma is a catecholamine-secreting tumor associated with hyperfunction of the adrenal medulla. Tumors located in the adrenal medulla produce both increased epinephrine and norepinephrine; those located outside the adrenal gland tend to produce epinephrine only. Excess catecholamine secretion produces hypertension, hypermetabolism, and hyperglycemia. Pheochromocytoma can occur at any age but is most common between ages 30 and 60 years. Approximately 5% of pheochromocytomas occur in children, more frequently in boys between 9 and 12 years of age. Most tumors are benign; 10% are malignant with metastasis.

◆ Assessment

1. Hypermetabolic and hyperglycemic effects produce excessive perspiration, tremor, pallor or facial flushing, nervousness, elevated blood glucose levels, polyuria, nausea, vomiting, diarrhea, abdominal pain, and paresthesias.
2. Hypertension may be paroxysmal (intermittent) or persistent (chronic). The chronic form mimics essential hypertension but does not respond to antihypertensives. Headaches and visual disturbances are common.
3. Emotional changes, including psychotic behavior, may occur.
4. Predisposing factors that may trigger symptoms include physical exertion, emotional upset, and allergic reactions.

◆ Diagnostic Evaluation

1. Elevated vanillylmandelic acid (VMA) and metanephrine (metabolites of epinephrine and norepinephrine) on 24-hour urine
2. Elevated epinephrine and norepinephrine in blood and urine while symptomatic
3. Clonidine suppression shows no significant decrease in catecholamines in patients with pheochromocytoma.

P

4. CT scan and MRI of the adrenal glands or entire abdomen to identify tumor

◆ Collaborative Management

Pharmacologic Interventions

1. Preoperatively, administer alpha-adrenergic blocking agents such as phentolamine to inhibit the effects of catecholamines on blood pressure.
   a. Effective control of blood pressure may take 1 or 2 weeks.
   b. Blood volume needs to be expanded as blood vessels dilate with inhibition of catecholamines.
   c. Surgery is delayed until blood pressure is controlled and blood volume has been expanded.
2. May give catecholamine synthesis inhibitors such as metyrosine preoperatively or for long-term management of inoperable tumors. Side effects include sedation and crystalluria leading to kidney stones.

Surgical Interventions

1. Surgery involves unilateral adrenalectomy or removal of nonadrenal tumor.
2. Bilateral adrenalectomy may be necessary if both adrenal glands are affected.
3. Manipulation of the tumor during surgery may cause release of stored catecholamines causing hypertension during and immediately after surgery.

◆ Nursing Interventions

Monitoring

1. Monitor blood pressure frequently while patient is symptomatic.
2. Monitor for orthostatic hypotension after administration of phentolamine.
3. Monitor vital signs, cardiac rhythm, arterial blood pressure, neurologic status, and urine output closely because immediate postoperative hypertension, then hypotension, may occur.

Supportive Care

1. Remain with the patient during acute episodes of hypertension.

2. Ensure bed rest and elevate the head of bed 45 degrees during severe hypertension.
3. Instruct the patient about use of relaxation exercises.
4. Reduce environmental stressors by providing calm, quiet environment. Restrict visitors.
5. Eliminate stimulants (coffee, tea, cola) from the diet.
6. Reduce events that precipitate episodes of severe hypertension—palpation of the tumor, physical exertion, emotional upset.
7. Administer sedatives as prescribed to promote relaxation and rest.
8. Encourage oral fluids and maintain IV infusion preoperatively to ensure adequate volume expansion going into surgery.
9. Maintain adequate hydration with IV infusion postoperatively to prevent hypotension.

NURSING ALERT
Because reduction of catecholamines postoperatively causes vasodilation and enlargement of vascular space, hypotension may occur.

10. Provide routine wound care and prevention of postoperative complications.

Family Education and Health Maintenance

1. Instruct the patient how to take metyrosine if being treated medically.
   a. May cause sedation and need to avoid taking other CNS depressants and participating in activities that require alertness
   b. Increase fluid intake to at least 2,000 mL/day to prevent kidney stones.
2. Inform patient regarding the need for continued follow-up for:
   a. Recurrence of pheochromocytoma
   b. Assessment of any residual renal or cardiovascular injury related to preoperative hypertension
   c. Documentation that catecholamines levels are normal 1 to 3 months postoperatively (by 24-hour urine).

P

3. Teach about corticosteroid replacement for rest of life if bilateral adrenalectomy was performed; or for a few weeks if one adrenal gland was removed, until the stress of surgery is over and the remaining gland can compensate.

Pituitary Tumors

Pituitary tumors are usually adenomas of unknown origin that arise primarily in the anterior pituitary. Symptoms reflect tumor effects on target endocrine tissues or on local structures surrounding the pituitary gland. Tumors may be classified by size as microadenoma (smaller than 10 mm) or macroadenoma (larger than 10 mm), or by functional status as hormone secreting or nonsecreting.

Pituitary tumors respond well to early diagnosis and treatment and rarely metastasize. Without treatment, however, death or severe disability caused by stroke, blindness, or target endocrine disorders result.

◆ Assessment

1. Effects of tumor on surrounding structures (mass effect)
   a. Headaches
   b. Possible nausea and vomiting
   c. Impairment of cranial nerves such as visual field defects and diplopia, which may indicate pressure from tumor on the optic chiasm
2. Hormone imbalances caused by tumor hypersecretion or diminished secretion (Table 13)

◆ Diagnostic Evaluation

1. Skull x-rays are usually normal but may show enlarged sella turcica.
2. Computed CT scan (usually enhanced with contrast media) and MRI show pituitary mass.
3. Serum hormone levels identify abnormalities suspected on clinical evaluation.
4. Provocative testing such as glucose tolerance test and

TABLE 13 Clinical Manifestations Associated with Hormone Effects of Pituitary Tumors

Hormone	Hyperpituitarism (increased secretion)	Hypopituitarism (diminished secretion)
Growth hormone (GH)	Gigantism (child) Acromegaly (adult)	Shortness of stature (child) Silent (adult)
Prolactin	Infertility and galactorrhea (female)	Postpartum lactation failure (female)
Adrenocorticotrophic hormone (ACTH)	Cushing's disease	Adrenocortical insufficiency
Thyroid-stimulating hormone (TSH)	Hyperthyroidism	Hypothyroidism
Luteinizing hormone (LH) and Follicle-stimulating hormone (FSH)	Gonadal dysfunction	Hypogonadism

dexamethasone suppression test detect abnormal hormone secretion.

◆ Collaborative Management

Therapeutic Interventions
1. Ablation of tumor and much of gland by cryogenic destruction or stereotaxic radiofrequency coagulation
2. Radiation therapy

Pharmacologic Interventions
1. Drug therapy with bromocriptine for prolactinomas and, in some instances, growth hormone–secreting tumors
2. Specific hormone replacement therapy is indicated for hypopituitarism after medical or surgical treatment.
   a. Hypothyroidism caused by lack of thyroid-stimulating hormone (TSH) is treated with thyroxine-based medications.
   b. Adrenocortical insufficiency requires immediate hormone replacement with adrenocorticotropic hormone (ACTH) or hydrocortisone.

    c. In women, menstruation ceases and infertility occurs almost always after total or near-total ablation; estrogen and progesterone may be indicated to prevent osteoporosis.

    d. Transient or permanent diabetes insipidus may occur because of deficient antidiuretic hormone (ADH) secretion requiring desmopressin administration.

Surgical Interventions

1. Transsphenoidal hypophysectomy: direct approach through the sinus and nasal cavity to sella turcica
2. Frontal craniotomy: uncommon approach except where tumor occupies broad area (see p. 226)
3. Manipulation of the posterior pituitary during surgery may cause transient syndrome of secretion of inappropriate ADH (SIADH) with excessive ADH secretion, requiring diuretics and fluid restriction.

◆ Nursing Interventions

Monitoring

1. After transsphenoidal hypophysectomy, monitor vital signs, visual acuity, and neurologic status frequently for signs of cerebrospinal fluid leak or infection.
2. Monitor for and report increased urine output and low urine specific gravity, indicating diabetes insipidus.
3. Monitor serum electrolytes (hyponatremia) and serum osmolality (low) for SIADH.

Supportive Care

1. Provide emotional support through the diagnostic process and answer questions about treatment options.
2. Prepare the patient for surgery or other treatment by describing nursing care thoroughly.
3. Stress likelihood of positive outcome with ablation therapy.
4. Assess for signs of sinus infection before transsphenoidal procedure, and administer antibiotics as prescribed.
5. Administer hydrocortisone preoperatively, because the source of ACTH is being removed, and surgery is a significant source of stress.
6. After transsphenoidal surgery:

a. Encourage deep breathing exercises.
b. Caution the patient to avoid coughing and sneezing postoperatively to prevent cerebrospinal fluid (CSF) leak.
c. Check incision within inner aspect of upper lip for drainage or bleeding.
d. Note frequency of nasal dressing changes and character of drainage. Prepare the patient for packing removal 1 to several days postoperatively.
e. Encourage the use of a humidifier to prevent drying from mouth breathing.
f. Report appearance of persistent clear fluid from nose and increasing headache; could signal cerebrospinal fluid leak.

Patient Education and Health Maintenance

1. Advise the patient on temporary limitations in activities outlined by surgeon.
2. Teach the patient the nature of hormonal deficiencies posttreatment and the purpose of replacement therapy.
3. Instruct the patient in the early signs and symptoms of cortisol or thyroid hormone deficiency or excess and the need to report them.
4. Describe and demonstrate the correct method of administering prescribed medications.
5. Teach the patient the need for frequent initial follow-up and lifelong medical management when on hormonal therapy.
6. If applicable, advise the patient on the need for postsurgery radiation therapy and periodic follow-up MRI and visual field testing.
7. Teach the patient to notify health care provider if signs of thyroid or cortisol imbalance become evident.
8. Advise the patient to wear medical alert tag.

Pneumonia

Pneumonia is inflammation of the terminal airways and alveoli caused by acute infection by various agents. Pneu-

P

monia is usually classified according to its causative agent, which can be bacterial (*Streptococcus, Staphylococcus, H. influenzae, Klebsiella*), viral (*Legionella*), fungal, or caused by *Pneumocystis carinii, Mycoplasma*, or another agent. The infective agent enters the lungs through the airways (inhalation), the bloodstream, or through surgery or trauma.

Bacterial pneumonia may occur in persons who are experiencing underlying diseases (cancer, drug abuse, AIDS) or therapies (immunosuppressants, chemotherapy, radiation therapy) that impair the immune response. Such persons may develop an overwhelming infection. In a healthy person, bacterial pneumonia may result from an underlying viral illness.

Aspiration pneumonia is an acute inflammatory condition that results from aspiration of oropharyngeal secretions or stomach contents into the lungs. Patients at risk include those with loss or impairment of swallowing or coughing reflexes caused by altered state of consciousness, alcohol or drug overdose, or motor disease of the esophagus; those undergoing nasogastric or endotracheal intubations, or childbirth; or those with GI conditions such as hiatal hernia or intestinal obstruction.

Complications of pneumonia include pleural effusion, septic shock, pericarditis, bacteremia, meningitis, delirium, atelectasis, and delayed resolution.

◆ Assessment

1. Sudden onset; shaking chill; rapidly rising fever of 39.5° to 40.5°C. (101°–105°F). Aspiration pneumonia produces a fever, but no chills.
2. Cough, often with purulent sputum. In aspiration pneumonia, sputum is pink, frothy, and foul-smelling, resembling that of acute pulmonary edema
3. Pleuritic chest pain, aggravated by respiration and coughing
4. Tachypnea, respiratory grunting, nasal flaring, use of accessory muscles of respiration. Cyanosis is evident in aspiration pneumonia.
5. Anxious, flushed appearance, splinting of affected side, hypoxia, confusion, disorientation. May indicate worsening condition

6. Auscultation shows crackles overlying affected lung; bronchial breath sounds when *consolidation* (filling of airspaces with exudate) is present
   a. In aspiration pneumonia, rhonchi and wheezing are also present.
   b. Absent breath sounds caused by atelectasis from mucous plugs
7. Mental status changes, indicating hypoxemia.

NURSING ALERT
Pneumonia may present as mental status change and cough in the elderly without fever or leukocytosis. Presentation may be subtle or dramatic.

8. Predisposing factors that may interfere with normal lung drainage include tumor, general anesthesia and postoperative immobility, CNS depression, intubation or respiratory instrumentation, and neurologic disease, increasing risk of aspiration.

GERONTOLOGIC ALERT
Persons older than 65 years have a high mortality rate, even with appropriate antimicrobial therapy.

NURSING ALERT
Recurring pneumonia often indicates underlying disease such as cancer of the lung or multiple myeloma.

◆ Diagnostic Evaluation

1. Chest x-ray to detect infiltrates, atelectasis, and consolidation. In aspiration pneumonia, films may be clear initially, but later show consolidation and other abnormalities.
2. Sputum specimens for Gram stain and culture and sensitivity studies to detect infectious agent

3. Arterial blood gas analysis to evaluate oxygenation and acid–base status
4. Blood cultures to detect bacteremia
5. Blood, sputum, and urine samples for immunologic tests to detect microbial antigens
6. Laryngoscopy/bronchoscopy to determine if airways are blocked by solid material

◆ Collaborative Management

Therapeutic Interventions

1. Oxygen therapy if patient has inadequate gas exchange:
   a. Avoid high O_2 concentrations in patients with COPD; use of high O_2 may worsen alveolar ventilation by removing the patient's remaining ventilatory drive.
   b. Mechanical ventilation may be necessary if adequate ABG values cannot be maintained.
2. Intercostal nerve block to obtain pain relief
3. In aspiration pneumonia, clear the obstructed airway.
   a. If a foreign body becomes lodged in the patient's throat, remove it with forceps.
   b. Place the patient in tilted head-down position on right side (right side more frequently affected if patient has aspirated solid particles).
   c. Suction the trachea or endotracheal tube, to remove any particulate matter.
4. Correct hypotension in aspiration pneumonia with fluid volume replacement.

Pharmacologic Interventions

1. Appropriate antimicrobial therapy, based on culture and sensitivity when possible. Be aware that fatal complications may develop during early stages of antimicrobial treatment.
2. Cough suppressants when coughing is nonproductive, debilitating, or when coughing paroxysms cause serious hypoxemia
3. Analgesics to relieve pleuritic pain. However, avoid narcotics in patients with a history of COPD.

GERONTOLOGIC ALERT

Sedatives, narcotics, and cough suppressants are generally contraindicated in the elderly, because of their tendency to suppress cough and gag reflexes and respiratory drive. Expectorants and bronchodilators may be more helpful.

NURSING ALERT

Restlessness, confusion, aggressiveness may be caused by cerebral hypoxia; if so, do not treat with sedatives.

◆ Nursing Interventions

Monitoring

1. Monitor temperature, pulse, respiration, and blood pressure at regular intervals to assess the patient's response to therapy.
2. Follow results of ABGs to determine oxygen need and acid–base balance.
3. Employ special nursing surveillance for patients with the following conditions:
   a. Alcoholism, COPD, immunosuppression; these persons, as well as elderly patients, may have little or no fever.
   b. Chronic bronchitis; it is difficult to detect subtle changes in condition, because the patient may have seriously compromised pulmonary function
4. Assess these patients for unusual behavior, alterations in mental status, stupor, and signs and symptoms of congestive heart failure.
5. Assess for resistant or recurrent fever, indicating bacterial resistance to antibiotics.
6. In aspiration pneumonia, closely monitor patients at risk for lung abscess, empyema, and necrotizing pneumonia.

Supportive Care

1. Place the patient in semi-Fowler's position for resting and breathing, to obtain greater lung expansion and

P

improve aeration. Encourage frequent position changes.

2. Encourage the patient to cough; provide suction as needed.

3. Demonstrate to the patient how to splint the chest while coughing, and advise against suppressing a productive cough.

4. Encourage increased fluid intake, unless contraindicated, to thin mucus, promote expectoration, and replace fluid losses from fever, diaphoresis, dehydration, and dyspnea. Also humidify room air or institute oxygen therapy.

5. Employ chest wall percussion and postural drainage when appropriate, to loosen and mobilize secretions.

6. Auscultate the chest for crackles to gauge effectiveness of percussion and drainage.

7. Apply heat or cold to chest as prescribed to relieve pleuritic pain.

8. Encourage modified bed rest during febrile period.

9. Watch for abdominal distention or ileus, which may be caused by swallowing of air during intervals of severe dyspnea. Insert a nasogastric or rectal tube as directed, to relieve distension.

10. In aspiration pneumonia, feed patients with impaired swallowing slowly, and ensure that no food is retained in mouth after feeding. Give enteral feedings if indicated.

   a. Give tube feedings slowly, with patient sitting up in bed.

   b. Check position of tube in stomach before feeding.

   c. Check seal of cuff of tracheostomy or endotracheal tube before feeding.

11. Keep the patient with aspiration pneumonia in a fasting state before anesthesia (at least 8 hours).

❖

NURSING ALERT
The morbidity and mortality rates of aspiration pneumonia remain high even with optimum treatment. Prevention is the key to the problem.

P

Patient Education and Health Maintenance

1. Encourage chair rest after fever subsides; gradually increase activities to bring energy level back to pre-illness stage.

2. Encourage breathing exercises to clear lungs and promote full expansion and function after the fever subsides.

3. Advise smoking cessation. Cigarette smoking destroys mucociliary action, and inhibits function of alveolar scavenger cells (macrophages).

4. Advise the patient to keep up natural resistance with good nutrition and adequate rest. A single episode of pneumonia may predispose the patient to recurring respiratory infections.

5. Instruct the patient to avoid sudden extremes in temperature and excessive alcohol intake, which lower resistance to pneumonia.

6. Encourage yearly influenza immunization and immunization for *Streptococcus pneumoniae,* if indicated (major cause of bacterial pneumonia).

7. Tell the patient to avoid persons who have upper respiratory infections for several months after pneumonia.

Pneumothorax

Pneumothorax is an accumulation of air in the pleural space that occurs spontaneously or as a result of trauma. In patients with chest trauma, it usually follows laceration of the lung parenchyma, tracheobronchial tree, or esophagus. If left untreated, acute respiratory failure may ensue.

In *spontaneous pneumothorax*, air suddenly enters the pleural space, deflating the lung on the affected side. Usually caused by rupture of a subpleural bleb, it may occur secondary to chronic respiratory diseases or idiopathically. It may also strike healthy patients (risk is high in thin white males and those with family history of pneumothorax).

In *open pneumothorax* (sucking chest wound), trauma to the chest wall creates an opening large enough for air to pass freely between the thoracic cavity and the outside

P

of the body. With each attempted respiration, part of the tidal volume moves back and forth through the open wound instead of the trachea.

In *tension pneumothorax*, air builds up under pressure in the pleural space, which interferes with filling of both the heart and lung vessels. Cardiovascular collapse may occur.

◆ Assessment

1. Mild to moderate dyspnea and chest discomfort with spontaneous pneumothorax
2. Air hunger, agitation, hypotension, and cyanosis with open or tension pneumothorax
3. Reduced mobility of affected half of thorax and possible tracheal deviation away from affected side (tension pneumothorax)
4. Diminished breath sounds and hyperresonance

◆ Diagnostic Evaluation

1. Chest x-ray to confirm presence of air in pleural space, evaluate possible lung collapse, and check for tracheal deviation away from affected side

◆ Collaborative Management

Therapeutic Interventions

1. In spontaneous pneumothorax:
   a. Observe and allow for spontaneous resolution for less than 50% pneumothorax in otherwise healthy patient.
   b. With greater than 50% pneumothorax, needle aspiration or chest tube drainage if needed to reexpand collapsed lung
2. In tension pneumothorax:
   a. Immediate decompression with thoracentesis, thoracostomy, or chest tube insertion to vent trapped air and prevent cardiovascular collapse
   b. Basic and advanced life support if cardiovascular collapse occurs
   c. Maintenance of chest tube drainage with underwater-seal suction, to allow full lung expansion and healing

3. In open pneumothorax:
   a. Immediate closure of wound with a pressure dressing (petrolatum gauze secured with elastic adhesive) to restore adequate ventilation and respiration
   b. The patient should inhale and exhale gently against a closed glottis (Valsalva maneuver) as pressure dressing is applied. This maneuver helps to expand a collapsed lung.
   c. Chest tube insertion and underwater-seal suction, to permit escape of fluid and air and allow lung to reexpand.

Surgical Interventions

1. For spontaneous recurrent pneumothorax:
   a. Pleurodesis: intrapleural instillation of a chemical irritant causing the visceral and parietal pleura to adhere
   b. Thoracotomy with pleural abrasion or pleurectomy
2. For traumatic pneumothorax—repair chest trauma

◆ Nursing Interventions

Monitoring

1. Monitor vital signs and respiratory status continuously until lung has been reinflated.
2. Monitor oxygenation with oximetry and regular ABG readings.
3. Monitor chest tube patency and drainage.

Supportive Care

1. Maintain patent airway; apply suction as needed.
2. Maintain patency of chest tubes.
   a. Check tubing connections and prevent kinking of tube.
   b. Milk the tube periodically if directed.
   c. Ensure fluctuation in the water seal chamber until lung is reexpanded.
   d. Report excessive bubbling in water seal chamber, which may indicate leak in system.
3. Position the patient upright if possible, to allow greater chest expansion.
4. Assist patient to splint chest while turning or coughing, and administer pain medications as needed.

P

5. Instruct and encourage patient to use an inspiratory spirometer to improve gas exchange.
6. Provide oxygen as needed.

Family Education and Health Maintenance

1. Instruct patient to continue use of the inspiratory spirometer at home.
2. Patients with spontaneous pneumothorax are at risk for repeat occurrence; encourage these patients to report sudden onset of dyspnea immediately.

Poisoning, Acute Ingested

Poisoning by ingestion refers to the oral intake of a harmful substance that, even in small amounts, can damage tissues, disturb bodily functions, and possibly cause death. Immediate injury results when the poison excoriates soft tissues, as with a strong acid or alkali.

Substances commonly ingested include over-the-counter medications (such as acetaminophen or iron supplements; Table 14), household cleaning products, or parts of houseplants. Ingested poisoning may be accidental or intentional. In some cases, a poison may be secreted in breast milk to an infant.

Ingestion poisonings occur most often in children younger than age 5 years, with peak incidence at age 2 years. More than 80% of these poisonings occur in the home. Ingested poisoning accounts for approximately 10% to 20% of emergency room visits; a high proportion of these are children. Permanent multiorgan damage may result from initial loss of airway, breathing, and circulation, and from specific organ toxicity.

◆ Assessment

1. Possible altered level of consciousness and abnormal vital signs

❖❖

NURSING ALERT
Be prepared to initiate emergency respiratory and circulatory support at any time.

TABLE 14 Two Commonly Ingested Poisons

Poison	Clinical Manifestations	Treatment Considerations
Acetaminophen Common drug poisoning agent in children because of its availability and palatability. Ingestion by adolescents is frequently intentional. Results in cell necrosis of the liver. Children younger than age 6 are unlikely to develop significant toxicity even with large doses because of their ability to metabolize; adolescents have higher incidence of toxicity.	**First 24 hours after ingestion:** May be asymptomatic or anorexia, nausea, vomiting, diaphoresis, malaise, pallor **Second 24 hours:** Above symptoms diminish or disappear. Development of right upper quadrant pain. elevated liver function tests, oliguria **Days 3–8:** Peak liver function abnormalities; anorexia, nausea, vomiting, and malaise may reappear. **Days 4–14:** Liver failure with overwhelming toxicity or recovery with blood chemistry return to normal.	1. Administration of syrup of ipecac 2. Gastric lavage 3. Charcoal administration 4. n-acetylcysteine (Mucomyst) as antidote. If charcoal is given, lavage it out before giving Mucomyst.
Iron Occurs frequently in children because of prevalence of iron-containing preparations. Severity is related to the amount of elemental iron absorbed. The range of potential toxicity is approximately 50 to 60 mg/kg.	**30 minutes to 2 hours after ingestion:** Local necrosis and hemorrhage of GI tract; nausea and vomiting (including hematemesis), abdominal pain, diarrhea (often bloody), severe hypotension Symptoms subside after 6–12 hours. **6–24 hours:** Period of apparent recovery. **24–40 hours:** Systemic toxicity with cardiovascular collapse, shock, metabolic acidosis, hepatic and renal failure, seizures, coma, and possible death **2–4 weeks after ingestion:** Pyloric and duodenal stenosis; hepatic cirrhosis	1. Administration of syrup of ipecac 2. Gastric lavage 3. Deferoxamine for severe cases. This drug binds with iron and is usually administered IV or IM.

2. Gastrointestinal symptoms common in metallic acid, alkali, and bacterial poisoning: nausea and vomiting, diarrhea, abdominal pain or cramping, anorexia
3. Seizures (especially with CNS depressants such as alcohol, chloral hydrate, barbiturates) and behavioral changes. Dilated or pinpoint pupils may be noted.
4. Dyspnea (especially with aspiration of hydrocarbons) and cardiopulmonary depression or arrest. Cyanosis, especially in cyanide and strychnine ingestion.
5. Skin irritation, rash, burns to the mouth, esophagus, and stomach, eye inflammation, stains or odor around the mouth, lesions of the mucous membranes

◆ Diagnostic Evaluation

1. Blood and urine toxicology screening
2. Gastric contents may also be sent for toxicology screening in serious ingestions.

◆ Collaborative Management

Therapeutic Interventions

1. Identify the poison when possible.
2. Call the nearest poison control center to identify the toxic ingredient and obtain recommendations for emergency treatment.
3. Save vomitus, stool, and urine for analysis.
4. Maintain an open airway, because some ingested substances may cause soft tissue swelling and constrict the airway.
5. If needed, obtain venous access, maintain safety during seizure activity, and treat shock.
6. Gastric lavage, forced diuresis, hemoperfusion, dialysis, or exchange transfusions may be necessary.

Pharmacologic Interventions

1. Administration of syrup of ipecac orally or by nasogastric tube to induce vomiting
2. Administration of antidotes, if known, such as charcoal

PEDIATRIC ALERT
Because charcoal inactivates ipecac, give charcoal only *after* ipecac has induced vomiting.

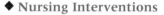

◆ **Nursing Interventions**

Monitoring
1. Continue to monitor airway, breathing, and circulation.
2. Monitor level of consciousness, pupil reactivity, and motor activity.
3. Monitor vital signs.
4. Monitor for fluid and electrolyte imbalance after vomiting or diuresis.

Supportive Care
1. To assist the family by telephone management, obtain and record the following information:
   a. Name, address, and telephone number of caller
   b. Immediate severity of the situation
   c. Age, weight, and signs and symptoms of the child, including neurologic status
   d. Route of exposure
   e. Name of the ingested product, approximate amount ingested, and the time of ingestion
   f. Brief medical history
   g. Caller's relationship to victim
2. Instruct the caller regarding appropriate emergency actions based on institution protocol.
   a. To remove poison from the body, dilute with 6 to 8 ounces of water, based on poison.
   b. For skin or eye contact, remove contaminated clothing and flush with water for 15 to 20 minutes.
   c. For inhalation poisons, remove from the exposed site.
   d. Induce vomiting unless contraindicated.

NURSING ALERT

Do *not* induce vomiting if patient is convulsing, semiconscious, or comatose; if the poison is likely to cause rapid decrease in consciousness; or if the poison is a strong acid or alkali, strychnine, iodide, silver nitrate, or a hydrocarbon (eg, lighter fluid, gasoline, kerosene, paint or nail polish remover). Strong acids or alkalis may damage the esophagus for a second time during emesis, and hydrocarbons can cause severe pneumonia if aspirated.

3. Direct the caller or patient to the nearest emergency department or have them call 911 for ambulance as necessary.

4. Instruct the caller to clear the child's mouth of any unswallowed poison.
5. Identify what treatments have already been initiated.
6. Instruct the parents to save vomitus, unswallowed liquid or pills, and the container and to bring them to the hospital as aids in identifying the poison.
7. While assisting with emergency care in the acute care facility, reassure child and family that therapeutic measures are being taken immediately.
8. Discourage anxious parents from holding, caressing, and overstimulating the child.
9. Avoid administering sedatives or narcotics to avoid CNS depression and masking of symptoms.
10. Have artificial airway and tracheostomy set available in case respiratory depression develops.
11. Administer oxygen as directed.
12. Maintain IV therapy as directed to prevent shock.
13. Avoid hypothermia or hyperthermia because control of body temperature is impaired in many types of poisoning.
14. Counsel parents, who often feel guilty about the accident.
15. Involve the young child in therapeutic play to determine how he or she views the situation. Explain the child's treatment and correct misinterpretations in a manner appropriate for age.
16. Initiate a community health nursing referral. A home assessment should be made so that underlying problems are recognized and appropriate help is provided.

Family Education and Health Maintenance.

1. Teach measures to prevent accidental poisonings in the home:
   a. Keep medicines and chemicals out of reach of children; use childproof containers, locked cabinets, and high shelves.
   b. Keep potentially toxic substances in original containers away from food.
   c. Teach children not to taste unfamiliar substances.
   d. Read all labels carefully before each use.
   e. Never refer to drugs as candy or bribe children with such inducements.

f. Teach adults not to take drugs in front of children, because children mimic behavior.
2. Reinforce the need for supervision of infants and young children.
3. Instruct parents and family to have syrup of ipecac and poison control center number readily available in the home.

Polycythemia Vera

Polycythemia vera is a chronic myeloproliferative disorder involving hyperplasia of all bone marrow elements. This causes increased red blood cell mass, blood volume and viscosity, decreased marrow iron reserve, and splenomegaly. Hyperviscosity may also lead to complications such as deep vein thrombophlebitis, myocardial and cerebral infarction, pulmonary embolism, and thrombotic occlusion of the splenic, hepatic, portal and mesenteric veins. Other complications include congestive heart failure, gout, spontaneous hemorrhage, and, possibly, myelofibrosis or acute leukemia in late stages of the disorder.

Polycythemia vera usually occurs in patients who are middle-aged or older. The underlying cause is unknown.

◆ Assessment

1. Headache, fullness in head, dizziness, visual abnormalities, weakness and fatigue resulting from hypervolemia and hyperviscosity
2. Reddish-purple hue of skin and mucosa; pruritus
3. Painful fingers and toes from arterial and venous insufficiency
4. Altered mentation from disturbed cerebral circulation
5. Splenomegaly and hepatomegaly
6. Bleeding tendency

◆ Diagnostic Evaluation

1. CBC shows elevated red blood cells, hemoglobin, and hematocrit.

P

2. Bone marrow aspiration and biopsy to check for hyperplasia

◆ Collaborative Management

Therapeutic Interventions

1. Phlebotomy (withdrawal of blood) is performed to treat hyperviscosity at intervals determined by CBC results, to reduce red cell mass. Generally, 250 to 500 mL is removed at a time.

Pharmacologic Interventions

1. Myelosuppressive therapy for marrow hyperplasia
   a. IV radioactive phosphorus (^{32}P)
   b. Alkylating agent such as hydroxyurea
2. Allopurinol to treat hyperuricemia

◆ Nursing Interventions

Monitoring

1. Monitor for signs of bleeding or thromboembolism.
2. Monitor for hypertension and signs and symptoms of congestive heart failure, including shortness of breath, distended neck veins.
3. Monitor complete blood counts.

Supportive Care and Patient Education

1. Encourage or assist with ambulation.
2. Educate the patient about risk of thrombosis; encourage maintenance of normal activity patterns and avoiding long periods of bed rest.
3. Advise the patient to avoid taking hot showers or baths because rapid skin cooling worsens pruritus; use skin emollients; take antihistamines as prescribed.
4. Instruct the patient to take only prescribed medications.
5. Encourage the patient to report at prescribed intervals for follow-up blood studies (hematocrit).

Premenstrual Syndrome

Premenstrual syndrome (PMS) is a group of symptoms related to onset of menstruation. The cause is unclear but may be linked to hormonal imbalances, prostaglandins, endorphins, psychological factors such as attitudes and beliefs related to menstruation, and environmental factors such as nutrition and pollution. PMS is usually self-limiting without complications.

◆ Assessment

1. Symptoms may begin 7 to 14 days before onset of menstrual flow; diminish 1 to 2 days after menses begins.
2. Physical: edema of extremities, abdominal fullness, breast swelling and tenderness, headache, vertigo, palpitations, acne, backache, constipation, thirst, weight gain
3. Behavioral: irritability, fatigue, lethargy, depression, anxiety, crying spells
4. Diagnosis based on clinical manifestations; usually no diagnostic evaluation necessary

◆ Collaborative Management

Therapeutic Interventions

1. Restrict sodium, caffeine, tobacco, alcohol, and refined sweets.
2. Aerobic exercise daily during symptomatic period helps reduce tension.
3. Counseling to help reduce emotional and behavioral symptoms

Pharmacologic Interventions

1. Vitamin B6 supplements may help reduce tension and irritability.
2. Progesterone replacement therapy may relieve symptoms.
3. Prostaglandin inhibitors such as ibuprofen are used.
4. Diuretics decrease fluid retention and weight gain.
5. Anxiolytic agents may be necessary.
6. Fluoxetine, an antidepressant, has been studied with success for relief of the psychological symptoms of PMS.

◆ Nursing Interventions

Supportive Care

1. Provide emotional support for patient and significant others.

P

2. Encourage patient to keep a diary for several consecutive months including dates, cycle days, stressors, and symptoms and their severity to determine if therapy is effective.

Patient Education and Health Maintenance

1. Instruct patient in the use and side effects of prescribed medications.
2. Teach patient possible causes of PMS and nonpharmacologic methods to alleviate distress, such as dietary modifications, exercise, and rest.
3. Teach stress reduction techniques such as imagery and deep breathing.
4. Refer for counseling and to support groups as needed.

Prostate Cancer
See Cancer, Prostate

Prostatic Hyperplasia, Benign

Benign prostatic hyperplasia (BPH) is enlargement of the prostate that constricts the urethra, causing urinary symptoms. One of every four men who reach the age of 80 years will require treatment for BPH. This disorder results from the effects of aging and the presence of circulating androgens. Complications of BPH may include involuntary bladder contractions, bladder diverticula, cystolithiasis, vesicoureteral reflux, hydronephrosis, and urinary tract infection.

◆ Assessment

1. In early or gradual prostatic enlargement, there may be no symptoms, because the detrusor musculature can initially compensate for increased urethral resistance.
2. Obstructive symptoms include hesitancy, diminution in size and force of urinary stream, terminal dribbling,

sensation of incomplete emptying of the bladder, urinary retention.
3. Irritative voiding symptoms include urgency, frequency, and nocturia.
4. Enlarged prostate on rectal examination

◆ Diagnostic Evaluation

1. Urinalysis to rule out hematuria and infection
2. Serum creatinine and blood urea nitrogen (BUN) to evaluate renal function
3. Serum prostate-specific antigen (PSA) to rule out cancer; however, PSA may also be elevated in BPH
4. Additional diagnostic studies for further evaluation:
    a. Urodynamics, to measure peak urine flow rate, voiding time, and volume, and to evaluate the bladder's ability to effectively contract
    b. Measurement of postvoid residual urine by ultrasound or by catheterization
    c. Cystourethroscopy to inspect the urethra and bladder and evaluate prostatic size

◆ Collaborative Management

Therapeutic Interventions
1. Patients with mild symptoms (in the absence of significant bladder or renal impairment) are followed annually; BPH does not necessarily worsen in all men.
2. Balloon dilation of the prostatic urethra provides temporary relief of symptoms.

Pharmacologic Interventions
1. Alpha-adrenergic blockers such as doxazosin or terazosin, to relax smooth muscle of bladder base and prostate to facilitate voiding
2. Finasteride may be ordered for its anti-androgen effect on prostatic cells, which can reverse or prevent hyperplasia.

Surgical Interventions
1. Transurethral resection of the prostate (TURP) or transurethral incision of the prostate (TUIP)
2. Open prostatectomy (usually by suprapubic approach) may be required to remove a very large prostate.

P

3. Newer approaches include laser surgery; insertion of prostatic stents or coils; and microwave hyperthermia treatments.

◆ **Nursing Interventions**

Supportive Care

1. To facilitate urinary elimination, provide privacy and time for the patient to void.
2. Assist with catheter insertion via guide wire or suprapubic cystotomy as indicated, and maintain catheter patency.
3. Administer medications as ordered; teach the patient about reportable side effects:
   a. Alpha-adrenergic blockers: hypotension, orthostatic hypotension, syncope (especially after first dose); impotence; blurred vision; rebound hypertension if discontinued abruptly
   b. Finasteride (Proscar): hepatic dysfunction; impotence; interference with PSA testing
4. Assess for and teach patient to report hematuria, signs of infection.
5. Be aware of and teach patient drugs that may exacerbate obstruction as BPH worsens—antidepressants, anticholinergics, decongestants, tranquilizers, and alcohol.

Patient Education and Health Maintenance

1. Advise patient to report urinary retention or signs of infection immediately.
2. After surgery, teach the patient do perform perineal (Kegel) exercises to help gain control over voiding:
   a. Contract the perineal muscle as if to stop stream of urine or control flatus, hold for 10 to 15 seconds, then relax.
   b. Repeat approximately 15 times (one set); do 15 sets per day.
3. Advise the patient that irritative voiding symptoms do not immediately resolve after obstruction is relieved, but that symptoms diminish over time.
4. Tell the patient to avoid sexual intercourse, straining

at stool, heavy lifting, and long periods of sitting, for 6 to 8 weeks after surgery until prostatic fossa is healed.
5. Advise follow-up visits after treatment because urethral stricture may occur and regrowth of prostate is possible after transurethral resection.

Prostate Surgery

Prostate surgery may be done to treat benign prostatic hyperplasia (BPH) or prostate cancer. The surgical approach depends on the size of the gland, severity of obstruction, the patient's age and underlying health, and the nature of the disease. There are two basic procedures.

Transurethral resection of the prostate (TUR or TURP) is the most common procedure. In TURP, superficial lesions (early carcinomas, benign papillomas) are removed from the bladder wall using a scope inserted through the urethra.

Open prostatectomy includes three approaches. Suprapubic prostatectomy (incision into the suprapubic area and through the bladder wall) is commonly used to treat BPH. Perineal prostatectomy (incision between the scrotum and rectal area) is used to treat prostate cancer. Because it has the highest incidence of urinary incontinence and impotence, it is usually used in patients who are no longer sexually active. Retropubic prostatectomy (incision at level of symphysis pubis) is done for BPH if the gland is too large for TURP, also for prostate cancer when the entire prostate must be removed. This approach preserves innervation related to sexual function in 50% of patients.

◆ Potential Complications

1. Urinary incontinence
2. Retrograde ejaculation and sexual dysfunction
3. Wound infection and dehiscence
4. Urinary obstruction and infection
5. Hemorrhage
6. Thrombophlebitis and pulmonary embolism

P

◆ Collaborative Management

Preoperative Care

1. Explain the nature of the procedure and the expected postoperative care, including catheter drainage, irrigation, and monitoring of hematuria.
2. Discuss complications of surgery and how patient will cope.
   a. Incontinence or dribbling of urine for up to 1 year after surgery; perineal (Kegel) exercises help regain urinary control.
   b. Retrograde ejaculation: seminal fluid released into bladder and eliminated in the urine rather than through prostatic fluid during intercourse. (Impotence is usually not a complication of TURP but is often a complication of open prostatectomy.)
3. Administer preoperative bowel preparation as prescribed, or instruct the patient in home administration and fasting after midnight.
4. Ensure that optimal cardiac, respiratory, and circulatory status have been achieved to decrease risk of complications.
5. Administer prophylactic antibiotics as ordered.

Postoperative Care

1. Maintain patency of urethral catheter placed after surgery.
   a. Monitor flow of three-way closed irrigation and drainage system if used.
   b. Using aseptic technique, perform manual irrigation with 50 mL irrigating fluid. Avoid overdistending the bladder, which could lead to hemorrhage.
2. Administer anticholinergic drugs, as ordered, to reduce bladder spasms.
3. Assess degree of hematuria and any clot formation; drainage should become light pink within 24 hours.
   a. Report any arterial bleeding (bright red, with increased viscosity): may require surgical intervention.
   b. Report any increase in venous bleeding (dark red): may require catheter traction to apply pressure to the prostatic fossa with inflated catheter balloon.
   c. Prepare for blood transfusion if bleeding persists.

4. Administer IV fluids as ordered and encourage oral fluids when tolerated to ensure hydration and urine output.

5. Maintain bed rest for the first 24 hours; frequently monitor vital signs, intake and output, and observe condition of incisional dressing, if present (no incision in TURP).

6. After 24 hours, encourage ambulation to prevent venous thrombosis, pulmonary embolism, and hypostatic pneumonia.

7. Observe urine for cloudiness or odor and obtain urine for evaluation of infection as ordered.

8. Report any testicular pain, swelling, and tenderness, which could indicate epididymitis from spreading infection.

9. Assist with perineal care if perineal incision is present to prevent contamination by feces.

10. Administer pain medication or monitor patient-controlled analgesia (PCA) as directed.

11. Position for comfort and tell the patient to avoid straining, which will increase pelvic venous congestion and may cause hemorrhage.

12. Administer stool softeners to prevent discomfort from constipation.

13. Make sure catheter is well secured to the patient's thigh to prevent traction on catheter, which will cause pain and potential hemorrhage.

❖

NURSING ALERT
Avoid rectal temperatures, enemas, or rectal tubes postoperatively to prevent hemorrhage or disruption of healing.

Patient Education and Health Maintenance

1. Tell patient to avoid sexual intercourse, straining at stool, heavy lifting, and long periods of sitting for 6 to 8 weeks after surgery, until prostatic fossa is healed.

2. Advise follow-up visits after treatment because urethral stricture may occur, and regrowth of prostate is possible after TURP.

3. Reassure patient that urinary incontinence, frequency,

P

urgency, and dysuria are expected after the catheter is removed, and that these effects should gradually subside.

   a. If the patient is sent home catheterized, advise that catheter will be removed in about 3 weeks, when cystogram confirms healing.

   b. Discuss the use of absorbent products to contain urine leakage.

   c. Advise that incontinence is more pronounced when abdominal pressure is increased, such as coughing, laughing, straining.

4. Teach measures to regain urinary control.

   a. Have patient imagine there is an egg in his rectum, then squeeze the muscles to try to "break" it; hold the position, then relax. Caution on using abdominal muscles, which increases incontinence.

   b. Tell patient to stop urinary stream while voiding, hold for few seconds, then continue. Practice this while not voiding 10 to 20 times an hour.

5. Reinforce the surgeon's discussion of risk of impotence. Remind patient that erectile function may not return for as long as 6 months.

6. Encourage patient to express fears and anxieties related to potential loss of sexual function, and to discuss concerns with partner.

7. Advise that options such as penile implant are available to restore sexual function if impotence persists.

Pulmonary Edema

Pulmonary edema is marked by accumulation of excess fluid in the lung, either in the interstitial spaces or in the alveoli. Fluid accumulation in the alveoli impairs gas exchange, especially oxygen movement into pulmonary capillaries. This disorder is a common complication of cardiac disorders, including acute left ventricular failure, myocardial infarction, aortic stenosis, severe mitral valve disease, hypertension, and congestive heart failure.

Pulmonary edema also may result from lung injuries, such as smoke inhalation, shock lung, pulmonary embolism, or infarct; from CNS injuries, such as stroke or head trauma; from allergies; and from infection (such as infectious pneumonia) and fever. It also can follow circulatory overload resulting from transfusions and infusions; adverse drug reactions, drug hypersensitivity, narcotic overdose, or poisoning; it also may be a complication in patients who have undergone cardioversion, anesthesia, or cardiopulmonary bypass procedures. The disorder may progress to dysrhythmias or respiratory failure.

◆ Assessment

NURSING ALERT
Acute pulmonary edema is a true medical emergency, a life-threatening condition.

1. Premonitory symptoms of cough and restlessness
2. Dyspnea, orthopnea, labored and rapid respirations, use of accessory muscles and retractions
3. White- or pink-tinged frothy sputum, inspiratory and expiratory wheezing, and bubbling sounds with respirations
4. Anxiety and panic because of suffocating feeling
5. Cyanosis with profuse perspiration, distended neck veins, and tachycardia

◆ Diagnostic Evaluation

1. Chest x-ray shows interstitial edema
2. Echocardiagram to detect underlying valvular disease, and additional tests to determine cause
3. Pulmonary artery catheterization to help differentiate cause

◆ Collaborative Management

Therapeutic Interventions
1. Oxygen in high concentration—to relieve hypoxia, hypoxemia, and dyspnea

P

2. Intubation and ventilatory support may be necessary to improve hypoxemia and prevent hypercarbia.

Pharmacologic Interventions

1. Morphine intravenously in small titrated intermittent doses, to reduce anxiety, promote venous pooling of blood in the periphery, and reduce vascular resistance and cardiac workload.
   a. *Do not* give morphine if pulmonary edema is caused by stroke or occurs in the presence of chronic pulmonary disease or cardiogenic shock.
   b. Have morphine antagonist available to treat respiratory depression.
2. Diuretics IV to reduce blood volume and pulmonary congestion by producing prompt diuresis
3. Vasodilators if patient fails to respond to therapy
4. Positive inotropic agents such as digoxin and dopamine, to enhance myocardial contractility and reduce fluid backup into the lungs
5. Aminophylline to prevent bronchospasm associated with pulmonary congestion, which may enhance myocardial contractility.

◆ Nursing Interventions

Monitoring

1. Auscultate lung fields frequently. Note inspiratory and expiratory wheezes, rhonchi, moist fine crackles appearing initially in lung bases and extending upward.
2. Monitor for presence of third heart sound (may be difficult to hear because of respiratory sounds) caused by volume overload or increasing heart failure.
3. Monitor for signs/symptoms of hypoxia: restlessness, confusion, headache.
4. Monitor hemodynamic status in response to therapy. Check blood pressure frequently and pulmonary artery pressure and cardiac output, as indicated.

NURSING ALERT
Watch for decreasing blood pressure, increasing heart rate, and decreasing urinary output—indications that the total body circulation is not tolerating diuresis and that hypovolemia may develop.

5. Monitor for respiratory depression and hypotension during morphine therapy.
6. Monitor potassium levels, daily weights, and intake and output while on diuretic therapy.

Supportive Care

1. Place patient in upright position, with head and shoulders up, feet and legs hanging down, to favor pooling of blood in dependent extremities and decrease venous return.
2. Help reduce the patient's anxiety by remaining with and reassuring the patient. Explain in a calm manner all therapies administered and the reason for their use. (Arterial vasoconstriction diminishes when anxiety is relieved.)
3. Explain to the patient importance of wearing oxygen mask to improve breathing, but be aware of fear of suffocation.
4. Evaluate for side effects of therapy—dysrhythmias, hypotension, headache.
5. Continually evaluate the patient's response to therapy and report findings.

Patient Education and Health Maintenance

1. Teach the patient about the pathogenesis of pulmonary edema to help prevent recurrence.
2. Help the patient to recognize and promptly report early symptoms of acute pulmonary edema.
3. If productive (wet) coughing develops, advise the patient to sit upright with legs dangling over the bedside to reduce symptoms.
4. See additional measures for heart failure, p. 393.

Pulmonary Embolism

Pulmonary embolism is obstruction of one or more pulmonary arteries by thrombi that are dislodged and carried to the lungs from their usual sites in the deep leg veins or in the right side of the heart. The obstruction restricts or cuts off blood flow, causing ventilation–perfusion mismatch and possible pulmonary infarction. Pulmonary emboli vary in size and seriousness of consequences; massive pulmonary embolism is a life-threatening emergency. Respiratory failure is the primary complication.

> **NURSING ALERT**
> Be aware of risk factors for pulmonary embolism—immobilization, trauma to pelvis (especially surgical) and lower extremities (especially hip fracture), obesity, history of thromboembolic disease, varicose veins, phlebitis, pregnancy, congestive heart failure (CHF), myocardial infarction, malignant disease, postoperative period, estrogen therapy, advancing age.

◆ Assessment

1. Sudden onset of severe dyspnea
2. Signs of hypoxia—headache, restlessness, apprehension, pallor, cyanosis, behavioral changes, tachypnea
3. Pleuritic chest pain (worsens with coughing and deep breathing). Pain is accompanied by apprehension and a sense of impending doom when most of the pulmonary artery is obstructed.
4. Pleural friction rub, crackles, rhonchi, and wheezing
5. Splitting of second heart sound, indicating increased right ventricular workload

> **NURSING ALERT**
> Have a high index of suspicion for pulmonary embolus if there is a subtle deterioration in the patient's condition and unexplained cardiovascular and pulmonary findings.

6. Cyanosis, distended neck veins, tachydysrhythmias, syncope, and circulatory collapse in massive pulmonary embolism

◆ Diagnostic Evaluation

1. Arterial blood gases show decreased PaO_2 caused by abnormal lung perfusion.

2. Chest x-rays may show a possible wedge-shaped infiltrate.
3. Ventilation–perfusion (V/Q) lung scan to evaluate regional blood flow and presence of perfusion defects. Ventilation may be abnormal with large perfusion defects.
4. Pulmonary angiography (most definitive test) in which emboli are shown as "filling defects"

◆ Collaborative Management

Therapeutic Interventions

1. Emergency measures in massive pulmonary embolism, to stabilize cardiorespiratory status
   a. Oxygen to relieve hypoxemia, respiratory distress, and cyanosis
   b. IV to open a route for drugs and fluids
   c. Mechanical ventilation may be necessary.

NURSING ALERT
Massive pulmonary embolism is a medical emergency; the patient's condition tends to deteriorate rapidly. There is a profound decrease in cardiac output, with an accompanying increase in right ventricular pressure.

Pharmacologic Interventions

1. Vasopressors, inotropic agents such as dopamine, or antidysrhythmic agents, to support circulation if the patient is unstable.
2. Small doses of morphine IV to relieve anxiety, alleviate chest discomfort (which improves ventilation), and ease adaptation to mechanical ventilator, if this is necessary.
3. After stabilization, heparin is given IV to stop further thrombus formation and extend clotting time.
   a. Follow IV loading dose with continuous pump or drip infusion or give intermittently every 4 to 6 hours.
   b. Adjust dosage to maintain activated partial throm-

P

boplastin time (PTT) at 1.5 to 2 times pretreatment value (if the value was normal).
   c. Protamine sulfate may be given to neutralize heparin in event of severe bleeding.
4. Thrombolytic agents such as urokinase and streptokinase may be used if patient has massive pulmonary embolism.
   a. Give IV in a loading dose followed by constant infusion.
   b. Bleeding may result from fibrinolysis.
   c. Newer clot-specific thrombolytics (tissue plasminogen activator, streptokinase activator complex, single-chain urokinase) activate plasminogen only within thrombus itself rather than systematically, thus minimizing generalized fibrinolysis and subsequent bleeding.

NURSING ALERT
Discontinue thrombolytic therapy in the event of severe, uncontrolled bleeding.

5. Oral anticoagulant for follow-up anticoagulant therapy
   a. Control dosage by monitoring serial prothrombin time (PT); desired PT is 1.2 to 1.5 times control value.
   b. PT is reported as international normalized ratio (INR) of 1.2 to 1.5 by most laboratories.

GERONTOLOGIC ALERT
Consider the patient's age and other medications in dosing of anticoagulation therapy—usually will need a decreased dosing regimen.

Surgical Interventions
1. Indications for surgery include contraindications to anticoagulation, recurrent embolization, or serious complications from drug therapy.

2. Embolectomy, or prophylactic procedures including interruption of inferior vena cava or placement of filter in vena cava, may be done.

◆ Nursing Interventions

Monitoring

1. Monitor vital signs, cardiac rhythm, oximetry, and ABG levels for adequacy of oxygenation.
2. Monitor for signs of shock—decreasing blood pressure, tachycardia, cool, clammy skin, decreasing urine output.
3. Monitor for bleeding related to anticoagulant or thrombolytic therapy. Perform stool guaiac test and monitor platelet count to detect heparin-induced thrombocytopenia.
4. Monitor patient's response to IV fluids/vasopressors.

Supportive Care

1. Prepare the patient for assisted ventilation when hypoxemia occurs.
2. Position the patient with the head of bed slightly elevated (unless contraindicated by shock) and with chest splinted for deep breathing and coughing.
3. Correct dyspnea and relieve physical discomfort to help reduce anxiety. Give prescribed morphine and monitor for pain relief and signs of respiratory depression.
4. Minimize risk of bleeding by performing essential ABGs on upper extremities. Apply digital compression at puncture site for 30 minutes, apply pressure dressing to previously involved sites, check site for oozing.
5. Maintain patient on strict bed rest during thrombolytic therapy and avoid unnecessary handling to reduce risk of rebleeding.

Patient Education and Health Maintenance

1. Advise patient of the possible need to continue taking anticoagulant therapy for 6 weeks up to an indefinite period.
2. Teach about signs of bleeding, especially of gums, nose, bruising, blood in urine and stools.
3. Warn against taking medications unless approved by

P

health care provider, because many drugs interact with anticoagulants.

4. Instruct patient to tell dentist about taking an anticoagulant.
5. Warn against inactivity for prolonged periods or sitting with legs crossed to prevent recurrence.
6. Warn against sports/activities that may cause injury to legs and predispose to a thrombus.
7. Encourage wearing a medical alert bracelet identifying patient as anticoagulant user.
8. Instruct patient to lose weight if applicable; obesity is a risk factor for women.
9. Discuss contraceptive methods with patient if applicable; advise female patients to avoid taking oral contraceptives.

Pyelonephritis

Pyelonephritis is an acute inflammation and infection of the renal pelvis, tubules, and interstitial tissue. The disease typically results from infection by enteric bacteria (most commonly *Escherichia coli*) that have spread from the bladder to the ureters and kidneys secondary to vesicoureteral reflux. Other causes of pyelonephritis include urinary obstruction or infection, trauma, blood-borne infection, other renal disease, pregnancy, or metabolic disorders. Complications include renal insufficiency and possible chronic renal failure, hypertension, renal abscess, or perinephric abscess.

◆ Assessment

1. Fever, chills, nausea and vomiting
2. Costovertebral angle tenderness, flank pain (with or without radiation to groin)
3. Infants may display irritability and failure to thrive.

GERONTOLOGIC ALERT
Elderly patients may exhibit gastrointestinal or pulmonary symptoms and not show the usual febrile response to pyelonephritis.

◆ Diagnostic Evaluation

1. Urinalysis to identify leukocytes, bacteria or pus in urine, gross or microscopic hematuria
2. Urine culture to identify antibody-coated bacteria (ACB) in urine. Bacteria invading the kidney induce an antibody response that coats the bacteria; this differentiates renal infection from bladder infection, in which bacteria are not coated.
3. Intravenous pyelography (IVP) and other urologic tests may be ordered to evaluate urinary tract obstruction and other causes.

◆ Collaborative Management

Pharmacologic Interventions

1. Organism-specific antimicrobial therapy:
   a. Usually begun immediately to cover prevalent gram-negative pathogens, then adjusted according to urine culture results
   b. Treatment for 2 weeks or more is needed.
2. Inpatient treatment with parenteral antimicrobial therapy if the patient cannot tolerate oral intake and is dehydrated or acutely ill
3. Percutaneous drainage or prolonged antibiotic therapy are needed to treat renal or perinephric abscess.
4. Maintenance therapy for chronic or recurring infections to preserve renal function:
   a. Continuous treatment with urine-sterilizing agents after initial antibiotic treatment
   b. Continue for months to years until there is no evidence of inflammation, causative factors have been treated or controlled, and renal function is stabilized.
   c. Serial urine cultures and evaluation studies must be done for an indefinite period.
   d. Blood counts and serum creatinine determinations are required during long-term therapy.

◆ Nursing Interventions

Monitoring

1. Assess vital signs frequently for impending sepsis if patient is elderly or acutely ill.

P

2. Monitor intake and output.
3. Monitor renal function through urinalysis and serum blood urea nitrogen (BUN) and creatinine.

Supportive Care

1. Administer or teach self-administration of antibiotics and analgesics as prescribed and monitor for effectiveness and side effects.
2. Administer antiemetic medications to control nausea and vomiting and antipyretics, as indicated.
3. Take measures to decrease body temperature if indicated (cooling blanket, application of ice to armpits and groin, etc.)
4. Use comfort measures such as positioning and heat to locally relieve flank pain.
5. Correct dehydration by replacing fluids, orally if possible, or IV.

Family Education and Health Maintenance

1. Explain to the patient possible causes of pyelonephritis and its signs and symptoms; review also signs and symptoms of lower urinary tract infection.
2. Review antibiotic therapy and stress importance of completing prescribed treatment regimen and having follow-up urine cultures.
3. Encourage follow-up (may be for 2 years after acute infection) to ensure eradication of infection and stabilization of kidney function.
4. Explain to the patient and family preventive measures including adequate fluid intake, healthy personal hygiene measures, and voiding habits.

Pyloric Stenosis, Hypertrophic

Hypertrophic pyloric stenosis is congenital, progressive hypertrophy of the muscle of the pylorus, which causes narrowing or obstruction of the pyloric lumen. Constriction of the lumen dilates the stomach, delaying gastric emptying and leading to vomiting after feeding. The disorder has no known cause, and is the second most common condition (after inguinal hernia) that requires surgery during the first 2 months of life. It is more common among females and Caucasians. Severe cases may lead to dehydration, severe electrolyte imbalance, hematemesis, and starvation.

◆ Assessment

1. Onset is within the first 2 months after birth, usually at about 3 weeks of age.
2. Vomiting—onset may be gradual and intermittent, or sudden and forceful. May be occasional and nonprojectile, gradually increasing in frequency and intensity; or projectile vomiting, not bile stained.
3. Constipation—decreased quantity of stools
4. Loss of weight or failure to gain weight
5. Visible gastric peristaltic waves, left to right
6. Excessive hunger—willingness to eat immediately after vomiting
7. Dehydration—electrolyte disturbance with alkalosis
8. Palpable pyloric mass ("olive") in upper right quadrant of abdomen, to the right of the umbilicus, and best felt during feeding or immediately after vomiting

◆ Diagnostic Evaluation

1. Palpation shows pyloric mass in conjunction with persistent, projectile vomiting with associated alkalosis.
2. Blood specimens show metabolic alkalosis.
   a. Sodium—decreased
   b. Chloride—decreased
   c. Potassium—decreased
   d. pH—increased above 7
   e. CO_2—increased
   f. Hematocrit and hemoglobin—elevated because of hemoconcentration
3. Urine becomes alkaline and concentrated.
4. X-rays of abdomen show dilated, air-filled stomach; nondilated pyloric canal.
5. Barium swallow shows narrowed pyloric canal, delayed gastric emptying, enlarged stomach, increased peristaltic waves, and gas distal to stomach.
6. Ultrasound evaluation shows thick hyperechoic ring in the region of the pylorus.

◆ Collaborative Management

Therapeutic Interventions

1. Initial treatment aims to rehydrate to correct electrolytes, correct metabolic alkalosis.
2. Replacement of body fat and protein stores depends on severity of depletion and may require total parenteral nutrition for several days or weeks before surgery to improve surgical risk.

Surgical Interventions

1. Pyloromyotomy (Fredet–Ramstedt procedure)
   a. Hypertrophy of the pyloric muscle regresses to normal size by approximately 12 weeks postoperatively.
   b. Gastroesophageal reflux may be a complication of surgery.

◆ Nursing Interventions

Monitoring

1. Carefully observe output, including amount and characteristics of urine (including specific gravity), also emesis and stools.
2. Accurately measure daily weight as a guide for calculating need for parenteral fluid.
3. Monitor laboratory data for serum electrolytes.
4. Monitor vital signs as indicated by condition. Watch for tachycardia, hypotension, change in respirations.

NURSING ALERT

Irregular respiratory rate with apnea is a sign of severe alkalosis.

5. Monitor blood glucose levels to prevent hypoglycemia.
6. Observe for drainage or signs of inflammation at surgical incision site.

Supportive Care

Preoperative care

1. Administer IV therapy as ordered to treat dehydration, metabolic alkalosis, and electrolyte deficiency.

2. Apply appropriate restraints on infants to prevent interference with fluid therapy
3. Maintain NPO status with indwelling nasogastric tube as ordered. Ensure proper functioning of tube and note drainage.
4. If oral feedings are to be continued, do the following:
   a. Provide small, frequent feedings; give slowly.
   b. Bubble frequently, before, during, and after feeding.
   c. Thicken formula if ordered.
   d. Allow breast-feeding as tolerated.
5. Prop the patient in upright position.
   a. Elevate head of bed, mattress, or infant seat at 75- to 80-degree angle.
   b. Place slightly on right side to aid gastric emptying.
6. Provide mouth care and wet lips frequently if NPO.
7. Let the infant suck on a pacifier.
8. Provide for physical contact or nearness without excessive stimulation.
9. Provide for audio and visual stimulation that may be soothing.
10. Do not palpate pyloric "olive," to decrease risk of postoperative wound infection from bruising abdominal wall and excoriation of tissue in operative site.
11. Administer analgesics as ordered.
12. Assess parents' understanding of diagnosis and plan of care. Provide specific information and clarify any misconceptions.
13. Prepare the parents for the surgery of their child; prepare them for the expected postoperative appearance of the infant.
14. Allow them to hold the infant to maintain bonding.
15. Reassure them that surgery is considered curative, and normal feeding should resume shortly afterward.

Postoperative care
1. Elevate head slightly.
2. Maintain patent nasogastric tube to prevent gastric distention. Record losses.
3. Administer IV fluids until adequate intake has been established.
4. Resume oral feeding 2 to 8 hours after surgery when infant is alert or as ordered.
5. Start with small, frequent feedings of glucose water

and slowly advance to full-strength formula and regular diet, as tolerated.

6. Report any vomiting—the amount and characteristics. Feeding schedule may be withheld 4 hours and then restarted.

7. Feed slowly and bubble frequently.

8. Increase the amount of feeding because the time between feedings is lengthened.

9. Allow breast-feeding to resume as tolerated; begin with limited nursing of 5 to 8 minutes and gradually increase.

10. Continue to elevate the infant's head and shoulders after feeding for 45 to 60 minutes, for several feedings after surgery. Place on right side to aid gastric emptying.

11. Expect that regurgitation may continue for a short period after surgery. Clamped nasogastric tube may be maintained for length of time, as determined by provider.

12. Administer analgesics as ordered and as indicated by behavior of infant.

13. Involve parents in care of infant postoperatively to prepare them for care after discharge.

Family Education and Health Maintenance

1. Teach proper care of the operative site, including watching for signs of infection. Provide specific care of site as ordered by health care provider.

2. Teach feeding technique to be continued at home; length of feeding technique varies, depending on wound healing, nutritional status, and growth. Advise that poor nutritional status may delay wound healing.

3. Provide written and verbal instructions regarding infant's care and follow-up schedule.

4. Review with family when medical attention is needed and appropriate resource:
   a. Signs of infection
   b. Frequent vomiting or poor feeding with signs of dehydration
   c. Abdominal distention

Raynaud's Disease

Raynaud's disease (vasospastic disorder) refers to a condition of increased or unusual sensitivity to cold or emotional factors. It is a form of intermittent arteriolar vasoconstriction that results in coldness, pain, and pallor of fingertips, toes, or the tip of the nose. The cause of Raynaud's disease is unknown, but symptoms must last at least 2 years to confirm the diagnosis. If the disorder is primary, it is called Raynaud's disease; if it is secondary to connective tissue disorders such as polymyositis, systemic lupus erythematosus, and scleroderma, it is called Raynaud's phenomenon or syndrome. Complications include atrophy of skin and muscle of involved digits or ulceration and possible gangrene.

◆ Assessment

1. Characteristic color changes (white to blue to red):
   a. White: blanching, dead-white appearance if vasospasm is severe
   b. Blue: cyanotic, relatively stagnant blood flow
   c. Red: a reactive hyperemia on rewarming; may be accompanied by pain
2. Warmth brings about symptom relief, but it may be delayed.

◆ Diagnostic Evaluation

1. Immunologic tests such as antinuclear antibody (ANA) to rule out connective tissue diseases
2. Arterial Doppler study to rule out acute arterial occlusion if vasospasm is severe

R

◆ Collaborative Management

Therapeutic Interventions

1. Smoking cessation; smoking increases vasoconstriction
2. Protection of extremities from cold
3. Optimal management of underlying disorder

Pharmacologic Interventions

1. Calcium channel–blocking agents to prevent or reduce vasospasm
2. Nitroglycerin or sympatholytics such as reserpine to cause vasodilation. Side effects include headache, dizziness, and orthostatic hypotension, which may necessitate discontinuation.
3. Antiplatelet agents such as aspirin or ticlopidine, or the xanthine derivative pentoxifylline to prevent total occlusion.

Surgical Interventions

1. Sympathectomy (removal of the sympathetic ganglia or division of their branches) in selected cases to maintain vasodilation

◆ Nursing Interventions

Monitoring

1. Monitor condition of toes and fingertips for ulceration and infection.
2. Monitor orthostatic hypotension if vasodilators are used.

Supportive Care and Patient Education

1. Administer and teach the patient about drug therapy.
   a. Stress importance of taking prescribed drugs every day to prevent or minimize symptoms.
   b. Advise the patient to prevent orthostatic hypotension by changing positions slowly if on sympatholytics.
2. Explain to the patient that pain may be experienced when spasm is relieved—hyperemic phase.
3. Administer or teach self-administration of analgesics.
4. Advise the patient that a vasospastic episode may be terminated by placing the hands (or feet) in warm water.

5. Reassure the patient that pain is temporary. However, advise the patient to report persistent pain, ulceration, or signs of infection.
6. Help the patient learn to avoid trigger/aggravating factors of vasoconstriction:
   a. Prevent exposure to cold
   b. Stop smoking
   c. Avoid stressful situations
7. Advise the patient to avoid injuring fingers and hands (eg, needle pricks, knife cuts), which may introduce infection and cause impaired healing.

Rectocele/Enterocele

Rectocele is displacement (protrusion) of the rectum into the vagina. *Enterocele* is displacement of a segment of the intestine into the vagina. These conditions may result from weakening of the posterior vaginal wall caused by obstetric trauma and childbirth, pelvic surgery, or aging.

◆ Assessment

1. Pelvic pressure or heaviness, backache, perineal burning; aggravated by standing for long periods
2. Constipation—may have difficulty in fecal evacuation; the patient may insert fingers into vagina to push feces up so defecation may take place
3. Fecal incontinence and flatus may occur with tear between rectum and vagina.
4. Visible protrusion into vagina when patient bears down or stands

◆ Diagnostic Evaluation

1. Vaginal examination to detect condition
2. May use Sims speculum to uplift cervix and fully evaluate condition

◆ Collaborative Management

Therapeutic and Pharmacologic Interventions

1. Vaginal pessary to insert into vagina to temporarily support pelvic organs

R

a. Prolonged use may lead to necrosis and ulceration.
b. Should be removed and cleaned every 1 to 2 months
2. Estrogen therapy after menopause to decrease genital atrophy

Surgical Interventions

1. If rectocele is large and interferes with bowel functioning, may do posterior colpoplasty (perineorrhaphy)—repair of posterior vaginal wall

◆ Nursing Interventions

Supportive Care

1. Encourage periods of rest with legs elevated to relieve pelvic strain and teach Kegel exercises.
2. Encourage use of mild analgesics as needed.
3. Provide postoperative care:
   a. Suggest low Fowler's position to decrease edema and discomfort.
   b. Administer perineal care to the patient after each voiding and defecation.
   c. Employ a heat lamp to help dry the incision line and enhance the healing process.
   d. Use ice packs locally to relieve congestion and discomfort.
   e. Administer analgesics and stool softeners as ordered.
4. Teach the patient to increase fluid and fiber in diet.
5. Encourage use of stool softeners or bulk laxatives to make passage of stool easier.
6. Enema may be necessary to prevent straining.

Patient Education and Health Maintenance

1. Advise the patient to avoid straining and obesity, which may cause return of rectocele or enterocele.
2. Encourage patient to follow-up and report bowel problems.

Regional Enteritis
See Crohn's Disease

Renal Cell Carcinoma
See Cancer, Renal Cell

Renal Failure, Acute

Acute renal failure (ARF) is a sudden decline in renal function, usually marked by increased serum concentrations of urea (azotemia) and creatinine; oliguria (less than 500 mL urine in 24 hours); hyperkalemia; and sodium retention. ARF has many causes, which are classified as prerenal, postrenal, and intrarenal. Prerenal failure results from conditions that interrupt the renal blood supply, thereby reducing renal perfusion (hypovolemia, shock, hemorrhage, burns, impaired cardiac output, diuretic therapy). Postrenal failure results from obstruction of urine flow. Intrarenal failure results from injury to the kidneys themselves (ischemia, toxins, immunologic processes, systemic and vascular disorders).

Whatever the cause, ARF progresses through three clinically distinct phases (oliguric–anuric, diuretic, and recovery), distinguished primarily by changes in urine volumes and serum blood urea nitrogen (BUN) and creatinine levels. The disorder can be reversed with medical treatment. Untreated ARF progresses to chronic renal failure, end-stage renal disease, and death from uremia or related causes.

◆ Assessment

1. Oliguric–anuric phase: urine volume less than 400 mL/ 24 hours; increase in serum creatinine, urea, uric acid, organic acids, potassium, and magnesium; lasts 3 to 5 days in infants and children, 10 to 14 days in adolescents and adults
2. Diuretic phase: begins when urine output exceeds 500 mL/24 hours, ends when BUN and creatinine levels stop rising; length is variable
3. Recovery phase: asymptomatic; lasts several months to 1 year
4. In prerenal disease, note decreased tissue turgor, dryness of mucous membranes, weight loss, hypotension.
5. In postrenal disease, note difficulty in voiding; changes in urine flow.
6. In intrarenal disease, note fever, skin rash, edema.

7. Nausea, vomiting, diarrhea, and lethargy may also occur.

◆ Diagnostic Evaluation

1. Urinalysis shows proteinuria, hematuria, casts. Urine chemistry distinguishes various forms of ARF (prerenal, postrenal, intrarenal).
2. Serum creatinine and BUN levels elevated; arterial blood gases, serum electrolytes may be abnormal.
3. Renal ultrasonography, to estimate renal size and to rule out treatable obstructive uropathy

◆ Collaborative Management

Preventive Interventions

1. Identify patients with preexisting renal disease.
2. Initiate adequate hydration before, during, and after operative procedures.
3. Avoid exposure to various nephrotoxins. Be aware that most drugs or their metabolites are excreted by the kidneys. Ensure that dosages are adjusted to the degree of renal impairment of individual patients.
4. Avoid chronic analgesic abuse—causes interstitial nephritis and papillary necrosis.
5. Prevent and treat shock with blood and fluid replacement. Prevent prolonged periods of hypotension.
6. Monitor urinary output and central venous pressure hourly in critically ill patients to detect onset of renal failure at the earliest moment.
7. Schedule diagnostic studies requiring dehydration so that there are "rest days," especially in elderly patients who may not have adequate renal reserve.
8. Pay special attention to draining wounds, burns, etc., which can lead to dehydration, sepsis, and progressive renal damage.
9. Avoid infection; give meticulous care to patients with indwelling catheters and intravenous lines.
10. Take every precaution to ensure that the right person receives the right blood, to avoid severe transfusion reactions, which can precipitate renal complications.

Therapeutic Interventions

1. Surgical relief of obstruction may be necessary.
2. Correction of underlying fluid excesses or deficits
3. Correction and control of biochemical imbalances
   a. Hyperkalemia: give glucose and insulin to shift potassium into cells; cation exchange resin orally or by enema to promote rectal excretion of potassium
   b. Acidosis: give sodium bicarbonate; be prepared for mechanical ventilation
4. Restoration and maintenance of blood pressure through IV fluids and vasopressors
5. Maintenance of adequate nutrition: low-protein diet with supplemental amino acids and vitamins
6. Initiation of hemodialysis, peritoneal dialysis, or continuous renal replacement therapy for patients with progressive azotemia and other life-threatening complications

◆ Nursing Interventions

Monitoring

1. Monitor 24-hour urine volumes to follow clinical course of the disease.
2. Monitor BUN, creatinine, and electrolytes.
3. Monitor for signs and symptoms of hypovolemia or hypervolemia because regulating capacity of kidneys is inadequate.
4. Monitor urine specific gravity; measure and record intake and output, including urine, gastric suction, stools, wound drainage, perspiration (estimate).
5. Report signs and symptoms of hyperkalemia.
   a. Notify health care provider of value above 5.5 mEq/L.
   b. Watch for electrocardiographic (ECG) changes indicating hyperkalemia: tall, tented T waves; depressed ST segment; wide QRS complex.
6. Monitor ABGs as necessary to evaluate acid–base balance.
7. Weigh the patient daily to provide an index of fluid balance; expected weight loss is 0.25 to 0.5 kg ($\frac{1}{2}$ to 1 lb) daily.
8. Measure blood pressure at various times of the day

with patients in supine, sitting, and standing positions.

9. Monitor for all signs of infection. Be aware that renal failure patients do not always demonstrate fever and leukocytosis.

10. Watch for and report mental status changes: somnolence, lassitude, lethargy, and fatigue progressing to irritability, disorientation, twitching, seizures.

Supportive Care

1. Adjust fluid intake to avoid volume overload and dehydration.
   a. Fluid restriction is not usually initiated until renal function is quite low.
   b. Give only enough fluids to replace losses during oliguric–anuric phase (usually 400–500 mL every 24 hours plus measured fluid losses).
   c. Fluid allowance should be distributed throughout the day.
   d. Restrict sodium and water intake if there is evidence of extracellular excess.

❖

NURSING ALERT
Avoid restricting fluids for prolonged periods for laboratory and radiologic examinations, because dehydrating procedures are hazardous to patients who cannot produce concentrated urine.

2. Watch for cardiac dysrhythmias and congestive heart failure from hyperkalemia, electrolyte imbalance, or fluid overload. Have resuscitation equipment available in case of cardiac arrest.

3. If ordered, prepare for dialysis when rapid lowering of potassium is needed. Administer blood transfusions during dialysis to remove excess potassium.

4. Watch for signs of urinary tract infection, and remove bladder catheter as soon possible.

5. Employ intensive pulmonary hygiene, because incidence of pulmonary edema and infection are high.

6. Provide meticulous wound care.

7. Work with the dietician to regulate protein intake according to the type of renal impairment. Protein

and potassium are usually restricted. Be aware that food and fluids containing large amounts of sodium and phosphorus may need to be restricted.

8. Offer high-carbohydrate feedings, because carbohydrates have a greater protein-sparing power and provide additional calories.

9. Prepare for hyperalimentation when adequate nutrition cannot be maintained through the GI tract. Nutrients can also be added through dialysate.

10. To prevent or treat gastric bleeding caused by stress ulcers:
    a. Examine all stools and emesis for gross and occult blood.
    b. Administer H_2-receptor antagonists or antacids as prophylaxis for gastric stress ulcers. If H_2-receptor antagonist is used, care must be taken to adjust the dose for the degree of renal impairment.
    c. Prepare for endoscopy when GI bleeding occurs.

11. Employ seizure precautions. Provide padded side rails and have airway and suction equipment at the bedside.

12. Encourage and assist the patient to turn and move, because drowsiness and lethargy may reduce activity.

Family Education and Health Maintenance

1. Explain that the patient may experience residual defects in kidney function for a long time after acute illness.

2. Encourage the patient to report for routine urinalysis and follow-up examinations.

3. Advise avoidance of *any* medications unless specifically prescribed.

4. Recommend resuming activity gradually, because muscle weakness will be present from excessive catabolism.

Renal Failure, Chronic

Chronic renal failure (CRF, end-stage renal disease, ESRD) is a progressive deterioration of renal function, which ends fatally in uremia (an excess of urea and other nitrogenous wastes in the blood) and its complications unless dialysis or a kidney transplantation is performed. Typically, the disease produces few signs and symptoms until approximately 75% of renal function (glomerular filtration) has already been lost.

Causes of CRF include prolonged, severe hypertension; diabetes mellitus; polycystic disease; glomerulopathies and hereditary renal disease (common causes in children aged 5–15 years); interstitial nephritis; obstructive uropathy; and developmental or congenital disorders (common causes in children younger than 5 years).

As renal function deteriorates, the disease may progress through four stages: 1) decreased renal reserve; 2) renal insufficiency; 3) renal failure; and 4) end-stage renal disease, leading to uremia.

◆ Assessment

1. Cardiovascular manifestations: hyperkalemic ECG changes, hypertension caused by increased aldosterone secretion, congestive heart failure (CHF), pericarditis, pericardial effusion, pericardial tamponade
2. Respiratory manifestations: pulmonary edema, pleural effusions, pleural friction rub
3. GI manifestations: anorexia, nausea, vomiting, hiccoughs, ulceration of GI tract, hemorrhage
4. Neuromuscular manifestations: fatigue, sleep disorders, headache, lethargy, muscular irritability, peripheral neuropathy, seizures, coma
5. Metabolic and endocrine manifestations: glucose intolerance, hyperlipidemia, and sex hormone disturbances causing decreased libido, impotence, and amenorrhea
6. Fluid, electrolyte, and acid–base balance: usually salt and water retention but may be sodium loss with dehydration, acidosis, hyperkalemia, hypomagnesemia, hypocalcemia (Table 15)
7. Dermatologic manifestations: pallor, hyperpigmentation, pruritus, ecchymoses, uremic frost
8. Skeletal manifestations: renal osteodystrophy resulting in osteomalacia
9. Hematologic manifestations: anemia caused by re-

TABLE 15 Signs and Symptoms of Fluid and Electrolyte Imbalances

	Deficit	Excess
Volume	Acute weight loss (>5%), drop in body temperature, dry skin and mucous membranes, postural hypotension, longitudinal wrinkles or furrows of tongue, oliguria or anuria	Acute weight gain (>5%), edema, hypertension, distended neck veins, dyspnea, rales
Sodium	Abdominal cramps, apprehension, convulsions, fingerprinting on sternum, oliguria or anuria	Dry, sticky mucous membranes, flushed skin, oliguria or anuria, thirst, rough and dry tongue
Potassium	Anorexia, abdominal distention, intestinal ileus, muscle weakness, tenderness, and cramps	Diarrhea, intestinal colic, irritability, nausea, parasthesias, flaccid paralysis, cardiac arrhythmias and arrest
Calcium	Abdominal cramps, positive Chvostek and Trousseau signs, tingling of extremities, tetany	Anorexia, nausea, vomiting, abdominal pain and distention, mental confusion
Bicarbonate	Deep, rapid breathing (Kussmaul), shortness of breath on exertion, stupor, weakness (metabolic acidosis)	Depressed respirations, muscle hypertonicity, tetany (metabolic alkalosis)
Magnesium	Positive Chvostek's sign, seizures, disorientation, hyperactive deep tendon reflexes, tremor	Hypotension, flushing, lethargy, dysarthria, hypoactive deep tendon reflexes, respiratory depression

duced erythropoietin from kidney; reduced platelet quality, increased bleeding tendencies
10. Alterations in psychosocial functions: personality and behavior changes, alteration in cognitive processes
11. Developmental manifestations: growth retardation, delayed sexual maturation

◆ Diagnostic Evaluation

1. CBC shows anemia
2. Elevated serum creatinine or BUN, phosphorus
3. Decreased serum calcium, bicarbonate, and proteins, especially albumin
4. ABGs show low pH, high CO_2

◆ Collaborative Management

Therapeutic Interventions

1. Detect and treat reversible causes of renal failure:
   a. Control diabetes.
   b. Treat hypertension.
2. Initiate fluid restriction and diet therapy:
   a. Low-protein diet supplemented with essential amino acids or their keto-analogues to minimize uremic toxicity and prevent wasting and malnutrition
   b. Limit potassium intake.
   c. Decrease dietary phosphorus (chicken, milk, legumes, carbonated beverages).
3. Institute maintenance dialysis or kidney transplantation when symptoms can no longer be controlled with conservative measures.

Pharmacologic Interventions

1. Treat anemia with recombinant human erythropoietin, a synthetic kidney hormone that enhances red blood cell (RBC) formation.
2. Treat acidosis with oral or IV sodium bicarbonate to replace bicarbonate stores.
3. Administer a cation exchange resin to promote enteric excretion of potassium.
4. Administer phosphate-binding agents because they bind phosphorus in the intestinal tract.

5. Growth hormone administration to treat growth retardation

◆ Nursing Interventions

Monitoring

1. Evaluate for signs and symptoms of hyperkalemia and monitor serum potassium levels.
   a. Notify health care provider of value above 5.5 mEq/L.
   b. Watch for dysrhythmias and electrocardiographic (ECG) changes indicating hyperkalemia: tall, tented T waves; depressed ST segment; wide QRS complex.
2. Monitor arterial blood gases (ABGs) as necessary to evaluate acid–base balance.
3. Weigh the patient daily and maintain intake and output.
4. Monitor for edema and respiratory compromise from fluid volume excess.
5. Monitor hemoglobin and hematocrit.
6. Monitor for all signs of infection. Be aware that renal failure patients do not always demonstrate fever and leukocytosis.

Supportive Care

1. Administer parenteral nutrition or oral supplements if unable to maintain adequate diet
2. Keep skin clean while relieving itching and dryness.
   a. "Basis" soap
   b. Sodium bicarbonate added to bath water
   c. Oatmeal baths
   d. Adding bath oil to bath water
3. Apply ointments or creams for comfort and to relieve itching.
4. Keep nails short and trimmed to prevent excoriation.
5. Keep hair clean and moisturized.
6. Administer oral antipruritics, if indicated.
7. To prevent constipation caused by phosphate binders, encourage high-fiber diet, bearing in mind the potassium content of some fruits and vegetables.
   a. Commercial fiber supplements (Fiberall; Fiber-Med) may be prescribed.
   b. Employ stool softeners as prescribed.

   c. Avoid laxatives and cathartics that cause electrolyte toxicities (compounds containing magnesium or phosphorus).

   d. Increase activity as tolerated.

8. To help ensure safe activity level, assess patient's gait, range of motion, and muscle strength.

9. Administer analgesics as ordered and provide massage for severe muscle cramps.

10. Increase activity as tolerated; avoid immobilization, because it increases bone demineralization.

11. Explore alternatives that may reduce or eliminate side effects of treatment.

   a. Adjust schedule so rest can be achieved after dialysis.

   b. Smaller, more frequent meals to reduce nausea and facilitate medication taking

12. Contract with the patient for behavioral changes if patient is noncompliant with therapy or control of underlying condition.

Family Education and Health Maintenance

1. To promote adherence to the therapeutic program, teach the following:

   a. Weigh every morning to avoid fluid overload.

   b. Drink limited amounts *only* when thirsty.

   c. Measure allotted fluids and save some for ice cubes; sucking on ice is thirst quenching.

   d. Eat food before drinking fluids to alleviate dry mouth.

   e. Use hard candy, chewing gum—to moisten mouth.

2. Encourage strengthening of social support system and coping mechanisms to lessen the impact of the stress of chronic kidney disease.

3. Advise patient of financial and other support through social service agencies.

Respiratory Distress Syndrome

Respiratory distress syndrome (RDS, hyaline membrane disease) is a progressive and frequently fatal respiratory failure resulting from lack of alveolar surfactant, a lipoprotein that functions to maintain alveolar patency. The syndrome occurs most frequently in premature infants weighing between 1,000 and 1,500 g (2.2–3.3 lbs) and between 28 and 37 weeks' gestation; incidence increases with the degree of prematurity. Without vigorous treatment, alveolar collapse leads to atelectasis, hypoxia, acidosis, and death.

Respiratory distress syndrome is usually self-limiting; moderately ill infants or those who do not require assisted ventilation usually show slow improvement by approximately 48 hours and rapid recovery over the next 3 to 4 days with few complications. However, severely ill and very immature infants who require some ventilatory assistance usually demonstrate rapid deterioration. Ventilatory assistance may be required for several days, and chronic lung disease and other complications are common.

◆ Assessment

1. Symptoms of RDS are usually observed soon after birth.
2. Retractions (sternal, suprasternal, substernal, and intercostal), progressing to paradoxical seesaw respirations
3. Tachypnea, nasal flaring
4. Expiratory grunting or whining sounds when not crying (indicates an attempt to maintain positive end-expiratory pressure [PEEP] and prevent alveoli from collapsing)
5. Cyanosis with room air
6. Diminished breath sounds and presence of dry "sandpaper" breath sounds
7. As the disease progresses: marked abdominal protrusion on expiration, peripheral edema, decreased muscle tone, increasing cyanosis, hypothermia, apnea, bradycardia, pale and grayish skin color
   a. Lethargic or listless
   b. Activity and response to stimuli
8. Assess the infant's cry.
9. Assess the skin for cyanosis, jaundice, mottling, paleness or grayness, edema.

R

◆ Diagnostic Evaluation

1. Arterial blood gas (ABG) analysis:
   a. PCO_2: elevated
   b. PO_2: low
   c. pH: low because of respiratory or metabolic acidosis
2. Serum calcium: low
3. Chest x-ray shows diffuse, fine granularity reflecting fluid-filled alveoli and atelectasis of some alveoli, surrounded by hyperdistended bronchioles. This is known as "ground glass" appearance with prominent air bronchogram extending into periphery of lung fields.
4. Pulmonary function studies may be done to evaluate stiff lung with reduced effective pulmonary blood flow.

◆ Collaborative Management

Therapeutic Interventions

Supportive
1. Maintenance of oxygenation: PaO_2 at 60 to 80 mm Hg to prevent hypoxia; frequent arterial pH and blood gas measurements
2. Maintenance of respiration with ventilatory support if necessary—intermittent mandatory ventilations plus PEEP, or continuous positive airway pressure (CPAP)
3. Maintenance of normal body temperature
4. Constant observation for complications: pneumothorax, disseminated intravascular coagulation (DIC), patent ductus arteriosus (PDA) with heart failure, chronic lung disease

Aggressive
1. High-frequency ventilation: mechanical ventilation that uses rapid rates (can be greater than 900 breaths/min) and tidal volumes near and often less than anatomic dead spaces
   a. Jet ventilator delivers short burst of gases at high flow with passive exhalation. Necrotizing tracheitis is a significant complication.
   b. Oscillator ventilator delivers gases by vibrating columns of air with active exhalation. The child appears to shake on the bed, which may be frightening for parents.
2. Extracorporeal membrane oxygenation (ECMO):

modified heart–lung bypass machine used to allow gas exchange outside the body

  a. Blood is removed from the venous system by a catheter placed in the internal jugular vein or right atrium.

  b. Oxygen is added and carbon dioxide removed with a membrane oxygenator.

  c. Oxygenated blood is returned by way of the right common carotid (in venoarterial ECMO) or the femoral vein (in venovenous ECMO).

  d. The infant must be heparinized for the procedure, increasing the risk of intraventricular hemorrhage. For this reason, very-low-birth-weight (VLBW) infants or infants of decreased gestational age are usually not candidates for the procedure.

Pharmacologic Interventions

Supportive

1. Maintenance of fluid, electrolyte, and acid–base balance—sodium bicarbonate is given to buffer metabolic acidosis
2. Nutrition maintained with IV dextrose 10%
3. Antibiotics as needed to treat infection

Aggressive

1. Administration of exogenous surfactant into lungs early in the disease
   a. Especially beneficial in the very-low-birth-weight infant
   b. May be given preventively to VLBW infants at birth
   c. Available preparations: bovine (Survanta) and synthetic (Exosurf) surfactant
   d. Administered into the endotracheal tube; suction avoided for a few hours after instillation

◆ Nursing Interventions

Monitoring

1. Institute cardiorespiratory monitoring to continuously monitor heart and respiratory rates.
2. Monitor for complications related to respiratory therapy:
   a. Air leak: pneumothorax, pneumomediastinum, pneumopericardium, and pneumoperitoneum

    b. Pneumonia, especially gram-negative organisms
    c. Pulmonary interstitial emphysema
3. Measure and record oxygen concentration with mechanical ventilation every hour.
4. Monitor ABGs as appropriate. Obtain sample through indwelling catheter (usually placed in the umbilical artery), arterial puncture, or capillary puncture.
5. Institute pulse oximetry for continuous monitoring of oxygen saturation of arterial blood (SaO_2).
    a. Avoid using adhesive to secure the sensor when infant is active. Wrap the sensor snugly enough around the foot to reduce sensitivity to movement but not tight enough to constrict blood flow.
    b. If transcutaneous PO_2 monitoring ($TcPO_2$) is used, reposition the probe every 3 to 4 hours to avoid burns caused when the probe is heated to achieve sufficient vasodilation.
6. Observe the infant's response to oxygen.
    a. Observe for improvement in color, respiratory rate and pattern, and nasal flaring.
    b. Note response by improvement in arterial pH, PO_2, PCO_2, or capillary blood gas.
    c. Observe closely for apnea.

PEDIATRIC ALERT
Stimulate infant if apnea occurs. If unable to produce spontaneous respiration with stimulation within 15 to 30 seconds, initiate resuscitation.

---

7. If umbilical artery catheter is in place, monitor for bleeding.
8. When providing IV fluids or enteral nutrition, observe infusion rate closely to prevent fluid overload. Also monitor for hypoglycemia, which is especially common during stress. Maintain serum glucose greater than 45 mg/dL.
9. Monitor intake and output closely and weigh infant daily.

Supportive Care
1. Have emergency resuscitation equipment readily available for use in the event of cardiac or respiratory arrest.

2. Administer supplemental oxygen.
   a. Incubator with oxygen at prescribed concentration
   b. Plastic hood with oxygen at prescribed concentration when using radiant warmer
   c. CPAP if indicated via face mask, nasal prongs, or endotracheal tube
3. Assist with endotracheal intubation and maintain mechanical ventilation as indicated.
4. Position the infant to allow for maximal lung expansion.
   a. Prone position provides for a larger lung volume because of the position of the diaphragm; decreases energy expenditure; and increases time spent in quiet sleep.
   b. May be contraindicated when umbilical artery catheter is in place
   c. Change position frequently.

PEDIATRIC ALERT
Prone position may present several problems: turning head to side can compromise upper airway and increase air flow resistance; observation of chest is obstructed, retractions are more difficult to detect, and abdominal distension is more difficult to recognize.

---

5. Suction as needed because the gag reflex is weak and cough is ineffective.
6. Try to minimize time spent on procedures and interventions, and monitor effects on respiratory status. (Infants undergoing multiple procedures lasting 45 minutes to 1 hour have shown a moderate decrease in PO_2).
7. Provide adequate caloric intake (80–120 kcal/kg per 24 hours) through nasojejunal tube (best tolerated by VLBW infants), nasogastric tube, or parenteral nutrition.
8. Provide a neutral thermal environment to maintain the infant's abdominal skin temperature between 97° and 98°F (36° and 36.5°C) to prevent hypothermia, which may result in vasoconstriction and acidosis.

R

9. Adjust Isolette or radiant warmer to obtain desired skin temperature.
   a. For the infant weighing less than 1,250 g, the radiant warmer should be used with caution because of increased water loss and potential for hypoglycemia.
   b. Prevent frequent opening of Isolette.
10. Ensure that O_2 is warmed to 87.6° to 93.2°F. (32°–34°C) with 60% to 80% humidity.
11. Allow the parents to hold the infant as soon as possible and participate in care.
12. If the mother plans to breast-feed, assist her with pumping, and use the breast milk to feed the infant when enteral feedings are initiated.
13. If the infant has been transported to a tertiary care center immediately after birth, prepare the parents for the neonatal intensive care unit, and update them on the infant's condition until they are able to visit.
14. If the infant has siblings, advise the parents on how to discuss the infant's illness with them.
15. Help the parents work through their grief at the birth of a premature child.

Family Education and Health Management

1. Prepare the family for long-term follow-up as appropriate. Infants with bronchopulmonary dysplasia (BPD) may eventually go home on oxygen therapy.
2. Stress the importance of regular health care, periodic eye examinations, and developmental follow-up with the parents.
3. Ensure that the family receives information on routine well baby care.

Respiratory Failure

Respiratory failure is an alteration in the function of the respiratory system that causes the PaO_2 to decrease to below 50 mm Hg (hypoxemia) or the $PaCO_2$ to increase to above 50 mm Hg (hypercapnia), as determined by arterial blood gas (ABG) analysis.

This complex condition is more a dysfunction than a

disease, and occurs in several recognized forms. *Acute respiratory failure* (ARF) occurs rapidly, usually within minutes to hours or days, and is marked by hypoxemia or hypercapnia and acidemia (pH less than 7.35); *chronic respiratory failure* occurs over a period of months to years, allowing compensatory mechanisms to operate; it is marked by hypoxemia or hypercapnia with a normal pH (7.35–7.40). *Acute and chronic respiratory failure* may occur after an acute upper respiratory infection or pneumonia (or without obvious cause) and is marked by an abrupt increase in hypoxemia or hypercapnia in patients with preexisting chronic respiratory failure.

Respiratory failure results from three physiologic conditions that increase the work of breathing and decrease respiratory drive: oxygenation failure, ventilatory failure in normal lungs, and ventilatory failure in intrinsic lung disease.

Causes of *oxygenation failure* include cardiogenic pulmonary edema and adult respiratory distress syndrome (ARDS) from shock of any cause, infections, trauma, near drowning, inhaled toxins, severe hematologic conditions, and metabolic disorders.

Causes of *ventilatory failure in normal lungs* include narcotic overdose, general anesthesia, cerebral vascular insufficiency, brain tumor or trauma, increased intracranial pressure, neuromuscular disease, chest wall trauma (multiple fractures), or spinal cord trauma.

Causes of *ventilatory failure in intrinsic lung disease* include chronic obstructive pulmonary disease (COPD; chronic bronchitis, emphysema, cystic fibrosis) and severe asthma.

Complications of respiratory failure include oxygen toxicity from the prolonged high fractional inspired oxygen (FIO_2) required, barotrauma from mechanical ventilation, or death.

◆ Assessment

1. Diaphoresis, rapid shallow breathing, abdominal paradox (inward movement of abdominal wall during inspiration), and intercostal retractions suggest inability to maintain adequate minute ventilation.

2. Diminished or absent sounds indicating inability to ventilate the lungs sufficiently to prevent atelectasis
3. Crackles caused by secretions and interstitial fluid and wheezing indicating bronchospasm
4. Confusion, restlessness, agitation, disorientation, delirium, and loss of consciousness signify hypoxemia; headache, somnolence, dizziness, and confusion signify hypercapnia.

◆ Diagnostic Evaluation

1. Arterial blood gases (ABGs) show deviations in PaO_2, $PaCO_2$, and pH from patient's normal; or PaO_2 less than 50 mm Hg, $PaCO_2$ greater than 50 mm Hg, and pH less than 7.35.
2. Pulse oximetry to detect decreasing SaO_2
3. End-tidal CO_2 monitoring (capnography) shows increase.
4. CBC, serum electrolytes, urinalysis, and cultures (blood, sputum) to determine underlying cause and patient's condition
5. Chest x-ray may show underlying disease.

Therapeutic Interventions

1. Oxygen therapy to maintain PaO_2 of 60 mm Hg or $SaO_2 > 90\%$. Use aerosol mask, partial rebreathing mask, or non-rebreathing mask to provide high oxygen concentration.

Pharmacologic Interventions

1. Antibiotics, cardiac medications, and diuretics to treat underlying disorder
2. Bronchodilators to reduce bronchospasm and corticosteroids to reduce airway inflammation; given orally, IV, or by nebulization
3. IV fluids and mucolytics to reduce sputum viscosity

◆ Nursing Interventions

Monitoring

1. Monitor fluid balance by measuring intake and output, urine specific gravity, daily weights, and pulmonary capillary wedge pressures to detect hypovolemia or hypervolemia.

R

2. Monitor vital capacity (VC), respiratory rate, minute ventilation (V_E), and negative inspiratory force (NIF). Values indicating need for mechanical ventilation:
   a. VC <10 to 15 mL/kg
   b. Respiratory rate > 35 breaths/min
   c. V_E >10 L/min
   d. NIF < −20 to −25 cm H_2O
3. Monitor ABGs and compare with previous values.
   a. If the patient cannot maintain a minute ventilation sufficient to prevent CO_2 retention, the pH will decrease.
   b. Mechanical ventilation may be needed if the pH decreases to <7.30.

NURSING ALERT

Obtain ABGs whenever the history or signs and symptoms suggest the patient is at risk for developing respiratory failure. Initial and subsequent values should be recorded on a flow sheet so that comparisons can be made over time. Need for ABG can be decreased by using an oximeter to continuously monitor the SaO_2.

Supportive Care

1. Provide measures to prevent atelectasis and promote chest expansion and secretion clearance, such as chest physiotherapy, pursed-lip breathing, incentive spirometry.
2. If the patient becomes increasingly lethargic, cannot cough or expectorate secretions, cannot cooperate with therapy, or if pH decreases to below 7.30, despite use of the above therapy, report and prepare to assist with intubation and initiation of mechanical ventilation.
3. Suction frequently to prevent buildup of secretions that will interfere with oxygenation, but avoid prolonged episodes of suctioning while on mechanical ventilation to prevent hypoxia.
4. Provide meticulous care while intubated to prevent infection.

5. Provide calm, confident care and reassurance during the weaning process to prevent dependence on mechanical ventilation.

Patient Education and Health Maintenance

1. Instruct patient with preexisting pulmonary disease to seek early intervention for infections to prevent acute respiratory failure.
2. Encourage patients at risk, especially the elderly and those with preexisting lung disease, to get yearly influenza and one-time pneumococcal pneumonia immunizations.

Respiratory Infections in Children

Respiratory tract infections are a common cause of acute illness in infants and children. Many pediatric infections are seasonal. Response of the child to the infection will vary based on the age of the child, causative organism, general health of the child, and existence of chronic medical conditions, as well as the degree of contact with other children. Information about specific respiratory infections, including bacterial pneumonia, viral pneumonia, *Pneumocystis* pneumonia, *Mycoplasma* pneumonia, bronchiolitis, croup, and epiglottitis may be found in Table 16.

◆ Assessment

1. Infants: poor feeding, vomiting, diarrhea, fever, tachypnea, grunting, nasal flaring, retractions
2. Older children: runny nose, headache, anorexia, fever, dry cough
3. Possible pharyngitis and otitis
4. Possible crackles and wheezes

◆ Diagnostic Evaluation

1. Chest x-ray shows patchy or disseminated infiltrate with pneumonia
2. Sputum cultures may isolate organism.
3. Complete blood count may show increased white

blood cells of predominantly neutrophils or lymphocytes based on cause.
4. Lateral neck x-ray shows subglottic edema in croup,
severely narrowed airway and pseudomembrane in
bacterial tracheitis, and epiglottic edema in epiglottitis.

◆ Collaborative Management

See Table 16.

◆ Nursing Interventions

Monitoring

1. Monitor for inspiratory stridor and retractions in epiglottis and report immediately.
2. Monitor for increasing respiratory difficulty signifying
need for oxygen, intubation, and respiratory support.
3. Observe the child's response to antibiotic therapy, including drug sensitivity.
4. Check temperature regularly to determine effectiveness of antipyretic medications.
5. Record the child's intake and output and monitor urine
specific gravity to identify dehydration.

Supportive Care

1. Provide a humidified environment enriched with oxygen to combat hypoxia and to liquefy secretions.
2. Use a Croupette with cool mist or ultrasonic mist in
tent to moisten airway, minimize fluid loss from lungs,
liquefy and mobilize respiratory secretions, and allow
for oxygen therapy up to 40% concentration.

PEDIATRIC ALERT
At no time should the mist be allowed to become so dense
that it obscures clear visualization of the child's respiratory
pattern.

---

3. Place the child in a comfortable position to promote
easier ventilation.
   a. Semi-Fowler's: use pillows, infant seat, or elevate
   head of bed.

(text continues on page 736)

TABLE 16 Common Pediatric Respiratory Infections

Condition and Description	Treatment
Pneumococcal pneumonia: Caused by gram-positive *Streptococcus pneumoniae*. Mild upper respiratory infection (URI) with sudden symptom onset. This type of bacterial pneumonia is most frequent in children, especially with cystic fibrosis or lack of spleen. Occurs from birth to age 2, primarily in winter and spring	1. Penicillin G or other antibiotics, including erythromycin, clindamycin, chloramphenicol, cephalosporins, ampicillin, trimethoprim-sulfamethoxazole 2. Bronchodilators 3. Monitor for complications of otitis media, sinusitis, empyema, bacteremia.
Streptococcal pneumonia Caused by gram-positive, beta-hemolytic *Streptococcus* group A Primarily occurs at ages 3–5 years, commonly superimposed on a viral infection.	1. Penicillin G 2. Cephalosporins 3. Monitor for complications of empyema, pneumatocele, pneumothorax, and permanent pulmonary fibrosis.
Staphylococcal pneumonia Caused by gram-positive, coagulase-positive *Staphylococcus aureus*. Occurs from birth to age 2, primarily from October to May Predisposing factors include maternal infection, cystic fibrosis, immunodeficiency.	1. Methicillin or other antibiotics, including chloramphenicol, penicillin G; ampicillin if organism is not resistant 2. Rapid treatment is important. 3. Methicillin-resistant *S. aureus* poses a real threat to other hospitalized children; take care to prevent nosocomial infection. 4. Monitor for complications of empyema, pneumothorax, lung abscess, osteomyelitis, pericarditis, and bronchiectasis.
Haemophilus influenzae pneumonia (Type B) Occurs from age 6 months to 3 years	1. Chloramphenicol, ampicillin, cephalosporins 2. Cough suppressant

Commonly associated infections include otitis media, meningitis, and epiglottitis.

3. Monitor for signs of associated upper respiratory tract impairment (stridor, dusky color, drooling in the older child).

4. Respiratory isolation should be instituted until 24 hours after appropriate antibiotic therapy is initiated.

Viral Pneumonia

Most commonly caused by respiratory syncytial virus (RSV); also by parainfluenza virus types 1, 2, and 3; adenoviruses; influenza viruses

Occurs from birth to age 2 years, usually in winter and early spring; affects more boys than girls

Gradual onset follows an upper respiratory infection.

Infants with RSV have significant respiratory distress and apneic spells.

Parainfluenza virus causes coryza and pharyngitis.

Adenovirus causes pharyngitis and cervical adenitis.

1. Broad-spectrum antibiotic therapy initiated until causative organism isolated.

2. Aerosolized ribavirin for RSV

3. Monitor the infant closely for respiratory fatigue; may need supplemental oxygen or intubation for ventilatory support.

4. RSV may be a life-threatening disease for the infant or young child with chronic cardiac or respiratory disease.

5. Institute respiratory and contact isolation for child with RSV.

Pneumocystis Pneumonia

Caused by *Pneumocystis carinii*, a sporozoan parasite. Predisposing factors include premature or debilitated infant, infectious disease, cystic fibrosis, immunosuppressive therapy, HIV-positive status, immunodeficiency disease. Onset is slow, peaking in 3 to 6 weeks.

1. Trimethoprim-sulfamethoxazole is drug of choice.

2. Pentamidine may be used, either IV or via nebulizer.

3. Supplemental oxygen

4. Supplemental immunoglobulin IV may be given.

5. Institute respiratory isolation for 48 hours after initiation of therapy

6. Monitor for concomitant bacterial pneumonia and sepsis.

(continued)

TABLE 16 *(Continued)*

Condition and Description	Treatment
Mycoplasma Pneumonia Caused by *M. pneumoniae*, which has characteristics of both bacteria and viruses. Occurs at ages 10 to 15 years. Onset is slow, requiring 2- to 3-week incubation period. May be fatal if infection becomes systemic or child has preexisting lung disease.	1. Erythromycin or other macrolide antibiotic 2. Tetracycline for children older than age 9 3. Institute secretion precautions.
Bronchiolitis Inflammation of bronchioles. Caused by RSV, adenovirus, parainfluenza virus types 1 or 3, influenza virus, and *M. pneumoniae*. Most common in infants younger than age 6 months; may occur in children up to age 2 Onset gradual after exposure to individual with respiratory infection. Occurs primarily in winter and spring; incidence rising in day-care centers.	1. Broad-spectrum antibiotic therapy initiated until causative organism isolated 2. Bronchodilators via nebulizer 3. Ribavirin through aerosol for RSV 4. Humidified oxygen and ventilatory assistance may be needed.
Croup (Laryngotracheo-bronchitis) Caused by parainfluenza virus types 1, 2, 3 (most common virus), RSV, rhinovirus, adenovirus. Occurs at ages 3 months to 3 years; peak incidence is at age 18 months, and in late fall to early winter. Onset is usually gradual and progresses slowly, occurring 1 to several days after a URI.	1. Nebulized racemic or L-epinephrine 2. Corticosteroids may be used. 3. Provide cool humidified mist with supplemental oxygen as needed. 4. Severe airway edema may require intubation and mechanical ventilation. 5. May be managed at home: sit in steamy bathroom with the child until cough lessens, then use cool air vaporizer.

R

Bacterial Tracheitis (Pseudomembranous Croup)

Caused by *S. aureus, H. influenzae,* or beta-hemolytic *Streptococcus.* Occurs at variable ages; no seasonal variation. Onset is rapid.

1. Antibiotic therapy (usually ampicillin); also cephalosporins, oxacillin
2. Provide humidified oxygen as required.
3. Intubation and mechanical ventilation may be required.
4. Monitor respiratory status closely; assess for signs of respiratory failure.
5. Tracheostomy may be required.

Epiglottitis

Caused by *H. influenzae* type B (most common). *S. pneumoniae,* or beta-hemolytic *Streptococcus.* Occurs at ages 3 to 10 years, peak incidence at ages 1 to 5. Most commonly occurs during winter. Incidence has decreased significantly since *H. influenzae* vaccination became routine. Onset and progression are rapid (6–24 hours).

1. *Medical emergency:* Avoid agitating the child; prepare to move the child to the operating room for intubation by skilled personnel.
2. Before OR, observe child closely and keep emergency tracheostomy set at bedside.
3. If epiglottitis is strongly suspected, do not place anything in child's mouth.
4. Intubation and mechanical ventilation are required for 2–3 days.
5. Chloramphenicol usually used.
6. Temporary tracheostomy is sometimes required in complete airway obstruction.

   b. Occasional side or abdominal position will aid drainage of liquefied secretions.
   c. Do not position the child in severe respiratory distress in a supine position; allow the child to assume a position of comfort.
4. Provide measures to improve ventilation of affected portion of the lung.
   a. Change position frequently.
   b. Provide postural drainage if prescribed.
   c. Relieve nasal obstruction that contributes to breathing difficulty. Instill saline solution or prescribed nose drops, and apply nasal suctioning.
   d. Quiet prolonged crying, which can irritate the airway, by soothing the child; however, crying may be an effective way to ventilate the lungs.
   e. Realize that coughing is a normal tracheobronchial cleansing procedure, but temporarily relieve coughing by allowing the child to sip water; use extreme caution to prevent aspiration.
   f. Insert a nasogastric tube as ordered to relieve abdominal distension, which can limit diaphragmatic excursion.
5. Ensure that compressed air or oxygen is supplied when using a mist tent to avoid excess CO_2 concentrations and increased respiratory rate.

❖ NURSING ALERT

To minimize spasm and sudden blockage of airway, avoid the following: making the child lie flat, forcing the child to drink, and looking down the child's throat.

---

6. For cases of severe respiratory distress, assist with intubation or tracheostomy and mechanical ventilation.
   a. Tracheostomy tubes are generally not cuffed for infants and small children because the tube itself is big enough relative to the size of the trachea to act as its own sealer.
   b. Position the infant with a tracheostomy with neck extended by placing a small roll under the shoulders to prevent occlusion of the tube by the chin.

Support the head and neck carefully when moving the infant to avoid dislodging the tube.

c. When feeding, cover the tracheostomy with a moist piece of gauze, or use a bib for older infants or young children.

7. To promote hydration, administer intravenous (IV) fluids at the prescribed rate.

8. To prevent aspiration, hold all oral food and fluids if the child is in severe respiratory distress.

9. Offer the child small sips of clear fluid when the respiratory status improves.

a. Note any vomiting or abdominal distention after the oral fluid is given.

b. As the child begins to take more fluid by mouth, notify the health care provider and modify the IV fluid rate to prevent fluid overload.

c. Do not force the child to take fluids orally, because this may cause increased distress and possibly vomiting. Anorexia will subside as condition improves.

10. To provide adequate rest, disturb the child as little as possible by organizing nursing care, and protect child from unnecessary interruptions.

11. Encourage the parents to stay with the child as much as possible to provide comfort and security for the child.

12. Provide opportunities for quiet play as the child's condition improves.

13. Provide a quiet, stress-free environment.

14. Provide frequent change of clothing and linen for child in tent to promote comfort; provide socks, booties, cap, if necessary to keep child warm (temperature in mist tent is usually 6° to 15°F below room temperature).

Family Education and Health Maintenance

1. Advise parents to use ultrasonic nebulizer at home and encourage fluids as tolerated.

2. Teach the importance of good hygiene. Include information on handwashing and appropriate ways to handle respiratory secretions at home.

3. Teach methods to isolate sick from well children in the home. Teach the family when it is appropriate to keep

the child home from school (any fever, coughing up secretions, significant runny nose in toddler age or younger).

4. Teach methods to keep the ill child well hydrated.
   a. Provide small amounts of fluids frequently.
   b. Offer clear liquids such as Pedialyte.
   c. Avoid juices with a high sugar content.
5. Teach ways to assess the child's hydration status at home.
   a. Decreased number of wet diapers or number of urinations in a day
   b. Decreased activity level
   c. Dry lips and mucous membranes
   d. No tears when the child cries
6. Teach parents when to contact their health care provider: signs of respiratory distress, recurrent fever, decreased appetite and activity.
7. Teach about medications and follow-up.
8. If tracheostomy was required, teach home care of the tracheostomy.

Retinal Detachment

Retinal detachment results from separation of layers of rod and cone cells of the retina from the pigmented epithelial layers beneath. It may occur spontaneously because of degenerative changes in the retina or vitreous humor, or from trauma to the eye, inflammation, or other problems. Rare in children, the disorder most commonly occurs after age 40 years. Untreated retinal detachment may result in blindness.

◆ Assessment

1. Initially, the patient complains of flashes of light, floating spots or filaments in the vitreous, or blurred, "sooty" vision. Most of these phenomena result from traction between the retina and the vitreous.
2. As detachment progresses, the patient may report a veil-like curtain or shadow obscuring portions of the visual field. The veil appears to come from above,

below, or from one side; the patient may initially mistake the obstruction for a drooping eyelid or elevated cheek.

3. Straight-ahead vision may be unaffected in early stages, but as detachment progresses, there will be loss of central as well as peripheral vision.

◆ Diagnostic Evaluation

1. Binocular ophthalmoscopy with full pupil dilation shows retina as gray or opaque in detached areas. The retina is normally transparent.

◆ Collaborative Management

Therapeutic Interventions

1. Preoperatively, sedation, bed rest, and eye patches may be used to restrict eye movements.

Surgical Interventions

1. Surgical intervention aims to reattach the retinal layer to the epithelial layer and has a 90% to 95% success rate. Techniques include:
   a. Photocoagulation, in which a laser or xenon arc "spot welds" the retina to the pigment epithelium
   b. Electrodiathermy, in which a tiny hole is made in the sclera to drain subretinal fluid, allowing the pigment epithelium to adhere to the retina
   c. Cryosurgery or retinal cryopexy, another "spot weld" technique that uses a supercooled probe to adhere the pigment epithelium to the retina
   d. Scleral buckling, in which the sclera is shortened to force the pigment epithelium closer to the retina

◆ Nursing Interventions

Supportive Care

1. Prepare the patient for surgery.
   a. Instruct the patient to remain quiet in prescribed position, to keep the detached area of the retina in dependent position.
   b. Patch both eyes.
   c. Wash the patient's face with antibacterial solution.

    d. Instruct the patient not to touch eyes, to avoid contamination.

    e. Administer preoperative medications as ordered.

2. Take measures to prevent postoperative complications.

    a. Caution the patient to avoid bumping head.

    b. Encourage the patient not to cough or sneeze or to perform other strain-inducing activities that will increase intraocular pressure.

    c. Assist the patient with activities as needed.

3. Encourage ambulation and independence as tolerated.

4. Administer medications for pain, nausea, and vomiting as prescribed.

5. Provide quiet diversional activities such as radio, audio books.

Patient Education and Health Maintenance

1. Teach proper technique for giving eye medications.

2. Suggest applying a clean, warm, moist, washcloth to eyes and eyelids several times a day for 10 minutes, to provide soothing and relaxing comfort.

3. Advise the patient to avoid rapid eye movements for several weeks, as well as straining and bending the head below the waist.

4. Advise the patient that driving is restricted until cleared by ophthalmologist and that light activities are resumed gradually within 3 weeks; heavier activities and athletics may be restricted up to 6 weeks.

5. Teach the patient to recognize and immediately report symptoms that indicate recurring detachment, such as floating spots, flashing lights, progressive shadows.

6. Advise the patient to follow up. The first follow-up visit to the ophthalmologist should take place in 2 weeks, with other visits scheduled thereafter.

Retinoblastoma

Retinoblastoma is a malignant, congenital tumor arising in the retina of one or both eyes. Endophytic retinoblastomas arise in the internal nuclear layers of the retina and grow forward into the vitreous cavity. Exophytic tumors arise in the external nuclear layer and grow into the subretinal space, causing retinal detachment. Most retinoblastomas occur as a combination of these two types. The overall survival rate is high (90%); however, if untreated the tumor may involve the choroid, sclera, and optic nerve. Hematogenous spread of the tumor may occur to the bone marrow, skeleton, lymph nodes, and liver. Retinoblastoma is rare, and its cause is unknown, but it may be associated with inherited or noninherited genetic mutations. It is usually diagnosed in children before the age of 2 years.

◆ Assessment

1. "Cat's-eye reflex" (most common sign) is a whitish appearance of the pupil caused by the appearance of the tumor through the lens when light strikes the tumor mass.
2. Strabismus is second most common presenting sign.
3. Other occasional presenting signs include orbital inflammation, hyphema, fixed pupil, and heterochromia iridis (different colors of each iris, or in the same iris).
4. Vision loss is not a symptom, because young children do not complain of unilaterally decreased vision.

◆ Diagnostic Evaluation

1. Bilateral indirect ophthalmoscopy under general anesthesia to evaluate tumor
2. CT scan or MRI may be done of head and eyes to visualize tumor.
3. Bone marrow aspiration and lumbar puncture under anesthesia to determine metastasis

◆ Collaborative Management

Therapeutic Interventions

1. Unilateral tumors in stages I, II, or III are usually treated with external beam irradiation to eradicate the tumor(s) and preserve useful vision. Radiation is usually administered over a period of 3 to 4 weeks.
2. Radioactive applicators, light coagulation, and cryotherapy are sometimes used to treat small, localized tumors.

Pharmacologic Interventions

1. Chemotherapy is used to treat extraocular regional or distant metastases. Drugs commonly used include cyclophosphamide, vincristine, dactinomycin, doxorubicin, ifosfamide, methotrexate, cisplatin, and teniposide.

Surgical Interventions

1. Enucleation is the treatment of choice for advanced tumor growth, especially with optic nerve involvement.
2. Bilateral disease often requires enucleation of the severely diseased eye and irradiation of the least affected eye.
   a. Every attempt is made to salvage remaining vision.
   b. Bilateral enucleation is indicated with extensive bilateral retinoblastoma if vision cannot be salvaged.

◆ Nursing Interventions

Monitoring

1. Monitor for postoperative complications, including hemorrhage, infection, or implant extrusion.

Supportive Care

1. Sedate the child for irradiation, if necessary.
2. Observe for possible side effects of irradiation and prepare the parents for their occurrence, including skin changes at the temples, loss of lashes, fat atrophy with ptosis, delayed wound healing, dry eye, permanent radiation dermatitis, and impaired bone growth.
3. To prevent irritation of irradiated skin, use soap sparingly in these areas, avoid exposure to the sun, and apply a nonirritating lubricant.
4. Encourage the parents to "room in" and participate in the child's care to minimize separation anxiety.
5. Describe the surgery and anticipated postoperative appearance of the child. Draw pictures or use a doll if available.
   a. A ball implant is put in at the time of enucleation.
   b. An eyelid conformer is inserted to maintain integrity of the lids.
   c. The child's face may be edematous and ecchymotic after the procedure.

    d. In 4 to 6 weeks after surgery, the patient will receive an ocular prosthesis.

6. Offer the family the opportunity to talk with another parent who has gone through the experience or to see pictures of another child with an artificial eye.

7. Explain that the prosthesis will be made for the child and will look like the removed eye.

8. Tell parents to expect the child to grieve the loss and to help the child by talking about it, but treating the child as the same person.

9. Provide postoperative care:
   a. Instill medications, usually antibiotic and steroid ointments, to prevent infection.
   b. Apply pressure/ice dressings as ordered to reduce swelling.
   c. Irrigate eyelid conformer area to reduce mucous.
   d. Cleanse eyelid to reduce chance of infection.

10. To minimize the effect of vision loss, maintain a safe, uncluttered environment for the child.

11. Assist patient in adjusting to monocular vision—especially with loss of peripheral vision and depth perception.
   a. Hold the child frequently and stand close, within his or her field of vision, while speaking or providing care.
   b. Encourage the use of touch and other senses for exploring.

12. Set environmental limits so the child feels safe and can obtain help easily.

13. Suggest genetic counseling if applicable.
   a. Risk for parents ranges from approximately 1% to 10% for having another affected child, and risk for patient's offspring is 1% to 50%, depending on family history and whether the affected child had unilateral or bilateral disease.
   b. Among affected offspring, there is a high probability (greater than 50%) of bilateral disease.

Family Education and Health Maintenance

1. Teach care of the orbit.

2. Teach care of the prosthesis—initial instructions are provided by the ocularist and should be reinforced by the nurse.

a. Inspecting eye and lid
b. Instillation of medication
c. Irrigating site to remove mucus
d. Removing and inserting the prosthesis

3. Advise protection of the remaining eye from accidental injury, such as wearing safety glass for sports, keeping sharp objects away from eye, treating eye infections promptly.

4. Encourage maintenance of routine checkups for eye and medical care.

5. Stress need to have subsequent children carefully evaluated for retinoblastoma.

   a. An ophthalmologic examination under anesthesia is usually recommended at about 2 months of age.

   b. The child should receive frequent examinations thereafter until judged safe from developing retinoblastoma, usually about age 3 years.

Reye's Syndrome

Reye's syndrome is an acute multisystem disease that causes encephalopathy and fatty degeneration of the viscera, mainly affecting the liver, kidneys, and heart. The syndrome usually follows an acute viral infection, such as influenza B, varicella (chicken pox), gastroenteritis, or upper respiratory tract infection. Incidence peaks in winter and spring, often accompanying a flu outbreak. The syndrome may be linked to use of drugs such as salicylates and phenothiazines during a prodromal viral infection. Genetic and environmental factors also may contribute, and there is some evidence that the syndrome may have an autoimmune component.

Hepatic dysfunction results in hyperammonemia, hypoglycemia, and increased fatty acids, leading to encephalopathy. Fatty infiltration also develops in brain tissue, renal tubules, and the heart. Reye's syndrome progresses through five definite stages, marked by increasing CNS depression, cerebral edema, and coma. Death usually results from cerebral edema or respiratory arrest. Other complications include mental retardation, motor impairment, syndrome of inappropriate antidiuretic hormone (SIADH), and diabetes insipidus.

◆ Assessment

1. Prodromal viral illness that is usually improving
2. Sudden onset of intractable vomiting—fever usually not present
3. Irrational behavior
4. Altered sensorium—from mild lethargy to progressive stupor and coma
5. Hyperventilation, tachypnea
6. Hepatomegaly
7. Cerebral edema
8. Hypoglycemia
9. Generally, the more rapid the progression through the following National Institutes of Health consensus stages, the poorer the prognosis.
   a. Stage I: lethargy, follows verbal commands, normal posture, purposeful response to pain, brisk pupillary light reflex, normal oculocephalic reflex (doll's eye sign)
   b. Stage II: combative or stuporous, inappropriate verbalizing, normal posture, purposeful or nonpurposeful response to pain, sluggish pupillary reflexes, conjugate deviation on doll's eye maneuver
   c. Stage III: comatose, decorticate posture, decorticate response to pain, sluggish pupillary response, conjugate deviation on doll's eye maneuver
   d. Stage IV: comatose, decerebrate posture and decerebrate response to pain, sluggish pupillary reflexes, inconsistent or negative oculocephalic reflex (absent doll's eye sign)
   e. Stage V: comatose, flaccid, no response to pain, no pupillary response, negative oculocephalic reflex

◆ Diagnostic Evaluation

PEDIATRIC ALERT
Early diagnosis is critical because of the rapidly fatal course of the disease.

1. Differential diagnosis must rule out acute toxic encephalopathy, hepatic coma, hepatitis, meningitis, or encephalitis.
2. Laboratory tests:
   a. Serum ammonia—elevated
   b. Liver enzymes (aspartate transaminase [AST], alanine transaminase [ALT])—elevated
   c. Clotting factors (prothrombin time [PT] and partial thromboplastin time [PTT])—prolonged
   d. Serum glucose—decreased
   e. Creatinine—elevated
   f. BUN—elevated
   g. Amino acids, free fatty acids—elevated
   h. Acid–base status—acidemia
   i. Serum levels of salicylates, acetaminophen, phenothiazines, toxins to rule out other causes
   j. CBC, electrolytes, serum osmolality may be performed to monitor condition.
3. Lumbar puncture may be performed if cerebrospinal fluid is needed to rule out other diagnoses.

❖

NURSING ALERT

If increased intracranial pressure (IICP) is suspected, lumbar puncture should not be done until a CT scan is obtained to evaluate risk of rapid decompression resulting in brain herniation.

4. Liver biopsy may be performed to show microvesicular fatty degeneration of liver.

◆ Collaborative Management

Therapeutic Interventions

1. Care of the comatose child to prevent complications of immobility

Pharmacologic Interventions

1. Control of IICP
   a. Muscle relaxant—pancuronium bromide while on mechanical ventilator
   b. Sedative—diazepam, chloral hydrate
   c. Osmotic diuretic—mannitol, glycerol

   d. Barbiturate therapy—thiopental, phenobarbital
   e. Analgesia as appropriate
2. Vitamin K to combat coagulation defects and prevent bleeding
3. During stages I or II, maintain serum glucose at 150 to 200 mg/dL through IV hypertonic glucose infusion
4. During stages III, IV, or V, maintain serum glucose at 200 to 300 mg/dL and serum osmolality at 300 to 310 mOsm/L through glucose infusion.

◆ Nursing Interventions

Monitoring

1. Keep strict intake and output record and monitor weight at least daily. Measure urine specific gravity every 4 hours.
2. Observe for fluid volume deficit—hemoconcentration, decreased urinary output, decreased mean arterial pressure.
3. Observe for fluid overload—elevated central venous pressure (6–8 cm H_2O), decreased urine output (less than 2 mL/kg/h), edema.
4. During stages I or II, provide hourly neurologic checks using Glasgow Coma Scale.
5. During stages III, IV, or V, monitor intracranial pressure frequently. Goal is to maintain intracranial pressure within normal range of 10 to 15 torr and to maintain cerebral perfusion pressure of at least 50 mm Hg.
6. Monitor arterial blood gases to maintain $PaCO_2$ of approximately 25 mm torr and PaO_2 at 100 to 150 torr.
7. Maintain continuous EEG monitoring if instituted.
8. Monitor nasogastric drainage; give an antacid every 2 to 4 hours to maintain gastric pH above 4. Neomycin may be given by nasogastric tube to aid in reduction of ammonia.

Supportive Care

1. Provide supportive care of the child in stage I or II (noncomatose).
2. Provide intensive care management of the child in stage III, IV, or V (comatose).
   a. Provide routine care for a child who is intubated

and mechanically ventilated, to correct acidosis and provide optimal cerebral blood flow.

   b. Monitor and maintain core body temperature at 97.7° to 98.6°F (36.5° to 37°C).

   c. Position the patient supine with head of bed elevated 30 degrees; keep head midline to promote intracranial venous drainage.

   d. Monitor nursing activities that may cause IICP: suctioning, turning, chest physical therapy, painful (intrusive) procedures, conversation at bedside about diagnosis.

3. Be aware of any activity, noise, and distractions that increase intracranial pressure.

4. Insert a nasogastric tube and measure drainage.

5. Administer nothing by mouth.

6. Limit fluid intake—peripheral IV fluids given at a rate of $\frac{2}{3}$ maintenance because of potential cerebral edema and IICP. Calculate administered medications as part of fluid intake.

7. Provide emotional support to the patient and family.

   a. Educate the patient and family concerning the course of the disorder.

   b. Explain all procedures to the patient and family, and answer their questions.

   c. Help the patient and family to express their feelings of fear and anxiety about what is happening.

8. Initiate referrals to the chaplain, social worker, and other resources as needed.

Family Education and Health Maintenance

1. Ensure that the parents understand the importance of medical follow-up, especially related to any complications associated with the illness.

2. Encourage parents to become involved in community education to help caretakers recognize early signs and symptoms suggestive of Reye's syndrome.

3. For additional resources and support, refer parents to agencies such as:

   The National Reye's Syndrome Foundation
   PO Box 829
   Bryan, Ohio 43506
   800-233-7393

Rheumatic Fever, Acute

Acute rheumatic fever (ARF) is a systemic disease character-ized by inflammatory lesions of connective tissue and endothelial tissue. The pathogenesis is thought to be an autoimmune response to group A beta-hemolytic streptococcus. There is a cross-reactivity between cardiac tissue antigens and streptococcal cell wall components. The unique pathological lesion of rheumatic fever is the Aschoff body, a collection of reticuloendothelial cells sur-rounding a necrotic center on some structure of the heart.

ARF is commonly seen in children 5 to 15 years of age, during winter months, and in poorer living conditions. There is a high recurrence rate, and 75% of those with ARF progress to rheumatic heart disease in adulthood. Complications include significant CHF, pericarditis, peri-cardial effusions, aortic/mitral valve regurgitation, and permanent cardiac damage.

◆ Assessment

1. History of streptococcal phyaryngitis or upper respira-tory infection 2 to 6 weeks before onset of illness
2. Jones Criteria established by the American Heart Asso-ciation: the presence of two major criteria, or one major and two minor criteria, plus evidence of a pre-ceding streptococcal infection, are required to establish a diagnosis.
3. Major manifestations:
   a. Carditis: manifested by significant murmurs, signs of pericarditis, cardiac enlargement, or CHF
   b. Polyarthritis: almost always migratory and mani-fested by swelling, heat, redness and tenderness, or by pain and limitation of motion of 2 or more joints
   c. Chorea, a CNS disorder that lasts 1 to 3 months: purposeless, involuntary, rapid movements often associated with muscle weakness, involuntary fa-cial grimaces, speech disturbances, emotional la-bility
   d. Erythema marginatum: an evanescent nonpruritic, pink rash. The erythematous areas have pale cen-ters and round or wavy margins, vary greatly in

R

size, and occur mainly on the trunk and extremities. Erythema is transient, migrates from place to place, and may be brought out by the application of heat.

  e. Subcutaneous nodules—firm, painless nodules seen or felt over the extensor surface of certain joints, particularly elbows, knees, and wrists, in the occipital region, or over the spinous processes of the thoracic and lumbar vertebrae; the skin overlying them moves freely and is not inflamed.

4. Minor manifestations
  a. History of previous rheumatic fever or evidence of preexisting rheumatic heart disease
  b. Arthralgia: pain in one or more joints without evidence of inflammation, tenderness to touch, or limitation of motion
  c. Fever: temperature in excess of 38°C (100.4°F).
  d. Erythrocyte sedimentation rate (ESR)—elevated
  e. C-reactive protein—positive
  f. ECG changes—mainly PR interval prolongation
  g. White blood cell (WBC) count—elevated (leukocytosis)

◆ Diagnostic Evaluation

1. Throat culture for group A beta-hemolytic streptococci and blood sample for titer of streptococcal antibodies (antistreptolysin O, or ASO titer) to support evidence of recent streptococcal infection
2. CBC, ESR, and C-reactive protein for changes described above
3. Baseline ECG and echocardiogram may be done to evaluate valve function.

◆ Collaborative Management

Pharmacologic Interventions

1. Antibiotics to treat streptococcal infection—generally IM penicillin or erythromycin in penicillin allergy
2. Corticosteroids for patients with carditis to prevent permanent cardiac damage
3. Salicylates for patients with arthritis (but not while on high-dose corticosteroids because of risk of GI bleeding) and antipyretics to control fever, after diagnosis has been established.

◆ Nursing Interventions

Monitoring

1. Monitor temperature frequently, and patient's response to antipyretics.
2. Monitor the patient's pulse frequently, especially after activity to determine degree of cardiac compensation.
3. Auscultate the heart periodically for development of new heart murmur or pericardial or pleural friction rub.
4. Observe for adverse effects of salicylate therapy such as stomach upset, tinnitus, headache, GI bleeding, and altered mental status.
5. Monitor salicylate blood levels as directed.
6. Monitor for adverse effects of corticosteroid therapy such as emotional disturbance, weight gain, hypertension caused by sodium retention, Cushingoid appearance, and GI bleeding.
7. Monitor the child's response to long-term activity restriction.

Supportive Care

1. Administer salicylates with milk or antacids to reduce stomach irritation.
2. Prepare the family for expected side effects of steroid therapy, such as rounding facial contour, acne, excessive hair, weight gain.
3. Restrict sodium and fluids and obtain daily weights as indicated.
4. Be aware that steroids diminish the child's resistance to infection and may mask symptoms of infection.

PEDIATRIC ALERT
Do not place a child with an infectious disease in the room with the child with rheumatic fever. Restrict visitors and personnel with infectious diseases from contact with the child on steroid therapy.

---

5. Administer medications punctually and at regular intervals to achieve constant therapeutic blood levels.
6. Explain to the child the need for rest (usually pre-

R

scribed for 4 to 12 weeks, depending on the severity of the disease and health care provider's preference) and assure the child that bed rest will be imposed no longer than necessary (usually until the ESR returns to normal).

7. Organize nursing care to provide periods of uninterrupted rest and assure the child that needs will be met by responding to call light promptly.

8. Assist the child to resume activity very gradually once asymptomatic at rest and indicators of acute inflammation have become normal.

9. Provide comfort measures such as use of a bed cradle over painful joints, supporting inflamed joints, providing meticulous skin care, maintaining the body in good alignment, changing positions frequently to decrease stiffness and prevent skin breakdown, and elevating the back of the bed and support the arms with pillows when child is dyspneic.

10. Provide a safe, supportive environment for the child with chorea.
    a. Place the child in a bed with padded side rails, especially if uncontrolled body movements are severe.
    b. Feed the child slowly and carefully because of incoordinate movements of the head, mouth, and swallowing muscles. Avoid the use of sharp eating utensils, and do not use straws.
    c. Provide frequent feedings that are high in calories, protein, vitamins, and iron, because constant movements cause the child to burn calories at a rapid rate.
    d. Spend time talking with the child even though speech may be defective. If severe, use other methods of communication.
    e. Assess the need for sedation.
    f. Keep the environment calm and provide increased periods of rest because movements increase with fatigue and increased excitement.

11. Observe for the development or disappearance of any major or minor manifestations of the disease and report signs of increased rheumatic activity as salicylates or steroids are being tapered.

Family Education/Health Maintenance

1. Explain rheumatic fever in age-appropriate terminology. Reassure child that he or she has not had a heart attack, and have child listen to heart with stethoscope to understand that heart is still functioning.
2. Ensure that the child's school has been notified and that some tutoring will be available. Initiate referrals for home nursing or social services as indicated.
3. To prevent a recurrence or an additional case of rheumatic fever within the family, advise all family members to have throat cultures, be treated if necessary, and be alert to specific symptoms of streptococcal infections.
4. Encourage continuous prophylactic antimicrobial therapy (throughout the childhood years and well into adult life, often indefinitely) to prevent recurrence.
5. Advise on additional prophylaxis for prevention of infective endocarditis according to the American Heart Association.

Rheumatoid Arthritis

Rheumatoid arthritis (RA) refers to an autoimmune inflammatory diseases of the joints and various organ systems. In this disorder, synovial inflammation produces antigens and inflammatory by-products leading to destruction of joint cartilage, edema, and production of granulation tissue (pannus) (Fig. 23). The pannus forms adhesions on joint surfaces and supporting structures such as ligaments and tendons, causing contractures and ruptures that degrade joint structure and mobility. Bilateral symmetric arthritis affects any diarthrodial joint but most often involves the hands, wrists, knees, and feet.

The cause of RA is unknown, but it may result from a combination of environmental, demographic, infectious, and genetic factors. An infectious agent has not been identified, but many infectious processes can produce a polyarthritis similar to RA. Women are affected more frequently than men.

R

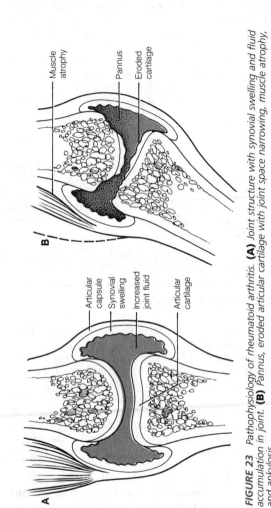

FIGURE 23 *Pathophysiology of rheumatoid arthritis.* **(A)** *Joint structure with synovial swelling and fluid accumulation in joint.* **(B)** *Pannus, eroded articular cartilage with joint space narrowing, muscle atrophy, and ankylosis.*

Labels for (B): Muscle atrophy, Pannus, Eroded cartilage

Labels for (A): Articular capsule, Synovial swelling, Increased joint fluid, Articular cartilage

◆ Assessment

1. Warm, tender, painful joints with stiffness lasting longer than 30 minutes after arising
2. Fever, fatigue, weight loss
3. Skin manifestations
   a. Rheumatoid nodules: elbows, occiput, sacrum
   b. Vasculitic changes: brown, splinterlike lesions in fingers or nail folds
4. Cardiac manifestations
   a. Acute pericarditis
   b. Conduction defects
   c. Valvular insufficiency
   d. Coronary arteritis
   e. Cardiac tamponade (rare)
5. Pulmonary manifestations
   a. Asymptomatic pulmonary disease
   b. Pleural effusion
   c. Interstitial fibrosis
   d. Laryngeal obstruction caused by involvement of the cricoarytenoid joint (rare)
6. Neurologic manifestations
   a. Mononeuritis multiplex
   b. Wrist drop
   c. Foot drop
   d. Carpal tunnel syndrome
   e. Compression of spinal nerve roots
7. Presence of deformities
   a. Swan neck: proximal interphalangeal (PIP) joints hyperextend
   b. Boutonniere: PIP joints flex
   c. Ulnar deviation: fingers point toward ulna
8. Altered functional status
   Class I: no restriction of ability to perform normal activities
   Class II: moderate restriction, but adequate for normal activities
   Class III: marked restriction, inability to perform most duties of usual occupation or self-care
   Class IV: incapacitation or confinement to bed or wheelchair

◆ Diagnostic Evaluation

1. CBC: decreased hemoglobin and hematocrit with normal indices

2. Rheumatoid factor: positive in a large percentage of patients
3. Erythrocyte sedimentation rate (ESR): elevated
4. Synovial fluid analysis: turbid, yellow color; WBC count 2,000 to 75,000/mm^3; low viscosity
5. X-rays:
   a. Hands and wrists: marginal erosions of the PIP, metacarpophalangeal (MCP), and carpal bones, generalized osteopenia
   b. Cervical spine: erosions producing atlantoaxial subluxation
6. MRI scan shows spinal cord compression resulting from C1–C2 subluxation and compression of surrounding vascular structures
7. Bone scan shows "increased uptake" in the joints involved
8. Synovial biopsy may be done to rule out other causes of polyarthritis by noting the absence of other pathologic findings.

◆ Collaborative Management

Therapeutic Interventions

1. Application of heat and cold to relieve pain and inflammation
2. Use of splints to prevent contractures
3. Use of transcutaneous electrical nerve stimulation (TENS) unit to treat chronic pain
4. Iontophoresis (delivery of medication through the skin using direct electrical current) to relieve pain
5. Behavior modification, biofeedback, and relaxation techniques

Pharmacologic Interventions

1. NSAIDs to relieve pain and inflammation
2. Disease-modifying antirheumatic drugs (DMARDs) to reduce disease activity, such as oral or injectable gold, hydroxchloroquine, or penicillamine
3. Corticosteroids to reduce inflammatory process

Surgical Interventions

1. Synovectomy
2. Arthrodesis (joint fusion)
3. Total joint replacement

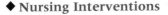

◆ Nursing Interventions

Monitoring

1. Monitor length of stiffness on arising.
2. Monitor pain control measures.
3. Monitor for signs and symptoms indicating adverse reaction to medications, such as rash, visual symptoms, GI distress.
4. Monitor functional ability.

Supportive Care

1. Apply local heat or cold to affected joints for 15 to 20 minutes three to four times daily.
   a. Avoid temperatures likely to cause skin or tissue damage by checking temperature of warm soaks or covering cold packs with a towel.
2. Administer or teach self-administration of pharmacologic agents. Advise the patient on when to expect pain relief based on mechanism of action of the drug.
3. Encourage use of adjunctive pain control measures.
   a. Progressive muscle relaxation
   b. TENS
   c. Biofeedback
4. Encourage warm bath or shower in the morning on arising to decrease morning stiffness and improve mobility.
5. Encourage measures to protect affected joints:
   a. Perform gentle range-of-motion exercises.
   b. Use splints.
   c. Assist with activities of daily living if necessary.
6. Encourage exercise consistent with degree of disease activity.
7. Refer to physical therapy and occupational therapy.
8. Provide pain relief before self-care activities.
9. Schedule adequate rest periods.
10. Help the patient obtain appropriate assistive devices such as raised toilet seats, special eating utensils, and zipper pulls.
11. Be aware of potential problems in job, child care, maintenance of home, and social and family functioning that may result from RA.
12. Encourage the patient to ventilate problems and feelings.

13. Assist with problem-solving approach to explore options and gain control of problem areas.
14. Refer to social worker or mental health counselor as needed.

Patient Education and Health Maintenance

1. Instruct the patient and family in the nature of disease.
2. Advise that there is no cure for RA; avoid "miracle cures" and quackery.
3. Educate about pharmacologic agents.
   a. Medication must be taken consistently to achieve maximum benefit.
   b. Most medications used in the treatment of RA require periodic laboratory testing to monitor for potential adverse reactions.
   c. Advise the patient of possible adverse reactions of medications and need to report these to health care provider.
4. Advise frequent follow-up for monitoring of CBC and urinalysis while on gold and penicillamine therapy, and ophthalmologic examinations while taking hydroxchloroquine.
5. Reinforce to the patient the need for lifelong treatment.

Rheumatoid Arthritis, Juvenile

Juvenile rheumatoid arthritis (JRA) is a chronic, inflammatory, systemic disease of unknown cause that involves the joints, connective tissues, and various organs throughout the body. Genetic or autoimmune factors are thought to play a role in this disorder, which affects approximately 250,000 children in the United States.

The disease causes inflammation involving the synovial membranes, joint capsules, and ligaments. Eventually the articular cartilage is destroyed; inflamed and overgrown synovial tissue eventually fills the joint space, leading to narrowing, fibrous ankylosis, and bony fusion. Adjacent tendons, tendon sheaths, and muscles may also become involved. Complications of JRA include crippling bony deformities from progressive polyarthritis, cervical spine and temporomandibular jaw problems, iridocyclitis leading to cataracts, glaucoma, or blindness; and pericarditis.

Three major forms of JRA are known: systemic, polyarticular, and pauciarticular. Depending on the form, JRA may occur from age 1 year throughout childhood. *Systemic JRA* accounts for approximately 20% of cases; incidence peaks at ages 1 to 3 years and again at ages 8 to 10 years and is more common in boys than girls. It can occur in any joint and is characterized by high intermittent fever, as well as involvement of other organs such as the liver, spleen, and lymph nodes. *Polyarticular JRA* involves five or more joints, most commonly small joints of the hands and fingers; 80% to 90% of cases are girls. There are two major subtypes, one positive for rheumatoid factor, the other negative. *Pauciarticular JRA* accounts for approximately 40% of cases. It involves fewer than five joints—usually knees, ankles, or elbows. There are two major subtypes: type I with iridocyclitis (inflammation of the iris and ciliary body) affects mostly girls, and type II with iridocyclitis and sacroillitis affects mostly boys.

Although JRA is a painful disease of long duration, the outlook for remission is good in 70% of cases.

◆ Assessment

1. Juvenile rheumatoid arthritis is characterized by exacerbations and remissions. Infections, injuries, or surgical procedures often precipitate exacerbations.
2. Involved joints become inflamed with morning stiffness (gelling), swelling, warmth, pain, and impaired movement. This may occur gradually or suddenly.
3. In systemic JRA:
   a. High intermittent fever (39°C [102°F]), malaise
   b. Maculopapular rash
   c. Pleuritis
   d. Pericarditis
   e. Splenomegaly, hepatomegaly
   f. Lymphadenopathy
4. In polyarticular JRA:
   a. Minimal systemic signs, such as low-grade fever, malaise, lymphadenopathy.

759

R

    b. Severe arthritis (occurs in >50% in rheumatoid-factor–positive type)
5. In pauciarticular JRA:
    a. Type I: chronic iridocyclitis (eye redness, pain, photophobia, decreased visual acuity, and nonreactive pupils). May be unilateral or bilateral, and lead to blindness
    b. May progress to polyarthritis in 20% of cases
    c. Type II: iridocyclitis, sacroillitis
    d. May progress to ankylosing spondylitis
6. Rheumatoid nodules are uncommon in children.

◆ Diagnostic Evaluation

1. C-reactive proteins (CRP) are elevated in all types.
2. Erythrocyte sedimentation rate (ESR) is elevated in all types.
3. Anemia and leukocytosis in systemic JRA
4. Rheumatoid factor negative in all types except RF-positive polyarticular JRA
5. Serum antinuclear antibodies (ANA):
    a. 25% positive in RF-negative polyarticular JRA
    b. 75% positive in RF-positive polyarticular JRA
    c. 90% positive in pauciarticular type I JRA
    d. Negative in pauciarticular types I,II, and systemic JRA
6. Human leukocyte antigen (HLA) studies:
    a. Positive in RF-positive polyarticular JRA and in pauciarticular types I and II
    b. Unknown in other types
7. Possible alteration in serum proteins (increased alpha and gamma; decreased albumin)
8. X-rays show changes in bone; initially nonspecific
9. Slit-lamp examinations of eye to rule out iridocyclitis

◆ Collaborative Management

Therapeutic Interventions
1. There is no specific cure; treatment is supportive.
2. Physical therapy is used to promote joint movement.

Pharmacologic Interventions
1. The goal of drug therapy is to reduce inflammation and relieve pain.

2. NSAIDs include aspirin, ibuprofen, and naproxen. Aspirin is the drug of choice, preferably enteric coated to avoid gastrointestinal complications.

R

COMMUNITY CARE CONSIDERATIONS
Because of the increased association of aspirin treatment of viral illness with incidence of Reye's syndrome, advise the family to contact the health care provider when the child has a viral illness. Aspirin may be discontinued and another treatment for JRA substituted until the viral illness is over.

3. Disease-modifying antirheumatic drugs (DMARDs) such as gold preparations or hydroxychloroquine may be added to the regimen when NSAIDs have been ineffective.
   a. Injectable gold salts are used sparingly because of the high risk of toxic side effects (skin rash, nephritis with hematuria or proteinuria, thrombocytopenia, neurotoxicity, gastric upset, leukopenia, anemia, and mucosal ulcers).
   b. An oral gold, auranofin, is being studied for use in children.
   c. Hydroxychloroquine or chloroquine may cause gastric upset, retinal toxicity, and corneal and retinal changes leading to blindness.
4. Cytotoxic drugs, such as cyclophosphamide, azathioprine, chlorambucil, and methotrexate, are reserved for patients with severe debilitating disease and those who have responded poorly to NSAIDs and DMARDs.
5. Corticosteroids, the most potent antiinflammatory agents available, are used for life-threatening disease, incapacitating systemic disease not responsive to other antiinflammatory therapy, and iridocyclitis.
   a. Administered in the lowest effective dose, on alternate days (rather than daily). Steroid use does not prevent complications of severe arthritis or influence ultimate prognosis.
   b. Tuberculin test should be done before starting steroid therapy, because corticosteroids can blunt skin test results.
6. Gamma globulin use is being investigated.

Surgical Interventions

1. Synovectomy may be used to maintain function when extensive synovitis develops, especially around wrists.
2. Joint replacement may be needed in severe destructive arthritis (ankylosing spondylitis).

◆ Nursing Interventions

Monitoring

1. Monitor serum levels of aspirin (keep at 20–30 mg/dL) for antiinflammatory effectiveness and to avoid toxicity. Therapeutic response may take weeks or even months. Signs of toxicity may include rapid or deep breathing or tinnitus.
2. Monitor steroid use for glucosuria and other side effects such as weight gain, edema, acne, and fatigue.

Supportive Care

1. Administer and teach parents to administer analgesic and antiinflammatory drugs as prescribed and based on child's response.
2. Provide daytime heat to joints with tub baths, whirlpools, paraffin baths, and warm moist pads; nighttime warmth with a sleeping bag, thermal underwear, or heated waterbed.
3. Immobilize any acutely inflamed joints with pillows, splints, or slings.
4. Encourage compliance with physical therapy regimen to strengthen muscles and mobilize joints. Assist with range of motion exercises as indicated.
5. Splint joints to maintain proper position (joint extension) and to decrease pain and deformity.
6. Encourage prone position with thin or no pillow and firm mattress.
7. Encourage therapeutic play (eg, swimming, throwing, riding bike).
8. Encourage child to do own activities of daily living (ADLs) to maintain joint mobility.
9. Refer to occupational therapy for provision of adaptation devices to facilitate completion of ADLs (eg, Velcro closures, utensils and self-care implements with enlarged handles).

10. Positively reward child for task completion.
11. Schedule rest periods to maximize energy; discourage bed rest and lengthy inactivity because it increases stiffness.
12. Offer pain medications and treatments before ADLs.
13. Encourage child and family to verbalize feelings.
14. Refer to community resources and support groups.
15. Encourage school attendance as much as possible, participation in activities, and socialization with peers.
16. Remind parents to devote time to other children, themselves, and each other, because this disease affects the whole family.

Family Education and Health Maintenance

1. Educate and motivate parents and child in continuing program of treatment at home. Compliance with prescribed treatment will minimize crippling and allow the child to grow and develop to full potential. Avoid unorthodox and unproven treatments.
2. Teach the family that daily exercises such as swimming help to maintain full range of motion. Avoid exercises that cause overtiring and joint pain.
3. Urge the parents to keep the school nurse informed of child's condition to ensure continuity of care even at school. Tell the parents to inform child's teacher of need for hourly movement, side effects of medications, and application of special equipment.
4. Teach the family about a nutritionally balanced diet to prevent obesity, which puts additional stress on joints.
5. Stress the need for routine follow-up care, ophthalmologic evaluation, and prompt attention to infections or other illness that may prompt exacerbations.

COMMUNITY CARE CONSIDERATIONS

Review child's immunization record for completeness because specialty focus may have caused parents and health care providers to overlook primary care needs. Advise child to get flu vaccine each year to decrease stress caused by the flu and risk of Reye's syndrome from salicylate intake.

6. Refer the family to agencies such as:

American Juvenile Arthritis Foundation
1314 Spring St., NW
Atlanta, GA 30309
(404) 872-7100

Rhinitis, Allergic

Allergic rhinitis is an inflammation of the nasal mucosa caused by an allergen. Airborne allergens such as pollen (seasonal) or dust, mold, or animal dander (perennial) cause a type I hypersensitivity reaction with local vasodilation and increased capillary permeability. Allergic rhinitis affects 8% to 10% of the population. Other types of rhinitis include *nonallergic rhinitis,* also called *vasomotor rhinitis,* and rhinitis caused by viral infection.

◆ Assessment

1. Mucous membrane congestion, edema, and itching; rhinorrhea, sneezing
2. Conjunctival edema, itching, and burning; increased lacrimation; dark circles under eyes (allergic shiners)
3. Itching and congestion of ears
4. Itching of palate and throat; nonproductive cough

◆ Diagnostic Evaluation

1. Increased eosinophils on nasal smear
2. Skin testing confirms hypersensitivity to specific allergens
3. Radioallergosorbent test (RAST): measurement of immunoglobulin (Ig) E antibodies in serum samples after a panel of allergens have been added

◆ Collaborative Management

Therapeutic Interventions
1. Minimize contact with offending allergens.

Pharmacologic Interventions
1. Antihistamines block the effects of histamine and relieve symptoms.

2. Topical or oral decongestants shrink mucous membranes by causing vasoconstriction.
3. Intranasal cromolyn sodium, a mast cell stabilizer, hinders the release of chemical mediators and prevents acute symptoms.
4. Corticosteroids used intranasally or orally for short course reduces inflammation; also works for nonallergic rhinitis
5. Immunotherapy: serial injections of increasing amounts of specific allergens to decrease sensitivity and reduce symptoms

NURSING ALERT
Immunotherapy should not be given to patients taking beta-adrenergic blocking agents, because they may mask a systemic reaction.

◆ Nursing Interventions

Supportive Care
1. Reassure patient that suffocation will not occur because of nasal obstruction; mouth breathing will occur.
2. Use a bedside humidifier and increase oral fluids to prevent drying of mucous membranes from mouth breathing.
3. Observe patient after immunotherapy injection for 30 minutes for severe local or systemic reaction.

NURSING ALERT
Always have epinephrine 1:1,000 available for injection should anaphylaxis occur after allergy shot.

Family Education and Health Maintenance
1. Teach the proper use of nasal inhalers: clear mucus from nose first, exhale, then inhale while releasing medication.
2. Advise caution with driving and other situations that

require alertness while taking potentially sedating antihistamines.

3. Advise limiting over-the-counter nasal decongestants to 2 to 3 days to prevent rebound effect causing mucosal edema.

4. Instruct patient on environmental control measures:
   a. Use nonallergic bedding materials and cover mattress and pillows with plastic covers.
   b. Use washable curtains and throw rugs.
   c. Avoid stuffed animals and other dust-collecting items.
   d. Damp-dust daily and wear a mask while doing it.
   e. Keep windows closed and use an air conditioner while allergens are prevalent outside.
   f. Change furnace filter frequently and use air filtering system if possible.
   g. If allergic to animal dander, keep pets outside, or at least out of bedroom.
   h. Keep damp areas well cleaned and dehumidified to avoid mold.

Ruptured Disk

See Herniated Intervertebral Disk (Ruptured disk)

Schizophrenia, Schizophreniform, and Delusional Disorders

Schizophrenia, schizophreniform, and delusional disorders are defined by psychotic symptoms. Psychotic symptoms are produced by a loss of ego boundaries and severe impairment of reality testing and include prominent hallucinations and delusions, disorganized speech, and grossly disorganized or catatonic behavior.

Schizophrenia may result from a complex combination of genetic, neurobiologic, and psychological factors. The *Diagnostic and Statistical Manual,* 4th Edition, recognizes five types of schizophrenia: paranoid, disorganized, residual, catatonic, and undifferentiated. Symptoms in each of these forms must be evident for at least 6 months. *Schizophreniform disorder* is a syndrome that resembles schizophrenia in many respects, but lasts less than 6 months. Schizophrenia may affect up to 2% of the general population, and it occurs primarily during adolescence or early adulthood.

In a *delusional disorder*, there are no symptoms of schizophrenia. The patient manifests false beliefs (delusions) that may have a plausible basis in reality. The delusions do not result from another mental disorder or disease process. Little has been established about the cause of delusional disorders; there is no demonstrated genetic linkage. It is possible that psychosocial stressors play a role in some persons. Delusional disorders are more common in middle-aged or older patients.

◆ Assessment

Positive symptoms of schizophrenia

These symptoms reflect aberrant mental activity and are usually present early in the first phase of the schizophrenic illness.

1. Delusion: false, fixed belief that is not amenable to change by reasoning. The most frequently elicited delusions include ideas of reference, delusions of grandeur, delusions of jealousy, delusions of persecution, and somatic delusions.
2. Loose associations: The thought process becomes illogical and confused.
3. Neologisms: made-up words that have a special meaning to the delusional person
4. Concrete thinking: an overemphasis on small or specific details and an impaired ability to abstract
5. Echolalia: pathologic repeating of another's words

6. Clang associations: the meaningless rhyming of a word in a forceful way
7. Word salad: a mixture of words that are meaningless to the listener
8. Hallucinations: sensory perceptions that have no external stimulus. The most common are auditory, visual, gustatory, olfactory, and tactile.
9. Loss of ego boundaries: The patient lacks a sense of the body and how he or she relates to the environment.
   a. Depersonalization is a nonspecific feeling or sense that a person has lost his or her identity or is unreal.
   b. Derealization is the false perception by a person that the environment has changed.
10. Bizarre behavioral patterns
    a. Motor agitation or restlessness
    b. Automatic obedience or robotlike movement
    c. Negativism
    d. Stereotyped behaviors
    e. Stupor
    f. Waxy flexibility
11. Agitated or impulsive behavior

Negative symptoms of schizophrenia

Reflect a deficiency of mental functioning
1. Alogia: inability to speak
2. Anergia: inability to react
3. Anhedonia: inability to experience pleasure
4. Avolition: inability to choose or decide
5. Poor social functioning
6. Poverty of speech
7. Social withdrawal
8. Thought blocking

Associated symptoms of schizophrenia
1. Chemical use, abuse, or dependence
2. Depression
3. Fantasy
4. Violent or aggressive behavior
5. Water intoxication
6. Withdrawal

◆ Diagnostic Evaluation

1. Clinical diagnosis is developed on historical information and thorough mental status examination.
2. No laboratory findings have been identified that are diagnostic of schizophrenia.
3. Routine battery of laboratory tests may be useful in ruling out possible organic causes.
4. Rating scale assessment
   a. Scale for the Assessment of Negative Symptoms (SANS)
   b. Scale for the Assessment of Positive Symptoms (SAPS)

◆ Collaborative Management

Therapeutic Interventions

1. Electroconvulsive therapy may be indicated for catatonic schizophrenia.
2. Psychosocial treatments in schizophrenia or schizophreniform disorder include:
   a. Supportive individual psychotherapy that is reality oriented and pragmatic
   b. Structured group psychotherapy
   c. Family therapy
   d. Psychoeducation group
   e. Support groups in community
   f. Community-based partial hospitalization programs
   g. Psychiatric home care nursing
3. Vocational and social skills education
4. In delusional disorders, individual psychotherapy
5. Hospitalization for comprehensive assessment for diagnostic purposes or if suicidal or homicidal

Pharmacologic Interventions

1. Antipsychotics (neuroleptic)
2. Adjunctive pharmacologic agents: anxiolytics, lithium, antidepressants, propranolol, carbamazepine

◆ Nursing Interventions

Monitoring

1. Monitor and document the patient's response to antipsychotic medication regimen.

2. Monitor the nonrestrained patient for behaviors that indicate increased anxiety.
3. Frequently monitor the restrained patient within the guidelines of the institution's policy on restrictive devices and assess the patient's level of agitation.
4. Monitor for side effects of orthostatic hypotension and extrapyramidal reactions.

Supportive Care

1. Encourage the patient to talk about feelings.
2. Provide the patient with honest and consistent feedback in a nonthreatening manner.
3. Avoid challenging the content of the patient's behaviors.
4. Focus interactions on the patient's behaviors.
5. Use simple and clear language when speaking with the patient.
6. Explain all procedures, tests, and activities to the patient before starting them, and provide written or video material for learning purposes.
7. Provide opportunities for socialization and encourage participation in group activities.
8. Be aware of the patient's personal space and use touch in a judicious manner.
9. Assist the patient to identify behaviors that alienate significant others/family members.
10. Collaborate with the patient and occupational and physical therapy specialists to assess the patient's ability to perform activities of daily living.
11. Collaborate with the patient to establish a daily, achievable routine within any physical limitations.
12. Teach strategies to manage side effects of antipsychotics:
    a. Change positions slowly.
    b. Gradually increase physical activities.
    c. Limit overexertion in hot, sunny weather.
    d. Use sun precautions.
    e. Use caution in activities if extrapyramidal symptoms develop.
13. Encourage the patient to explore adaptive behaviors that increase the patient's abilities and success in socializing and accomplishing activities of daily living.
14. Decrease environmental stimuli.

15. Collaborate with the patient to identify anxious behaviors, as well as the causes.
16. Tell the patient that you will help him or her maintain control.
17. Establish consistent limits on the patient's behaviors and clearly communicate these limits to the patient, family members, and health care providers.
18. Secure all potential weapons and articles that could be used to inflict an injury from the patient's room and the unit environment.
19. To prepare for possible continued escalation, form a psychiatric emergency assist team and designate a leader to facilitate an effective and safe aggression management process.
20. Determine the need for external control, including seclusion or restraints. Communicate the decision to the patient and put plan into action.
21. When the patient's level of agitation begins to decrease and self-control is regained, establish a behavioral agreement that identifies specific self-control behaviors against reescalating agitation.

Patient Education and Health Maintenance

1. Teach about the disease process and how to recognize and cope with relapse symptoms.
2. Instruct about the uses, actions, and side effects of any prescribed medications.
3. Advise about community resources, support groups, and possible use of psychiatric home care nursing.
4. For additional information and support, refer to:

> **National Alliance for Research on Schizophrenia and Depression (NARSAD)**
> 60 Cutter Mill Rd.
> Suite 200
> Great Neck, NY 11021
> 516-829-0091

Scleroderma

Scleroderma (systemic sclerosis) is a generalized connective tissue disorder of unknown cause characterized by hardening or thickening of the skin, blood vessels, synovium, skeletal muscles, and internal organs. Fibrotic, degenerative, and inflammatory changes including vascular insufficiency are most likely caused by overproduction of collagen by fibroblasts. The disorder affects three to four times as many women as men.

Complications include skin ulcers, malabsorption, esophageal adenocarcinoma, pulmonary hypertension, renal failure, congestive heart failure, and death.

◆ Assessment

1. Skin-related manifestations:
   a. Bilateral symmetric swelling of the hands and sometimes the feet
   b. Hardening and thickening of skin after edematous phase
   c. Digits, dorsum of hand, neck, face, and trunk are involved.
   d. Normal landmarks in skin are absent (no skin folds).
   e. Increased or decreased skin pigmentation
   f. Skin changes may regress after several years.
   g. Telangiectasias on tongue, face, fingers, and lips
   h. Areas of calcinosis in late disease
   i. Raynaud's phenomenon
2. Gastrointestinal manifestations:
   a. Esophageal dysmotility resulting in reflux and esophagitis
   b. Distal esophageal dilation and esophagitis
   c. Barrett's metaplasia may predispose to adenocarcinoma of the esophagus.
   d. Duodenal atrophy and dilation may cause postprandial abdominal pain, malabsorption, diarrhea, and abdominal distension.
   e. Colonic hypomotility resulting in constipation
3. Musculoskeletal manifestations:
   a. Joint pain
   b. Polyarthritis (large and small joints affected)
   c. Carpal tunnel syndrome
   d. Flexion contractures
   e. Inflammatory muscle atrophy
4. Cardiac manifestations:
   a. Left ventricular dysfunction

   b. Congestive heart failure and atrial and ventricular arrhythmias

   c. Right ventricular involvement secondary to pulmonary disease

5. Pulmonary manifestations:
   a. Interstitial fibrosis
   b. Restrictive lung disease
   c. Pulmonary hypertension

6. Renal manifestations:
   a. Scleroderma renal crisis—rapid malignant hypertension with encephalopathy

7. CREST Syndrome: *C*alcinosis, *R*aynaud's phenomenon, *E*sophageal Dysmotility, *S*clerodactyly, *T*elangiectasia

8. Linear and morphea scleroderma: Localized scleroderma with lesions appearing as streaks or bands in linear scleroderma, or purple-bordered lesions of several centimeters in diameter in morphea scleroderma. There is generally no visceral involvement.

◆ Diagnostic Evaluation

1. CBC and erythrocyte sedimentation rate: usually normal

2. Rheumatoid factor is positive in approximately 30% of patients

3. Antinuclear antibodies: generally present

4. Scl 70 positive in diffuse cutaneous disease

5. Anti–centromere antibody highly specific for limited cutaneous disease

6. X-rays of hands and wrists show muscle atrophy, osteopenia, osteolysis

7. Barium swallow shows esophageal dysmotility

8. Multigated angiogram (MUGA) scans may be done to determine left ventricular function.

9. Pulmonary function tests show decreased diffusion capacity and vital capacity, restrictive lung disease.

10. Endoscopy may be done to obtain biopsy specimen for Barrett's metaplasia.

11. Esophageal manometry may be done to determine contractile capacity of esophageal muscles.

◆ Collaborative Management

Therapeutic Interventions

1. Application of prescribed skin lubricants
2. Avoidance of factors associated with exacerbation of Raynaud's phenomenon
3. Use of biofeedback

Pharmacologic Interventions

1. Penicillamine to decrease disease activity
2. Calcium channel–blocking agents for Raynaud's phenomenon
3. NSAIDs to control pain of arthralgias and polyarthritis
4. Histamine H_2 blockers and omeprazole for reflux
5. Antibiotics for malabsorption caused by bacterial overgrowth
6. Antihypertensive agents
7. Metoclopramide for intestinal dysmotility

◆ Nursing Interventions

Monitoring

1. Monitor for evidence of adverse reactions related to medications such as stomach upset, GI bleeding, decreased hemoglobin and hematocrit, and proteinuria.
2. Monitor nutritional intake and weigh the patient weekly.
3. Inspect the skin daily for cracking, ulceration, and signs of infection.

Supportive Care

1. Teach the patient to recognize Raynaud's phenomenon and to reduce factors associated with precipitation or exacerbation.
2. Protect ulcerated digits and observe for signs of infection.
3. Apply moisturizers to skin daily.
4. Advise the patient to avoid use of drying soaps and detergents.
5. Use protective padding (eg, elbow pads) to protect the skin from friction or trauma.
6. Provide small, frequent, well-balanced meals.
7. Encourage the patient to remain upright after meals

for 45 to 60 minutes and raise head of bed during sleep to avoid reflux and aspiration.

8. Encourage good oral hygiene and frequent dental visits.
9. Advise to use lubricating agents, if necessary, to treat dry mouth and teach stretching exercises of mouth to maintain aperture.
10. Refer to social worker for supportive services and for counseling as needed.

Patient Education and Health Maintenance

1. Explain all diagnostic tests and their purpose in detecting GI, pulmonary, renal, or cardiac involvement.
2. Teach about drug treatments, including adverse reactions.
3. Advise on fluid and sodium restriction if congestive heart failure has been identified.
4. Advise on modifying activity and using oxygen to prevent dyspnea caused by restrictive lung disease.
5. Encourage regular follow-up and prompt attention to worsening symptoms.

Scoliosis

Scoliosis is a lateral curvature of the spine resulting from rotation and deformity of vertebrae. Three forms of structural scoliosis are recognized. *Idiopathic scoliosis* is the most common form and is classified into three groups: infantile, which presents from birth to age 3 years; juvenile, which presents from ages 3 to 10 years; and adolescent, which presents after age 10 years (most common age). *Congenital scoliosis* results in the malformation of one or more vertebral bodies. In *neuromuscular scoliosis,* the child has a neuromuscular condition (such as cerebral palsy, spina bifida, or muscular dystrophy) that directly contributes to the deformity. Additional but less common causes of scoliosis include osteopathic conditions such as fractures, bone disease, arthritic conditions, and infections. In severe scoliosis, progressive changes in the thoracic cage may cause respiratory and cardiovascular compromise.

S

◆ Assessment

1. Poor posture, uneven shoulder height
2. One hip more prominent than the other
3. Crooked neck, lump on back (rib hump)
4. Uneven waistline (pelvis) or hemline
5. Uneven breast size
6. Back pain may be present but is not a routine finding in idiopathic scoliosis.

PEDIATRIC ALERT
The adolescent who presents with back pain and a scoliosis warrants close consideration to rule out other conditions, such as a tumor, disk pathology, or intraspinal anomalies.

◆ Diagnostic Evaluation

1. X-rays of the spine in the upright position, preferably on one long (36 in) cassette, show characteristic curvature.
2. MRI, myelograms, or CT with or without three-dimensional reconstruction may be indicated for children with severe curvatures who have a known or suspected spinal column anomaly, before management decisions are made.
3. Pulmonary function tests detect compromised respiratory status.
4. Clinical photographs to assist with documenting the appearance of the spine over time (*Note:* Consent for photographs must be obtained from the child's legal guardian.)

◆ Collaborative Management

Therapeutic Interventions

1. Periodic physical and radiographic examinations to detect curve progression
2. Brace management to prevent progression of spinal curvature
   a. Requires child's faithful compliance to succeed
   b. Some curves progress despite brace wear.
   c. Recommended wearing time is 23 hours per day.

3. Types of braces include:
   a. Boston orthosis for low thoracic and thoracolumbar curves. This is an underarm molded orthosis.
   b. Milwaukee brace for thoracic or double major curves. Standard brace has neck ring with chin rest.
   c. Charleston bending brace has been tried for nighttime use in selected patients. Results have been positive in some centers, but brace is not yet widely accepted.
4. Exercise therapy has been promoted to help maintain spinal flexibility and prevent muscle atrophy during prolonged bracing.

Surgical Interventions

1. Stabilization of the spinal column is usually accomplished with a spinal fusion and one of several methods of instrumentation.
   a. Harrington instrumentation and posterior spinal fusion
   b. Multiple-level (segmental fixation) systems such as the TSRH or Cotrel-Dubousset
   c. Luque technique, which includes dual rods with sublaminar wire segmental fixation (usually reserved for children with preexisting neurologic compromise, because of increased risk of neurologic damage from sublaminar wires)
   d. Anterior procedures, which include staple and cable or rod systems such as the Dwyer or Anterior TSRH
2. Indications for surgical correction vary, but generally include the following:
   a. Progression of the curve over a short period in a curve greater than 45 degrees despite bracing
   b. Skeletal immaturity
   c. Bracing not possible
3. Preoperative traction or casting may be used to help gain correction and increase flexibility.
4. Postoperative protection of the fusion mass by means of a cast or brace is usually required.

◆ Nursing Interventions

Supportive Care

1. Prepare the child for casting or immobilization procedure by showing materials to be used and describing procedure in age-appropriate terms.

2. Promote comfort with proper fit of brace or cast.
3. Provide opportunity for the child to express fears and ask questions about deformity and brace wear.
4. Assess skin integrity under and around the brace or cast frequently.
5. Provide good skin care to prevent breakdown around any pressure areas.
6. Care of child undergoing surgery is similar to care of patient with herniated disc (see p. 428).

Family Education and Health Maintenance

1. Instruct the patient to examine brace daily for signs of loosening or breakage. An orthotist should be contacted for necessary repairs.
2. Instruct patient to wear cotton shirt under brace to avoid rubbing.
3. Instruct as to which previous activities can be continued in the brace. Usually all but contact sports and certain gymnastic activities
4. Provide a peer support person when possible so the child can associate positive outcomes and experiences from others.

Seizure Disorder

Seizures (also known as convulsions, epileptic seizures and, if recurrent, epilepsy) are thought to result from abnormal, recurrent, uncontrolled electric discharges of neurons in the brain. The pathophysiology of seizures is poorly understood but seems to be related to metabolic and electrochemical factors at the cellular level. Predisposing factors include head or brain trauma; tumors; cranial surgery; metabolic disorders (hypocalcemia, hypo/hyperglycemia, hyponatremia, anoxia); CNS infection; circulatory disorders; drug toxicity; drug withdrawal states (alcohol, barbiturates); and congenital neurodegenerative disorders.

Seizures are classified as *partial* or *generalized* by the origin of the seizure activity and associated clinical manifestations. Simple partial seizures manifest motor, somatosensory, and psychomotor symptoms without impairment of consciousness. Complex partial seizures manifest impairment of consciousness with simple partial symptoms.

Generalized seizures manifest a loss of consciousness with convulsive or nonconvulsive behaviors and include tonic–clonic, myoclonic, atonic, and absence seizures. Simple partial seizures can progress to complex partial seizures, and complex partial seizures can secondarily become generalized.

Seizures affect all ages. Most cases of epilepsy are identified in childhood, and several seizure types are particular to children. Complications include status epilepticus (see Box 6), cerebral impairment caused by anoxia with generalized seizures, and injuries caused by falls.

S

◆ Assessment

1. Generalized tonic–clonic (grand mal) seizure
   a. Sudden onset with loss of consciousness
   b. Rigid muscle contraction in tonic phase with clenched jaw and hands; eyes open with pupils dilated; lasts 30 to 60 seconds
   c. Rhythmic, jerky contraction and relaxation of all muscles in clonic phase with incontinence and frothing at the lips; may bite tongue or cheek; lasts several minutes
   d. Sleeping or dazed post-ictal state for up to several hours
2. Absence (petit mal) seizure
   a. Loss of contact with environment for 5 to 30 seconds
   b. Appears to be daydreaming or may roll eyes, nod head, move hands, or smack lips
   c. Resumes activity and is not aware of seizure
3. Myoclonic seizure
   a. Seen in children or in infants (infantile spasms), caused by cerebral pathology, often with mental retardation
   b. Infantile spasms usually disappear by 4 years of age, but child may develop other type of seizures
   c. Brief, sudden, forceful contractions of the muscles of the trunk, neck, and extremities
   d. May cause children to drop or throw something
   e. Cause episodes of laughing and smiling in infants

S

■ BOX 6   EMERGENCY MANAGEMENT OF STATUS EPILEPTICUS

Status epilepticus (acute, prolonged, repetitive seizure activity) is a series of generalized seizures without return to consciousness between attacks. The term has been broadened to include continuous clinical or electrical seizures lasting at least 5 minutes, even without impairment of consciousness.

Status epilepticus is considered a serious neurologic emergency. It has a high mortality and morbidity rate (permanent brain damage; severe neurologic deficits).

Factors that precipitate status epilepticus include medication withdrawal, fever, metabolic or environmental stresses, alcohol withdrawal, sleep deprivation, etc., in patient with preexisting seizure disorder.

■ Interventions

1. Establish an airway and maintain blood pressure.
2. Obtain blood studies for glucose, blood urea nitrogen, electrolytes, and anticonvulsant drug levels to determine metabolic abnormalities and serve as a guide for maintenance of biochemical homeostasis.
3. Administer oxygen—there is some respiratory arrest at height of each seizure, which may produce venous congestion and hypoxia of brain.
4. Establish IV lines and keep open for blood sampling, drug administration, and infusion of fluids.

(continued)

> ■ **BOX 6** *(Continued)*
>
> 5. Administer intravenous anticonvulsant (lorazepam [Ativan], phenytoin [Dilatin]) give *slowly* to ensure effective brain tissue and serum concentrations.
>   a. Additional anticonvulsants given as directed—effects of lorazepam are of short duration.
>   b. Anticonvulsant drug levels monitored regularly.
> 6. Monitor the patient continuously; depression of respiration and blood pressure induced by drug therapy may be delayed.
> 7. Use of mechanical ventilation as needed.
> 8. If initial treatment is unsuccessful, general anesthesia may be required.
> 9. Assist with search for precipitating factors.
>   a. Monitor vital and neurologic signs on a continuing basis.
>   b. Use electroencephalographic monitoring to determine nature and abolition (after diazepam administration) of epileptic activity.
>   c. Determine (from family member) if there is a history of epilepsy, alcohol/drug use, trauma, recent infection.

4. Atonic seizure (drop attacks)
    a. Sudden, transient loss of muscle tone causes falling.
    b. Hundreds of episodes may occur per day.
    c. Common in children 3 to 12 years old
5. Partial (focal) motor seizure
    a. Rhythmic twitching of muscle group, usually hand or face
    b. May spread to involve entire limb, other extremity, and face on that side; known as Jacksonian seizure
6. Partial (focal) somatosensory seizure

a. Numbness and tingling in a part of the body
b. May also be visual, taste, auditory, or olfactory sensation

7. Partial psychomotor (temporal lobe) seizure
   a. May be aura of abdominal discomfort or bad odor or taste
   b. Auditory or visual hallucinations, déjà vu feeling, or sense of fear or anxiety
   c. Repetitive purposeless movements (automatisms) may occur, such as picking at clothes, smacking lips, chewing, and grimacing.
   d. Lasts seconds to minutes
   e. More common in adults than children

8. Complex partial seizures: begin as partial seizures and progress to impairment of consciousness or impaired consciousness at onset

9. Febrile seizure
   a. Generalized tonic–clonic seizure with fever over 101.8°F (38.8°C)
   b. Occur in children younger than 5 years of age
   c. Treatment is to decrease temperature, treat source of fever, and control seizure.
   d. Long-term treatment to prevent recurrent seizures with fever is controversial.

◆ Diagnostic Evaluation

1. EEG with or without video monitoring, to locate epileptic focus, spread, intensity, and duration; helps classify seizure type
2. CT or MRI to identify lesion that may be cause of seizure
3. Single photon emission computed tomography (SPECT) or positron emission tomography (PET) or additional tests to identify seizure foci
4. Neuropsychological studies to evaluate for behavioral disturbances
5. Serum electrolytes, glucose, and toxicology screen to determine cause of first seizure

◆ Collaborative Management

Therapeutic Interventions

1. Maintain good nutrition and sleep hygiene and avoid stress to help decrease frequency of seizures.

2. A ketogenic diet has been used for seizure control in some patients, when medications fail or adequate dosage of medication causes toxicity.
   a. The diet consists of precisely calculated portions of protein and fat without carbohydrates. As fats are metabolized for energy, ketones are formed, which are thought to inhibit seizures.
   b. IV fluids should be dextrose free, and all medications should be in sugar-free suspensions.
3. Biofeedback may help prevent seizures in the patient with reliable auras.

Pharmacologic Interventions

1. Commonly prescribed drugs include clonazepam, ethosuximide, primidone, carbamazepine, felbamate, gabapentin, phenytoin, and valproic acid.
   a. It may take several months to obtain the desired clinical effect.
   b. Combination drug therapy may be necessary to avoid toxicity or intolerable adverse reactions.
2. A wide variety of adverse reactions may occur, including hepatic and renal dysfunction, visual disturbances, ataxia, anemia, leukopenia, thrombocytopenia, psychotic symptoms, skin rash, stomach upset, and idiosyncratic reactions.

PEDIATRIC ALERT
There is some evidence that long-term treatment of children with some anticonvulsants may cause intellectual impairment. Therefore, medication may be withdrawn if child is seizure free for 2 years.

Surgical Interventions

1. Surgical treatment of brain tumor or hematoma may relieve seizures caused by these.
2. Temporal lobectomy, extratemporal resection, corpus callosotomy, or hemispherectomy may be necessary in medically intractable seizure disorders.

◆ Nursing Interventions

Monitoring

1. Monitor the entire seizure event, including prodromal signs, seizure behavior, and postictal state.
2. Monitor serum levels for therapeutic range of medications.

S

> **NURSING ALERT**
> Noncompliance, as well as toxicity of antiepileptic medications, can increase seizure frequency. Review serum drug levels before implementing medication changes.

3. Monitor the patient for toxic side effects of medications.
4. Monitor complete blood count, urinalysis, and liver function studies for toxicity caused by medications.
5. Monitor emotional and intellectual development in children with seizures.

Supportive Care

1. Provide a safe environment by padding side rails and removing clutter.
2. Place the bed in a low position.
3. Do not restrain the patient during a seizure.

> **COMMUNITY CARE CONSIDERATIONS**
> Ensure that the home environment is safe, especially for children. Remove toys with sharp edges or parts and small pieces that could be choked on, and cover very hard surfaces that the child could fall against.

4. Do not put anything in the patient's mouth during a seizure.
5. Maintain a patent airway until the patient is fully awake after a seizure. An oral airway may be placed at the start of a seizure or the airway suctioned if necessary.
6. Provide oxygen during the seizure if the patient becomes cyanotic.

7. Place the patient on side during a seizure to prevent aspiration.
8. Protect the patient's head during a seizure. Provide a helmet to the patient who may fall during a seizure.
9. Stay with the patient who is ambulating or in a confused state during a seizure.
10. Consult with social worker for community resources for vocational rehabilitation, counselors, support groups.
11. Teach stress reduction techniques that will fit into the patient's lifestyle.
12. Initiate appropriate consultation for management of behaviors related to personality disorders and possible brain damage secondary to chronic epilepsy.

Family Education and Health Maintenance

1. Encourage the patient to determine existence of trigger factors for seizures, such as skipped meals, lack of sleep, emotional stress.
2. Remind the family of the importance of following medication regimen and maintaining regular immunizations, medical checkups, and dental and visual examinations.
3. Tell the patient to avoid alcohol because it interferes with metabolism of antiepileptic medications.
4. Encourage the patient and family to discuss feelings and attitudes about epilepsy.
5. Encourage the patient to wear a medical alert card or bracelet.
6. Encourage a moderate lifestyle routine, including exercise, mental activity, and nutritious diet.
7. Correct myths about epilepsy and reassure family that epilepsy is not contagious, not proven to be hereditary, and not associated with insanity.
8. For the surgical candidate, reinforce instructions related to surgical outcome of the specific surgical approach.
9. Refer the patient and family to:

> **Epilepsy Foundation of America**
> 4351 Garden City Dr.
> Landover, MD 20785
> 301-459-3700

(text continues on page 788)

TABLE 17 Sexually Transmitted Diseases

Disorder, Cause, Incubation	Clinical Manifestations	Diagnosis and Treatment
Herpes Genitalis Caused by herpes simplex virus, type II in most cases; incubation is 5–20 days.	Clustered vesicles on erythematous, edematous base that rupture, leaving shallow, painful ulcer that eventually crusts; mild lymphadenopathy; recurrent and may be brought on by sunburn, fever, stress, infection, menses, pregnancy.	Diagnostic tests include Tzanck smear, viral culture, antibody tests. No cure, but symptomatic period is diminished by acyclovir started with each recurrence; or recurrences reduced or prevented by continuous therapy. Analgesics and sitz baths promote comfort.
Condyloma Acuminatum (Genital Warts) Caused by human papilloma virus (HPV); incubation is 3 weeks to 3 months, possible years before grossly visible	Single or multiple, soft, fleshy, flat or vegetating, nonpainful growths that may occur on external genitalia, anal area, or internally in the vagina, cervix, or urethra	Diagnosed by appearance, Pap smear, or biopsy. Topical therapy with podofilox 0.5%, podophyllin 10%–25%, or trichloroacetic acid 80%–90%—may require multiple applications. Cryotherapy, electrodissection, electrocautery, carbon dioxide laser, or surgical excision may be necessary.

S

S

Syphilis Caused by the spirochete *Treponema pallidum*; incubation is 10 to 90 days for primary, up to 6 months after chancre for secondary	Primary: nontender, shallow, indurated, clean, dry ulcer; mild regional lymphadenopathy. Secondary: maculopapular rash including palms and soles; mucous patches and condalomatous lesions; fever, generalized lymphadenopathy	VDRL or rapid plasma reagin (RPR) blood test with confirmation by specific treponemal antibody test. Preferred treatment is benzathine penicillin G 2.4 million units in single dose. Oral doxycycline, tetracycline, or erythromycin may be used.
Gonorrhea Caused by *Neisseria gonorrhoeae*; incubation is 2–5 days	Urethritis in men: dysuria, thin clear or yellow discharge; may develop into epididymitis or prostatis. Cervicitis in females: asymptomatic or mucopurulent discharge, dysuria, pelvic pain; may progress to pelvic inflammatory disease (PID). In both sexes: pharyngitis, conjunctivitis, proctitis, or disseminated arthritis and skin lesions	Diagnosed by Gram stain, culture, or antigen detection test. IM or oral antibiotic therapy with penicillinase—resistant penicillins, some cephalosporins, and quinolones; one large-dose treatment is effective for cervicitis and urethritis.
Chlamydia Caused by *Chlamydia trachomatis*; incubation period is 7–10 days or longer	Urethritis in men: asymptomatic or clear to whitish discharge, dysuria; may progress to epididymitis. Cervicitis: asymptomatic or clear to creamy discharge, bleeding, dysruia, pelvic discomfort; may progress to PID or infertility.	Antigen detection tests. One dose to 7 days of therapy with doxycycline, azithromycin, ofloxacin, or erythromycin.

Senile Dementia of the Alzheimer Type
See Alzheimer's Disease

Sexually Transmitted Diseases

Sexually transmitted diseases (STDs) include a wide variety of viral, bacterial, and other infections transmitted through sexual contact, usually through genital secretions and direct contact with lesions. STDs include gonorrhea, chlamydia, genital herpes, genital warts, syphilis, trichomonas (p. 867), human immunodeficiency virus and acquired immunodeficiency syndrome (p. 867), viral hepatitis (p. 417), scabies, and pubic lice. Rarer STDs include chancroid, lymphogranuloma venereum (LGV), and granuloma inguinale. Table 17 describes common STDs and their management.

◆ Nursing Interventions and Patient Education

1. Explain transmission of STDs and preventive measures such as male or female condoms, abstinence, and mutual monogomy.
2. Stress the need for sexual abstinence or the use of condoms until treatment of both patient and partner is complete and follow-up has determined cure. In recurrent herpes genitalis, intercourse should be avoided from the first sign of outbreak to complete resolution of symptoms; however asymptomatic shedding still occurs in some patients.
3. Encourage women to have routine Pap smears because herpes simplex virus (HSV) and human papilloma virus (HPV) may cause cervical changes leading to cancer.
4. Ensure that pregnant women are tested and treated for STDs because risk to fetus occurs during pregnancy and delivery.
5. For further information and support, refer to:

    STD National Hotline
    1-800-227-8922

Shock

Shock is inadequate tissue prefusion that occurs as a result of failure of one or more of the following: the heart as a pump, blood volume, arterial resistance vessels, and the capacity of venous beds. Shock is classified as:

Hypovolemic shock: occurs when a significant amount of fluid (blood, plasma, electrolytes) is lost from the intravascular space. May result from hemorrhage, burns, or fluid shifts

Cardiogenic shock: occurs when the heart fails as a pump, primarily because of myocardial infarction, serious cardiac dysrhythmias, and depressed myocardial contractility. Secondary causes include mechanical restriction or venous obstruction, as in cardiac tamponade, vena cava obstruction, or tension pneumothorax.

Septic shock: occurs as a result of bacteria and their toxins, primarily vasoactive mediators released by gram-negative bacteria. Any infection has the potential to produce septic shock and compromise every physiologic system.

Neurogenic shock: occurs as a result of failure of arterial resistance caused by loss of thoracic spinal nerve control, as in spinal cord injury or spinal anesthesia

◆ Assessment

1. Decreased level of consciousness
   a. Confusion, irritability, anxiety, inability to concentrate—early signs
   b. Progresses to lethargy, obtundation, and coma
2. Cool, pale extremities and capillary refill greater than 2 seconds
3. Change in blood pressure
   a. May initially increase because of compensation
   b. Narrow pulse pressure seen early because of increase in diastolic pressure
   c. Decrease in systolic pressure eventually occurs: deviation from normal or systolic below 80 mm Hg or mean below 60 mm Hg
4. Tachycardia, weak thready pulse
5. Decreased urine output: less than 25 mL/h in adults; less than 1 mL/kg/h in children

◆ Diagnostic Evaluation

1. Condition is diagnosed by clinical signs, and treatment is begun immediately.
2. Diagnostic testing is done to determine cause of sepsis (cultures of blood, urine, wounds, sputum, etc.) as well as body's response to shock (electrolytes, complete blood count, kidney function tests, etc.).

◆ Collaborative Management

Therapeutic Interventions

1. Oxygen therapy by non-rebreather face mask to augment oxygen-carrying capacity of arterial blood
2. Intubation and assisted ventilation if necessary
3. Military antishock trousers (MAST) to facilitate blood flow to vital organs
4. Fluid resuscitation for hypovolemic shock, preferably through two large-bore or central lines, initially with Ringer's lactate solution
5. Blood product replacement as indicated
6. Hemodynamic monitoring with Swan-Ganz catheter, especially for cardiogenic shock
7. Hypothermia blanket in septic shock to cool patient

Pharmacologic Interventions

1. Vasopressors such as dopamine, norepinephrine, and metaraminol to cause vasoconstriction and raise blood pressure
2. Positive inotropic agents in cardiogenic shock such as isoproterenol, digoxin, dobutamine, and amrinone to increase cardiac contractility and raise cardiac output
3. Diuretics may be given in cardiogenic shock to decrease pulmonary congestion.
4. Broad-spectrum antibiotics and antipyretics in septic shock

◆ Nursing Interventions

Monitoring

1. Maintain ongoing monitoring of blood pressure, heart rate, central venous pressure, and cardiac rhythm.
2. Monitor respiratory rate, effort, and breath sounds.

3. Monitor temperature in septic shock.
4. Monitor pulmonary artery pressure, pulmonary capillary wedge pressure, and cardiac output in cardiogenic shock.
5. Monitor hourly urinary output.
6. Monitor arterial blood gases for acidosis associated with poor perfusion.
7. Monitor hemoglobin and hematocrit to assess hemorrhage.

Supportive Care

1. Maintain patient in supine position with legs elevated.

> **NURSING ALERT**
> Trendelenberg position for shock is no longer recommended because of potential for respiratory compromise from pressure of abdominal organs.

2. Stay with patient and provide reassurance.
3. Report changes in blood pressure and clinical condition immediately.
4. Maintain NPO status until condition is stable and patient is fully alert with good bowel sounds.
5. Titrate vasopressors to desired blood pressure and within prescribed parameters.
6. Keep family informed of patient's condition.
7. After stabilization, provide for periods of uninterrupted rest.

Family Education and Health Maintenance

1. Explain effects of shock on all body systems so patient understands seriousness of illness.
2. Ensure the proper follow-up for underlying cause as well as residual effects of shock (such as renal impairment).
3. Teach about medications the patient may be maintained on, such as antibiotics or digoxin.
4. Encourage follow-up blood work for hemoglobin and hematocrit, electrolytes, kidney function tests, digoxin level, and other tests as indicated.

Sickle Cell Disease

Sickle cell disease (sickle cell anemia) is a severe, chronic, hemolytic anemia occurring in persons who are homozygous for the abnormal hemoglobin-S (sickle) gene. The clinical course is marked by episodes of pain caused by the occlusion of small blood vessels by malformed or "sickled" red blood cells (RBCs), brought on by hypoxia, acidosis, and dehydration. Persons heterozygous for the sickling gene are said to possess *sickle cell trait*, which does not progress to sickle cell anemia.

Sickled RBCs are fragile and are rapidly destroyed in the circulation; they live 6 to 20 days versus 120 days for normal RBCs. Anemia results when the rate of destruction of RBCs is greater than the rate of production. Increased sequestration of red cells also occurs in the spleen.

Approximately 8% of African Americans have sickle cell trait; approximately 1 of every 600 African American infants has sickle cell disease. Life expectancy is variable but improving with new forms of treatment. The greatest risk of death is in children younger than age 5 years, mainly from overwhelming sepsis or RBC sequestration.

◆ Assessment

1. Children do not become symptomatic until late in the first year of life, then symptoms are sporadic.
2. Anemia may last 1 to 2 weeks and subside spontaneously. The child may have a hemoglobin of 6 to 9 g/dL with loss of appetite, pallor, weakness, fever, irritability, and jaundice.
3. Crisis may be precipitated by dehydration, infection, trauma, strenuous physical exertion, extreme fatigue, cold exposure, hypoxia, or acidosis.
4. *Vasoocclusive (painful) crisis*—most common form of crisis:
   a. Osteoporosis or ischemic necrosis of bones
   b. Bone pain; painful and swollen large joints
   c. Dactylitis ("hand–foot" syndrome): aseptic infarction of metacarpals and metatarsals causing symmetric swelling and pain; often first vasoocclusive crisis seen in infants and toddlers

    d. Abdominal pain and splenomegaly

    e. Cerebral occlusion causing stroke, hemiplegia, retinal damage leading to blindness, seizures

    f. Pulmonary infarction

    g. Altered renal function: enuresis, hematuria

    h. Impaired liver function

    i. Priapism: abnormal, recurrent, prolonged, painful erection of the penis

5. *Splenic sequestration crisis:* Spleen becomes massively enlarged because of pooling of blood.

    a. Sudden decrease in RBC count

    b. Signs of circulatory collapse develop rapidly.

    c. Frequent cause of death in infant with sickle cell disease

6. *Aplastic crisis:* Bone marrow ceases to produce RBCs.

    a. Low reticulocyte count

    b. Pallor, lethargy, dyspnea

    c. Possible coma

7. Chronic symptoms related to organ damage:

    a. Jaundice

    b. Gallstones

    c. Progressive impairment of kidney function

    d. Fibrotic spleen resulting in high susceptibility to *Haemophilus influenzae, Streptococcus pneumoniae,* osteomyelitis, and pneumococcal septicemia

    e. Growth retardation of the long bones and spine deformities

    f. Aseptic necrosis of bones, especially the femoral and humoral heads

    g. Delayed puberty

    h. Cardiac decompensation related to chronic anemia

    i. Chronic, painful leg ulcers related to decreased peripheral circulation and unrelated to injury; may take months to heal or may not heal without intense therapy, including blood transfusions and grafting

    j. Decreased life span

◆ Diagnostic Evaluation

1. Sickle cell preparation (sickling test)

    a. Blood from heel or finger stick is deoxygenated, and

observed under the microscope for evidence of sick-led RBCs.

b. Test does not distinguish between persons with sickle cell trait and disease or other sickle hemoglobinopathies.

2. Sickledex test

a. Combines blood sample in test tube with solution containing a chemical reducing agent. Clouded solution indicates hemoglobin-S.

b. Also does not distinguish between persons with sickle cell trait and disease or other sickle hemoglobinopathies

3. Hemoglobin electrophoresis

a. Requires venipuncture

b. Hemoglobin is subjected to an electric current that separates the various types and determines the amounts present.

c. Used to diagnose both sickle cell trait and sickle cell disease if two types of hemoglobin are demonstrated in approximately equal amounts

d. A person is diagnosed as having sickle cell disease if most of his or her hemoglobin is S-type. The test may also diagnose other sickle hemoglobinopathies, including sickle-C, sickle-G thalassemia, or other hemoglobin variants.

4. Antenatal diagnosis is available to the high-risk group through amniocentesis or chorionic villi sampling, with DNA analysis.

5. CBC indicates:

a. RBCs: decreased

b. WBCs: elevated

c. Platelets: elevated

d. Erythrocyte sedimentation rate: decreased

e. Serum iron: increased

f. RBC survival time: decreased

g. Hemoglobin: low or normal

◆ Collaborative Management

Therapeutic Interventions

1. Prevention of sickling by promoting adequate oxygenation and hemodilution

a. Encourage increased fluid intake: 150 mL/kg/day or 2,250 mL/m^2 per day.
b. Avoid high altitudes and other low-oxygen environments.
c. Avoid strenuous physical exertion.
d. Administer oxygen for pulse oximetry of 90% or less.

2. *Aplastic episode:* usually requires a blood transfusion starting at 10 mL/kg

3. *Splenic sequestration:* usually requires a blood transfusion to release trapped RBCs in severe cases. Plasma volume expanders also may be used to correct hypovolemia.

4. *Hemolytic episode:* usually requires only hydration. May occur with splenic sequestration, aplastic, and painful episodes, which are then treated accordingly. Transfusions are required if there is a significant decrease in hemoglobin.

5. *Vasoocclusive (painful) episode:* must be distinguished from underlying illness (infection) or other inflammatory condition.
a. Hydration is provided by increased oral and parenteral fluid intake of up to one and one-half or twice fluid maintenance needs.
b. Electrolytes and acid–base balance must be maintained.

6. In vasoocclusive (painful) episode, nonpharmacologic pain management techniques may include behavior modification programs, relaxation therapy, hypnosis, and transcutaneous electrical nerve stimulation (TENS).

Pharmacologic Interventions

1. Analgesics: administered on fixed schedule, not to extend beyond the duration of the pharmacologic effect
a. IV narcotics such as morphine are preferred for severe pain, either as a continuous infusion or on a patient-controlled analgesia (PCA) pump to reach desired effects.
b. Other agents such as NSAIDs and acetaminophen are used for milder pain or to increase the analgesic effects of narcotics.

2. Investigational drugs include alpha butyrate and hy-

droxyurea, which increase fetal hemoglobin, thereby preventing sickling.

3. Prevention of infection—major cause of morbidity and mortality—is accomplished through regular immunizations as well as pneumococcal, influenza, and hepatitis immunizations.

4. Antibiotics may be given prophylactically.

Surgical Interventions

1. One or more episodes of splenic sequestration may require splenectomy.

◆ Nursing Interventions

Monitoring

1. Obtain pulse oximetry reading frequently. Arterial blood gases should be done for correlation and to evaluate acid–base status.

2. Monitor pain relief and adjust dose or time interval for adequate control.

3. Monitor for respiratory depression, hypotension, and drowsiness with narcotic analgesics.

4. Monitor fluid intake and output, daily weight, and urine specific gravity, to determine fluid balance and hydration status.

Supportive Care

1. Employ effective pain relief measures, such as:
   a. Carefully position and support painful areas.
   b. Hold or rock the infant; handle gently.
   c. Distract the child by singing, reading stories, providing play activities.
   d. Provide familiar objects; encourage visits by familiar persons.
   e. Bathe the child in warm water, applying local heat or massage.
   f. Give suitable medications. *DO NOT* give aspirin, because it enhances acidosis.
   g. Maintain bed rest during crisis.

PEDIATRIC ALERT
Avoid giving analgesia intramuscularly if possible, because children associate a great deal of pain with shots and may deny pain to avoid getting the shot.

---

2. Share effective methods of reducing pain with other staff members and family.
3. Administer oxygen via tent, face mask, or nasal cannula, depending on age of patient.
4. Give meticulous care to leg ulcers and other open wounds.
5. Use good handwashing and fastidious technique in all procedures.
6. Maintain adequate hydration before and after surgery and observe the child closely for signs of infection postoperatively, especially of the respiratory tract, to prevent crisis.
7. Maintain bed rest during crisis, then increase activity gradually to increase endurance.
8. Encourage good eating habits, sleep, and relaxation.
9. Provide emotional support to the child and family.
10. Help the child and family to express their feelings of fear and anxiety about what is happening.
11. Assure adolescents that although sexual development is delayed, they will eventually catch up with their peers.
12. Stress the normalcy of the child despite sickle cell.
    a. Disease does not affect intelligence; the child should go to school and keep up with classwork while stable.
    b. Between periods of crisis the child can usually participate in peer group activities, with the exception of some strenuous sports.
    c. The child needs discipline and limit setting, as do other children in family.

Family Education and Health Maintenance

1. Discuss the genetic implications of sickle cell disease and offer genetic counseling to the family.
2. Instruct the parents in ways that they can help their child to avoid precipitating factors of sickling episodes.
3. Encourage parents to seek prompt treatment of cuts, sores, mosquito bites, etc. and to notify the health care provider if the child is exposed to a communicable disease.
4. Encourage good dental hygiene and frequent dental checkups to avoid dental infections.

5. Instruct on preventive care, including all of the normal childhood immunizations and a tuberculin test every 2 to 3 years. In addition, children older than age 2 years should receive the pneumococcal, *Haemophilus* type b, meningococcal, recombinant hepatitis B (series of 3), and trivalent influenza (yearly) vaccines.
6. Teach the child to avoid undue emotional stress.
7. Warn against trips to the mountains or in not well-pressurized airplanes that will decrease oxygen concentration.
8. Provide sexually active adolescents with information on contraception and sexually transmitted disease.
9. Teach parents to recognize and manage a mild crisis. Hospitalization may be required for the child if pain becomes severe or if IV hydration is required.
10. Teach the signs of severe crisis and whom to notify. Immediately report fever of 102°F (38.9°C).
11. Instruct the parents to have emergency information available to those involved in the child's care (school nurse, teacher, babysitter, family members, etc.).
12. Stress the benefit of wearing a medical alert tag.
13. For additional information and support, refer to:

> **Sickle Cell Foundation**
> 4401 Crenshaw Blvd. Suite 208
> Los Angeles, CA 90043
> 213-299-3600

Sinusitis

Sinusitis is an inflammation of the mucous membranes of one or more paranasal sinuses (Fig. 24). Occurring in acute and chronic forms, sinusitis is usually precipitated by congestion from a viral upper respiratory infection or nasal allergy, leading to obstruction of the sinus ostia and retention of secretions. *Chronic sinusitis* is a suppurative inflammation of the sinuses that produces irreversible changes in the mucous membranes. Complications of sinusitis include orbital cellulitis, cranial osteomyelitis, cavernous sinus thrombosis, meningitis, and brain abscess.

S

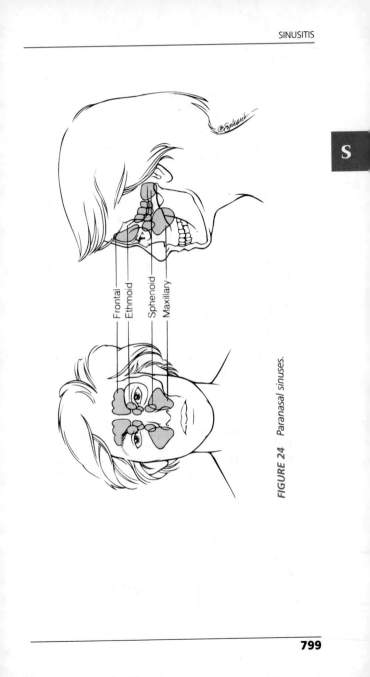

FIGURE 24 *Paranasal sinuses.*

Frontal
Ethmoid
Sphenoid
Maxillary

♦ **Assessment**

1. Acute sinusitis:
   a. Stabbing or aching pain over the infected sinus. Pain in forehead intensified by bending forward indicates *frontal sinusitis*. Aching pain in facial region, and from inner canthus of the eye to the teeth, indicates *maxillary sinusitis*. Frontal or orbital headache indicates *ethmoid sinusitis*. Headache referred to top of head and deep to the eyes indicates *sphenoid sinusitis*.
   b. Nasal congestion, discharge, postnasal drip, and anosmia (lack of smell) may or may not be present.
   c. Fever may be present.
   d. Nasal mucosa appears red and edematous.
   e. Percussion over involved sinus may produce tenderness, and transillumination will produce dullness.
2. Chronic sinusitis:
   a. Persistent nasal obstruction; chronic nasal discharge, clear but becomes purulent when acutely infected
   b. Feeling of facial fullness or pressure
   c. Cough produced by chronic postnasal drip
   d. Headache (more noticeable in the morning), fatigue

♦ **Diagnostic Evaluation**

1. Sinus x-rays or CT: may show air–fluid level, thickened mucous membranes, or complete opacification
2. Antral puncture and lavage to provide culture material to identify infectious organism; also a therapeutic modality to clear sinus of bacteria, fluid, and inflammatory cells (acute sinusitis)
3. Endoscopy of nose with CT imaging to show mucosal changes in chronic sinusitis

♦ **Collaborative Management**

Pharmacologic Interventions

1. Topical decongestant spray or drops or systemic decongestants for mucosal shrinkage to enhance sinus drainage. Topical therapy should not be used for more than 3 successive days.

2. In chronic sinusitis, nasal corticosteroids may be used to promote drainage.

3. Antibiotics such as penicillinase-resistant penicillin, trimethroprim-sulfamethoxazole, macrolide preparations, or cephalosporins are used for purulent sinusitis. Therapy may be extended for 6 weeks or more in chronic sinusitis.

Surgical Interventions

1. Endoscopic sinus surgery—endoscopic removal of diseased tissue from affected sinus; used to treat chronic sinusitis of maxillary, ethmoid, and frontal sinuses

2. Nasal antrostomy (nasal–antral window): surgical placement of an opening under inferior turbinate to provide aeration of the antrum and to allow drainage of purulent materials in chronic sinusitis

◆ Nursing Interventions

Monitoring

1. Be alert for possible extension of infection to the orbital contents and eyelids.

NURSING ALERT

Watch for lid edema, edema of ocular conjunctiva, drooping lid, limitation of extraocular motion, visual loss. May indicate orbital cellulitis, which requires immediate treatment.

2. Monitor response to therapy and for adverse reactions to antibiotics.

3. After surgery, monitor for bleeding, fever caused by local infection, and aspiration.

Supportive Care

1. After surgery, keep head elevated at night to reduce swelling and encourage fluids and use of humidifier while nasal packing in place and patient is mouth breathing.

2. Encourage use of cold compresses over incisional area or involved sinus to reduce bleeding and swelling.

3. Encourage frequent mouth care and change of any external dressings when saturated.

4. Advise follow-up for removal of packing approximately 48 hours after surgery.
5. Encourage blotting of nose with tissue rather than blowing or picking at crusts.

Family Education and Health Maintenance

1. Advise use of over-the-counter analgesics and warm compresses over sinuses to relieve acute pain.
2. Advise patient to promptly seek medical attention for acute sinus infection to prevent chronic sinus disease.
3. Discourage swimming or diving, which may cause contaminated water to be forced into a sinus (usually frontal).
4. Stress the importance of complying with antibiotic therapy; 2 to 3 weeks usually necessary for acute infection, longer for chronic infection
5. Advise the patient with asthma that sinusitis has been associated with exacerbation of asthma symptoms; warn the patient to seek treatment for increased wheezing, chest tightness, or cough.

Sjögren's Syndrome

Sjögren's syndrome is a chronic inflammatory autoimmune process of unknown cause that affects the lacrimal and salivary glands. It is thought that antibodies directed at exocrine glands are produced, causing lymphocytic infiltration and impairing function of the involved tissue. The disease occurs primarily in middle-aged women and can be primary or secondary. Secondary Sjögren's syndrome is seen most commonly in rheumatoid arthritis (RA) but can be seen in systemic lupus erythematosus (SLE) and some other connective tissue diseases.

The syndrome may cause a variety of complications, such as corneal disease, tooth loss, pulmonary fibrosis or hypertension, obstructive airway disease, chronic atrophic gastritis, chronic pancreatitis, abnormal liver or kidney function, and dementia.

◆ Assessment

1. Decreased tear production leading to keratoconjunctivitis, photophobia

2. Dry mouth (xerostoma), mucosal ulcers, stomatitis, salivary gland enlargement (unilateral or bilateral), dysphagia
3. Nasal dryness, epistaxis, nasal ulcers
4. Dryness of bronchial tree, hoarseness, recurrent otitis media, pneumonia, and bronchitis
5. Skin dryness (xerodermia), urticaria, purpura
6. Pancreatitis, hypochlorhydria or achlorhydria, autoimmune liver disease
7. Renal tubular acidosis, nephrogenic diabetes insipidus
8. Trigeminal neuropathy (Bell's palsy), polymyopathy, sensory and motor neuropathy, seizures, multiple sclerosis–like syndrome
9. Autoimmune thyroiditis
10. Raynaud's phenomenon, vasculitis; babies born to mothers with Sjögren's syndrome may have congenital heart block.
11. Vaginal dryness, dyspareunia
12. Nonerosive polyarthritis

◆ Diagnostic Evaluation

1. CBC: mild anemia; leukopenia present in 30% of patients
2. Erythrocyte sedimentation rate: Elevated in 90% of patients
3. Rheumatoid factor: positive in 75% to 90% of patients
4. Antinuclear antibody (ANA): positive in 70% of patients; speckled and nucleolar patterns are most common
5. Antibodies to SSA/SSB: to detect antibodies to specific nuclear proteins
   a. SSA: positive in patients with Sjögren's syndrome and SLE
   b. SSB: positive in 60% of patients with Sjögren's syndrome; can also be positive in patients with SLE
   c. Organ-specific antibodies: antibodies directed against specific organ tissues, including gastric, thyroid, smooth muscle, salivary glands, and lacrimal glands, have been found.
6. Salivary scintigraphy to evaluate salivary gland function

7. X-rays of affected joints to rule out erosive arthritis
8. Salivary gland biopsy may be done to determine lymphocytic infiltration of tissue.

◆ Collaborative Management

Therapeutic Interventions

1. Provide symptomatic relief of dryness:
   a. Artificial tears
   b. Saliva substitutes
   c. Frequent use of nonsugar liquids, gums, and candies
   d. Vaginal lubricants
   e. Use of occlusive goggles at bedtime to prevent drying
2. Encourage dental care—frequent brushing and flossing, topical fluoride treatments, avoidance of high-sucrose foods

Pharmacologic Interventions

1. Corticosteroids and immunosuppressants such as cyclophosphamide are used in severe cases.
2. Antifungal agents therapeutically or prophylactically for superimposed fungal infections of mouth or vagina

◆ Nursing Interventions

Supportive Care

1. Inspect oral mucosa for oral candida, ulcers, saliva pools, and dental hygiene.
2. Instruct or assist the patient in proper oral hygiene.
3. Encourage frequent intake of noncaffeinated nonsugar liquids. Keep pitcher filled with cool water.
4. Instruct or assist the patient with daily inspection of skin for areas of trauma or potential breakdown.
5. Apply lubricants to skin daily.
6. Avoid shearing forces and encourage or perform frequent position changes.
7. Increase liquid intake with meals.
8. Assist or instruct the patient to avoid choosing spicy or dry foods from menu choices.
9. Suggest smaller, more frequent meals.
10. Weigh weekly and review diet history for basic nutrient deficiencies.

11. Advise on proper use of water-soluble vaginal lubrication.
12. Suggest alternate positioning and practices to prevent dyspareunia.
13. Teach the patient to recognize and report symptoms of vaginitis because infection may result from altered mucosal barrier.

Health Maintenance and Patient Education

1. Advise the patient of commercially available artificial saliva preparations, artificial tears, moisturizing nasal sprays, artificial vaginal moisturizers.
2. Encourage frequent dental visits. Dental cavities are more frequent in Sjögren's syndrome.
3. Advise the patient to check with health care provider before using any medications because many cause mouth dryness (eg, diuretics, tricyclic antidepressants, antihistamines).
4. Advise the patient to wear protective eyewear while outdoors.

Skin Cancer
See Cancer, Skin

Somatoform Disorders
See Anxiety, Somatoform, and Dissociative Disorders

Spina Bifida

Spina bifida refers to malformations of the spine in which the posterior portion of the vertebral laminae fails to close. These malformations are thought to result from incomplete or defective closure of the neural tube during the 4th to 6th weeks of embryonic life.

Three major types of spina bifida are recognized (Fig.

25). In *spina bifida occulta,* the most common type, the defect involves only the vertebrae; the spinal cord and meninges are normal. However, the spinal cord and its meninges may be connected with a fistulous tract extending to and opening onto the surface of the skin. Neurologic problems are rare.

In *meningocele,* the meninges protrude through the opening in the spinal canal, forming a cyst filled with cerebrospinal fluid and covered with skin. The defect may occur anywhere on the spinal cord. Higher defects (from thorax and upward) are usually meningoceles. As in spina bifida occulta, neurologic problems are rare.

In *myelomeningocele,* both the spinal cord and meninges protrude through the defect in the vertebral column and are protected by a thin, membranous sac. Various forms of permanent neurologic deficit are present. The sac may leak in utero or may rupture after birth, allowing free drainage of cerebrospinal fluid. This renders the child highly susceptible to meningitis. Myelomeningocele occurs four to five times more frequently than meningocele. In the absence of treatment, most infants with meningomyelocele die soon after birth.

Spina bifida is the most common developmental defect of the central nervous system and occurs in approximately 1 per every 1,000 live births in the United States. The condition may have other congenital anomalies associated with it, especially hydrocephalus.

◆ Assessment

1. Spina bifida occulta
   a. Most patients have no symptoms. A dimple in the skin or hair growth may appear over the malformed vertebra.
   b. With growth, the child may develop foot weakness or bowel and bladder sphincter disturbances.
2. Meningocele
   a. Physical examination shows a saclike outpouching in the spinal cord, usually in the midline.
   b. Seldom evidence of weakness of the legs or lack of sphincter control
3. Myelomeningocele
   a. Physical examination shows a round, raised, and

S

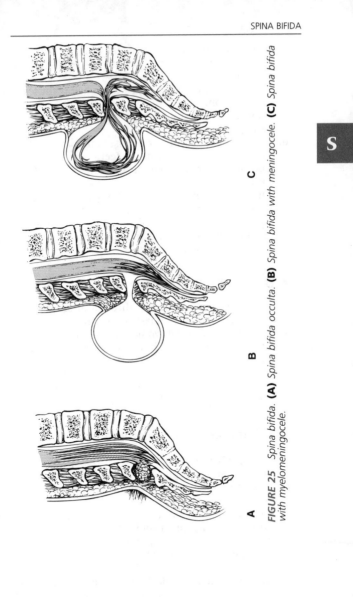

FIGURE 25 Spina bifida. **(A)** Spina bifida occulta. **(B)** Spina bifida with meningocele. **(C)** Spina bifida with myelomeningocele.

poorly epithelialized area, usually in the lumbosacral area. Lesion may occur at any level of the spinal column.
b. Loss of motor control and sensation below the level of the lesion.
c. A low thoracic lesion may cause total flaccid paralysis below the waist.
d. A small sacral lesion may cause only patchy spots of decreased sensation in the feet.
e. Contractures may occur in the ankles, knees, or hips.
f. Clubfoot commonly occurs; thought to be related to position of paraplegic feet in the uterus
g. Urinary incontinence and retention and fecal incontinence and constipation occur because of impairment of sacral nerves.

◆ Diagnostic Evaluation

1. Prenatal detection is possible through amniocentesis and measurement of alpha-fetoprotein. This testing should be offered to all women at risk (women who are affected themselves or have had other affected children).
2. Diagnosis is primarily based on clinical manifestations.
3. CT scan and MRI may be performed to further evaluate the brain and spinal cord.

◆ Collaborative Management

Therapeutic Interventions

1. A coordinated team approach will help maximize the physical and intellectual potential of each affected child.
   a. The team may include a neurologist, neurosurgeon, orthopedic surgeon, urologist, primary care provider, social worker, physical therapist, a variety of community-based and hospital staff nurses, the child, and family.
   b. Numerous neurosurgical, orthopedic, and urologic procedures may be necessary to help the child achieve maximum potential.

Pharmacologic Interventions

1. Imipramine or ephedrine may be used to help retain urine rather than dribbling, along with Credé's maneuver or self-catheterization to facilitate elimination.
2. Antibiotics to prevent or treat urinary tract infection
3. Stool softeners, suppositories, and enemas may be necessary to achieve bowel movements.

Surgical Interventions

1. In meningocele and myelomeningocele, laminectomy and closure of an open lesion or removal of the sac usually can be done soon after birth.
2. Surgery is done to prevent further deterioration of neural function, to minimize danger of rupture of sac and meningitis, to improve cosmetic effect, and to facilitate handling of infant.
3. For those children who cannot achieve urinary continence through intermittent catheterization, options include surgically implanted mechanical urinary sphincters, bladder pacemakers, or urinary diversion.

◆ Nursing Interventions

Monitoring

1. Monitor and report immediately any signs of infection.
   a. Oozing of fluid or pus from the sac
   b. Fever
   c. Irritability or listlessness
   d. Seizure
2. Monitor urine elimination and report concentrated or foul-smelling urine, indicating urinary tract infection.
3. Monitor for signs of hydrocephalus and report immediately.
   a. Irritability
   b. Feeding difficulty, vomiting, decreased appetite
   c. Temperature fluctuation
   d. Decreased alertness
   e. Tense fontanel
   f. Increased head circumference
4. Frequently monitor temperature, pulse, respirations, color, and level of responsiveness postoperatively, based on the infant's stability.

S

Supportive Care

Preoperative care in neonatal period

1. Use prone positioning with hips only slightly flexed to decrease tension on the sac; check position at least once every hour.

2. Do not place diaper or any covering directly over the sac.

3. Observe the sac frequently for evidence of irritation or leakage of cerebrospinal fluid.

4. Place padding between the infant's legs to maintain the hips in abduction and to prevent or counteract subluxation.

5. Use a foam or fleece pad to reduce pressure of the mattress against the infant's skin.

6. Allow the infant's feet to hang freely over pads or mattress edge to avoid aggravating foot deformities.

7. Provide meticulous skin care to all areas of the body, especially ankles, knees, tip of nose, cheeks, and chin.

8. Provide passive range-of-motion exercises for those muscles and joints that the infant does not use spontaneously. Avoid hip exercises because of common hip dislocation, unless otherwise recommended.

9. Avoid pressure on infant's back during feeding by holding the infant with your elbow rotated to avoid touching the sac, or feeding while infant is lying on side or prone on your lap. Encourage parents to use these positions to provide infant stimulation and bonding.

10. Keep the buttocks and genitalia scrupulously clean; infection of the sac is most commonly caused by contamination by urine and feces.
    a. Do not diaper the infant if the defect is in the lower portion of the spine.
    b. Use a small plastic drape taped between the defect and the anus to help prevent contamination.

11. Apply a sterile dressing over the sac only as directed and change frequently to prevent adhesion to sac and maintain sterility.

12. To promote urinary elimination, use Credé's method to empty the bladder (unless contraindicated by vesicoureteral reflux), and teach parents the technique.

Continue the procedure as long as urine can be manually expressed.

13. Ensure fluid intake to dilute the urine.

Postoperative care in infancy and childhood

1. Use an Isolette or infant warmer to prevent temperature fluctuation.
2. Prevent respiratory complications.
   a. Periodically reposition the infant to promote lung expansion.
   b. Watch for abdominal distension, which could interfere with breathing.
   c. Have oxygen available.
3. Maintain hydration and nutritional intake.
   a. Administer IV fluids as ordered; keep accurate intake and output log.
   b. Administer gavage feedings as ordered.
   c. Begin bottle feeding when infant responsive and tolerating feedings.
4. Be aware that children with spina bifida are susceptible to latex allergy. Symptoms include hives, itching, wheezing, and anaphylaxis.
   a. Limit or prevent direct contact of child with such products as blood pressure cuffs, tourniquets, tape, Foley catheters, gloves, and IV tubing injection ports.

COMMUNITY CARE CONSIDERATIONS

Toys and equipment for children such as nipples, pacifiers, and elastic on the legs of some clothing also contain latex. The home environment should be surveyed for latex and substitute products obtained, if possible. Teach the parents how to recognize latex allergy and notify the child's health care provider.

5. Teach parents that continence can usually be achieved with clean, intermittent self-catheterization.
   a. Children can generally be taught to catheterize themselves by age 6 to 7 years.
   b. Parents can catheterize younger children.
   c. Red rubber catheters are used rather than latex catheters.

> **COMMUNITY CARE CONSIDERATIONS**
> The family can be taught to clean and reuse urinary catheters. The catheter should be washed in warm, soapy water and rinsed well in warm water. The catheter should be air dried and, when completely dried, placed in a clean jar or plastic bag. A catheter should be replaced when it becomes dry, cracked, stiff, or if the child develops a urinary tract infection.

6. Teach the signs of urinary tract infection (concentrated, foul-smelling urine, burning, and fever) and the proper administration of antibiotics either prophylactically or when prescribed for infection.
7. Assist with bowel training program, including high-fiber, high-fluid diet, bowel medication, and regular elimination time.
8. To foster positive body image in an older child, emphasize rehabilitation that uses the child's strengths and minimizes disabilities.
9. Continually reassess functional abilities and offer suggestions to increase independence. Periodically consult with physical or occupational therapists to help maximize function.
10. Encourage the use of braces and specialized equipment to enhance ambulation, while minimizing the appearance of the equipment.
11. Encourage participation with peer group and in activities that build on strengths such as cognitive abilities, interest in music, or art.
12. Periodically reassess bowel and bladder programs. The ability to stay dry for reasonable intervals is one of the greatest factors in enhancing self-esteem and positive body image.

Family Education and Health Maintenance

1. Teach special techniques that may be required for holding and positioning, feeding, caring for the incision, emptying the bladder, and exercising muscles.
2. Alert the parents to safety needs of the child with decreased sensation, such as protection from prolonged pressure, risk of burns from bath water that is too

warm, and avoidance of trauma from contact with sharp objects.

3. Reinforce that parents need to notify the health care provider for signs of associated problems such as hydrocephalus, meningitis, urinary tract infection, and latex sensitivity.

4. Urge continued follow-up and health maintenance, including immunizations and evaluation of growth and development.

5. Advise parents that children with paralysis are at risk for becoming overweight because of inactivity, so they should provide a low-fat, balanced diet; control snacking; and encourage as much activity as possible.

6. For additional resources, refer families to agencies such as:

> **The Spina Bifida Association of America**
> 4590 MacArthur Blvd. NW, Suite 250
> Washington, DC 20007
> 800-621-3141

Spinal Cord Injury

Spinal cord injury is caused by mechanical displacement of the vertebral column through trauma that impinges on the spinal cord and its nerve roots. The injury may vary from a mild cord concussion with transient numbness to complete cord transection causing immediate and permanent quadriplegia. The most common sites of injury are the cervical areas C5, C6, and C7, and the junction of the thoracic and lumbar vertebrae, T12 and L1.

Clinical manifestations vary with the location and severity of cord damage. In general, complete transection causes loss of all function below the level of the lesion, and incomplete cord damage results in a variety of regional deficits (Table 18). Complications include shock, respiratory or cardiac arrest, thromboembolism, infections, and autonomic dysreflexia.

◆ Assessment

1. Motor and sensory deficits that determine the level of the spinal cord lesion. Widening deficits may be attributable to edema and hemorrhage.

S

TABLE 18 Incomplete Cord Syndromes

Lesion	Mechanism of Injury	Preserved	Impaired
Anterior cord syndrome (dorsal columns of the spinal cord are spared)	Flexion	Light touch Vibratory sensation Proprioception	Motor function Pain and temperature sensation
Posterior cord syndrome (anterior columns of the cord are spared)	Extension	Motor function Pain and temperature sensation	Light touch Vibratory sensation Proprioception
Central cord syndrome (central gray matter of the cord is injured)	Flexion or extension	Motor function of lower extremities	Motor function of upper extremities
Brown-Séquard syndrome (hemisection of the cord)	Penetrating trauma	Contralateral—pain and temperature sensation Ipsilateral—movement, light touch, proprioception	Contralateral—movement, light touch, proprioception Ipsilateral—pain and temperature

(Neff J., Kidd P. [1993]. *Trauma Nursing. The Art and Science*, Chicago: Mosby.)

2. Signs of autonomic dysfunction:
   a. Respirations: unusual patterns, distress, signs of hypoxia. Diaphragmatic or abdominal breathing may indicate cervical spine injury.
   b. Cardiovascular function: hypotension caused by vasodilation and blood pooling in lower extremities; bradycardia from unopposed vagal influence
3. Decreased rectal sphincter tone and bowel and bladder dysfunction

◆ Diagnostic Evaluation

1. X-rays of spinal column, including open mouth studies for adequate visualization of C1 and C2, may show fracture.
2. MRI of spine to detect soft tissue injury, bony injury, hemorrhage, edema
3. Nerve conduction testing and electromyogram to determine function of neural pathways

◆ Collaborative Management

Therapeutic Interventions

1. Immediate posttrauma phase (<1 hour): immobilize the patient, including the head, body, and hips.
2. In the acute phase (1–24 hours), maintain pulmonary stability through intubation and mechanical ventilation or diaphragmatic pacing, if needed. Maintain cardiovascular stability and ensure perfusion of spinal cord by restoring blood pressure and implementing localized cord cooling.
3. During the subacute phase (within 1 week), the vertebral column and ligamentous injuries are stabilized using traction (such as skull tongs or halo vest) or surgical intervention.
4. During chronic phase (beyond 1 week), emphasis is on rehabilitation, including physical therapy, urologic evaluation, and occupational therapy.

Pharmacologic Interventions

1. Methylprednisolone is given IV as soon as possible to reduce spinal cord edema.
2. Naloxone is given during acute stage to maintain spinal cord perfusion.

3. Histamine (H_2) receptor blockers are given to prevent gastric irritation and hemorrhage.
4. Anticoagulants are given in small doses to reduce risk of thrombophlebitis and pulmonary emboli.

◆ Nursing Interventions

Monitoring

1. For patients with high-level lesions, continuously monitor respirations and maintain a patent airway. Be prepared to intubate if respiratory fatigue or arrest occur.
2. Monitor results of arterial blood gases, chest x-ray, and sputum cultures for possible respiratory infections.
3. Monitor fluid intake and output.
4. Monitor neurologic changes; report change in skin sensation, loss or gain of muscle strength, which may indicate worsening or resolving lesion.
5. Monitor for spinal shock—may cause loss of all reflex, motor, sensory and autonomic activity below the level of the lesion; eventually resolves
6. Monitor for autonomic dysreflexia (exaggerated autonomic response to stimuli below the level of the lesion in patients with lesions at or above T6).

NURSING ALERT
Autonomic dysreflexia is a medical emergency that may result in convulsions and death without prompt treatment. Be alert to signs such as pounding headache, profuse sweating, nasal congestion, piloerection (goose bumps), bradycardia, and severe hypertension. Immediately place the patient in a sitting position to help lower blood pressure and diminish intracranial pressure. Remove possible causative stimuli; administer antihypertensive medication as ordered; and monitor blood pressure every 3 to 5 minutes until the condition resolves.

7. Monitor blood pressure with position changes in a patient with lesions above midthoracic area to prevent orthostatic hypotension.

Supportive Care

1. Frequently assess cough and vital capacity. Teach effective coughing if the patient is able.
2. Provide fluids and humidified air or oxygen to loosen secretions. Implement chest physiotherapy to assist pulmonary drainage and prevent infection.
3. Suction as needed; observe for vagal response, which causes bradycardia (should be temporary).
4. Turn the patient frequently, maintaining alignment, or transfer the patient to a turning table or rotating bed when stable.
5. Keep skin clean and dry and well lubricated. Inspect for pressure sore development every 2 hours when turning patient, including the back of head, ears, heels, elbows, etc.
6. Provide meticulous skin care at pin sites of skull tongs or halo device to prevent infection.
7. Perform range-of-motion exercises to prevent contractures and maintain rehabilitation potential. Encourage physical therapy and practicing of exercises as tolerated.
8. Encourage weight-bearing activity to prevent osteoporosis and risk of kidney stones.
9. Apply elastic support hose and administer anticoagulants as ordered, to reduce the risk of thrombophlebitis.
10. Replace an indwelling catheter with intermittent catheterization as soon as possible to minimize risk of infection. Avoid overdistension of the bladder.
    a. If reflex voiding is present, monitor for urinary retention by percussing the suprapubic area for dullness, or catheterizing for residual urine after voiding.
    b. Train the patient in reflex voiding by encouraging fluids at 2-hour intervals, then applying pressure to the suprapubic area $\frac{1}{2}$-hour later in attempt to void. Avoid giving fluids in the evening to prevent nocturnal dribbling and overdistension.
11. Assess bowel sounds and note abdominal distention. Paralytic ileus is common immediately after injury.
    a. Initiate nasogastric suction as necessary.
    b. Encourage high-calorie, high-protein, and high-

fiber diet when bowel sounds return and the patient tolerates food.

12. Institute a bowel program as early as possible to manage defecation. Observe for loose stool oozing from rectum and check for fecal impaction; remove if necessary.

13. Protect the patient from possible stimuli for autonomic dysreflexia, including:

   a. Bowel or bladder distention caused by fecal impaction, urinary retention, or a kinked indwelling catheter

   b. Abnormal skin stimulation such as lying on wrinkled sheets, hot or cold stimulation, or pain from constricting clothing

   c. Distention or contraction of visceral organs such as gastric distention or emptying an overdistended bladder too fast

   d. Infection, especially of the urinary tract

COMMUNITY CARE CONSIDERATIONS
Alert caregivers that autonomic dysreflexia is a complication that may occur for 5 to 6 years after a spinal cord injury. Teach patient and caregivers how to prevent autonomic dysreflexia, identify it, and implement emergency measures.

14. Praise patient for accomplishments; minimize deficits.

15. Ensure adequate rest and discuss stress management techniques such as relaxation therapy, counseling, and problem solving.

Family Education and Health Maintenance

1. Teach patient and family about the physiology of nerve transmission and how spinal injury has affected normal function.

2. Reinforce that rehabilitation is lengthy and involves compliance with therapy to increase bodily function.

3. Explain that spasticity may develop 2 weeks to 3 months after injury and may interfere with routine care and activities of daily living (ADL).

   a. Teach measures to manage spasticity such as maintaining a calm, stress-free environment; allowing plenty of time for activities; performing range of motion slowly and smoothly; and avoiding temperature extremes.

b. Advise reporting spasms to health care provider for possible treatment with muscle relaxants.

4. Teach protection from pressure sore development by frequent inspection of skin, repositioning while in bed, weight-shifting and lift-offs every 15 minutes while in a wheelchair, and avoidance of shear forces and friction.

5. Encourage sexual counseling, if indicated, to promote satisfaction in personal relationships.

Spinal Cord Tumor

Tumors of the spinal cord and canal cause compression of the spinal cord and nerves, progressing to paralysis if untreated. Spinal tumors vary widely in type and location—they may be extradural (existing outside the dural membranes) and may spread to the vertebral bodies; intradural–extramedullary (within the subarachnoid space), including meningiomas and schwannomas; or intramedullary (within the spinal cord), including astrocytomas, ependymomas, and oligodendrogliomas. Complications include spinal cord infarction, hydrocephalus, and infection.

◆ Assessment

1. Pain may be localized or radiating, depending on location and type of tumor.
2. Weakness of extremities, abnormal reflexes, and sensory changes
3. Abnormal autonomic function relative to level of lesion—abnormal pupillary responses, orthostatic hypotension, or bladder or bowel dysfunction indicates tumor in the cauda equina)

◆ Diagnostic Evaluation

1. CT or MRI to show cord compression and tumor location

2. Lumbar puncture to analyze cerebrospinal fluid for increased protein levels and presence of cancer cells
3. Myelography before surgery to pinpoint the level of the tumor

◆ Collaborative Management

Therapeutic Interventions
1. Radiation therapy with or without surgery

Surgical Interventions
1. Surgical excision of the tumor
2. Laminectomy and decompression if tumor cannot be excised

◆ Nursing Interventions

Monitoring
1. Monitor intake and output to evaluate urinary retention.
2. After surgery, monitor site for bleeding, CSF drainage, signs of infection.

Supportive Care
1. Administer analgesics or instruct the patient in the use of patient-controlled analgesia, as necessary and as ordered.
2. Instruct the patient with painful paresthesias in appropriate use of ice, massage, exercise, or rest.
3. Instruct the patient in relaxation techniques such as deep breathing, distraction, or imagery.
4. Instruct the patient with sensory loss to visually scan the extremity during use to avoid injury related to lack of tactile input. Pad the bed rails or chair to prevent injury.
5. Encourage fluid intake to maintain urinary elimination pattern. Teach Credé's maneuver or self-catheterization as indicated.
6. Assess for urinary retention by percussing the bladder for dullness or catheterizing for residual after voiding.
7. Support the weak or paralyzed extremity in a functional position, to prevent contractures.
8. Refer the patient to physical therapy for assistance with activities of daily living (ADLs), ambulation.

9. Promote periods of rest to enhance coping skills.
10. Reassure the postoperative patient that the degree of sensory/motor impairment may decrease during the recovery period as surgical edema decreases.
11. Keep surgical dressings clean and dry, and cleanse surgical site as ordered.
12. Position the patient to keep pressure off postoperative surgical site.

Patient Education and Health Maintenance

1. Encourage the patient with motor impairment to use adaptive devices.
2. Demonstrate proper positioning and transfer techniques.
3. Instruct the patient with sensory losses about dangers of extreme temperatures, and the need for adequate foot protection at all times.
4. Refer the patient and family to cancer and spinal cord lesion support groups as needed.

Sprains, Strains, and Contusions

A *sprain* is an injury to ligamentous structures surrounding a joint; it is usually caused by a wrench or twist resulting in a decrease in joint stability. A *strain* is a microscopic tearing of muscle or tendon caused by excessive force, stretching, or overuse. A *contusion* is an injury to the soft tissue produced by a blunt force (blow, kick, or fall).

◆ Assessment

1. Sprain: rapid swelling caused by extravasation of blood within tissues; pain on passive movement of joint; increasing pain during first few hours caused by continued swelling
2. Strain: swelling, tenderness; pain with isometric contraction; may be associated spasm
3. Contusion: hemorrhage into injured part (ecchymosis); pain, swelling; hyperkalemia may be present with extensive contusions, resulting from destruction of body tissue and loss of blood

◆ Diagnostic Evaluation

1. X-ray of affected part may be done to rule out fracture.

◆ Collaborative Management

Therapeutic Interventions

1. Immobilize the affected part in splint, elastic wrap, or compression dressing to support weakened structures and control swelling.
2. Apply ice first 24 hours.

Pharmacologic Interventions

1. Analgesics usually include NSAIDs.

Surgical Interventions

1. Severe sprains may require surgical repair or cast immobilization.

◆ Nursing Interventions

Supportive Care

1. Elevate the affected part. Maintain splint or immobilization as prescribed.
2. Apply cold compresses for the first 24 hours (20–30 minutes at a time) to produce vasoconstriction, decrease edema, and reduce discomfort.
3. Apply heat to affected area after 24 hours (20–30 minutes at a time) four times a day to promote circulation and absorption.
4. Assess neurovascular status of distal extremity if significant swelling occurs.
5. Ensure correct use of crutches or other mobility aid with or without weight bearing as prescribed.

Family Education and Health Maintenance

1. Instruct the patient on use of pain medication as prescribed.
2. Educate on need to rest injured part for about a month to allow for healing.
3. Teach the patient to resume activities gradually.
4. Advise the patient to avoid excessive exercise of injured part.

5. Teach the patient to avoid reinjury by "warming up" before exercise.

Status Asthmaticus
See Asthma

Stomach Cancer
See Cancer, Gastric

Stroke
See Cerebrovascular Accident

Subdural Hematoma in Children

Subdural hematoma refers to an accumulation of fluid, blood, and its degradation products between the dura mater and subarachnoid membrane. Hematoma results from direct or indirect trauma to the head, such as birth trauma; accidents; purposeful injury, as in cases of child abuse; or a disease process such as meningitis. Subdural hematomas may be acute (evident within 24 to 48 hours of injury) or chronic (most common, evident after days or weeks). It is often difficult to delineate the exact time and type of injury, because the precipitating episode may appear relatively insignificant. The lesion may arrest spontaneously at any point, or it may enlarge and, if unrelieved, ultimately cause cerebral atrophy or death of compression and herniation.

Treatment is usually successful and subsequent development is normal when the diagnosis is made early, before cerebral atrophy and a fixed neurologic deficit have occurred. With delayed treatment, complications include mental retardation, ocular abnormalities, seizures, spasticity, and paralysis. Mortality in massive, acute subdural bleeding is very high, even if promptly diagnosed.

S

◆ Assessment

Acute subdural hematoma
1. Continuous unconsciousness from time of injury or lucid interval followed by unconsciousness
2. Progressive hemiplegia
3. Focal seizures
4. Signs of brain stem herniation: pupillary enlargement, changes in vital signs, decerebrate posturing, and respiratory failure

Chronic subdural hematoma
1. In infants, early signs include anorexia, difficulty feeding, vomiting, irritability, low-grade fever, retinal hemorrhages, failure to gain weight
2. In infants, later signs include: enlargement of head, bulging and pulsation of anterior fontanel, glossy scalp with dilated scalp veins, strabismus, pupillary inequality, hyperactive reflexes, seizures, retarded motor development
3. In older children, early signs include: lethargy, anorexia, and signs of increased intracranial pressure (IICP) such as vomiting, irritability, headache, increased pulse pressure, and change in respirations
4. In older children, later signs include: seizures and coma

◆ Diagnostic Evaluation

1. CT scan is the procedure of choice for diagnosing subdural hematomas.
2. Bilateral subdural taps may provide the diagnosis as well as give immediate relief of IICP.
3. Skull x-rays may be obtained if abuse is suspected.

◆ Collaborative Management

Surgical Interventions

1. In acute subdural hematoma, the clot is evacuated through a burr hole or craniotomy.
2. In chronic subdural hematoma, repeated subdural taps are done to remove the accumulating fluid.
   a. In infants, the needle can be inserted through the fontanel or suture line.
   b. In older children, the needle is inserted through bur holes into the skull.

   c. The subdural taps may be the only treatment required if the fluid disappears entirely and symptoms do not recur.

   d. Concurrent treatment is instituted to correct anemia, electrolyte imbalance, and malnutrition.

3. A shunting procedure may be done if repeated taps fail to significantly reduce the volume or protein content of the subdural collections. Shunting is usually to the peritoneal cavity.

S

◆ Nursing Interventions

Monitoring

1. Monitor vital signs, for changes indicating IICP.
2. Monitor level of consciousness and behavior for changes.
3. Monitor urine output and specific gravity daily to ensure adequate hydration.
4. Monitor electrolyte and protein levels to prevent imbalances.
5. After subdural tap:
   a. Observe the child frequently for signs of shock.
   b. Observe for drainage from the site of the tap; report purulent drainage.
   c. Monitor temperature frequently and monitor for signs of developing infection.
6. Monitor for signs of respiratory or urinary infection related to immobility.

Supportive Care

1. Maintain a quiet environment without sudden changes in position, to avoid IICP.
2. Organize nursing activities to allow for long periods of uninterrupted rest.
3. Carefully regulate fluid administration to avoid danger of fluid overload.
4. Administer laxatives or suppositories to prevent straining during a bowel movement, which may increase ICP.
5. Assist with subdural taps.
   a. Hold the child securely to avoid injury caused by sudden movement.
   b. Apply firm pressure over the puncture site(s) for

a few minutes after the tap has been completed, to prevent fluid leakage along the needle tract.

  c. Note whether there is serous drainage or frank blood.

  d. Reinforce the dressing as needed to prevent contamination of the wound.

6. Have emergency equipment available for resuscitation.

7. Change the child's position frequently and provide meticulous skin care to prevent hypostatic pneumonia and decubitus ulcers.

8. Perform passive range-of-motion exercises on all extremities and support the child's body in good alignment using splints as necessary to prevent contractures.

9. Apply suction as necessary to remove secretions in the mouth and nasopharynx.

10. Keep the child's eyes well lubricated to prevent corneal damage while unconscious.

11. Provide nutrition and fluids through nasogastric feedings as ordered. Observe for gastric distension.

12. Maintain good mouth care even if child is not eating.

13. Encourage the parents to care for and hold the child as much as possible.

14. Encourage the parents to bring diversional materials from home for the recovery period.

15. Provide emotional support to the parents; reassure them that the prognosis is favorable with adequate treatment.

16. Act nonjudgmentally in cases caused by intentional or accidental trauma.

PEDIATRIC ALERT
Ensure that cases of suspected child abuse have been reported to the appropriate agency and that parents have been referred for counseling.

Family Education and Health Maintenance

1. Reinforce explanations regarding the child's condition, causes of the child's specific symptoms, rationale for treatment, and postoperative recovery expectations.

2. Encourage parents to keep all follow-up appointments for medical evaluation and physical and occupational therapy.
3. Teach parents safety measures to prevent injuries in the future.
4. Assist parents in seeking additional support and resources through social work department, church groups, community agencies, or private counseling.

Systemic Sclerosis
See Scleroderma

Testicular Cancer
See Cancer, Testicular

Thoracic Surgeries

Thoracic surgeries are operative procedures that are performed to aid in the diagnosis and treatment of certain pulmonary conditions. Procedures include thoracotomy, lobectomy (Fig. 26), pneumonectomy, segmental resection, and wedge resection. Except with pneumonectomy, these procedures require chest drainage immediately after surgery. Chest drainage is usually not used after pneumonectomy, because it is desirable that the empty hemithorax fill with an effusion, which eventually obliterates the space.

Indications for thoracic surgeries include biopsy of sus-

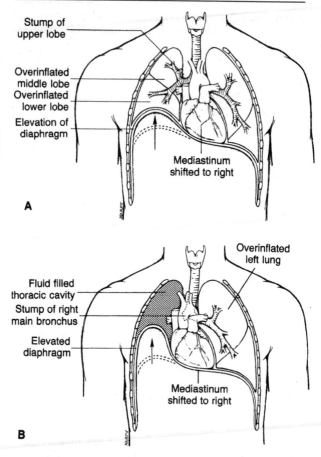

FIGURE 26 *Operative procedures.* **(A)** *Lobectomy.* **(B)** *Pneumonectomy.*

picious masses, chest trauma, benign and malignant tumors, giant emphysematous blebs, bronchiectasis, fungal infections, abscesses, and extensive tuberculosis.

◆ Potential Complications

1. Hypoxia
2. Postoperative bleeding
3. Atelectasis and pneumonia
4. Bronchopleural fistula from disruption of a bronchial suture or staple; bronchial stump leak
5. Cardiac dysrhythmias (usually occurring on the 3rd to the 4th postoperative day)
6. Myocardial infarction or heart failure

◆ Collaborative Management

Preoperative Care

Goal is to maximize respiratory function to improve the outcome postoperatively and reduce risk of complications.

1. Encourage the patient to stop smoking to restore bronchial ciliary action and to reduce the amount of sputum and likelihood of postoperative atelectasis or pneumonia.
2. Teach an effective coughing technique:
   a. Sit upright with knees flexed and body bending slightly forward (or lie on side with hips and knees flexed if unable to sit up).
   b. Splint the incision with hands or folded towel.
   c. Take three short breaths, followed by a deep inspiration, inhaling slowly and evenly through the nose.
   d. Contract abdominal muscles and cough twice forcefully.
3. Humidify the air to loosen secretions.
4. Administer bronchodilators if bronchospasm occurs.
5. Administer antimicrobials to reduce risk of infection.
6. Encourage deep breathing with the use of incentive spirometer to prevent atelectasis postoperatively.
7. Teach diaphragmatic breathing.
8. Evaluate cardiovascular status for risk and prevention of complication.
9. Encourage activity to improve exercise tolerance.

10. Correct anemia or dehydration with blood transfusions and intravenous infusions, as indicated.
11. Orient the patient to events that will occur in the postoperative period—coughing and deep breathing, suctioning, chest tube and drainage bottles, oxygen therapy, ventilator therapy, pain control, leg exercises and range-of-motion exercises for affected shoulder.
12. Ensure that patient fully understands surgery and is emotionally prepared for it; verify that informed consent has been obtained.

Postoperative Care

1. Auscultate chest for adequacy of air movement—to detect bronchospasm, consolidation, atelectasis.
2. Obtain arterial blood gases (ABGs) and pulmonary function measurements as ordered.
3. Monitor level of consciousness and inspiratory effort closely. If mechanically ventilated, begin weaning from ventilator as soon as possible.
4. Suction frequently using meticulous aseptic technique because tracheobronchial secretions are increased because of trauma to the tracheobronchial tree during operation, diminished lung ventilation, and diminished cough reflex.

> **NURSING ALERT**
> Look for changes in color and consistency of sputum. Colorless or white, fluid sputum is not unusual; change in color or thickening of sputum may mean dehydration or infection.

5. Elevate the head of the bed 30 to 40 degrees when patient is oriented and blood pressure stabilized to improve movement of diaphragm.
6. Encourage coughing and deep breathing exercises and use of an incentive spirometer to prevent bronchospasm, retained secretions, atelectasis, and pneumonia.
7. Watch for and report restlessness, tachycardia, tachypnea, and elevated blood pressure, indicating hypoxia.

NURSING ALERT

Sudden onset of respiratory distress or cough productive of sero-sanguinous fluid may indicate bronchopulmonary fistula or leak after pneumonectomy. Position with operative side down and report immediately. Prepare for immediate chest tube insertion or surgical intervention.

8. Monitor heart rate and rhythm with auscultation and ECG, because dysrhythmias are frequently seen after thoracic surgery.

9. Monitor central venous pressure, if indicated, for prompt recognition of hypovolemia and for effectiveness of fluid replacement. Also note restlessness, anxiety, pallor, tachycardia, and hypotension, which may indicate postoperative bleeding.

10. Monitor cardiac output and pulmonary artery systolic, diastolic, and wedge pressures if Swan-Ganz catheter is in place. Watch for subtle changes, especially in the patient with underlying cardiovascular disease.

11. Assess chest tube drainage for amount and character of fluid.
    a. Chest drainage should progressively decrease after first 12 hours.
    b. Prepare for blood replacement and possible reoperation to achieve hemostasis if bleeding persists.

12. Maintain intake and output record, including chest tube drainage.

13. Monitor infusions of blood and parenteral fluids closely because patient is at risk for fluid overload if portion of pulmonary vascular system has been reduced (with pneumonectomy).

14. Give narcotics (usually by continuous IV infusion or by epidural catheter) for pain relief, as prescribed, to permit patient to breathe more deeply and cough more effectively.
    a. Severity of pain varies with type of incision and patient's individual pain tolerance. Usually a posterolateral incision is the most painful.
    b. Be alert for respiratory and CNS depression caused

by narcotics; patient should be alert enough to cough.

15. Assist with intercostal nerve block or cryoanalgesia (intercostal nerve freezing) for pain control as ordered.

16. Position for comfort and optimal ventilation (head of bed elevated 15–30 degrees); this also helps residual air to rise in upper portion of pleural space, where it can be removed by the chest tube.

   a. Vary the position from horizontal to semierect to prevent retention of secretions in the dependent portion of the lungs.

17. Encourage splinting of incision with pillow, folded towel, or hands, while turning.

18. Teach relaxation techniques such as progressive muscle relaxation and imagery to help reduce pain.

19. Begin range of motion of arm and shoulder on affected side immediately to prevent ankylosis of the shoulder ("frozen" shoulder).

   a. Perform exercises at time of maximal pain relief.

   b. Encourage patient to actively perform exercises three to four times daily, taking care not to disrupt chest tube or IV lines.

◆ Patient Education and Health Maintenance

1. Advise that there will be some intercostal pain for several weeks, which can be relieved by local heat and oral analgesia.

2. Advise that weakness and fatigability are common during the first 3 weeks after a thoracotomy, but exercise tolerance will improve with conditioning.

3. Suggest alternating walking and other activities with frequent short rest periods. Walk at a moderate pace and gradually extend walking time and distance.

4. Encourage continuing deep-breathing exercises for several weeks after surgery to attain full expansion of residual lung tissue.

5. Advise avoiding lifting more than 20 pounds for several months until complete healing has taken place.

6. Warn that any activity that causes undue fatigue, in-

creased shortness of breath, or chest pain should be discontinued.

7. Encourage to have an annual influenza injection and obtain a pneumococcal pneumonia vaccine. Also, avoid respiratory irritants and persons with respiratory infections.

8. Encourage to keep follow-up visits.

Thrombocytopenia

Thrombocytopenia is a decrease in circulating platelet count (less than $100,000/mm^3$), which is the most common cause of bleeding. It may be congenital or acquired, and results from 1) decreased platelet production, as in aplastic anemia, myelofibrosis, radiation therapy, or leukemia; 2) increased platelet destruction, as in certain infections, drug toxicity, or disseminated intravascular coagulation; 3) abnormal distribution or sequestration in spleen; or 4) dilutional thrombocytopenia after hemorrhage or red blood cell transfusions.

An idiopathic form of thrombocytopenia, *immune thrombocytopenic purpura (ITP)*, results from destruction of platelets by antiplatelet antibodies. Acute ITP typically follows a viral illness and is more common in children. Eighty to ninety percent of patients recover uneventfully. Chronic ITP (more than 6-month course) is most common at ages 20 to 40 years, and is more common in women than men.

Patients with thrombocytopenia are usually asymptomatic until the platelet count decreases to below $20,000/mm^3$. Severe thrombocytopenia may cause death of blood loss or bleeding into vital organs.

◆ Assessment

1. Asymptomatic until platelet count decreases to below 20,000

2. Signs of bleeding
   a. Petechiae: occur spontaneously
   b. Ecchymoses: occur at sites of minor trauma

    c. Bleeding: from mucosal surfaces, gums, nose, respiratory tract

    d. Menorrhagia

    e. Hematuria

    f. Gastrointestinal bleeding

3. Excessive bleeding after surgical and dental procedures

◆ Diagnostic Evaluation

1. CBC and platelet count show decreased hemoglobin, hematocrit, platelets.
2. Bleeding time, prothrombin time, and partial thromboplastin time are prolonged.
3. Assay for platelet autoantibodies is sometimes helpful in diagnosing ITP.

◆ Collaborative Management

Therapeutic Interventions

1. Treat underlying cause.
2. Administer platelet transfusions and institute bleeding control.

Pharmacologic Interventions

1. Corticosteroids or IV immunoglobulins may be helpful in selected patients.
2. Immunosuppressants, danazol, and the cancer chemotherapeutic agents vincristine and vinblastine may be used to treat ITP.

Surgical Interventions

1. Splenectomy may be done to decrease destruction of platelets in ITP.

◆ Nursing Interventions

Monitoring

1. When administering blood products, monitor for signs and symptoms of allergic reactions, anaphylaxis, and volume overload.
2. Evaluate all urine and stool for gross and occult blood.
3. Monitor platelet count.

Supportive Care

1. Institute bleeding precautions.
   a. Avoid use of plain razor, hard toothbrush or floss, IM injections, tourniquets, rectal temperatures or suppositories.
   b. Administer stool softeners as necessary to prevent constipation.
   c. Discourage blowing of nose.
   d. Restrict activity and exercise when platelet count is less than $20,000/mm^3$ or when there is active bleeding.
2. Monitor pad count and amount of saturation during menses; administer or teach self-administration of hormones to suppress menstruation as ordered.
3. Administer blood products as ordered.

Family Education and Health Maintenance

1. Teach the patient bleeding precautions.
2. Tell the patient to take only prescribed medications and to avoid aspirin and nonsteroidal antiinflammatory agents, which may interfere with platelet function.
2. Demonstrate the use of direct, steady pressure at bleeding site if bleeding does develop.
3. Stress the importance of routine follow-up for platelet counts.

Thrombophlebitis and Related Conditions

Thrombophlebitis is a condition in which a clot forms in a vein secondary to phlebitis (inflammation of the vein wall) or because of partial obstruction of the vein. In general, the clotting is related to 1) stasis of blood, 2) injury to the vessel wall, and 3) altered blood coagulation (Virchow's triad).

Deep vein thrombosis (DVT) refers to thrombosis of deep rather than superficial veins. Deep veins of the lower extremities are most commonly involved.

Phlebitis is an inflammation in the wall of a vein. The term is used clinically to indicate a superficial and localized condition that can be treated with application of heat.

Venous thrombosis can result from many conditions,

such as venous stasis (after operations, childbirth, or any prolonged bed rest or sitting); direct trauma to veins from IV injections or indwelling catheters; extension of nearby infection to the vein; a complication of varicose veins; continuous pressure on the vessel, as from a tumor, aneurysm, or heavy pregnancy; unusual activity in a person who has been sedentary; hypercoagulability associated with malignant disease, or blood dyscrasias. Complications include pulmonary embolism and postphlebitic syndrome.

◆ **Assessment**

1. High-risk factors for thrombophlebitis include malignancy, previous venous insufficiency, conditions causing prolonged bed rest, leg trauma, general surgery (especially if the patient is older than 40 years of age), obesity, smoking.
2. Patient may be asymptomatic or have severe calf and leg pain.
3. Fever and chills may occur with DVT.
4. Asymmetry of the legs, venous distension or edema, taut skin, hardness to the touch, warmth of extremity, and redness and induration along a vein (venous cord)
5. Calf pain may be aggravated when foot is dorsiflexed with the knee flexed (positive Homan's sign).

   Note: Homan's sign is nonspecific and has a low sensitivity for detecting thrombophlebitis.
6. Contrast with signs of arterial occlusion (Table 19).

◆ **Diagnostic Evaluation**

1. Phlebography, involving x-rays and injection of contrast medium, shows venous obstruction.
2. Plethysmography, to measure changes in calf volume corresponding to changes in blood volume caused by temporary venous occlusion with a high-pressure pneumatic cuff (will not show characteristic decrease in calf circumference)
3. ^{125}I fibrinogen uptake test to detect clot formation with serial scanning and comparison of one leg with the other (most sensitive screen for acute calf vein thrombosis)

TABLE 19 Assessment of Acute Arterial Occlusion Versus Deep Vein Thrombosis

Factor	Acute Arterial Occlusion	Deep Vein Thrombosis
Onset	Sudden	Gradual
Color	Pale; later—mottled, cyanotic	Slightly cyanotic; rubescent
Skin temperature	Cold	Warm
Leg size—diameter	May be reduced from normal	Enlarged
Superficial veins	Collapsed	Appear enlarged and prominent
Arterial pulsation	Pulse deficit noted	Normal and palpable (except in marked edema)
Effect of elevating leg	Condition worsens	Condition improves

4. Prothrombin time (PT), partial thromboplastin time (PTT), and platelet count are obtained before anticoagulant treatment is initiated, to detect hidden bleeding tendencies.

◆ Collaborative Management

Therapeutic Interventions

1. Conservative measures for superficial thrombophlebitis, and as an adjunct to anticoagulation with DVT:
   a. Dry heat to the affected area with warm water bottles, thermostatically controlled heat cradle, ultrasound
   b. Moist heat using hydrotherapy, whirlpool baths, or warm compresses
   c. Pressure gradient therapy using compression devices and garments to promote vasodilation
   d. Bed rest to prevent muscle contraction with walking that may dislodge the clot

Pharmacologic Interventions

1. To prevent embolization in DVT, heparin is given subcutaneously or IV.

837

2. Oral anticoagulation with coumadin is given for 3 to 6 months after heparin therapy to prevent recurrence and embolization. Heparin may be continued for 4 to 5 days after oral anticoagulant is started because of delayed onset of therapeutic effectiveness with oral anticoagulants.

NURSING ALERT

Drug interactions can alter the effect of anticoagulants. Review the effect of other medications the patient may be taking during anticoagulant therapy.

Surgical Interventions

1. If the patient cannot tolerate prolonged anticoagulant therapy, a filter may be placed in the inferior vena cava to prevent pulmonary embolism.
2. Thrombectomy may be necessary for severely compromised venous drainage of the extremity.

◆ Nursing Interventions

Monitoring

1. Measure and record the patient's leg circumferences daily to monitor for venous obstruction.
2. With anticoagulant therapy, monitor PT and PTT daily or as ordered and check results before giving next anticoagulant dose. Dosage may be adjusted to achieve desired elevation of these levels.
   a. PTT monitors heparin therapy—should be 1.5 to 2 times the control
   b. PT monitors oral anticoagulant therapy—international normalized ratio (INR) should be greater than 2.0 to 2.5, or higher based on condition being treated.
3. Monitor for signs of pulmonary embolism—chest pain, dyspnea, apprehension—and report immediately.

Supportive Care

1. Elevate the patient's legs as directed to promote venous drainage, reduce swelling, and relieve pain.

2. Apply warm compresses or a heating pad as directed to promote circulation and reduce pain.

NURSING ALERT
Avoid massaging or rubbing the calf—this risks breaking up the clot, which can then circulate as an embolus.

3. Administer analgesic as prescribed and as needed. Avoid using aspirin and NSAID-containing products during anticoagulant therapy to prevent further risk of bleeding.
4. Prevent venous stasis by proper patient positioning in bed. Support the full length of the legs when they are to be elevated
5. Initiate active exercises, unless contraindicated, in which case use passive exercises.
6. Encourage adequate fluid intake, frequent changes of position, effective coughing, and deep-breathing exercises to prevent complications of bed rest.
7. After the acute phase (5–7 days), apply elastic stockings, as directed. Remove twice daily and check for skin changes and calf tenderness.
8. Encourage ambulation when allowed (usually after 5–7 days when clot has fully adhered to vessel wall).

Patient Education and Health Maintenance

1. Teach the patient to recognize and immediately report signs of recurrent thrombophlebitis and pulmonary embolism.
2. Provide thorough instructions about oral anticoagulation therapy.
3. Teach the patient to promote circulation and prevent stasis by applying elastic hosiery at home.

NURSING ALERT
Elastic hosiery has no role in managing the acute phase of deep venous thrombosis but is of value once ambulation has begun. Using hosiery will minimize or delay development of postphlebitic syndrome (venous insufficiency).

4. Advise against straining or any maneuver that increases venous pressure in the leg. Eliminate the necessity to strain at stool by increasing fiber and fluids in the diet.

5. Warn the patient of hazards of smoking and obesity: nicotine constricts veins, decreasing venous blood flow, and extra pounds increase pressure on leg veins. Arrange a consultation with a dietitian, if necessary.

COMMUNITY CARE CONSIDERATIONS

Practice preventive measures for bedridden patients who are prone to develop thrombosis:

1. Have the patient lie in bed in the slightly reversed Trendelenburg position because it is better for the veins to be full of blood than empty.

2. Place a footboard across the foot of the bed.

3. Instruct the patient to press the balls of the feet against the footboard, as if rising up on toes.

4. Then have the patient relax the foot.

5. Request that the patient do this 5 to 10 times each hour.

Thyroid Cancer
See Cancer, Thyroid

Thyroidectomy

Thyroidectomy involves the partial or complete removal of the thyroid gland to treat thyroid tumors, hyperthyroidism, or hyperparathyroidism.

◆ Potential Complications

1. Hemorrhage, glottal edema, laryngeal nerve damage
2. Hypocalcemic tetany resulting from parathyroid damage

3. Hypothyroidism occurs in 5% of patients in first post-operative year; increases at rate of 2% to 3% per year

4. Hypoparathyroidism occurs in approximately 4% of patients and is usually mild and transient. More severe cases require oral and IV calcium supplements.

◆ Collaborative Management

Preoperative Care

1. Administer thionamides to control hyperthyroidism and ensure that the patient is euthyroid at time of surgery.

2. Administer iodide to increase firmness of gland tissue and reduce its vascularity to control bleeding during surgery.

3. Maintain a restful and therapeutic environment and provide nutritious diet to counteract effects of hypermetabolism. Ensure that the patient has a good night's rest preceding surgery.

4. Advise the patient that speaking is minimized immediately after surgery and that oxygen and humidification may be administered to facilitate breathing.

5. Explain that, postoperatively, fluids may be given IV to maintain fluid, electrolyte, and nutritional needs; glucose may also be given IV before administration of anesthesia.

Postoperative Care

1. Administer humidified oxygen as prescribed to reduce irritation of airway and prevent edema.

2. Observe for signs of hemorrhage.
   a. Watch for repeated clearing of the throat or complaint of smothering or difficulty swallowing, which may be early signs of hemorrhage.
   b. Watch for irregular breathing, swelling of the neck, and choking—other signs pointing to the possibility of hemorrhage and tracheal compression.
   c. Observe for bleeding at sides and back of the neck, as well as anteriorly, when the patient is in dorsal position.
   d. Monitor vital signs frequently, watching for tachycardia and hypotension indicating hemorrhage

(most likely between 12 and 24 hours postoperatively).

3. Be alert for voice changes, which may indicate damage to laryngeal nerve.

4. Keep a tracheostomy set in the patient's room for 48 hours for emergency use.

5. Move the patient carefully; provide adequate support to the head so that no tension is placed on the sutures.

6. Place the patient in semi-Fowler's position with the head elevated and supported by pillows; avoid flexion of neck.

7. Reinforce dressing if indicated.

8. Watch for the development of tetany caused by removal or disturbance of parathyroid glands. Progression of signs and symptoms includes:

   a. Patient is apprehensive; reports tingling of toes and fingers and around the mouth

   b. Positive *Chvostek's sign:* tapping the cheek over the facial nerve causes a twitch of the lip or facial muscles (Fig. 27A).

   c. Positive *Trousseau's sign:* carpopedal spasm induced by occluding circulation in the arm with a blood pressure cuff (Fig. 27B).

9. Be prepared to treat tetany.

   a. Position the patient for optimal ventilation, with pillow removed to prevent the head from bending forward and compressing the trachea.

   b. Keep side rails padded and elevated, and position the patient to prevent injury if a seizure occurs. Avoid restraints, because they only aggravate the patient and may cause muscle strain or fractures.

   c. Have equipment available to treat respiratory difficulties: airway, suction equipment, tracheostomy tray.

   d. Have cardiac arrest equipment available.

   e. Monitor calcium levels: if level decreases to below 7 mg/100 mL (3 mEq) in 48 hours, administer calcium replacement (gluconate, lactate) IV. Administer slowly through large vein to avoid extravasation and necrosis.

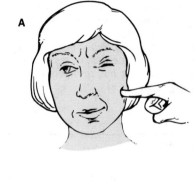

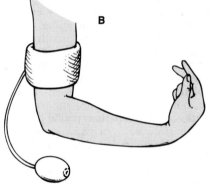

FIGURE 27 **(A)** *Chovstek's sign.* **(B)** *Trousseau's sign.*

❖

NURSING ALERT
Give IV calcium cautiously to a patient who has renal disease or who is receiving digitalis preparations; hypercalcemia may result.

◆ **Patient Education and Health Maintenance**

1. Ensure that patient understands the importance of follow-up blood work in evaluating thyroid hormone and calcium balance.

2. Teach patient about thyroid hormone replacement. It may not be necessary immediately postoperatively, but may become necessary later.
3. Advise proper rest, relaxation, and nutrition to facilitate healing. Patient may resume usual activities as soon as swelling has resolved and incision has adequately healed.

Thyroiditis

Thyroiditis is an inflammation of the thyroid gland that is more common in women than men. It takes several forms, depending on the cause. *Subacute thyroiditis* is an acute, self-limiting, painful inflammation usually associated with viral infections (eg, mumps). In approximately 10% of patients with this disorder, permanent hypothyroidism occurs and long-term thyroxine therapy is needed. A clinical variant of this disorder, called "silent thyroiditis," causes milder, nonpainful symptoms, and tends to occur within 6 months of the postpartum period in women.

Hashimoto's (lymphocytic) thyroiditis is a chronic progressive disease caused by infiltration of the gland by lymphocytes. This form of thyroiditis may be the most common cause of adult hypothyroidism and appears to be increasing in incidence. It is believed to be a heritable autoimmune disease, perhaps related to Graves' disease. Ninety-five percent of patients are women in their 40s or 50s. Untreated, it may progress to destruction of the thyroid parenchyma and hypothyroidism.

◆ Assessment

1. The thyroid gland is enlarged, and a bruit may be auscultated over gland.
2. In subacute thyroiditis, patient complains of pain and swelling of the gland, which lasts several weeks or months, then disappears. Pain may radiate to the ear, making swallowing difficult and uncomfortable. Gland is tender on palpation.
3. In Hashimoto's thyroiditis, there is no pain or tender-

ness, but the patient may note symptoms of compression: neck tightness, cough, hoarsenesss.
4. Sore throat, fever, and chills may be present in subacute thyroiditis.
5. Signs and symptoms of hyperthyroidism may occur initially with either type: nervousness, irritability, insomnia, weight loss, perspiration, heat intolerance.
6. Later, clinical hypothyroidism may develop.

◆ Diagnostic Evaluation

1. In subacute thyroiditis: low thyroid-stimulating hormone (TSH) level, elevated T_3 and T_4 levels, increased erythrocyte sedimentation rate (ESR), and low radioactive iodine uptake on thyroid scan.
2. In Hashimoto's thyroiditis: normal T_3 and T_4 levels initially, usually become subnormal as the disease progresses; elevated TSH levels; antithyroglobulin antibodies and antimicrosomal antibodies usually present; normal or high concentration of thyroglobulin binding protein

◆ Collaborative Management

Pharmacologic Interventions
1. For subacute thyroiditis, analgesics and mild sedatives are given along with beta-adrenergic blocking agents to reduce symptoms of hyperthyroidism.
   a. Corticosteroids may be necessary for pain, fever, and malaise.
   b. Aspirin or NSAIDs may be used in mild cases to treat the symptoms of inflammation.

NURSING ALERT
Aspirin should be avoided if the patient exhibits signs of hyperthyroidism, because it may increase the amount of free circulating hormone and exacerbate the symptoms of hyperthyroidism.

2. For Hashimoto's thyroiditis, thyroid hormones are given to maintain a normal level of circulating thyroid hormone; this is done to suppress production of TSH,

to prevent enlargement of the thyroid, and to maintain a euthyroid state.

Surgical Interventions

1. Thyroidectomy may be necessary if tracheal compression occurs (see p. 827).

◆ Nursing Interventions

T

Monitoring

1. Monitor carefully for episodes of hyperthyroidism and hypothyroidism.
2. Monitor for tracheal compression symptoms.
3. Monitor fever and pain control.

Supportive Care

1. Provide a restful environment and explain all testing and treatment regimens.
2. Administer or teach self-administration of thyroid hormone to suppress stimulation of gland and possibly reduce gland size in Hashimoto's thyroiditis.
3. Suggest wearing open-necked clothing, avoiding jewelry or scarves around neck, and avoiding excessive neck flexion or hyperextension, which may aggravate pain or feeling of compression.

Patient Education and Health Maintenance

1. Explain all medications the patient is to continue at home.
2. Reassure patient that subacute thyroiditis usually resolves spontaneously over weeks to months.
3. Teach the patient with subacute thyroiditis to recognize and report signs and symptoms of hypothyroidism (ie, fatigue and lethargy, weight gain, cold intolerance) that may occur as gland inflammation subsides.
4. Teach the patient with Hashimoto's thyroiditis to recognize and immediately report signs of tracheal compression (ie, difficulty breathing, cough, hoarseness).
5. Encourage follow-up to monitor thyroid function tests.

GERONTOLOGIC ALERT
Careful and regular follow-up of elderly patients with Hashimoto's thyroiditis is especially important because the progression to hypothyroidism is usually subtle in such patients.

Tonsillectomy and Adenoidectomy

Tonsillectomy and *adenoidectomy* are the surgical removal of the tonsillar and adenoidal structures, part of the lymphoid tissue that encircles the pharynx. These procedures are the most frequently performed pediatric surgeries, and are used primarily to treat obstructive sleep apnea resulting from excessive adenotonsillar swelling, as well as to treat chronic persistent tonsillitis or adenoiditis and chronic persistent otitis media, when these disorders do not respond satisfactorily to antibiotics. Tonsillectomy and adenoidectomy may be performed together or separately. Surgery is contraindicated in bleeding or coagulation disorders; uncontrolled systemic disorders (ie, diabetes, rheumatic fever, cardiac, renal disease); presence of upper respiratory infection in the child or immediate family; child younger than age 4 years (unless life-threatening situation); and in certain palate abnormalities (ie, cleft palate or submucus cleft palate).

◆ Potential Complications

1. Hemorrhage
2. Reactions to anesthesia
3. Otitis media
4. Bacteremia

◆ Collaborative Management

Preoperative Care

1. Conduct thorough ear, nose, and throat examination and collect appropriate cultures to determine presence and source of infection.
2. Obtain blood specimens for preoperative studies to de-

847

termine risk of bleeding: clotting time, smear for platelets, prothrombin time, partial thromboplastin time.
3. Conduct preoperative assessment.
   a. Assess the child's psychological preparation for hospitalization and surgery.

PEDIATRIC ALERT
The preschool child is especially vulnerable to psychological trauma as a result of surgical procedures or hospitalization.

T

   b. Obtain thorough nursing history from the parents to obtain any pertinent information that would impact on the child's care, such as recent infections (the child should be free of respiratory infection for at least 2–3 weeks); recent exposure to any communicable diseases; presence of any loose teeth that may pose the threat of aspiration; bleeding tendencies in child or family.
4. Assess hydration status.
5. Prepare the child specifically for what to expect postoperatively, using techniques appropriate to the child's developmental level (books, dolls, drawings).
6. Talk to the child about the new things to be seen in the operating room, and clear up any misconceptions.
7. Help the parents prepare their child by talking at first in general terms about surgery and progressing to more specific information.
8. Assure parents that complication rates are low and that recovery is usually swift.
9. Encourage parents to stay with child and help provide care.

Postoperative Care
1. Assess pain on a frequent basis and administer analgesics as indicated.
2. Assess frequently for signs of postoperative bleeding.
3. Have suction equipment and nasal packing material readily available in case of emergency.
4. While the child is still under the effects of anesthesia, position the child prone or semiprone with head turned to the side to prevent aspiration.

5. Allow the child to assume a position of comfort when alert. (Parent may hold the child.)

6. The child may vomit old blood initially. If suctioning is necessary, avoid trauma to oropharynx.

7. Remind the child not to cough or clear throat unless necessary.

8. Provide adequate fluid intake; give ice chips 1 to 2 hours after awakening from anesthesia. When vomiting has ceased, advance to clear liquids cautiously.

9. Offer cool fruit juices without pulp at first since they are best tolerated; then offer Popsicles and cool water for first 12 to 24 hours.

10. There is some controversy regarding intake of milk and ice cream the evening of surgery: it can be soothing and reduce swelling, but it does increase mucous production, which causes the child to clear throat more often, increasing risk of bleeding.

11. Provide ice collar to neck, if desired. (Remove ice collar if child becomes restless.)

12. Rinse mouth with cool water or alkaline solution.

13. Keep child and environment free from blood-tinged drainage to help decrease anxiety.

14. Encourage the parents to be with the child when the child awakens.

Family Education and Health Maintenance

1. Explain and provide written instructions for care of the child at home after discharge.
   a. Diet should still consist of large amounts of fluids as well as soft, cool, nonirritating foods.
   b. Eating helps promote healing because it increases the blood supply to tissues and prevents tightness of throat muscles.
   c. Bed rest should be maintained for 1 to 2 days, then daily rest periods for about a week. Resume normal eating and activities within 2 weeks after surgery.
   d. Avoid contact with persons with infections.
   e. Discourage the child from frequent coughing and clearing of throat.
   f. Avoid gargling. Mouth odor may be present for a few days after surgery; only mouth rinsing is acceptable.

2. Advise when to call health care provider. (Ensure that

T

parents have phone number of health care provider and emergency department.):
   a. Earache accompanied by fever
   b. Any bleeding, often indicated only by frequent swallowing; most common about 5th to 10th day when membrane sloughs from surgical site
3. Teach about medications prescribed or suggested for pain relief.
4. Guide parents in helping the child think of the experience as a positive one once surgery is over, to make subsequent health care experiences easier.

Total Joint Replacement
See Arthroplasty and Total Joint Replacement

Toxic Shock Syndrome

Toxic shock syndrome (TSS) is a potentially life-threatening condition caused by a bacterial toxin secreted by *Staphylococcus aureus* in the bloodstream. The cause is uncertain, but 70% of cases are associated with menstruation and tampon use. Research suggests that magnesium-absorbing fibers in tampons may lower magnesium levels in the body, thereby providing ideal conditions for toxin formation.

Toxic shock syndrome has also occurred in nonmenstruating individuals with conditions such as cellulitis, surgical wound infection, vaginal infections, subcutaneous abscesses, and with the use of contraceptive sponges, diaphragms, and tubal ligation. Death may result from cardiovascular collapse and renal failure caused by shock.

◆ Assessment

1. Sudden onset of high fever greater than 102°F (39°C)
2. Vomiting and profuse watery diarrhea
3. Rapid progression to hypotension and shock within 72 hours of onset
4. Mucous membrane hyperemia

850

5. Sometimes, sore throat, headache, and myalgia
6. Rash (similar to sunburn) that develops 1 to 2 weeks after onset of illness and is followed by desquamation, particularly of the palms and soles

◆ Diagnostic Evaluation

1. Blood, urine, throat, and vaginal/cervical cultures, and possibly cerebrospinal fluid culture, to detect or rule out infectious organism.
2. Additional tests may be required to rule out other febrile illnesses: Rocky Mountain spotted fever, Lyme disease, meningitis, Epstein–Barr, or Coxsackie viruses.

◆ Collaborative Management

Therapeutic Interventions
1. Fluid and electrolyte replacements to increase blood pressure and prevent renal failure
2. Supportive care to maintain cardiorespiratory functions

Pharmacologic Interventions
1. Vasopressors such as dopamine to treat shock
2. Antibiotics such as penicillinase-resistant penicillins or cephalosporins to decrease the rate of relapse
3. Antipyretics to treat fever
4. The use of corticosteroids and immunoglobulins is controversial.

◆ Nursing Interventions

Monitoring
1. Monitor core body temperature frequently.
2. Perform hemodynamic monitoring as indicated (ie, arterial line, central venous pressure, or pulmonary artery pressure).
3. Maintain strict intake and output measurement.
4. Insert indwelling catheter to monitor urine output.
5. Monitor respiratory status for pulmonary edema and respiratory distress syndrome caused by fluid overload from increased fluid replacement; diuretics may be necessary.

Supportive Care

1. Employ cooling measures such as sponge baths and hypothermia blanket, if indicated.
2. Tell the patient to expect desquamation of skin, as in peeling sunburn.
3. Protect skin and avoid using harsh soaps and alcohol, which cause drying.
4. Tell patient to apply mild moisturizer and avoid direct sunlight until healed.
5. Advise the patient that reversible hair loss may occur 1 to 2 months after TSS.

Patient Education and Health Maintenance

1. Tell the patient to expect fatigue for several weeks to months after TSS.
2. Tell the patient to avoid using tampons to reduce risk of recurrence.
3. Encourage follow-up visits for examination and cultures.
4. Teach prevention of TSS:
   a. Alternate use of pads with tampons, avoid superabsorbent tampons.
   b. Change tampons frequently and do not wear one longer than 8 hours; 4 hours maximum during heavy menses.
   c. Be careful of vaginal abrasions that can be caused by some applicators.
   d. Recognize and report symptoms of TSS.

Tuberculosis

Tuberculosis is an infectious disease caused by the bacteria *Mycobacterium tuberculosis,* which are usually spread from person to person by droplet nuclei through the air. The lung is the usual infection site, but the disease can occur elsewhere in the body. Typically, the bacterium forms lesions (tubercles) in the alveoli. The lesions damage additional lung tissue; they are either self-limiting or may extend to adjacent tissues, through the bloodstream, the lymphatic system, or the bronchi. Most individuals who become infected do not develop clinical illness, because the body's immune system brings the infection under control. However, the incidence of tuberculosis (especially drug-resistant varieties) is rising. Patients infected with the human immunodeficiency virus (HIV) are especially at risk. Complications include pneumonia and pleural effusion.

◆ Assessment

1. Constitutional symptoms:
   a. Fatigue, anorexia, weight loss, low-grade fever, afternoon temperature elevation, night sweats, indigestion
   b. Some patients have acute febrile illness, chills, generalized influenzalike symptoms.
   c. Some patients may be asymptomatic or may have insidious symptoms that are ignored.
2. Pulmonary signs and symptoms:
   a. Cough (insidious onset) progressing in frequency and producing mucoid or mucopurulent sputum
   b. Hemoptysis; pleuritic chest pain; dyspnea (indicates extensive involvement)
   c. Crackles on auscultation of lungs
3. Extrapulmonary forms of tuberculosis: lesions in any organ in the body including pleurae, lymph nodes, genitourinary tract, bones and joints, peritoneum, central nervous system

◆ Diagnostic Evaluation

1. Tuberculin skin test (PPD or Mantoux) to detect *M. tuberculosis* infection (past or present, active or inactive)
2. Sputum for smears and cultures to confirm the infection by *M. tuberculosis*
3. Chest x-rays, bone x-rays, and other tests to determine presence and extent of disease

◆ Collaborative Management

Therapeutic Interventions

1. Isolation precautions if hospitalized, including use of negative pressure room, universal precautions, and masks

2. Adequate nutrition and alcohol detoxification for malnourished, alcoholic patient

Pharmacologic Interventions

1. Combination of drugs to which the organism is susceptible to destroy viable bacilli as rapidly as possible and to protect against the emergence of drug-resistant organisms
   a. Current recommended regimen for treating uncomplicated pulmonary tuberculosis is 2 months of bactericidal drugs: isoniazid, rifampin, and pyrazinamide followed by 4 months of isoniazid and rifampin.
   b. Second-line drugs such as capreomycin, kanamycin, ethionamide, para-aminosalicylic acid, and cycloserine are used in patients with resistant strains, for retreatment, and in those intolerant to other agents. Patients taking these drugs should be monitored by health care providers experienced in their use.
2. Once treatment is instituted, obtain sputum smears every 2 weeks until they are negative; sputum cultures do not become negative for 3 to 5 months.
3. Pyridoxine (vitamin B6) is given to prevent peripheral neuropathy in patients taking isoniazid.

◆ Nursing Interventions

Monitoring

1. Monitor breath sounds, respiratory rate, sputum production, respiratory effort, and fever.
2. Monitor compliance with long course of antibiotic therapy.
3. Monitor daily weight to assess nutritional status.
4. If patient is on isoniazid, assess for liver dysfunction.
   a. Question the patient about loss of appetite, fatigue, joint pain, fever, abdominal pain, nausea and vomiting, rash, and dark urine.
   b. Monitor results of periodic liver function studies.

Supportive Care

1. Encourage rest and avoidance of exertion.
2. Provide supplemental oxygen as ordered.

3. Take measures to prevent spread of infection.
   a. Provide care for hospitalized patient in a negative-pressure room to prevent respiratory droplets from leaving room when door is opened.
   b. Enforce that all staff and visitors use standard dust/mist/fume masks (class C) for any contact with patient.
   c. Use high-efficiency particulate masks such as Hepa-filter masks for high-risk procedures such as suctioning, bronchoscopy, or pentamadine treatments.
   d. Use universal precautions for additional protection: gowns and gloves for any direct contact with patient, linens, or articles in room, meticulous hand-washing, etc.
4. Teach the patient measures to control spread of infection through secretions.
5. Stress the importance of eating a nutritious diet to promote healing and improve defense against infection.
6. Provide small frequent meals and liquid supplements during symptomatic period.
7. Participate in observation of medication taking, weekly pill counts, or other programs designed to increase compliance with treatment for tuberculosis.

COMMUNITY CARE CONSIDERATIONS
Patient compliance remains a major problem in eradicating tuberculosis. Therefore, it may be helpful or necessary to have the patient take medication in an observed setting throughout therapy.

8. Investigate living conditions, availability of transportation, financial status, alcohol and drug abuse, and motivation, which may affect compliance with follow-up and treatment. Initiate referrals to a social worker for interventions in these areas.

Patient Education and Health Maintenance
1. Educate the patient about the disease and stress the importance of continuing to take medications for the prescribed time.
2. Review the side effects of drug therapy and tell patient to immediately report experiencing any of these.

3. Review symptoms of recurrence (persistent cough, fever, or hemoptysis). Urge the patient to report symptoms.

4. Advise the patient to avoid job-related exposure to excessive amounts of silicone (working in foundry, rock quarry, sand blasting), which increases chance of reactivation.

5. Encourage the patient to report at specified intervals for bacteriologic (smear) examination of sputum to monitor therapeutic response and compliance.

6. Teach patient about basic hygiene practices and investigate living conditions, because crowded conditions contribute to development and spread of tuberculosis.

7. Encourage follow-up chest x-rays for rest of life to evaluate for recurrence.

8. Instruct on prophylaxis with isoniazid for persons infected with the tubercle bacillus without active disease to prevent disease from occurring, or to individuals at high risk of becoming infected. Prophylaxis is recommended for the following groups:

   a. Household members and other close associates of potentially infectious tuberculosis cases

   b. Newly infected persons (positive skin test within 2 years)

   c. Persons with past tuberculosis who have not received adequate therapy

   d. Persons with significant reactions to tuberculin skin test and who are in special clinical situations (silicosis, diabetes, B-cell malignancies, end-stage renal disease, severe malnutrition, immunosuppression, HIV positive)

   e. Tuberculin skin reactors younger than 35 years of age with none of the aforementioned risk factors

Ulcerative Colitis

Ulcerative colitis is a chronic inflammatory disease of the mucosa and, less frequently, the submucosa of the colon and rectum. Its exact cause is unknown, but theories include viral or bacterial infections, immune mechanisms, allergy (causes release of inflammatory histamine), enzyme overproduction (ulcerates mucous membranes), psychosomatic factors and stress, and genetic predisposition. The disease usually begins in the rectum and sigmoid and spreads upward, eventually involving the entire colon. There is a tendency for the patient to experience remissions and exacerbations.

Ulcerative colitis affects women slightly more than men and occurs mostly in persons between 20 and 40 years of age. The disease is associated with a very high frequency of secondary colon cancers. Other complications include perforation, hemorrhage, toxic megacolon, abscess formation, stricture and obstruction, anal fistula, malnutrition, and anemia.

◆ Assessment

1. Diarrhea is the prominent symptom; may be bloody or contain pus or mucus. Tenesmus (painful straining), urgency, and cramping may be associated with bowel movements.
2. Crampy abdominal pain may be prominent and brought on by certain foods or milk.
3. May be increased bowel sounds, and left lower abdomen may be tender on palpation
4. As the disease progresses, there may be anorexia, nausea and vomiting, weight loss, fever, dehydration, hypokalemia, and cachexia.
5. There may be associated systemic manifestations such as arthritis, iritis, skin lesions, and liver disease.

◆ Diagnostic Evaluation

1. Stool evaluation for culture and ova and parasites to rule out other causes of diarrhea. Tests for blood are positive during active disease.
2. Blood tests may show low hemoglobin and hematocrit caused by bleeding; increased white blood cells; and decreased potassium, magnesium, and albumin.
3. Proctosigmoidoscopy or colonoscopy with biopsy is necessary to confirm diagnosis.
4. Barium enema determines extent of disease and detects pseudopolyps, carcinoma, and strictures.

◆ Collaborative Management

Therapeutic Interventions

1. During acute exacerbations, bed rest, IV fluids containing potassium and vitamins, and clear liquid diet are indicated.
2. When resuming oral fluids and foods, select those that are mechanically, thermally, and chemically bland. If this fails, a low-residue diet may be necessary to rest the lower intestinal tract. Avoid dairy products if patient is lactose intolerant.
3. For severe dehydration and excessive diarrhea, hyperalimentation may be necessary to rest the intestinal tract and restore nitrogen balance.

Pharmacologic Interventions

1. Iron supplements are necessary to treat anemia from chronic bleeding; blood replacement for massive bleeding.
2. Sulfasalazine is the mainstay drug for acute and maintenance therapy.
3. If patient does not tolerate sulfasalazine, oral salicylates such as mesalamine appear to be as effective as sulfasalazine.
4. Mesalamine enema is available for proctosigmoiditis; suppository for proctitis.
5. Corticosteroids may be used IV, orally, or by enema to manage inflammatory disease and induce remission.
6. Antidiarrheal medications may be prescribed to control diarrhea, rectal urgency and cramping, abdominal pain; their use is not routine.

Making the internal pouch

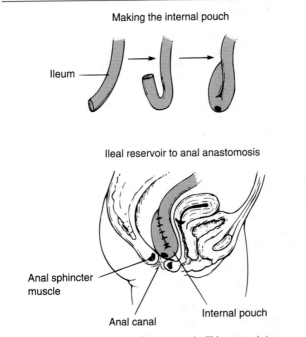

Ileum

Ileal reservoir to anal anastomosis

Anal sphincter
muscle

Anal canal

Internal pouch

FIGURE 28 *Ileal reservoir–anal anastomosis. This reservoir is constructed of two loops of small intestine forming a J configuration (J pouch).*

Surgical Interventions

1. Surgery is recommended when patient fails to respond to medical therapy, if clinical status is worsening, for severe hemorrhage, or for signs of toxic megacolon. Surgery aims to remove entire colon and rectum to cure patient of ulcerative colitis (see Gastrointestinal Surgeries, p. 350). Procedures include:
   a. Subtotal colectomy and ileostomy and Hartmann's pouch
   b. Total proctocolectomy with end-ileostomy
   c. Total colectomy with continent ileostomy
   d. Total colectomy with ileal reservoir–anal anastomosis (Fig. 28)

◆ Nursing Interventions

Monitoring

1. Monitor intake and output, including liquid stools.
2. Monitor serum or fingerstick glucose of patient on corticosteroids or hyperalimentation and report elevations.
3. Weigh patient daily; rapid increase or decrease may relate to fluid imbalance, slower change related to nutritional status.
4. Monitor patient's response to therapy. Observe for adverse reactions. Dose-related side effects of sulfasalazine include vomiting, anorexia, headache, skin discoloration, dyspepsia, and lowered sperm count.
5. Observe for complications such as sudden abdominal distension and pain, which may indicate perforation or toxic megacolon.
6. Observe for signs of dehydration—decreased skin turgor, dry skin, oliguria, decreased temperature, weakness, and increased hemoglobin, hematocrit, blood urea nitrogen (BUN), and specific gravity.

Supportive Care

1. Provide comfort measures and assess the need for sedatives and tranquilizers, to facilitate rest and slow peristalsis.
2. Observe for pressure sores caused by malnourishment and enforced inactivity, especially if patient is thin.
   a. Cleanse the skin gently after each bowel movement.
   b. Apply a protective emollient such as petroleum jelly, skin sealant, or moisture-barrier ointment.
3. Reduce physical activity to a minimum or provide frequent rest periods.
4. Provide commode or bathroom next to bed, because urgency of movements may be a problem.
5. Determine which foods agree with this patient and which do not. Modify diet plan accordingly.
6. Avoid cold fluids and discourage smoking because they increase intestinal motility.
7. Encourage the patient to talk; listen and offer psychological support. Answer questions about the perma-

nent or temporary ileostomy, if appropriate. Refer for psychological counseling, as needed.

Patient Education and Health Maintenance

1. Teach patient about chronic aspects of ulcerative colitis and each component of care prescribed.
2. Encourage self-care in monitoring symptoms, seeking annual checkup, and maintaining health.
3. Alert patient to possible postoperative problems with skin care, aesthetic difficulties, and surgical revisions.
4. Warn patients to report immediately any early indications of relapse, such as bleeding or increased diarrhea, so that steroid treatment may be initiated.
5. Facilitate referral to local chapter of the United Ostomy Association or:

U

> **Crohn's and Colitis Foundation of America**
> 444 Park Ave. South
> New York, NY 10016
> 212-685-3440

Urinary Tract Infection, Lower

A *urinary tract infection* (UTI) may occur in the bladder, where it is called *cystitis,* or in the urethra, where it is called *urethritis*. Most UTIs result from ascending infections by bacteria that have entered through the urinary meatus. Urinary tract infections are much more common in women than men because the shorter female urethra makes them more vulnerable to entry of organisms from surrounding structures (vagina, periurethral glands, and rectum). Acute infection in women is most often caused by organisms of the patient's own intestinal flora (*Escherichia coli*). In men, obstructive abnormalities (strictures, prostatic hyperplasia) are the most frequent cause.

Upper urinary tract disease may occasionally cause recurrent bladder infection. In children, UTIs are also caused by congenital obstruction, vesicoureteral reflux, and urinary stasis.

Recurrent UTIs may indicate *relapse* (recurrent infection with an organism that has been isolated during a prior infection), or *reinfection* (recurrent infection with an organism distinct from previous infecting organism). Untreated UTIs may lead to pyelonephritis and sepsis.

◆ Assessment

1. Dysuria, frequency, urgency, nocturia
2. Suprapubic pain and discomfort
3. Hematuria
4. Children may experience fever and enuresis or dribbling.
5. May be asymptomatic

◆ Diagnostic Evaluation

1. Obtain urine specimens for urine dipstick test: may react positively for blood, white blood cells (WBC), and nitrates, indicating infection.
2. Urine microscopy shows red blood cells and many white blood cells per field without epithelial cells.

NURSING ALERT

Urinalysis showing many epithelial cells is likely contaminated by vaginal secretions in women and is therefore inaccurate in indicating infection. Urine culture may be reported as contaminated as well. Obtaining a clean-catch midstream specimen is essential for accurate results.

---

3. Obtain urine specimens for urine culture to detect presence of bacteria and for antimicrobial sensitivity testing. Bacteriuria (10^5 bacteria/mL of urine or greater) generally indicates infection.
4. In asymptomatic bacteriuria, organisms are found in urine, but the patient has no symptoms.
5. Urologic workup with renal ultrasound, intravenous pyelogram, and voiding cystourethrogram, and other studies may be done to evaluate cause of recurrent infections.

◆ Collaborative Management

Pharmacologic Interventions

1. Women with uncomplicated UTIs are usually treated with a 2- to 3-day course of antibiotics such as trimethoprim-sulfamethoxazole, ofloxacin, or nitrofurantoin.
2. Children and men are treated with 7 to 10 days of antibiotic therapy.
3. Analgesic or antispasmodic if pain is severe
4. Follow-up culture is recommended to prove effectiveness, especially for pregnant women, children with severe or recurrent infection, and men.

◆ Nursing Interventions

Supportive Care

1. Administer or teach self-administration of prescribed antibiotic and antispasmodic.
2. Apply heat to the abdomen to relieve bladder spasms.
3. Encourage rest during the acute phase if symptoms are severe.
4. Encourage plenty of fluids to promote urinary output and to flush out bacteria from urinary tract.
5. Encourage frequent voiding (every 2–3 hours) and emptying the bladder completely. This enhances bacterial clearance, reduces urine stasis, and prevents reinfection.

COMMUNITY CARE CONSIDERATIONS
Patients with indwelling catheters or who intermittently self-catheterize are at increased risk for UTIs; review methods of handling catheters and drainage bags at home.

Family Education and Health Maintenance

1. For women with recurrent UTIs, give the following instructions on preventative measures:
   a. Reduce vaginal introital concentration of pathogens by hygienic measures: wash genitalia in shower or while standing in bathtub; cleanse around the perineum and urethral meatus after each bowel move-

  ment, with front-to-back cleansing to minimize fecal contamination of periurethral area.

  b. Drink liberal amounts of water to lower bacterial concentrations in the urine.

  c. Avoid urinary irritants—coffee, tea, alcohol, cola drinks.

  d. Decrease the entry of microorganisms into the bladder during intercourse by voiding immediately after sexual intercourse.

  e. Avoid external irritants such as bubble baths and perfumed vaginal cleansers or deodorants.

2. Advise patients with persistent bacteria who are on long-term antimicrobial therapy to:

  a. Take antibiotic at bedtime after emptying bladder to ensure adequate concentration of drug during overnight period, because low rates of urine flow and infrequent bladder emptying predispose to multiplication of bacteria.

  b. Use self-monitoring tests (dip sticks) at home to monitor for urinary tract infection.

3. Advise women with recurrent uncomplicated UTIs to discuss with health care provider the possibility of self-administered 2- to 3-day antibiotics when symptoms begin, or single-dose antibiotic treatment after intercourse.

4. Advise parents to avoid giving child bubble baths that may act as irritant and enhance bacteria to ascend the urethra.

5. Teach young girls to wipe from front to back after using the bathroom.

Uterine Cancer
See Cancer, Uterine

Uterine Prolapse

Uterine prolapse refers to an abnormal position of the uterus, in which the organ herniates through the pelvic floor and protrudes into the vagina (prolapse) and possibly beyond the introitus (procidentia). This condition usually results from obstetric trauma and overstretching of musculofascial supports. Three degrees of uterine prolapse are recognized. In first-degree prolapse, the cervix appears at the introitus without straining or traction. In second-degree prolapse, the cervix extends over the perineum. In third-degree prolapse, the entire uterus (or most of it) protrudes. Complications include cervical or uterine necrosis.

◆ Assessment

1. Backache or abdominal pain; pressure and heaviness in vaginal region
2. Symptoms aggravated by obesity, standing, straining, coughing, or lifting a heavy object, because of increased intraabdominal pressure
3. Bloody discharge caused by cervix rubbing against clothing or inner thighs
4. Protrusion and ulceration of cervix on examination

◆ Diagnostic Evaluation

1. Pelvic examination identifies condition; spread labia gently, do not attempt to insert speculum

◆ Collaborative Management

Therapeutic Interventions
1. Vaginal pessary to insert into vagina to support pelvic organs if surgery cannot be done
   a. Prolonged use may lead to necrosis and ulceration.
   b. Should be removed and cleaned every 1 to 2 months

Pharmacologic Interventions
1. Estrogen cream to decrease genital atrophy

Surgical Interventions
1. Surgical correction is recommended treatment with an anterior and posterior repair; effective and permanent
2. Abdominal sarcopexy may be done to anchor the vagina.
3. Hysterectomy may be necessary for necrosis.

◆ Nursing Interventions

Supportive Care

1. Encourage sitz baths to relieve discomfort.
2. Provide heating pad for low back or lower abdomen.
3. Administer pain medications as ordered.
4. Increase fluid intake and encourage the patient to void frequently to prevent bladder infection.
5. For second- and third-degree prolapse, apply saline compresses frequently.
6. Provide postoperative care:
   a. Administer perineal care to the patient after each voiding and defecation.
   b. Employ a heat lamp to help dry the incision line and enhance healing process.
   c. If urinary retention occurs, catheterize or use indwelling catheter until bladder tone is regained.
   d. Apply an ice pack locally to relieve congestion.
   e. Promote ambulation but prevent straining to reduce pelvic pressure.
7. Explain to the patient that sexual intercourse is possible with pessary; however, vaginal canal may be shortened.

Patient Education and Health Maintenance

1. Reinforce surgeon's instructions postoperatively about waiting to have vaginal penetration.
2. Encourage the patient to explore with partner ways to engage in sexual activity without strain and with greatest comfort.
3. Instruct the patient on care of vaginal pessary—removal for cleaning every 1 to 2 months.

U

Vaginitis

Vaginitis is inflammation of the vagina caused by infection from a variety of organisms, and is commonly marked by vaginal discharge and discomfort. Five major types of vaginitis are recognized.

In *simple (contact) vaginitis,* inflammation results from poor hygiene, irritation (eg, from contact allergens, tampons or diaphragm that have been retained in the vaginal canal for too long), and invading organisms.

In *nonspecific vaginitis (bacterial vaginosis),* inflammation results from infection by *Gardnerella vaginitis,* a gram-negative bacillus that is not considered sexually transmitted. The infection is benign (When discharge is wiped away, underlying tissue is healthy and pink.).

In *Trichomonas vaginitis,* inflammation results from infection by a protozoan, *T. vaginalis,* which thrives in alkaline environments and is sexually transmitted. This organism may spread to the urinary tract, where it is hard to eradicate. Men are usually asymptomatic carriers. In *Candida vaginitis,* inflammation results from infection by a fungus, *C. albicans,* a normal inhabitant of the gastrointestinal (GI) tract. Because this fungus thrives in an environment rich in carbohydrates, it commonly occurs in patients with poorly controlled diabetes and in patients who have been on prolonged antibiotic or steroid therapy.

The last type, *atrophic vaginitis,* commonly occurs in postmenopausal women, because of atrophy of the vaginal mucosa secondary to decreased estrogen levels.

Urethritis and vulvitis often accompanies vaginitis because of the proximity to the vagina.

◆ Assessment

1. Vaginal itching, irritation, burning
2. Odor, increased or unusual vaginal discharge

3. Dyspareunia, pelvic pain, dysuria
4. Possible history of unprotected intercourse with a new or infected partner

◆ Diagnostic Evaluation

1. Physical examination including vaginal speculum examination to obtain vaginal discharge specimens
2. Wet smear for microscopic examination
   a. Saline slide: discharge mixed with saline; useful in detecting *Gardnerella* and *Trichomonas*
   b. Potassium hydroxide (KOH): useful in detecting *C. albicans*. If fishy odor is noted when KOH mixed with discharge, suspect *Gardnerella*.
3. Vaginal pH: use Nitrazie paper:
   a. Normal pH: 4.0 to 4.5
   b. *Gardnerella:* 5.0 to 5.5
   c. *Trichomonas:* 5.5+
4. Pap smear: may detect any type of vaginitis
5. Chlamydia and gonorrhea cultures or DNA probe: to rule out chlamydia or gonorrhea cervicitis

◆ Collaborative Management

See Table 20.

◆ Nursing Interventions

Supportive Care

1. Instruct the patient to discontinue use of irritating agents, such as bubble baths, vaginal douches.
2. Suggest cool baths or sitz baths and pat dry or dry with hair dryer on low setting.
3. Encourage the patient to wear loose cotton undergarments.
4. Teach the patient to cleanse perineum before topically applying medication. Demonstrate application of prescribed medication.
5. Emphasize importance of taking prescribed medication for full length of therapy and as directed; teach the patient side effects.
6. Instruct the patient on the proper technique for douching.

(text continues on page 872)

TABLE 20 Specific Types of Vaginitis

Type	Clinical Manifestations	Management
Simple (contact) vaginitis	Increased vaginal discharge with itching, redness, burning, and edema Voiding and defecation aggravate symptoms	1. Enhance natural vaginal flora by administering a weak acid douche—15 mL vinegar to 1,000 mL water (1 T white vinegar to 1 qt water). 2. Stimulate growth of lactobacilli (Doderlein's bacilli) by administering beta-lactamase vaginal suppository; this dissolves with body heat, and the sugar then acts. 3. Foster cleanliness by meticulous care after voiding and defecation. 4. Discontinue use of causative agent.

(continued)

TABLE 20 *(Continued)*

Type	Clinical Manifestations	Management
Nonspecific vaginitis	Vaginal discharge with odor Itching and burning may suggest concomitant organisms present It is benign in that when discharge is wiped away, underlying tissue is healthy and pink Vaginal pH is between 5.0 and 5.5 May be asymptomatic	1. Metronidazole (Flagyl) taken orally for 7 days or topical clindamycin or metronidazole 2. Alcohol intake should be avoided during Flagyl treatment to avoid nausea and vertigo. Flagyl has been associated with teratogenic effects and should not be used in pregnant women during first trimester. 3. Treating partners is controversial unless the condition is recurrent; if so, Flagyl is usually prescribed.
Trichomonas vaginitis	Copious malodorous discharge; may be frothy and yellow-green May have pruritis, dyspareunia, and spotting Red, speckled (strawberry) punctate hemorrhages on the cervix May also have vulvar edema, dysuria, and hyperemia secondary to irritation of discharge	1. Destroy infective protozoa by taking metronidazole (Flagyl) orally, usually single dose of 2 g. NOTE: Flagyl is contraindicated in the first trimester of pregnancy. 2. Prevent reinfection by treating male concurrently with Flagyl. 3. Avoid alcohol during treatment.

V

Candida vaginitis

Vaginal discharge is thick and
irritating; white or yellow patchy,
cheeselike particles adhere to
vaginal walls

Itching is the most common
complaint

May also experience burning,
soreness, dyspareunia, frequency,
and dysuria

1. Eradicate fungus by applying
   antifungal vaginal cream, or
   vaginal suppository for 3 or 4
   nights as ordered.
2. Treat the symptomatic or
   uncircumcised partner by applying
   antifungal cream under the
   foreskin nightly for 7 nights.
3. For severe or recurrent cases can
   use systemic antifungal.

Atrophic vaginitis

Vaginal itching, dryness, burning,
dyspareunia, and vulvar irritation
May also have vaginal bleeding

1. Because this is a manifestation of
   general body estrogenic depletion,
   patient should be treated with oral
   or transdermal estrogen. The condition reverses itself under treatment,
   which must be maintained.
2. Vaginal estrogen cream may also be
   used.
3. If infection also present, this is
   treated.

❖

NURSING ALERT

In the postmenopausal woman, if
vaginal bleeding occurs, it must be
investigated promptly to determine if
cancer is the cause

V

7. Emphasize importance of abstinence until therapy is complete and sexual partner has been treated, if indicated.
8. Tell the patient that use of condoms may be protective but may produce irritation during treatment.
9. Instruct the patient in the use of water-soluble lubricant if vagina is dry and atrophic.

Patient Education and Health Maintenance

1. Teach causes of vaginitis and their symptoms so the patient can seek treatment promptly.
2. Teach the patient about all sexually transmitted diseases and means of prevention.
3. Teach measures to prevent vaginitis.
   a. Wipe from front to back after toilet use.
   b. Keep area clean and dry.
   c. Wear loose cotton clothing, to absorb moisture and provide good circulation.
   d. Change sanitary pads, tampons frequently so they do not become saturated.
   e. Avoid bubble baths, vaginal deodorants, sprays, and douches.
   f. If the patient insists on using douches, advise using a mild vinegar solution (2 tsp. white vinegar to 1 qt. water).
4. For recurrent *Candida* infections, encourage good control if diabetic, or encourage the patient to be tested for diabetes. Teach all patients to eliminate concentrated carbohydrates from diet to prevent recurrence.

Valvular Heart Disease, Acquired

Normal heart valves function to maintain the forward flow of blood from the atria to the ventricles and from the ventricles to the great vessels. *Valvular dysfunction* stems from three types of valvular damage: stenosis, or narrowing of the valve opening; incomplete valve closure causing regurgitation; or prolapse, in which valve leaflets drop down into the heart chamber. Valvular disorders may progress to congestive heart failure (CHF), possible right-sided heart failure, and various dysrhythmias. Acquired valvular disease occurs in several forms:

In *mitral stenosis*, valve cusps become progressively thickened and contracted, which narrows the orifice and impairs forward blood flow. Acute rheumatic valvulitis is a common cause. Because of increased workload, the left atrium becomes dilated and hypertrophied. As pulmonary circulation becomes congested, pulmonary arterial pressure increases, leading to right ventricular failure.

In *mitral insufficiency* or regurgitation, the mitral valve fails to close tightly during systole, which allows blood to flow back into the left atrium. Poor closure may be caused by valve distortion or damage to chordae tendinae or papillary muscles caused by mitral valve prolapse, chronic rheumatic heart disease, postinfarction mitral regurgitation, infective endocarditis, or trauma. Left atrial pressures increase because of inefficient atrial emptying, and left ventricular hypertrophy may develop because of inefficient emptying.

In *aortic stenosis*, the orifice between the left ventricle and the aorta is narrowed because of congenital anomalies, calcification, or rheumatic fever. Impaired aortic outflow increases left ventricular workload that results in hypertrophy and failure. Left atrial pressure also increases; the increased pulmonary vascular pressure may eventually cause right ventricular failure.

In *aortic insufficiency*, poor valve closure during diastole allows blood to flow back from the aorta into the left ventricle. This condition may be caused by rheumatic or infective endocarditis, congenital malformation, Marfan's syndrome, Ehler–Danlos syndrome, systemic lupus erythematosus, or by diseases that cause dilation or tearing of the ascending aorta (syphilis, rheumatoid spondylitis, dissecting aneurysm). The left ventricle contracts more forcefully to maintain adequate cardiac output and becomes hypertrophied as a result. Low aortic diastolic pressures result in decreased coronary artery perfusion.

In *tricuspid stenosis*, commissural fusion and fibrosis restricts the tricuspid valve orifice. This condition usually follows rheumatic fever, commonly accompanies mitral valve diseases, and can lead to right ventricular failure.

In *tricuspid insufficiency* or regurgitation, valve leaflets allow blood to flow back from the right ventricle into the

V

right atrium during ventricular systole. Commonly caused by a dilated right ventricle or rheumatic fever, this condition reduces cardiac output and eventually leads to right ventricular failure.

◆ Nursing Assessment

1. Possible symptoms of fatigue, weakness, dyspnea, cough, orthopnea, and nocturnal dyspnea
2. Hemoptysis (from pulmonary hypertension) and hoarseness (from compression of left recurrent laryngeal nerve) in in mitral stenosis
3. Hypotension, dizziness, syncope, angina, and CHF in aortic stenosis
4. Arterial pulsations visible and palpable over precordium and visible in neck; widened pulse pressure, and water-hammer (Corrigan's) pulse (pulse strikes palpating finger with a quick, sharp stroke and then suddenly collapses) in aortic insufficiency
5. Right-sided heart failure (edema, ascites, hepatomegaly) in tricuspid stenosis and insufficiency
6. Characteristic heart sounds:
    a. *Mitral stenosis:* accentuated first heart sound, usually accompanied by an "opening snap" (caused by sudden tensing of valve leaflets), and a low-pitched diastolic murmur (rumbling murmur). Murmur best heard at apex, with bell of stethoscope, with patient in left lateral recumbent position. Note duration of murmur (long duration indicates significant stenosis).
    b. *Mitral insufficiency:* diminished first heart sound and blowing systolic murmur (pansystolic if mild insufficiency), commencing immediately after first heart sound at apex, and radiating to axilla and left infrascapular area
    c. *Aortic stenosis:* prominent fourth heart sound, possible paradoxical splitting of second heart sound (suggestive of associated left ventricular dysfunction), and a midsystolic murmur heard best over the aortic area. Note harsh and rasping quality at base of heart and a higher pitch at apex of heart. Often associated with a palpable thrill.
    d. *Aortic insufficiency:* soft first heart sound and high-

pitched blowing de crescendo diastolic murmur along left sternal border. Accentuated with patient in sitting position leaning forward, and with patient holding breath at end of deep expiration.

e. *Tricuspid stenosis:* blowing diastolic murmur at the lower left sternal border (increases with inspiration); similar to that of rheumatic mitral disease

f. *Tricuspid insufficiency:* third heart sound (may be accentuated by inspiration) and a pansystolic, usually high-pitched murmur at the lower left sternal border

◆ Diagnostic Evaluation

1. 12-lead ECG to detect dysrhythmias
2. Echocardiogram to show structural/functional abnormalities of valves
3. Chest x-ray to detect cardiomegaly and pulmonary vascular congestion
4. Cardiac catheterization and angiocardiography to confirm diagnosis and determine severity of valvular disease

◆ Collaborative Management

Pharmacologic Interventions

1. Antibiotic prophylaxis for endocarditis before invasive procedures (eg, cardiac catheterization) for mitral regurgitation, rheumatic heart disease, and prosthetic cardiac valves
2. Treatment of heart failure with diuretics, vasodilators, and cardiac glycosides (see p. 393).

Surgical Interventions

1. Depending on condition, surgical procedures may include valvotomy, balloon valvuloplasty, annuloplasty (retailoring of the valve ring), or valve replacement with biologic or prosthetic valve (see p. 163).

◆ Nursing Interventions

Monitoring

1. Assess frequently for change in existing murmur or new murmur.

2. Assess for signs of left or right ventricular failure.
3. Maintain continuous ECG monitoring and watch for dysrhythmias, as indicated.
4. After cardiac catheterization, monitor blood pressure and apical pulse closely, check peripheral pulses in affected extremity, watch for hematoma formation at puncture site, assess for chest, back, thigh, or groin pain, and keep the patient in bed until the following morning.
5. Monitor response to therapy.

Supportive Care

1. Maintain bed rest while symptoms of congestive heart failure are present.
2. Allow the patient to rest between interventions.
3. Assist with or perform hygiene needs for patient to reserve patient's strength for ambulation.
4. Begin activities gradually, such as chair sitting for brief periods.
5. Monitor intake and output and dietary sodium intake, and enforce restrictions, as indicated.
6. Instruct the patient regarding the specific valvular dysfunction, possible causes, and therapies implemented to relieve symptoms. Explain to the patient the surgical intervention selected, if applicable.

Patient Education/Health Maintenance

1. Review activity restrictions and schedule with the patient and family.
2. Instruct the patient to report signs of impending/worsening heart failure: dyspnea, cough, increased fatigue, ankle swelling.
3. Review sodium or fluid restrictions.
4. Review medications: purpose, action, schedule, and side effects.
5. Advise of the need for antibiotic prophylaxis before some dental and other invasive procedures.

COMMUNITY CARE CONSIDERATIONS
Refer the patient to appropriate counseling services, if indicated (vocational, social work, cardiac rehabilitation).

Varicose Veins

Varicose veins result from poor venous valve function and dilation of weakened vein walls. This combination of vein dilation and valve incompetence produces the varicosity. The process is irreversible.

Primary varicose veins result from bilateral dilation and elongation of saphenous veins, whereas deeper veins are normal. Secondary varicose veins are obstructed deep veins. Most common in leg veins, varicose veins may occur elsewhere (eg, esophageal and hemorrhoidal veins) when blood flow or pressure is abnormally high. Complications include hemorrhage and ulceration and infection.

◆ Assessment

1. Predisposing factors include hereditary weakness of vein walls or valves; pregnancy, obesity, or prolonged standing (may cause chronic venous distention); elderly patient (loss of vessel elasticity with age).
2. Presenting symptoms include easy leg fatigue, feeling of heaviness in the legs, leg cramps, nocturnal muscle cramps, discoloration of calves or ankles, increased pain during menstruation.
3. Dilated, tortuous vessels of extremities
4. Manual compression test to assess severity. Place the fingertips of one hand on the dilated vein. With your other hand, compress firmly at least 20 cm (8 inches) higher on the leg. Feel for an impulse transmitted toward your lower hand. Competent saphenous valves should block the impulse. A palpable impulse indicates incompetent valves.
5. Ulceration (rare in primary varices), chronic venous insufficiency, or possible signs of infection

◆ Diagnostic Evaluation

1. Walking tourniquet test: to demonstrate presence or absence of valvular incompetence of communicating veins
   a. A tourniquet is snugly fastened around the lower extremity just above the highest noted varicosities.

    b. The patient is directed to walk briskly for 2 minutes.

    c. Failure of varicosities to empty suggests valvular incompetence of communicating veins distal to tourniquet.

2. Doppler ultrasound: rapidly detects presence or absence of venous reflux in deep or superficial vessels; noninvasive

3. Photoplethysmography: shows venous flow hemodynamics by noting changes in the blood content of the skin; noninvasive

4. Venous outflow and reflux plethysmography—detects deep venous occlusion; noninvasive

5. Ascending and descending contrast venography (an invasive test) to demonstrate secondary venous occlusion and patterns of collateral flow in deep veins

Therapeutic Interventions

1. Conservative measures such as encouraging weight loss if appropriate and avoiding activities that cause venous stasis by obstructing venous flow

Pharmacologic Interventions

1. Injection of a sclerosing agent to thicken and harden vessel walls (usually done for isolated varicosity). The sclerosed vessel is then compressed with a bandage for 6 weeks to bring inflamed endothelial surfaces together.

Surgical Interventions

1. To treat ulceration, bleeding, or for cosmetic purposes in selected patients, if patency of deep veins is ensured

    a. Ligation and stripping of the greater or lesser saphenous systems (most effective procedure)

    b. Multiple vein ligation or laser therapy may be tried in some cases.

◆ Nursing Interventions

Monitoring

1. Postoperatively, monitor neurovascular status of feet (color, warmth, capillary refill, sensation, pulses) to prevent circulatory compromise caused by swelling.

2. Monitor for signs of bleeding (especially the first 24 hours): blood soaking through bandages, increased

pain, hematoma formation, hypotension, and tachy-cardia.

Supportive Care

1. Maintain elastic compression bandages from toes to groin postoperatively.
2. Elevate legs approximately 30 degrees, providing support for the entire leg. Ensure that knee Gatch is positioned for straight incline.
3. Encourage mostly bed rest the first day with legs elevated. The second day, encourage ambulation for 5 to 10 minutes every 2 hours.
4. Advise ambulatory patient to avoid prolonged standing or sitting, or crossing or dangling legs to prevent obstruction. (Crossing legs reduces circulation by 15%).
5. If incisional bleeding occurs, elevate the leg above the level of the heart, apply pressure over the site, and notify the surgeon.
6. Be alert for complaints of pain over bony prominences of the foot and ankle; if the elastic bandage is too tight, loosen it—later, have it reapplied.
7. Maintain IV infusion for fluids and antibiotics as ordered.
8. Administer analgesics as prescribed.
9. After removal of compression bandages (approximately 7 days postoperatively), observe or teach patient to observe for signs of cellulitis or incisional infection.

Patient Education and Health Maintenance

Postoperatively, instruct the patient to:

1. Wear pressure bandages or elastic stockings as prescribed—usually for 3 to 4 weeks after surgery.
2. Elevate legs approximately 30 degrees and provide adequate support for entire leg during periods of rest.
3. Take analgesics for pain as ordered.
4. Report signs such as sensory loss, calf pain, or fever to the health care provider.
5. Avoid dangling the legs.
6. Walk as able.
7. Note that complaints of patchy numbness can be expected, but should disappear in less than a year.
8. Follow conservative management instructions to prevent recurrence:

a. Avoid activities that cause venous stasis.
b. Control excessive weight gain.
c. Wear firm elastic support as prescribed, from toe to thigh when in upright position.
d. Elevate the foot of the bed 15 to 20 cm (6–8 inches) for night sleeping, to encourage venous return.
e. Avoid injuring legs.

Vasospastic Disorder
See Raynaud's Disease

Von Willebrand's Disease

Von Willebrand's disease is an inherited (autosomal dominant) or acquired bleeding disorder characterized by decreased level of von Willebrand factor and prolonged bleeding time. Von Willebrand factor enhances platelet adhesion as the first step in clot formation, and also acts as a carrier of factor VIII in the blood. Von Willebrand's is the most common inherited bleeding disorder. It occurs both in females and males and presents in children unless mild, in which case it may not present until adulthood. The acquired form is rare and generally appears late in life, often in association with lymphoma, leukemia, multiple myeloma, or autoimmune disorders. Severe blood loss or bleeding into vital organs may be life-threatening in untreated disease.

◆ Assessment

1. Mucosal and cutaneous bleeding, such as bruising, gingival bleeding, epistaxis
2. Menorrhagia (heavy menstrual bleeding)
3. Prolonged bleeding from cuts or after dental and surgical procedures.
4. GI bleeding—bloody stools, hematemesis, or positive occult blood

◆ Diagnostic Evaluation

1. Bleeding time—prolonged
2. Partial thromboplastin time (PTT)—prolonged
3. von Willebrand factor—decreased
4. Factor VIII—generally decreased

◆ Collaborative Management

Pharmacologic Interventions

1. Replacement of factor VIII through infusions of cryoprecipitate, as needed
2. Antifibrinolytic medication, specifically aminocaproic acid, to stabilize clot formation before dental procedures and minor surgery
3. Desmopressin (DDAVP), a synthetic analogue of vasopressin, may be given to manage mild to moderate bleeding.

◆ Nursing Interventions

Monitoring

1. Monitor replacement therapy for signs and symptoms of allergic reactions, anaphylaxis, and volume overload.
2. Monitor pad count and amount of saturation during menses.
3. Monitor hemoglobin and hematocrit for anemia caused by blood loss.

Supportive Care

1. Institute bleeding precautions: avoid use of plain razor, hard toothbrush or floss, IM injections, tourniquets, rectal temperatures, or suppositories; administer stool softeners as necessary to prevent constipation; restrict activity and exercise when platelet count is less than 20,000/mm^3 or when there is active bleeding.
2. Administer or teach self-administration of hormones to suppress menstruation as prescribed.

Family Education and Health Maintenance

1. Teach bleeding precautions; also advise to avoid blowing nose, take only prescribed medications, avoid use

of aspirin and NSAIDs, which may interfere with platelet function.

2. Demonstrate the use of direct, steady pressure at bleeding site if bleeding develops.

3. Encourage routine follow-up for laboratory screening.

Vulvar Cancer
See Cancer, Vulvar

Wilms' Tumor

Wilms' tumor is a malignant neoplasm that arises in the fetal kidney. It generally grows to a large size before it is diagnosed, usually before the child reaches age 5 years. In most cases, the tumor expands the renal parenchyma, and the capsule of the kidney becomes stretched over the surface of the tumor. The tumor may metastasize to the perirenal tissues, lymph nodes, lungs, liver, the diaphragm, and abdominal muscles. Invasions of bone and brain are less common. With prompt treatment, overall survival rates for Wilms' tumor are the highest among all childhood cancers—greater than 85%.

Staging of Wilms' tumor is done on the basis of clinical and anatomic findings. It ranges from group I (tumor is limited to the kidney and is completely resected) to group IV (metastases are present in the liver, lung, bone, or brain). Group V includes those cases in which there is bilateral involvement either initially or subsequently.

◆ Assessment

1. A firm, nontender mass in the upper quadrant of the abdomen is usually the presenting sign; it may be on either side. (It is often detected by the parents.)

NURSING ALERT
Avoid indiscriminate manipulation of the abdomen both preoperatively and postoperatively to decrease the danger of metastasis. Because the tumor is soft and highly vascular, seeding may occur because of excessive palpation or handling of the child's abdomen.

2. Abdominal pain, which is related to rapid growth of the tumor
3. As the tumor enlarges, pressure may cause constipation, vomiting, abdominal distress, anorexia, weight loss, and dyspnea.
4. Less common manifestations are hypertension, fever, hematuria, and anemia.
5. Associated anomalies include aniridia (absence of the iris), hemihypertrophy of the vertebrae, and cryptorchidism.

◆ Diagnostic Evaluation

1. Abdominal ultrasound detects the tumor and assesses the status of the opposite kidney.
2. Chest x-ray and chest computed tomography may be done to identify metastases.
3. Magnetic resonance imaging or computed tomography of the kidney may be done to evaluate local spread to lymph nodes.
4. Urine specimens show hematuria; and no increase in vanillylmandelic acid (VMA) and homovanillic acid (HVA) levels as occurs with neuroblastoma
5. Blood chemistries, especially serum electrolytes, uric acid, renal function tests, and liver function tests are done for baseline measurements and to detect metastasis.

◆ Collaborative Management

Therapeutic Interventions

1. The tumor bed is irradiated postoperatively to render nonviable all cells that have escaped locally from the excised tumor. Radiation is usually indicated for children who have stage III and IV tumors or an unfavorable histology.
2. Whole-lung radiation is used to treat stage IV tumors with lung metastasis.
3. Late effects of radiation therapy to the abdomen include scoliosis and underdevelopment of soft tissues.

Pharmacologic Interventions

1. Chemotherapy is initiated postoperatively to achieve maximal killing of tumor cells. Drug combinations include vincristine and doxorubicin or vincristine and actinomycin D, depending on stage.

Surgical Interventions

1. Surgery is performed to determine the type of the tumor, the extent of invasiveness, and to excise as much of the lesion as possible immediately after diagnosis has been made.

◆ Nursing Interventions

Monitoring

1. Observe the surgical incision for erythema, drainage, or separation. Report any of these changes.
2. Monitor for elevated temperature or sign of infection postoperatively.
3. Monitor IV fluid therapy and intake and output carefully, including nasogastric drainage.

Supportive Care

1. Encourage the parents to ask questions and to understand fully the risks and benefits of surgery.
2. Prepare the child for surgery; explain procedures at the appropriate developmental level.
3. Continue supporting the parents during the postoperative period. They may be frightened and upset by the appearance of their child.
4. Insert a nasogastric tube as ordered. Many children

require gastric suction postoperatively to prevent distension or vomiting.

5. When bowel sounds have returned, begin administering small amounts of clear fluids.

6. Administer pain control medications as ordered in the immediate postoperative period.

7. Feed the child after he or she vomits. (Vomiting is not usually associated with nausea.)

8. Allow the child to participate in the selection of foods.

9. As the child recovers, encourage child to eat progressively larger meals.

10. If unable to eat because of radiation and chemotherapy, provide IV fluids, hyperalimentation, or tube feedings as indicated.

11. Prepare child and family for fatigue during recovery from surgery and with radiation treatments. Plan frequent rest periods between daily activities.

12. Prepare the child and parents for loss of hair associated with chemotherapy and encourage use of hat as desired; reassure that hair will grow back.

Family Education and Health Maintenance

1. Provide parents with written information regarding the child's needs—medications, activity, care of the incision, and follow-up appointments.

2. Teach the parents about radiation or chemotherapy treatments and their side effects.

3. Teach parents that children who have only one kidney should not play rough contact sports to avoid injuring the remaining kidney.

4. Inform parents to call with temperature of over 101°F (38.4°C), any bleeding, any signs of infections, or any exposure to chicken pox if the child has not had them.

5. Teach measures to prevent infection while immunosuppressed because of chemotherapy and radiation therapy, such as handwashing and isolation from children with communicable disease.

W

PART TWO

Maternity Nursing

THE USUAL CHILDBEARING EXPERIENCE

Prenatal Care

◆ Maternal Physiology During Pregnancy

Duration of Pregnancy

1. Averages 280 days or 40 weeks from the first day of the last normal menstrual period
2. Duration also may be divided into three equal parts, or trimesters, of slightly more than 13 weeks or 3 calendar months each.
3. *Estimated date of confinement* (EDC) is calculated by adding 7 days to the date of the first day of the last menstrual period and counting back 3 months (*Nägele's rule*).
   a. For example, if a woman's last menstrual period began on 9/10/91, her EDC would be 9/10/91 plus 7 days = 9/17/91, minus 3 months = 6/17/91.

Changes in Reproductive Tract

1. Enlargement of the uterus during pregnancy involves stretching and marked hypertrophy of existing muscle cells. There is an increase in fibrous tissue, elastic tissue, blood vessels, and lymphatics.
   a. By the end of the third month (12 weeks), the uterus is too large to be contained wholly within the pelvic cavity—it can now be palpated suprapubically.
   b. By 20 weeks' gestation, the fundus has reached the level of the umbilicus.
   c. By 36 weeks, the fundus has reached the xiphoid.
   d. During the last 3 weeks, the uterus descends

slightly—because of fetal descent into pelvis. Walls of uterus become thinner.

2. Changes in contractility occur—from the first trimester, irregular painless contractions occur (Braxton Hicks contractions). In latter weeks of pregnancy, these contractions become stronger and more regular.

3. Pronounced softening and cyanosis of the cervix occurs—caused by increased vascularity, edema, hypertrophy, and hyperplasia of the cervical glands. Clot of very thick mucus obstructs the cervical canal (cervical plug).

4. Chadwick's sign is noted as a characteristic violet color of the cervix and vagina caused by increased vascularity and hyperemia.

5. Vaginal walls prepare for labor: mucosa increases in thickness, connective tissue loosens, and smooth-muscle cells hypertrophy. Vaginal secretions increase, and pH becomes more acidic.

6. Breasts increase in size by second month because of hypertrophy of mammary alveoli. Nipples become larger, more deeply pigmented, and more erectile.

7. Colostrum may be expressed by second trimester.

8. Scattered through the areola are a number of small elevations (glands of Montgomery), which are hypertrophic sebaceous glands.

Metabolic Changes

1. Weight gain averages 11.5 to 16 kg (25–35 lb)

2. The average woman retains 6 to 8 liters extra water during the pregnancy, most of which increases blood volume.

3. Protein metabolism is increased to supply the fetus, uterus, breasts, and maternal blood, which is rich in protein.

4. Pregnancy can initiate diabetes or aggravate preexisting diabetes. Human placental lactogen (hPL or placental hormone) estrogen, progesterone, and an insulinase produced by the placenta oppose the action of insulin during pregnancy.

5. Total circulating red blood cells increase approximately 40% to 50% during pregnancy; therefore, iron requirements are increased to 20 to 40 mg daily. This often exceeds dietary intake.

Changes in Cardiovascular System

1. Diaphragm is progressively elevated during pregnancy; heart is displaced to the left and upward, with the apex moved laterally.
2. Exaggerated splitting of the first heart sound, loud third heart sound, and systolic murmurs may occur but disappear after delivery.
3. In the supine position, the large uterus compresses the venous return from the lower half of the body to the heart. This may cause arterial hypotension, referred to as the *supine hypotensive syndrome.* Cardiac output increases when the woman turns from her back to her left side.
4. Pulse rate usually increases 10 to 15 beats/min during pregnancy, and blood pressure decreases slightly during the first half of pregnancy.
5. Total volume of circulating red blood cells increases; hemoglobin concentration at term averages 12 g/dL.
6. Leukocyte count is elevated to 25,000 or more during labor—cause unknown; probably represents the reappearance in the circulation of leukocytes previously shunted out of active circulation.
7. Blood coagulation—fibrinogen levels increase 50%, and other clotting factors increase.

Changes in Respiratory Tract

1. Hyperventilation occurs—increase in respiratory rate, tidal volume (45%), and minute volume (40%)—causing mild respiratory alkalosis that is compensated for by lowering bicarbonate concentration.
2. Diaphragm is elevated and thoracic cage expands by means of flaring of the ribs—result of increased mobility of rib cartilage

Changes in Urinary Tract

1. Ureters become dilated and elongated during pregnancy because of mechanical pressure and perhaps the effects of progesterone.
2. Glomerular filtration rate (GFR) increases early in pregnancy, and the increase persists almost to term. Renal plasma flow (RPF) increases early in pregnancy and decreases to nonpregnant levels in the third trimester.

3. Glucosuria may be evident, because of the increase in glomerular filtration without increase in tubular resorptive capacity for filtered glucose.
4. Proteinuria does not occur normally, except for slight amounts during or just after vigorous labor.
5. Toward the end of pregnancy, pressure of the presenting part impedes drainage of blood and lymph from the bladder base, often leaving the area edematous, easily traumatized, and more susceptible to infection.

Changes in Gastrointestinal Tract

1. Gums may become hyperemic and softened and may bleed easily.
2. Stomach and intestines are displaced upward and laterally by the enlarging uterus. Heartburn is common, caused by reflux of acid secretions in the lower esophagus.
3. Tone and motility of gastrointestinal tract decrease, leading to prolongation of gastric emptying caused by large amount of progesterone produced by the placenta.
4. Hemorrhoids are common because of elevated pressure in veins below the level of the large uterus and constipation.
5. Distension of the gallbladder is common along with a decrease in emptying time and thickening of bile.
6. Liver function tests yield significantly different results during pregnancy.

Changes in Endocrine System

1. *Pituitary gland* enlarges slightly.
2. *Thyroid* is moderately enlarged because of hyperplasia of glandular tissue and increased vascularity, and basal metabolic rate increases progressively.
3. *Adrenal* secretions increase considerably.
4. *Pancreas:* Because of the fetal glucose needs for growth, there are alterations in maternal insulin production and usage.

Changes in Integumentary System

1. Pigmentary changes occur because of melanocyte-stimulating hormone, the level of which is elevated from the second month of pregnancy until term.
2. Striae gravidarum appear in later months of pregnancy

as reddish, slightly depressed streaks in the skin of the abdomen and occasionally over the breasts and thighs.

3. A brownish-black line of pigment is often formed in the midline of the abdominal skin—known as *linea nigra*.

4. Brownish patches of pigment may form on the face—known as *chloasma* or "mask of pregnancy."

5. Angiomas (vascular spiders), minute red elevations commonly on the skin of the face, neck, upper chest, and arms, may develop.

6. Reddening of the palms *(palmar erythema)* also may occur.

Changes in Musculoskeletal System

1. The increasing mobility of sacroiliac, sacrococcygeal, and pelvic joints during pregnancy is a result of hormonal changes.

2. This mobility contributes to alteration of maternal posture and to back pain.

3. Late in pregnancy, aching, numbness, and weakness in the upper extremities may occur because of lordosis, which ultimately produces traction on the ulnar and median nerves.

4. Separation of the rectus muscles caused by pressure of the growing uterus creates a diastasis recti. If this is severe, a portion of the anterior uterine wall is covered by only a layer of skin, fascia, and peritoneum.

◆ Maternal Assessment

Health History

1. Age is important because adolescents have an increased incidence of anemia, pregnancy-induced hypertension, preterm labor, small-for-gestational-age infants, cephalopelvic disproportion, and dystocia; older women have an increased incidence of hypertension, pregnancies complicated by underlying medical problems, and infants with genetic abnormalities.

2. Family history of congenital disorders; hereditary diseases; multiple pregnancies; diabetes; heart disease; hypertension; mental retardation

3. Woman's medical history
   a. Childhood diseases, especially rubella

   b. Major illnesses, surgery; blood tranfusions
   c. Drug, food, and environmental sensitivities
   d. Urinary infections; heart disease; diabetes, hypertension, endocrine disorders; anemias
   e. Use of oral or other contraceptives
   f. History of sexually transmitted diseases
   g. Menstrual history (menarche; length and regularity of menstrual cycle)
   h. Use of medications, other drugs, alcohol, tobacco, and caffeine

4. Woman's obstetric history
   a. Problems of infertility, date of previous pregnancies and deliveries—dates; infant weights; length of labors; types of deliveries; multiple births; abortions; maternal, fetal, and neonatal complications
   b. Woman's perception of past pregnancy, labor, and delivery for herself and impact on her family
   c. Gravidity; parity
   d. Date of last menstrual period (LMP)
   e. Estimated date of birth—expected date of confinement (EDC).
   f. Signs and symptoms of pregnancy—amenorrhea, breast changes, nausea and vomiting, fetal movement, fatigue, urinary frequency, skin pigmentary changes

5. Psychosocial status—emotional changes she is experiencing; woman's and family's reactions to current pregnancy; support system—family's and friends' willingness to provide support; woman's current coping with lifestyle changes caused by the pregnancy

Laboratory Data

1. Urinalysis—for glucose and protein
   a. Glucose may be present in small amounts
   b. Proteinuria should be reported because it may be a sign of a hypertensive disorder of pregnancy or renal problems.
   c. If the urine is cloudy and bacteria or leukocytes are present, a urine culture is done.

2. Hematocrit and hemoglobin levels and morphology of the red blood cells are done to find evidence of anemia.

3. Blood type, Rh factor, and antibody screen—if the

woman is found to be Rh negative or have a positive antibody screen, her partner is screened and a maternal antibody titer is drawn as indicated.

   a. Coomb's test: retested at 28 weeks in the Rh-negative woman for detection of antibodies

   b. Rh D immune globulin, RhoGAM, given at 28 weeks as indicated

4. Glucose: diabetic screening done at 24 to 28 weeks using 1-hour 50-g glucose load test

5. Alpha-fetoprotein (AFP): done at 15 to 18 weeks. High maternal levels after 18 weeks may indicate a neural tube defect (NTD) in the fetus; however, this test has high false-positive results.

6. Venereal Disease Research Lab (VDRL) or other tests for syphilis are done on the initial visit; repeated at 32 weeks as indicated.

7. Gonorrhea and chlamydia: cervical cultures or DNA test are usually done at the initial visit and when symptoms are present.

8. Herpes: all possible lesions are cultured, and the cervix is cultured weekly beginning 4 to 8 weeks before delivery if genital herpes is active.

9. Rubella titer: if nonimmune (less then 1:8), immunize postpartum

10. Hepatitis B surface antigen: for chronic hepatitis and carrier state

11. Human immunodeficiency virus (HIV): screen is done on high-risk women

12. Other tests

   a. Toxoplasmosis: done as indicated for women at risk

   b. Tuberculin skin tests: done as indicated

   c. Papanicolaou smear: done unless recent results available

Physical Assessment

1. Ask the woman to empty her bladder before the examination so that during vaginal examination her uterus and pelvic organs may be readily palpated.

2. Evaluate the woman's weight and blood pressure.

3. Examination of eyes, ears, and nose: nasal congestion during pregnancy may occur as a result of peripheral vasodilation.

4. Examination of the mouth, teeth, throat, and thyroid: gums may be hyperemic and softened because of increased progesterone; thyroid may be slightly enlarged.
5. Inspection of breasts and nipples: breasts may be enlarged and tender; nipple and areolar pigment may be darkened
6. Auscultation of heart for changes in heart sounds and murmurs
7. Auscultation and percussion of the lungs
8. Examination of the abdomen for scars or striations, diastasis, or umbilical hernia
9. Palpation of the abdomen for height of the fundus
10. Palpation of the abdomen for fetal outline and position—third trimester
11. Check of fetal heart tone (FHT): FHTs are audible with Doppler after 10 weeks and at 18 to 20 weeks with a fetoscope.
12. Record fetal position, presentation, and FHTs.

Pelvic Examination

1. Assist woman to lithotomy position.
2. Inspect external genitalia.
3. Vaginal examination is done to rule out abnormalities of the birth canal and to obtain cytologic smear
4. Cervix is examined for position, size, mobility, and consistency.
5. Ovaries are identified for size, shape, and position.
6. Rectovaginal exploration is done to identify hemorrhoids, fissures, herniation, or masses.
7. Pelvic inlet is evaluated: anteroposterior diameter of the pelvis by measuring the diagonal conjugate (distance between the lower margin of the symphysis pubis and sacral promontory)
8. Midpelvis is evaluated for prominence of the ischial spines.
9. Pelvic outlet is evaluated: distance between ischial tuberosities

Subsequent Prenatal Assessments

1. Uterine growth and estimated fetal growth (Fig. 29)
   a. A greater fundal height suggests multiple pregnancy, miscalculated due date, polyhydramnios

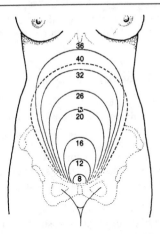

FIGURE 29 *Height of fundus (From Scott, J, DiSaia, PJ, Hammond, C. & Spellacy, WN, Danforth's Obstetrics and Gynecology, 7th ed. Philadelphia, JB Lippincott, 1994).*

      (excessive amniotic fluid), hydatidiform mole (degeneration of villi into grapelike clusters; fetus does not usually develop)

  b. A lesser fundal height suggests intrauterine fetal growth retardation, error in estimating gestation, fetal or amniotic fluid abnormalities, intrauterine fetal death

2. Fetal heart tones: normal is 120 to 160 beats/min
3. Weight: major increase in weight occurs during second half of pregnancy; usually between 0.22 kg (0.5 lb)/week and 0.44 kg (1 lb)/week. Greater weight gain may indicate fluid retention and hypertensive disorder.
4. Blood pressure: should remain near woman's normal baseline
5. Urinalysis: for protein, glucose, blood, and nitrates (indicates infection)
6. Edema: check the lower legs, face, and hands
7. Discomforts of pregnancy: fatigue, heartburn, hemorrhoids, constipation, and backache
8. Evaluate eating and sleeping patterns, general adjustment and coping with the pregnancy.

9. Evaluate concerns of the woman and her family.
10. Evaluate preparation for labor, delivery, and parenting.

◆ Health Education and Intervention

Backache and Leg Cramps

1. Teach good body mechanics, wear comfortable, low-heeled shoes with good arch support, try the use of a maternity girdle if desired.
2. Instruct in the technique for pelvic rocking exercises.
3. Encourage rest periods with legs elevated.
4. Encourage adequate calcium intake to decrease leg cramps.
5. Instruct on immediate relief of leg cramps: dorsiflex the foot while applying pressure to the knee to straighten the leg.

Breast Care

1. Advise wearing a fitted, supportive brassiere.
2. Instruct to wash breasts and nipples with water only.
3. Apply vitamin E or lanolin cream to nipples. Lanolin is contraindicated for women with allergies to lamb's wool.

Nausea, Heartburn, and Nutrition

1. Encourage low-fat, protein-containing foods and dry carbohydrates such as toast and crackers.
2. Encourage small frequent meals.
3. Advise not to brush teeth soon after eating.
4. Suggest getting out of bed slowly.
5. Encourage drinking liquids between meals to avoid stomach distension.
6. Instruct in the use of antacids; caution against the use of sodium bicarbonate because it results in the absorption of excess sodium and fluid retention.
7. Review the basic food groups with appropriate daily servings for good balanced nutrition.
   a. 7 servings of protein foods, including 1 serving of a vegetable protein
   b. 3 servings of milk or milk products
   c. 7 servings of grain products
   d. 1 serving of vitamin C–rich vegetable or fruit

  e. 4 servings of other fruits and vegetables
  f. 3 servings of unsaturated fats
8. Teach about appropriate weight gain (25–35 lbs); less for overweight women, and more for young adolescents, multiple pregnancy, and underweight women
9. Advise limiting the use of caffeine.
10. Inform that alcohol should be limited or eliminated during pregnancy; no safe level of intake has been established.
11. Stress that smoking should be eliminated or severely reduced during pregnancy; risk of spontaneous abortion, fetal death, low birth weight and neonatal death increases with increased levels of maternal smoking.
12. Advise that ingesting any drug during pregnancy may affect fetal growth and should be discussed with health care provider.

Urinary Frequency
1. Advise limiting fluid intake in the evening.
2. Encourage voiding before going to bed and after meals.

Constipation
1. Instruct on increasing fluid intake to at least 8 glasses of water a day. One to 2 quarts of fluid per day is desirable.
2. Teach about foods high in fiber.
3. Encourage regular patterns of elimination.
4. Encourage daily exercise such as walking.
5. Discourage the use of over-the-counter laxatives; bulk-forming agents may be prescribed if indicated.

Varicose Veins
1. Encourage frequent rest periods with legs elevated.
2. Advise on use of support stockings and to wear loose-fitting clothing for leg varicosities.
3. Instruct the woman to rest periodically with a small pillow under the buttocks to elevate the pelvis for vulvar varicosities.
4. Instruct the woman to avoid constipation, apply cold compresses, take sitz baths, and use topical anesthetics, such as witch hazel, for the relief of anal varicosities (hemorrhoids).
5. Provide reassurance that varicosities will totally or greatly resolve after delivery.

Preparation for Labor, Delivery, and Parenthood

1. Encourage the woman/couple to discuss their knowledge, perceptions, and expectations of the labor and delivery process.
2. Provide information on childbirth education classes and encourage participation.
3. Facilitate a tour of the birth facility.
4. Discuss coping and pain control techniques for labor and birth.
5. Encourage the woman/couple to discuss their perceptions and expectations of parenthood and their "idealized child."
6. Discuss the infant's sleeping, eating, activity, and response patterns for the first month of life.
7. Discuss physical preparations for the infant such as a sleeping space, clothing, feeding, changing, and bathing equipment.
8. Encourage discussion of feelings and concerns regarding the new role of mother and father.
9. Discuss physiologic causes for changes in sexual relationships such as fatigue, loss of interest, and discomfort from advancing pregnancy.
10. Teach the woman/couple that there are no contraindications to intercourse or masturbation to orgasm, provided the woman's membranes are intact, there is no vaginal bleeding, and she has no current problems or history of premature labor.

Fatigue

1. Advise 8 hours of rest at night. Inability to sleep may be caused by excessive fatigue during day.
2. Advise that, in the latter months of pregnancy, sleeping on the side with a small pillow under the abdomen may enhance comfort.
3. Encourage frequent 15- to 30-minute rest periods during the day to avoid overfatigue.
4. Suggest working while sitting with legs elevated whenever possible.
5. Discourage standing for prolonged periods, especially during the third trimester.
6. To promote placental perfusion, discourage lying flat

900

on back—the left lateral position provides the best placental perfusion.

Exercise

1. Explain that exercise during pregnancy should be in keeping with the woman's prepregnancy pattern and type of exercise.
2. Discourage activities or sports that have a risk of bodily harm (skiing, snowmobiling, horseback riding).
3. Explain that endurance during exercise may be decreased.
4. Recommend exercise classes for pregnant women that concentrate on toning and stretching to enhance physical condition, increase self-esteem, and provide socialization.

◆ Physiologic Changes in the Fetus

Fetal Growth and Development

1. First lunar month: fertilization to 2 weeks of embryonic growth
   a. Implantation occurs.
   b. Primary chorionic villi form.
   c. Embryo develops into two cell layers (bilaminar embryonic disc).
   d. Amniotic cavity appears.
2. Second lunar month: 3 to 6 weeks of embryonic growth
   a. At the end of 6 weeks of growth, the embryo is approximately 1.2 cm long.
   b. Arm and leg buds are visible; arm buds are more developed, with finger ridges beginning to appear.
   c. Rudiments of the eyes, ears, and nose appear.
   d. Lung buds and primitive intestinal tract are developing.
   e. Primitive cardiovascular system is functioning.
   f. Neural tube, which forms the brain and spinal cord, closes by the fourth week.
3. Third lunar month: 7 to 10 weeks of growth
   a. The middle of this period (8 weeks) marks the end of the embryonic period and the beginning of the fetal period.

     b. At the end of 10 weeks of growth, the fetus is 6.1 cm from crown to rump and weighs 14 g.

     c. Appearance of external genitalia

     d. By the middle of this month, all major organ systems have formed.

     e. The membrane over the anus has broken down, and rudimentary kidneys begin to secrete urine.

     f. The heart has formed four chambers (by seventh week), and bone ossification begins.

     g. The fetus assumes a human appearance.

4. Fourth lunar month: 11- to 14-week-old fetus

     a. At the end of 14 weeks of growth, the fetus is 12 cm crown to rump length and 110 g.

     b. Head is erect, and lower extremities are well developed.

     c. Hard palate and nasal septum have fused; eyelids are sealed.

     d. External genitalia of male and female can now be differentiated.

5. Fifth lunar month: 15- to 18 week-old fetus

     a. At the end of 18 weeks of growth, the fetus is 16 cm crown to rump length and 320 g.

     b. Ossification of fetal skeleton can be seen on x-ray.

     c. Ears stand out from head; fetus makes sucking motions and swallows amniotic fluid.

     d. Meconium is present in the intestinal tract.

     e. Fetal movements may be felt by the mother (end of month).

6. Sixth lunar month: 19- to 22-week-old fetus

     a. At the end of 22 weeks of growth, the fetus is 21 cm crown to rump length and 630 g.

     b. Vernix caseosa covers the skin; head and body hair (lanugo) form.

     c. Skin is wrinkled and red; nipples appear on breasts.

     d. Brown fat, an important site of heat production, is present in neck and sternal area.

7. Seventh lunar month: 23- to 26-week-old fetus

     a. At the end of 26 weeks of growth, the fetus is 25 cm crown to rump length and 1,000 g.

     b. Body is lean; fingernails present

     c. Eyes partially open; eyelashes present

    d. Bronchioles are present; primitive alveoli are forming.
    e. Skin begins to thicken on hands and feet.
    f. Startle reflex present; grasp reflex is strong.
8. Eighth lunar month: 27- to 30-week-old fetus
    a. At the end of 30 weeks of growth, the fetus is 28 cm crown to rump length and 1,700 g.
    b. Eyes open; skin slightly wrinkled; toenails present
    c. Ample hair on head; lanugo begins to fade
    d. Testes in inguinal canal, begin descent to scrotal sac
    e. Surfactant coats much of the alveolar epithelium.
9. Ninth lunar month: 31- to 34-week-old fetus
    a. At the end of 34 weeks of growth, the fetus is approximately 32 cm crown to rump length and 2,500 g.
    b. Fingernails reach fingertips; skin pink and smooth
    c. Testes in scrotal sac
10. 10th lunar month: 35- to 38-week-old fetus; end of this month is also 40 weeks from onset of last menstrual period
    a. End of 38 weeks of growth, fetus is approximately 36 cm crown to rump length and 3,400 g.
    b. Ample subcutaneous fat; lanugo almost absent
    c. Toenails reach toe tips; vernix caseosa mainly on back
    d. Testes in scrotum; breasts are firm

Fetal Circulation
1. Oxygenated blood from the placenta travels through the umbilical vein through the ductus venosus (bypassing the liver) to the inferior vena cava.
2. Blood from the inferior vena cava is shunted from the right atrium to the left atrium via the foramen ovale.
3. Blood enters the left ventricle and then is routed preferentially to the brain and upper extremities.
4. Blood drains from the upper body into the superior vena cava, and from the lower extremities into the inferior vena cava, which both empty into the right atrium.
5. Blood flows from the right atrium through the pulmonary artery, and to the aorta through the ductus arteriosus, bypassing the lungs.

6. Blood travels through the aorta to the lower extremities.
7. The lower aorta branches to the umbilical arteries and is returned to the placenta and maternal circulation for oxygenation.

◆ Assessment of Fetal Maturity and Well-Being

Fetal Heart Tones (FHTs)

1. Audible by Doppler at approximately 10 weeks' fetal gestation; fetoscope (fetal stethoscope) at approximately 20 weeks' fetal gestation. Electronic fetal monitoring may be done after 24 weeks.
2. Rate should be between 120 and 160 beats/min.
3. Location of heart sounds varies with presentation of fetus.
4. Failure to hear FHTs at the expected time may be caused by maternal obesity, polyhydramnios, error in date calculation, or fetal death.
5. Nursing/patient care considerations
   a. Explain the procedure and assist the woman to a side-lying or semi-Fowler's position; expose and drape the abdomen.
   b. Document findings on chart with date, time, activity level, medications, etc. and include monitor strip if applicable.

NURSING ALERT
Monitor tracings become part of the patient's chart and are legal documents. They may be used in litigation if certain health problems develop in years to come.

Fetal Movement

1. Fetal movements or "kick counts" may be evaluated daily by the pregnant woman to provide reassurance of fetal well-being.
2. Fetal movements are counted for 60 minutes three times a day, usually after meals.
3. The health care provider must be notified for:

a. Fewer than 10 movements in 12 hours
b. An increase of violent movements, followed by decreased movement
c. No movement for 8 hours
4. Nursing/patient care considerations
   a. Instruct the woman to lie on her side and place her hands on the largest part of her abdomen and concentrate on fetal movement.
   b. Instruct the woman to use a clock and record the movements felt.

Maternal Serum Alpha-Fetoprotein

1. Elevated AFP levels are associated with neural tube defects, Rh isoimmunization, multiple gestation, maternal diabetes mellitus, and fetoplacental dysfunction.
2. Decreased levels are associated with Down syndrome.
3. Follow-up for abnormal high or low levels includes ultrasound examination and amniocentesis.
4. Nursing/patient care considerations
   a. Obtain health and pregnancy history, including the date of the woman's last menstrual period and risk factors. Accurate dating of the pregnancy is crucial to interpret the results of the serum levels (done at 15–18 weeks).
   b. Obtain blood sample and discuss the woman's concerns.

Ultrasound

1. Uses in the first trimester of pregnancy include:
   a. Early confirmation of pregnancy and determination of the EDC
   b. Diagnosis of an extopic pregnancy
   c. Detection of an intrauterine device
   d. Evaluation of placental location
   e. Diagnosis of a multiple gestation
2. Uses in the second trimester include:
   a. Evaluation of fetal growth, weight, and gestational age
   b. Evaluation of the placenta for placenta previa or separation associated with vaginal bleeding
   c. Evaluation of fetal presentation and position
   d. Evaluation of fetal abnormalities and viability
   e. Determination of the Biophysical Profile Score

   f. Evaluation of amniotic fluid volume
   g. Guidance for amniocentesis
3. Nursing/patient care considerations
   a. Explain the purpose and procedure to the woman, emphasizing the need to remain still
   b. Instruct the woman to drink three to four glasses of water to ensure full bladder before procedure.
   c. Remove the lubricant from the woman's abdomen and allow her to void after the procedure.

Amniocentesis

1. Usually performed between 16 and 18 weeks' gestation, involves placement of a needle through the abdominal and uterine walls and into the amniotic sac to remove fluid
2. In determination of genetic or metabolic diseases, the procedure is useful for women 35 years of age or older, family history of metabolic disease, previous child with a chromosomal abnormality, family history of chromosomal abnormality, patient or husband with a chromosomal abnormality, or a possible female carrier of an X-linked disease.
3. In determination of lung maturity, the lecithin/sphingomyelin (L/S) ratio is analyzed (should be $2:1$ or greater).
4. In treatment of polyhydramnios, amniotic fluid is removed.
5. Nursing considerations before the procedure
   a. Reduce the parents' anxiety by determining their understanding of the procedure and the concerns they have about the procedure and the fetus.
   b. Correct misinformation they may have; make sure they know when the results will be available and how they may obtain the results as soon as possible.
   c. Ensure woman that local anesthetic will be given.
5. Nursing considerations during the procedure
   a. Have the woman empty her bladder if the fetus is more than 20 weeks' gestation to avoid injury to the woman's bladder. If the fetus is less than 20 weeks' gestation, the woman's full bladder will hold the uterus steady and out of the pelvis. The placenta is localized by ultrasound.
   b. Obtain maternal vital signs, and a 20-minute fetal

heart rate tracing to serve as a baseline to evaluate possible complications.

c. Have the woman lie comfortably on her back with her hands and a pillow under her head. Relaxation breathing may help.

d. Monitor the woman during and after the procedure for signs of premature labor or bleeding.

e. Tell the woman to report signs of bleeding, unusual fetal activity or abdominal pain, cramping, or fever while at home after the procedure.

Chorionic Villus Sampling (CVS)

1. Using an ultrasound picture, a catheter is passed vaginally into the woman's uterus, where a sample of CV tissue is snipped off or obtained by suction.
2. Can be performed earlier than amniocentesis; between 8 and 12 weeks of pregnancy
3. Results from CVS are available in 1 to 2 weeks.
4. Complications include rupture of membranes, intrauterine infection, spontaneous abortion, hematoma, fetal trauma, or maternal tissue contamination.
5. Incidence of fetal loss is approximately 2% to 5%.
6. Nursing/patient care considerations
   a. Obtain maternal vital signs.
   b. Instruct the woman to void.
   c. Inform the woman that a small amount of spotting is normal, but heavy bleeding or passing clots or tissue should be reported.
   d. Instruct the woman to rest at home after the procedure for a few hours.

Percutaneous Umbilical Blood Sampling (PUBS)

1. PUBS or cordocentesis involves a puncture of the umbilical cord for aspiration of fetal blood under ultrasound guidance.
2. It is used in the diagnosis of blood incompatibilities, anemias, and genetic studies or for blood transfusion.
3. Nursing/patient care considerations
   a. Explain the procedure and provide support during the procedure.
   b. Monitor the woman after the procedure for uterine contractions and the fetal heart rate for distress.

Nonstress Test (NST)

1. Used to evaluate fetal heart rate accelerations that normally occur in response to fetal activity. Accelerations are indicative of an intact central and autonomic nervous system.
2. Maternal indications include post dates, Rh sensitization, maternal age 35 years or older, chronic renal disease, hypertension, collagen disease, sickle cell disease, diabetes, premature rupture of membranes (PROM), history of stillbirth, vaginal bleeding in the second and third trimester.
3. Fetal indications include decreased fetal movement, intrauterine growth retardation, fetal evaluation after an amniocentesis, oligohydramnios, or polyhydramnios.
4. Criteria for a reactive NST include two accelerations in a 20-minute period, each lasting at least 15 seconds with a fetal heart rate increased by 15 beats/min above baseline in response to fetal activity. The test period should be a minimum of 40 minutes to allow for fetal rest cycle patterns.
5. In a nonreactive NST, the test period may be extended to allow for fetal rest cycles. Fruit juice may be given, or abdominal manipulation may stimulate the fetus.
6. Nursing/patient care considerations
   a. Explain the procedure and monitoring equipment.
   b. Assist the woman to a semi-Fowler's position in bed and apply the external fetal and uterine monitors.
   c. Instruct the woman to make a mark on the monitor strip each time fetal movement is felt. The nurse will do this if the woman cannot.
   d. Evaluate the response of the fetal heart rate immediately after fetal activity.
   e. Monitor the woman's blood pressure and uterine activity for deviations during the procedure.

Acoustic Stimulation Test (AST)

1. Vibroacoustic stimulation, using an artificial larynx, is used to stimulate the fetus and assess its reaction to the sound.
2. One method of evaluation indicates that a reactive acoustic stimulation test will have at least one acceleration of at least 15 beats/min lasting 2 minutes or two

accelerations with an increase of 15 beats/min lasting 15 seconds within 5 minutes of stimulation.

3. Nursing/patient care considerations
   a. Explain procedure and equipment to the woman.
   b. Assist woman to a semi-Fowler's position in bed.
   c. Apply external fetal monitors to the woman.
   d. Observe for reactivity.

Oxytocin Challenge Test (OCT)

1. OCT, also called stress test (ST) or contraction stress test, is used to evaluate the ability of the fetus to withstand the stress of uterine contractions as would occur during labor. It is used with decreasing frequency because it may stress an already compromised fetus.
2. Usually used when a woman has a nonreactive NST
3. Contraindicated in woman with third-trimester bleeding, multiple gestation, incompetent cervix, or PROM
4. Nursing/patient care considerations
   a. Obtain maternal vital signs and instruct the woman to void.
   b. Assist the woman to a semi-Fowler's or side-lying position in bed.
   c. Obtain a 30-minute strip of the fetal heart rate (FHR) and uterine activity for baseline data.
   d. Administer diluted oxytocin via an intravenous line infusion pump as indicated until three contractions occur within 10 minutes. This may take 1 to 2 hours.
   e. Discontinue the infusion when the test is complete.

Biophysical Profile (BPP)

1. Uses ultrasonography and NST to assess five variables in determining fetal well-being
   a. NST: looking for acceleration in relation to fetal movements
   b. Amniotic fluid volume: assessing for one or more pockets of amniotic fluid measuring 1 cm in two perpendicular planes
   c. Fetal breathing: one or more episodes lasting at least 30 seconds
   d. Gross body movements: three or more body or limb movements in 30 minutes
   e. Fetal tone: one or more episodes of active extension with return to flexion

3. For each variable, if the criteria are met, a score of 2 is given. For an abnormal observation, a score of 0 or 1 is given. A score of 8 to 10 is considered normal, 6 is equivocal, and 4 or less is abnormal.
4. Nursing/patient care considerations
   a. Explain the purpose and procedure to the woman.
   b. Instruct the woman to drink three to four glasses of water if the bladder is not full.
   c. Remove the lubricant from the woman's abdomen and allow her to void after the procedure.

Labor and Delivery

◆ The Labor Process

Events Preliminary to Labor

1. *Lightening* (the settling of the fetus in the lower uterine segment) occurs 2 to 3 weeks before term in the primigravida and later, during labor, in the multigravida.
   a. Breathing becomes easier as the fetus falls away from the diaphragm.
   b. Lordosis of the spine is increased as the fetus enters the pelvis and falls forward. Walking may become more difficult; leg cramping may increase.
   c. Urinary frequency occurs because of pressure on the bladder.
2. Vaginal secretions may increase.
3. Mucous plug is discharged from the cervix along with a small amount of blood from surrounding capillaries—referred to as "show" or "bloody show."
4. Cervix becomes soft and effaced (thinned).
5. Membranes may rupture.
6. False labor contractions may occur (Table 21).
7. Backache may increase.
8. Diarrhea may occur.
9. Weight loss of 1 to 3 lb
10. Sudden burst of energy is experienced by some women.

TABLE 21 True and False Labor Contractions

True Labor Contractions	False Labor Contractions
Result in progressive cervical dilation and effacement	Do not result in progressive cervical dilation and effacement
Occur at regular intervals	Occur at irregular intervals
Interval between contractions decreases	Interval between contractions remains the same or increases
Intensity increases	Intensity decreases or remains the same
Located mainly in back and abdomen	Located mainly in lower abdomen and groin
Generally intensified by walking	Generally unaffected by walking
Not affected by mild sedation	Generally relieved by mild sedation

Stages of Labor

1. First stage of labor (stage of cervical dilation): begins with the first true labor contractions and ends with complete effacement and dilation of the cervix (10 cm dilation)
   a. Averages 13.3 hours for a nullipara and 7.5 hours for a multipara
   b. Latent phase (early): dilation from 0 to 4 cm; contractions are usually every 5 to 20 minutes, lasting 20 to 40 seconds, and of mild intensity
   c. Active phase: dilation from 4 to 7 cm; contractions are usually every 2 to 5 minutes; lasting 30 to 50 seconds, and of mild to moderate intensity
   d. Transitional phase: dilates from 8 to 10 cm; contractions are every 2 to 3 minutes, lasting 50 to 60 seconds, and of moderate to strong intensity. Some contractions may last up to 90 seconds.
2. Second stage of labor, or stage of expulsion: begins with complete dilation and ends with birth of the baby
   a. May last from 1 to $1\frac{1}{2}$ hours in the nullipara and from 20 to 45 minutes in the multipara
3. Third stage of labor, or placental stage: begins with

delivery of the baby and ends with delivery of the placenta

a. May last from a few minutes up to 30 minutes

4. Fourth stage: begins after delivery of the placenta and ends when postpartum condition of the woman has become stabilized (usually 1 hour after delivery)

Mechanisms of Labor

1. If the woman's pelvis is adequate, size and position of the fetus are adequate, and uterine contractions are regular and of adequate intensity, the fetus will move through the birth canal.

2. The position and rotational changes of the fetus as it moves down the birth canal will be affected by resistance offered by the woman's bony pelvis, cervix, and surrounding tissues.

3. The events of engagement, descent, flexion, internal rotation, extension, external rotation, and expulsion overlap in time.

4. Engagement: when biparietal diameter of fetal head has passed through pelvic inlet:

   a. In primigravidas occurs up to 2 weeks before onset of labor

   b. In multigravidas usually occurs with onset of labor

   c. Because biparietal diameter is narrowest diameter of fetal head, and anteroposterior diameter is the narrowest diameter of pelvic inlet, the fetal head usually enters pelvis in a transverse position

5. Descent: occurs throughout labor and is essential for fetal rotations before birth

   a. Accomplished by force of uterine contractions on fetal portion in fundus; during second stage of labor, bearing down increases intraabdominal pressure, thus augmenting effects of uterine contractions

6. Station is the relationship of the level of the presenting part to the ischial spines. The degree of descent is described as floating (presenting part above pelvic inlet); fixed (presenting part has entered pelvis); engaged (presenting part has passed through pelvic inlet); station -1, -2, -3, or -4 (presenting part is 1, 2, 3, or 4 cm above the level of the ischial spines): station 0 (presenting part is at the level of the ischial

spines); station $+1$, $+2$, $+3$, or $+4$, (presenting part is 1, 2, 3, or 4 cm below the ischial spines). A station of $+4$ indicates that the presenting part is on the pelvic floor.

7. Flexion: resistance to descent causes head to flex so that the chin is close to the chest; this causes the smallest fetal head diameter to present through the canal.

8. Internal rotation: in accommodating to the birth canal, the fetal occiput rotates anteriorly from its original position toward the symphysis. This movement results from the shape of the fetal head, space available in the midpelvis, and contour of the perineal muscles. The ischial spines project into the midpelvis, causing the fetal head to rotate anteriorly to accommodate to the available space.

9. Extension: As the fetal head descends further, it meets resistance from the perineal muscles and is forced to extend. The fetal head becomes visible at the vulvovaginal ring; its largest diameter is encircled (crowning), and the head then emerges from the vagina.

10. External rotation: when the head emerges, the shoulders are undergoing internal rotation as they turn in the midpelvis to accommodate to the projection of the ischial spines. The head, now born, rotates as the shoulders undergo this internal rotation.

11. Expulsion: after delivery of the infant's head and internal rotation of the shoulders, the anterior shoulder rests beneath the symphysis pubis. The anterior shoulder is born, followed by the posterior shoulder and the rest of the body.

◆ Fetal Monitoring

Types of Monitoring

1. The purposes of *continuous fetal monitoring* during labor are to monitor the progress of a woman's contraction pattern and to monitor the condition of the fetus in response to the stress of uterine contractions.

2. *External monitoring* (indirect monitoring) uses separate transducers secured to the woman's abdomen: a tokodynamometer (tocotransducer) measures abdominal

tension, and an ultrasonic transducer transmits fetal heart sounds into electrical signals that record on a graph chart.

  a. Apply ultrasonic transducer over the area of the abdomen where the sharpest FHT is heard and lubricate with a thin layer of ultrasonic gel to aid in the transmission of sounds.

  b. Readjust transducer when the fetus changes positions.

  c. Apply the tokodynamometer over the fundus and adjust as the uterus descends during labor.

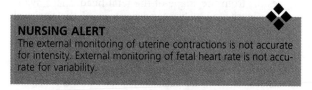

NURSING ALERT
The external monitoring of uterine contractions is not accurate for intensity. External monitoring of fetal heart rate is not accurate for variability.

3. *Internal monitoring* (direct monitoring) records intrauterine pressure and the FHR through internal measurements; it is more accurate than external monitoring.

  a. Fetal electrocardiograph: obtained by screwing a small spiral electrode into the presenting part. The membranes must be ruptured, the cervix dilated at least 2 to 3 cm, and the presenting part must be accessible and identifiable.

  b. Uterine contractions are recorded by means of a sterile water-filled catheter placed in the uterine cavity behind the presenting part. A transducer converts the pressure values to millimeters of mercury (mm Hg).

  c. Monitor strips record the fetal heart and uterine contraction simultaneously.

Interpretation

1. FHR is initially evaluated for the baseline rate when the fetus is not moving, between contractions, and when the fetus is not being stimulated. Fluctuations in the heart rate are either accelerations or decelerations.

2. Tachycardia is an FHR of 160 beats/min or more, or more than 30 beats/min above the normal baseline

rate for at least 10 minutes. It may be caused by early fetal hypoxia, fetal immaturity, maternal fever, maternal hyperthyroidism, maternal ingestion of parasympatholytic and beta-sympathomimetic drugs, amnionitis, fetal anemia, fetal cardiac arrhythmias, and fetal heart failure.

3. Bradycardia is a baseline FHR below 120 beats/min for at least 10 minutes. Bradycardia may be caused by late or profound fetal hypoxia, maternal hypotension, prolonged umbilical cord compression, hypothermia, maternal ingestion of beta-adrenergic blocking drugs, and anesthetics. Fetal bradycardia above 90 beats/min in the third stage of labor is not considered abnormal unless there is a loss of variability.

4. Variability refers to the beat-to-beat changes in FHR that result from the interplay between the sympathetic and parasympathetic nervous systems. It indicates normal neurologic function in relation to heart rate and also fetal reserve.
   a. Short-term variability: the beat-to-beat change in the FHR.
   b. Long-term variability: the rhythmic changes in the heart rate, usually three to five cycles/min.
   c. Short- and long-term variability tend to increase and decrease together.
   d. Variability is described as 0 to 2 beats/min, no variability; 3 to 5 beats/min, minimal variability; 6 to 25 beats/min, moderate variability (normal); greater than 25 beats/min, marked variability.

Accelerations and Decelerations

1. Accelerations are increases in the FHR caused most often by fetal movements or fetal stimulation; also seen with breech presentations, occiput posterior presentations, and uterine contractions
   a. Graphic configuration may or may not resemble the shape of the uterine contraction.
   b. Recovery varies, and if they occur with contractions, they may return to baseline as the uterine pressure decreases.
   c. Treatment: none, other than observe the tracing for late or variable decelerations later in labor

2. Early decelerations are decreases in FHR caused by

head compression from uterine contractions, vaginal examination, scalp stimulation; also frequently seen in women who are completely dilated.

a. Configuration mirrors the image of the contraction, and all look the same.

b. Onset is early in the contraction, with the peak being at the acme of the contraction.

c. Recovery: returns to baseline by the end of the contraction

d. Treatment: none

3. Late decelerations occur late in the contraction and are caused by uteroplacental insufficiency.

a. Configuration is a reverse mirror image of the contraction phase, and they remain uniform.

b. Onset: usually after the acme of the contraction, with the low point of the deceleration occurring well after the acme

c. Recovery: returns to baseline after the end of the contraction

d. Treatment is aimed at increasing uteroplacental perfusion: change maternal position to left lateral position; correct any hypotension through increasing the maintenance intravenous (IV) fluids; stop oxytocin; give oxygen by face mask at 8 to 12 L/min.

4. Variable decelerations are caused by cord compression that can result from maternal position, prolapsed cord, cord around a fetal part, a short cord, and a true knot in the cord.

a. Configuration is variable, and does not follow the uterine contraction; frequently are shaped like a "U" or "W."

b. Onset is variable, frequently preceded by an acceleration.

c. Recovery occurs rapidly, often followed by an acceleration.

d. Treatment involves changing of maternal position, observing that the return occurs quickly and that there is no loss of variability.

Unusual Patterns

1. The sinusoidal pattern is characterized by a waveform of rhythmic regular oscillations occurring evenly above and below the baseline.

2. Short-term variability is decreased or absent.
3. FHR ranges between 120 and 160 beats/min.
4. Seen in the presence of fetal anemia and fetal hypoxia
5. Seen after narcotic analgesic administration for a temporary period, and in this instance is not associated with a compromised fetal outcome

◆ Nursing Interventions When Labor Begins

Obtaining History and Baseline Data

1. Introduce yourself; ask for name of woman's health care provider and if he or she has been notified that the woman was coming to the hospital or birth center.
2. Establish baseline information:
   a. Gravidity, parity, expected date of delivery or confinement
   b. When contractions began; how far apart they are; how long they last
   c. If the membranes have ruptured; if so, what is the color, consistency, and amount of fluid leakage
   d. Presence of bloody show
   e. Level of discomfort the woman is experiencing
   f. Any problems in this or past pregnancies
   g. Blood type and Rh
3. Establish baseline maternal and fetal vital signs:
   a. Temperature: elevation suggests a possible infection or dehydration.
   b. Pulse: evaluate between contractions; may be slightly elevated over the resting rate
   c. Respirations: evaluated between contractions
   d. Blood pressure: evaluated between contractions
   e. Assess the FHR: if a fetal monitor is to be used, run a 30-minute strip for baseline data.
4. Obtain a urine specimen: test the urine for glucose and protein. Protein may be positive if the membranes have ruptured.

Assessing Fetal Heart Tones

1. Determine the position, presentation, and lie of the fetus by palpation. As internal rotation and descent occur, the location of the FHT changes, swinging gradually from the lateral to the medial area and dropping

until immediately before birth, when it is above the pubic bone

2. Place the fetoscope or doptone on the abdomen over the back or chest of fetus. Avoid friction noises caused by fingers on the abdominal surface area.

3. Differentiate between FHT and other abdominal sounds.
   a. *Fetal heart tone:* a rapid crisp or ticking sound
   b. *Uterine bruit:* a soft murmur, caused by the passage of blood through dilated uterine vessels; is synchronous with maternal pulse
   c. *Uterine souffle:* a hissing sound produced by passage of blood through the umbilical arteries; it is synchronous with the fetal heart rate

4. Listen and count the rate for 1 full minute; note the location and character when counting.

5. Check the rate before, during, and after a contraction to detect any slowing or irregularities.

6. Check the FHT immediately after the rupture of membranes; a sudden release of fluid may cause a prolapse of the umbilical cord.

Assessing Uterine Contractions

1. Place fingertips gently on the fundus. As contraction begins, tension will be felt under the fingertips. Uterus will become harder, then slowly soften.

2. Describe the intensity as follows:
   a. Mild: the uterine muscle is somewhat tense.
   b. Moderate: the uterine muscle is moderately firm.
   c. Strong (hard): the uterine muscle is so firm that it seems almost boardlike.

3. Determine frequency in minutes—represents the time from the beginning of one contraction until the beginning of the next

4. Determine duration of a contraction—time from the moment the uterus first begins to tighten until it relaxes again

5. Note the progression of labor—the character of the contractions changes and they last longer. When the cervix becomes completely dilated (the transition phase), the contractions become very strong, last for 60 seconds, and occur at 2- to 3-minute intervals.

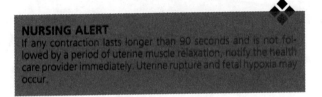

Performing Vaginal Examination

1. Place the woman in lithotomy position and conduct examination gently, under aseptic conditions.
2. Evaluate the condition of cervix:
   a. Hard or soft (in labor, cervix is soft)
   b. Effaced and thin or thick and long (in labor cervix is thin and effaced)
   c. Easily dilatable or resistant
   d. Closed or open (dilated); degree of dilation
3. Determine presentation:
   a. Breech, cephalic (head), or shoulder
   b. Caput succedaneum (edema occurring in and under fetal scalp) present (small or large)
   c. Station: engaged or floating
4. Evaluate position: for cephalic presentation identify sagittal suture and of its direction; locate posterior fontanelle (Fig. 30)
5. Determine if membranes are intact or ruptured.
   a. If ruptured, determine time of drainage of fluid or passage of meconium.
   b. Rupture usually increases frequency and intensity of uterine contractions.
   c. Manual rupture of membranes is contraindicated in presence of vaginal bleeding, premature labor, or abnormal fetal presentation or position.

Assessing Woman's/Couple's Expectations and Concerns

1. What are their concerns?
2. How anxious are they?
3. What has been their preparation for labor (type, by whom, and when)?
4. What is their understanding of the labor process?
5. What are their expectations of the labor and delivery

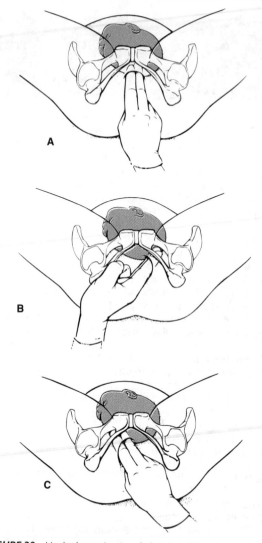

FIGURE 30 Vaginal examination. **(A)** Determining the station and palpating the sagittal suture. **(B)** Identifying the posterior fontanelle. **(C)** Identifying the anterior fontanelle.

process (prepared childbirth, anesthesia, analgesics, use of birthing room, etc.)?

6. How well are they coping and how well are they communicating with each other?

7. Review birth plan with the couple.

◆ Nursing Interventions During First Stage of Labor—Latent Phase

Providing Supportive Care

1. Provide clear liquids and ice chips as allowed.
2. Evaluate urine for ketones and glucose.
3. Administer IV fluids as indicated.
4. Encourage ambulation as tolerated if membranes are not ruptured and the presenting part is engaged. (This may vary according to health care provider).
5. Encourage comfort measures such as a warm shower, relaxation and diversion techniques, back rubs, and position changes.
6. Reposition external monitors as needed.
7. Inform the woman/couple of maternal status and fetal status and labor progress.

Monitoring Mother and Fetus

1. Monitor temperature every 4 hours, unless elevated or membranes ruptured, then every 2 hours.
2. Obtain pulse rate and respirations every hour unless receiving pain medication, then every 15 to 30 minutes or as indicated.
3. Check blood pressure every hour unless hypertension or hypotension exists or woman has received pain medication or anesthesia. Then evaluate more frequently based on findings or as indicated.
4. Monitor the FHR once per hour for 15 to 20 minutes for intermittent monitoring. Evaluate the monitor strip at least hourly with continuous monitoring. Evaluate immediately and after each of the next five contractions on rupture of the membranes.

Reviewing Breathing Techniques

1. Teach slow paced breathing: relax, take one deep breath and exhale slowly and completely. Breathe deeply, slowly, rhythmically throughout contraction.

Follow with another deep, complete breath. Take about six to nine breaths per minute.

2. Teach modified paced breathing: take one deep breath and exhale slowly and completely. Breathe regularly at more shallow level. When stronger contraction occurs, breathe more quickly with very light breaths. Then take deep breath and exhale slowly.

3. Teach patterned paced breathing (most often used during transition): concentrate on breathing in controlled manner. Take a deep breath and exhale slowly and completely. At beginning of contraction, take a fairly deep breath. Then engage in modified paced breathing. After a certain number of breaths, the woman exhales with a more forceful puff or blow. The number of breaths before the more forceful exhalation can range between two and six, or the ratio of breaths to blows may be constant.

◆ Nursing Interventions During First Stage of Labor—Active/Transition Phase

Monitoring Mother and Fetus

1. Monitor maternal temperature every 4 hours, unless elevated or membranes ruptured, then every 2 hours.

2. Monitor blood pressure, pulse, and respirations every 30 minutes unless receiving pain medication or epidural anesthesia; then at least every 15 minutes or more frequently as indicated until stable.

3. Evaluate the FHR every 30 minutes unless using continuous monitoring.

4. Evaluate FHR once per hour for 10 to 15 minutes with intermittent monitoring.

Providing Supportive Care

1. Provide intensive encouragement and support and involve the support person in the woman's care.

2. Assist the woman with breathing and relaxation techniques as needed.

3. Provide back, leg, and shoulder massage as needed.

4. Maintain IV fluids as indicated.

5. Encourage the woman to void every 2 hours at least 100 cc. Catheterize (in and out) if bladder becomes distended and unable to void.

6. Monitor intake and output.

Assisting With Regional Anesthesia

1. Administer IV fluid bolus of Ringer's lactate before epidural catheterization as indicated.
2. Assist with positioning the woman.
3. Monitor the fetal heart rate during the procedure and assess for a nonreassuring pattern.
4. Monitor the woman's blood pressure, pulse, and respirations every 2 to 3 minutes after the procedure, then every 15 minutes thereafter or as indicated.
5. Observe for hypotension, nausea and vomiting, and lightheadedness after epidural is initiated. If these occur:
    a. Increase the rate of the IV fluid.
    b. Flatten the head of the bed and elevate legs if necessary.
    c. Turn the woman to her left side.
    d. Administer oxygen face mask at 8 to 10 L/min.
    e. Have ephedrine available.

Minimizing Pain

1. Provide comfort measures, which may include back and leg rubs; a cool cloth to face, neck, abdomen, or back; ice chips to moisten mouth; clean pads and linens as needed; a quiet environment; and repositioning—either side is preferable—with pillow and blanket.
2. Administer prescribed analgesia after confirming that the woman has no known allergies to the drug.
    a. Evaluate maternal vital signs after drug administration.
    b. Evaluate FHR pattern. Decreased variability and a sinusoidal pattern are sometimes seen after narcotic administration to the mother.
3. Encourage the woman to deal with one contraction at a time and to alter her breathing techniques to maintain control. Provide reassurance and encouragement during each contraction.
4. Provide information on the contractions' ascent, peak, and descent.
5. Encourage resting between contractions.
6. Encourage the woman not to push with feelings of rectal pressure until complete cervical dilation has oc-

curred, to prevent cervical edema and lacerations. Assisting her with panting may be helpful.

Preventing Intrauterine Infection

1. Change the pads and linens when wet or soiled.
2. Provide perineal care after voiding and as needed.
3. Discourage the use of sanitary pads because they create a warm moist environment for bacteria.
4. Minimize vaginal examinations.
5. Report elevated maternal temperature and fetal tachycardia immediately; obtain complete blood count (CBC) and specimens for culture as directed.

◆ Nursing Interventions During Second Stage of Labor

Monitoring Mother and Fetus

1. Monitor blood pressure every 5 to 30 minutes, depending on the woman's status.
2. Monitor pulse and respirations every 15 to 30 minutes.
3. Monitor temperature every 2 hours once membranes have ruptured.
4. Monitor fetal heart rate and uterine contractions every 15 minutes in low-risk women and every 5 minutes in high-risk women.
   a. Early decelerations and some fetal bradycardia may occur because of head compression.
   b. There is normally no loss of variability during pushing.
   c. Contractions may become less frequent, but intensity does not decrease.

Providing Supportive Care

1. Explain procedures and equipment during pushing and delivery.
2. Keep the woman/couple informed of status.
3. Provide frequent, positive encouragement. Use of a mirror often allows the woman to see her progress.
4. Assist and instruct the woman in the pushing technique:
   a. Take a full cleansing breath, in through the nose and out through the mouth, at the beginning and end of each contraction.

    b. Push only during contractions.

    c. Push down toward the perineum with the abdominal muscles and try to keep the rest of the body relaxed.

    d. For each push, take a breath and push for 6 to 7 seconds while exhaling slightly.

5. Assist the woman to a comfortable position such as left or right lateral, squatting, or semi-sitting position.

    a. Assist the woman with pulling her legs back so that her knees are flexed.

    b. Teach the woman to put her chin to her chest so that her body forms a "C" shape while pushing.

6. Evaluate bladder fullness and encourage voiding or catheterize as needed.

Promoting a Safe Delivery

1. Prepare the birthing room or delivery room using aseptic technique, allowing ample time for setup before delivery.

2. Prepare the infant resuscitation area for delivery.

3. Prepare necessary items for newborn care.

4. Notify necessary personnel to prepare for delivery.

5. Transfer the primigravida to the delivery room when the fetal head is crowning. The multigravida is taken earlier, depending on fetal size and speed of fetal descent.

6. Place all side rails up before moving. Instruct the woman to keep her hands off the rails, and move from the bed to the delivery table between contractions.

7. Position the woman for delivery, using a large cushion for her head, back, and shoulders. Elevate the head of the bed. Stirrups or footrests may be used for leg or foot support. Pad the stirrups. Place both legs in the stirrups at the same time to avoid ligament strain, backache, or injury.

8. Cleanse the vulva and perineal areas once the woman is positioned for delivery.

    a. Cleanse from the mons to the lower abdomen.

    b. Then cleanse the groin to the inner thigh of each side.

    c. Then cleanse each labium.

    d. Finally, cleanse the introitus.

Assisting With Delivery

(Also see Box 7 for emergency delivery.)

1. When the fetal head is encircled by the vulvovaginal ring, an episiotomy may be performed to prevent tearing.
2. When the head is delivered, mucus is wiped from the face, and the mouth and nose are aspirated with a bulb syringe.
3. If loops of umbilical cord are found around the infant's neck, they are loosened and slipped from around the neck. If the cord cannot be slipped over the head, it is clamped with two clamps and cut between the two clamps.
4. After this step, the woman is asked to give a gentle push so the infant's body may be quickly delivered.
5. After delivery of the infant's body and cutting of the cord, the infant is shown to the parents and then placed on the maternal abdomen, or taken to the radiant warmer for inspection and identification procedures.

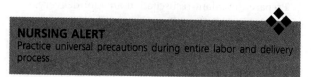

NURSING ALERT
Practice universal precautions during entire labor and delivery process.

◆ Nursing Interventions During Third Stage of Labor

Assisting With Placental Delivery

1. Ask the woman to bear down gently, or fundal pressure may be applied to facilitate delivery of the placenta on signs of separation. These include:
   a. The uterus rises upward in the abdomen.
   b. The umbilical cord lengthens.
   c. Trickle or spurt of blood appears.
   d. The uterus becomes globular in shape.
2. Evaluate the placenta for size, shape, and cord site implantation.
3. Check to see that the placenta and membranes are complete.
4. Evaluate and massage the uterine fundus until firm.

■ BOX 7 EMERGENCY DELIVERY

1. Provide reassurance and instruct the woman in a calm controlled manner while assisting her to a lithotomy position.
2. Wash hands and cleanse woman's perineum.
3. Exert gentle pressure against the head of the fetus to control its progress and prevent too rapid a delivery.
   a. Use a clean or sterile towel.
   b. This prevents undue stretching of the perineum and sudden expulsion through the vulva with subsequent infant and maternal complications.
4. Encourage the woman to pant at this time to prevent bearing down.
5. If membranes have not ruptured by the time the head has been delivered, tear them at the nape of the infant's neck.
6. Wipe the infant's face and mouth with a clean towel. Suction the mouth and nose with a bulb syringe if available.
7. Check to see if the cord is wrapped around the infant's neck or other body part. If the cord is too tight to permit slipping it over the infant's head, it must be clamped in two places and cut between the clamps before the rest of the body is delivered.
8. Hold the infant's head in both hands and gently exert downward pressure toward the floor, thus slipping the anterior shoulder under the symphysis pubis.
9. Support the infant's body and head as it is born.
10. Hold the infant with the head down to help drain mucus; wipe away excess mucus from the mouth and nose; gentle rubbing of the back may stimulate breathing.

continued

■ **BOX 7** *(Continued)*

11. Place the infant on the mother's abdomen, where she can see him or her after the infant cries.
12. Avoid touching the perineal area to prevent infection.
13. Avoid pulling on the cord, which might break and cause hemorrhage.
14. Watch for signs of placental separation
15. Do the following when the placenta is delivered:
    a. Clamp the cord with a cord clamp when the cord stops pulsating. If a clamp is not available, tie off the cord with any suitable material several centimeters from the infant's abdomen.
    b. Wrap the infant and placenta in a blanket; keep the infant warm and close to the mother.
16. Check fundal contractions; massage if indicated. Putting the baby to the breast may help the uterus to contract.
17. Place identification of some kind on the mother and infant.
18. Give the woman fluids.
19. Assist the woman to a suitable environment, if she is not in a bed or a place where she can lie down.
20. Do not leave the woman alone.
21. Teach the woman to massage her fundus; explain why the cord has not been cut.
22. Record the time and date of birth.

■ BOX 8   NEWBORN RESUSCITATION

1. Call for assistance if needed.
2. Place the infant in a warm radiant warmer in Trendelenburg position.
3. Suction the nose and mouth with a bulb syringe or wall suction.
4. Dry off the trunk with warmed towels and attempt to keep the infant warm.
5. Assess respiratory and cardiac status.
6. Begin bag and mask ventilation.
   a. Use an inspiratory pressure of 20–30 cm H_2O cm at a rate of 40–60 breaths/min.
   b. Observe chest movement and ausculate for air movement in all lung fields.
7. Begin external cardiac massage at a rate of 100–120 compressions/min if needed.
8. Assist with endotracheal intubation if needed.
9. Assist with insertion of an umbilical venous line for administration of medications and fluids if needed.
10. Transport when stable.

---

5. Evaluate vaginal bleeding.
6. Administer Pitocin as indicated to assist with maintaining uterine tone.
7. Reassure woman that repair of lacerations of the vagina and cervix are made by the birth attendant.

◆ Immediate Care of the Newborn

Promoting Respiratory Function

1. Wipe mucus from the face and mouth and nose. Aspirate with a bulb syringe. If meconium is present before the delivery, mechanical suctioning of the nasopharynx with an 8 or 10 French catheter will be done by the birth attendant when the head is delivered. See Box 8 for newborn resuscitation.

TABLE 22 Apgar Scoring Chart

Sign	0	1	2
Heart rate	Absent	Slow (less than 100)	Over 100
Respiratory effort	Absent	Slow, irregular	Good, crying
Muscle tone	Flaccid	Some flexion of extremities	Active motion
Reflex irritability	No response	Cry	Vigorous cry
Color	Blue, pale	Body pink, extremities blue	Completely pink

2. Assist with clamping the umbilical cord approximately 2.5 cm (1 inch) from the abdominal wall with a cord clamp (usually done by birth attendant). Count the number of vessels in the cord—fewer than three vessels have been associated with renal and cardiac anomalies.
3. Evaluate the newborn's condition by the Apgar scoring system (Table 22) at 1 and 5 minutes after birth.
   a. Newborns scoring 7 to 10 are free of immediate stress.
   b. Newborns scoring 4 to 6 are moderately depressed.
   c. Newborns scoring 0 to 3 are severely depressed.

Promoting Thermoregulation
1. Dry the newborn immediately after delivery. A wet, small newborn loses up to 200 calories/kg/min in the delivery room through evaporation, convection, and radiation. Drying the infant cuts this heat loss in half.
2. Cover the newborn's head with a cotton stocking cap to prevent heat loss.
3. Wrap the newborn in warm blankets.
4. Place the newborn under a radiant heat warmer, or place the newborn on the mother's abdomen with skin-to-skin contact.
5. Provide a warm, draft-free environment for the newborn.
6. Take the newborn's axillary temperature. A normal

temperature is between 36.4° and 37.2°C (97.5°–99.0°F).

Preventing Infection and Ensuring Safety

1. Administer prophylactic treatment against ophthalmia neonatorum (gonorrheal or chlamydial) by applying silver nitrate drops, or erythromycin or tetracycline antibiotic ophthalmic ointment or drops.
   a. If the mother has a positive gonococcal or chylamydial culture, the newborn will require further treatment.
   b. Treatment is mandatory in all states.
2. Administer injection of vitamin K to prevent neonatal hemorrhage during the first few days of life before the neonate begins to produce its own vitamin K.
3. Place matching identification bracelets on the mother's and the newborn's wrists or ankles.
   a. The father or significant other also may wear a bracelet matching the mother's.
   b. Information includes the mother's name, hospital number, newborn's sex, race, and date and time of birth.
4. Obtain fingerprints of the mother and footprints of the newborn per institution policy. If footprints are to be done, remove all vernix from the foot before inking to improve the quality of the footprint.
5. Complete all identification procedures before the infant leaves the delivery room.
6. Weigh and measure the infant:
   a. Normal newborn weight is 2,700 to 4,000 g (6–9 lbs).
   b. Normal newborn length is 48 to 53 cm (19–21 inches).
7. Administer hepatitis B vaccine—for all infants born in the United States, recommended within 12 hours after birth for the prevention of acute and chronic hepatitis B infection.

◆ Nursing Interventions During Fourth Stage of Labor

Preventing Hemorrhage

1. Monitor blood pressure, pulse, and respirations every 15 minutes for 1 hour, then every $\frac{1}{2}$ hour to 1 hour until stable or transferred to the postpartum unit.

2. Take temperature every 4 hours unless elevated, then every 2 hours.
3. Evaluate uterine fundal tone, height, and position. The uterus should be firm around the level of the umbilicus, at the midline.
4. Evaluate amount of vaginal bleeding:
   a. Scant: only blood on tissue when wiped, or less then 1-inch stain on peripad within 1 hour
   b. Small/light: less than 4-inch stain on peripad within 1 hour
   c. Moderate: less than 6-inch stain on peripad within 1 hour
   d. Heavy: saturated peripad within 1 hour
5. Observe perineum for edema, discoloration, bleeding, or hematoma formation.
6. Check episiotomy for intactness and bleeding.

Providing Supportive Care

1. Maintain intravenous fluids as indicated.
2. Provide oral fluids and a snack or meal as tolerated.
3. Apply a covered ice pack to the perineum for an episiotomy, perineal laceration, or edema.
4. Administer analgesics as indicated.
5. Assist the woman with a partial bath and perineal care, and change linens and pads as necessary.
6. Allow for privacy and rest periods between postpartum checks.
7. Provide warm blankets and reassure the woman that tremors are common during this period.
8. Encourage voiding and evaluate the bladder for distension. Provide privacy, the sound of running water, and the flow of water against the perineum, if necessary to facilitate voiding.
9. Catheterize the woman (in and out) if the bladder is full and she is unable to void.
   a. Birth trauma, anesthesia, and pain from lacerations and episiotomy may reduce or alter the voiding reflex.
   b. Bladder distension may displace the uterus upward and to the side, resulting in improper contraction and risk of hemorrhage.
10. Evaluate mobility and sensation of the lower extremities if regional anesthesia was given.

a. Remain with the woman and assist her out of bed for the first time. Evaluate her ability to support her weight and ambulate at this time.
b. Do not provide hot fluids if sensation is decreased.

Promoting Parenting

1. Show the newborn to the mother and father or support person immediately after birth when possible.
2. Encourage the mother or father to hold the baby as soon as possible.
3. Teach the mother/parents to hold the newborn close to their faces, approximately 8 to 12 inches when talking to the baby.
4. Have the mother/parents look at and inspect the baby's body to familiarize themselves with their child.
5. Assist the mother with breast-feeding during the first 2 hours after birth. This is often a period of quiet alert time for the newborn, and he or she will often readily take to the breast.
6. Provide quiet alone time in a low-lit room for the family to become acquainted.
7. Observe and record the reaction of the mother/parents to the newborn.

Postpartum and Newborn Care

◆ Physiologic Changes of the Puerperium

The *puerperium* is the period beginning after delivery and ending when the woman's body has returned as closely as possible to its prepregnant state; lasts approximately 6 weeks.

Uterine Changes

1. The fundus is usually midline and approximately at the level of the woman's umbilicus after delivery. Within 12 hours of delivery, the fundus may be 1 cm above the umbilicus. After this, the level of the fundus descends approximately 1 fingerbreadth (or 1 cm) each day until, by the 10th day, it has descended into the pelvic cavity and can no longer be palpated.

2. A vaginal discharge known as lochia, consisting of fatty epithelial cells, shreds of membrane, decidua, and blood, is red (*lochia rubra*) for approximately 2 to 3 days after delivery. It then progresses to a paler or more brownish color (*lochia serosa*), followed by a whitish or yellowish color (*lochia alba*) in the 7th to 10th day. Lochia usually ceases by 3 weeks, and the placental site is completely healed by the 6th week.

3. The vaginal walls, uterine ligaments, and muscles of the pelvic floor and abdominal wall regain most of their tone during the puerperium.

Breast Changes

1. With loss of the placenta, circulating levels of estrogen and progesterone decrease and levels of prolactin increase, thus initiating lactation in the postpartum woman.

2. *Colostrum*, a yellowish fluid containing more minerals and protein but less sugar and fat than mature breast milk and having a laxative effect on the infant, is secreted for the first 2 days postpartum.

3. Mature milk secretion is usually present by the third postpartum day but may be present earlier if a woman breast-feeds immediately after delivery.

4. Breast engorgement with milk, venous and lymphatic stasis, and swollen, tense, and tender breast tissue may occur between days 3 and 5 postpartum.

Changes in Blood Volume

1. Postpartum diuresis occurs between the second and fifth postpartum days, as extracellular water accumulated during pregnancy begins to be excreted.

2. A diuresis may also occur shortly after delivery if urinary output was obstructed because of the pressure of the presenting part or if IV fluids were given to the woman during labor.

Emotional and Behavioral Changes

1. After delivery, the woman may progress through Rubin's stages of "taking in" and "taking hold."

   a. "Taking in" may begin with a refreshing sleep after delivery. The woman exhibits passive, dependent behavior and is concerned with sleep and the intake of food, both for herself and for the infant.

b. With "taking hold," the woman begins to initiate action and to function more independently.

2. Some women may experience a euphoria in the first few days after delivery and set unrealistic goals for activities after discharge from the birthing place.

3. Many women may experience temporary mood swings during this period because of the discomfort, fatigue, and exhaustion after labor and delivery and because of hormonal changes after delivery.

4. Some mothers may experience "postpartum blues" about the third postpartum day and exhibit irritability, poor appetite, insomnia, tearfulness, or crying. This is a temporary situation. Severe or prolonged depression is usually a sign of a more serious condition.

5. Nursing research findings indicate that new mothers identified the following postpartum needs: Coping with
   a. The physical changes and discomforts of the puerperium, including a need to regain their pre-pregnancy figure
   b. Changing family relationships and meeting the needs of family members, including the infant
   c. Fatigue, emotional stress, feelings of isolation, and being "tied down"
   d. A lack of time for personal needs and interests

◆ Postpartum Nursing Interventions

Performing Postpartum Assessment

1. Check firmness of the fundus at regular intervals.

NURSING ALERT
The first hour after delivery of the placenta is a critical period; postpartum hemorrhage is most likely to occur at this time.

2. Inspect the perineum regularly for frank bleeding.
   a. Note color, amount, and odor of the lochia.
   b. Count the number of perineal pads that are saturated in each 8-hour period.

3. Assess vital signs at least every 4 hours for first 24 hours, then every 8 to 12 hours, as indicated.

a. Decreased respiratory rate below 14 to 16 breaths/min may occur after receiving epidural narcotics or narcotic analgesics.

b. Increased respiratory rate greater than 24 breaths/min may be attributable to increased blood loss, pulmonary edema, or a pulmonary embolus.

c. Increased pulse rate greater than 100 beats/min may be present with increased blood loss, fever, or pain.

d. Decrease in blood pressure 15 to 20 mm Hg below baseline pressures may indicate decreased fluid volume or increased blood loss.

4. Assess for bowel and bladder elimination.

5. Evaluate interaction and care skills of mother and family with infant.

6. Assess for breast engorgement and condition of nipples if breast-feeding.

7. Inspect legs for signs of thromboembolism, and assess for calf tenderness.

8. Assess incisions for signs of infection and healing.

9. If a patient is Rh negative, evaluate the need for Rho (D) immune globulin (RhoGAM). If indicated, administer the RhoGAM within 72 hours of delivery.

10. If the woman is not rubella immune, a rubella vaccination may be given, and pregnancy must be avoided for at least 3 months.

Preventing Hypotension

1. Evaluate for orthostatic blood pressure changes, and have the woman lie in bed if symptoms exist.

2. Evaluate lower extremity sensory and motor function before ambulation if the woman had regional anesthesia.

3. Encourage food and drink as tolerated.

4. Maintain IV line as indicated.

5. Monitor hemoglobin and hematocrit as indicated.

Encouraging Bladder Emptying

1. Palpate the abdomen for bladder distension if the woman is unable to void within 6 to 8 hours after delivery or complains of fullness after voiding.

a. Uterine displacement from the midline suggests bladder distension

b. Frequent voidings of small amounts of urine suggest urinary retention with overflow.

2. Catheterize the woman (in and out) if indicated.

3. Instruct the woman to void every several hours and after meals to keep her bladder empty. An undistended bladder may help decrease uterine cramping.

Promoting Bowel Function

1. Teach the woman that bowel activity is sluggish because of decreased abdominal muscle tone, anesthetic effects, effects of progesterone, decreased solid food intake during labor, and prelabor diarrhea. In addition, pain from hemorrhoids, lacerations, and episiotomies may cause her to delay her first bowel movement.

2. Review dietary intake and encourage daily adequate amounts of fresh fruit, vegetables, fiber, and at least 8 glasses of water.

3. Encourage frequent ambulation.

4. Administer stool softeners as indicated.

Reducing Fatigue

1. Provide a quiet and minimally disturbed environment.

2. Organize nursing care to keep interruptions to a minimum.

3. Encourage the woman to minimize visitors and phone calls.

4. Encourage the woman to sleep while the baby is sleeping.

Minimizing Pain

1. Instruct the woman to apply ice packs intermittently to the perineal area for the first 24 hours for perineal trauma or edema.

2. Initiate the use of sitz baths three times a day for 15 to 20 minutes for perineal discomfort after the first 24 hours.

3. Instruct the woman to contract her buttocks before sitting and to use pillows to reduce perineal discomfort.

4. Teach the woman to use a peri-bottle and squirt warm water against her perineum while voiding.

5. Provide pads such as witch hazel or topical anesthetic creams or ointments for perineum as indicated.

6. Administer pain medication as indicated.

7. If breasts are engorged and the woman is breast-feeding:
   a. Allow warm to hot shower water to flow over the breasts to improve comfort.
   b. Hot compresses on the breasts may improve comfort.
   c. Express some milk manually or by breast pump to improve comfort and make nipple more available for infant feeding.
   d. Nurse the infant.
8. If breasts are engorged and the mother is bottle-feeding:
   a. Wear a supportive bra night and day.
   b. Avoid handling the breasts because this stimulates more milk production.
   c. Suggest ice bags to the breasts to provide comfort.

Promoting Breast-Feeding

1. Have the mother wash her hands before feeding to help prevent infection.
2. Encourage the mother to assume a comfortable position such as sitting upright, tailor sitting, or lying on her side.
3. Have the woman hold the baby so that he or she is facing the mother. Common positions for holding the baby are the "cradle hold," with the baby's head and body supported against the mother's arm with buttocks resting in her hand; the "football hold" supports the baby's legs under the mother's arm while his or her head is at the breast resting in her hand; lying on the side with the baby lying on his or her side facing the mother.
4. Have the woman cup the breast in her hand in a "C" position with bottom of the breast in the palm of her hand and the thumb on top.
5. Have the woman place her nipple against the baby's mouth, and when the mouth opens guide the nipple and the areola into the mouth.
6. If the baby has "latched on" only to the nipple, have the mother take him/her off the breast by putting the tip of her finger in the corner of the baby's mouth to break the suction and then reposition on the breast to prevent nipple pain and trauma.

7. Encourage the woman to alternate the breast she begins feeding with at each feeding to ensure emptying of both breasts and stimulation for maintaining milk supply.

8. Advise the mother to use each breast at each feeding. Begin with about 5 minutes at each breast, then increase the time at each breast, allowing the infant to suck until he or she stops sucking actively.

9. Have the mother breast-feed frequently and on a demand schedule (every 2–4 hours) to help maintain the milk supply.

10. Have the mother air dry her nipples for approximately 15 to 20 minutes after feeding to help prevent nipple trauma.

11. Have the mother burp the infant at the end or midway through the feeding to help release air in the stomach.

12. Alert the mother that uterine cramping may occur, especially in multiparous women because of the release of oxytocin.

13. Teach the mother to provide for adequate rest and to avoid tension, fatigue, and a stressful environment, which can inhibit the letdown reflex and make breast milk less available at feeding.

14. Advise the woman to avoid taking medications and drugs, because many substances pass into the breast milk and may affect milk production or the infant.

Promoting Healing

1. Teach the woman to carry out perineal care—warm water over the perineum after each voiding, bowel movement, and routinely several times a day—to promote comfort, cleanliness, and healing.

2. Teach the woman to apply perineal pads by touching the outside only, thus keeping clean the portion that will touch her perineum.

3. Advise the woman that healing occurs within 4 weeks; however, evaluation by the health care provider 4 to 6 weeks postpartum is necessary.

4. Inform the woman that intercourse may be resumed when perineal and uterine wounds have healed. Review methods of contraception.

5. Inform the woman that menstruation usually returns

within 4 to 8 weeks if bottle-feeding; if breast-feeding, menstruation usually returns within 4 months, but may return between 2 and 18 months postpartum. Nursing mothers may ovulate even if experiencing amenorrhea, so a form of contraception should be used if pregnancy is to be avoided.

6. Counsel the woman to rest for at least 30 minutes after she arrives home from the hospital and to rest several times during the day for the first few weeks.

7. Advise the woman to confine her activities to one floor if possible and avoid stair climbing as much as possible for the first several days at home.

8. Counsel the woman to provide quiet times for herself at home and help her establish realistic goals for resuming her own interests and activities.

9. Encourage the couple to provide times to reestablish their own relationship and to renew their social interests and relationships.

Teaching Postpartum Exercises

1. Instruct the woman in exercises for the immediate postpartum period (can be performed in bed).

   a. Toe stretch (tightens calf muscles): While lying on back, keep legs straight and point toes away from body, then pull legs toward body and point toes toward chest. Repeat 10 times.

   b. Pelvic floor exercise (tightens perineal muscles): Contract buttocks for a count of 5 and relax. Contract buttocks and press thighs together for a count of 7 and relax. Contract buttocks, press thighs together, and draw in anus for a count of 10 and relax.

2. Teach exercises for the later postpartum period (after the first postpartum visit).

   a. Bicycle (tightens thighs, stomach, waist): lie on back on the floor, arms at sides, palms down. Begin rotating legs as if riding a bicycle, bringing the knees all the way in toward the chest and stretching the legs out as long and straight as possible. Breathe deeply and evenly. Do the exercises at a moderate speed and do not tire yourself.

   b. Buttocks exercise (tightens buttocks): lie on abdomen and keep legs straight. Raise left leg in the air, then repeat with right leg to feel the contraction in buttocks. Keep hips on the floor. Repeat 10 times.

c. Twist (tightens waist): stand with legs wide apart. Hold arms at sides, shoulder level, palms down. Twist body from side to front and back again to feel the twist in waist.

◆ Physiologic Changes in the Newborn

The first 24 hours of life constitute a highly vulnerable time during which the infant must make major physiologic adjustments to extrauterine life.

Respiratory Changes

1. The infant begins life with intense activity; diffuse, purposeless movements alternate with periods of relative immobility.
2. Respirations are rapid, as frequent as 80 breaths/min, accompanied by tachycardia, 140 to 180 beats/min.
3. Relaxation occurs and the infant usually sleeps, then awakes to a second period of activity. Oral mucus may be a major problem during this period.
4. Respirations are reduced to 35 to 50 breaths/min and become quiet and shallow; respiration is carried out by the diaphragm and abdominal muscles.
5. Period of dyspnea and cyanosis may occur suddenly in an infant who is breathing normally; this may indicate an anomaly or a pathologic condition.
6. Apnea is normal in the neonatal period and lasts 10 to 15 seconds.

Circulatory Changes

1. Blood volume is 85 to 100 mL/kg at birth; influenced by maternal blood volume, blood loss, and if cord is clamped and cut after pulsation ceases (increases blood volume)
2. Residual cyanosis in hands and feet for 1 to 2 hours after birth because of sluggish circulation.
3. Pulse rate may fluctuate with respiration; normal rate, 120 to 150 beats/min; may increase to 180 beats/min when the infant is crying or drop to 70 beats/min during deep sleep
4. Blood pressure averages 70/45 at birth, 100/50 by 10th day; rises with crying

5. Blood coagulability is temporarily diminished because of lack of bacteria in the intestinal tract that contributes to the synthesis of vitamin K.
6. Values for blood components in the neonate:
   a. Hemoglobin: 16 to 22 g
   b. Reticulocytes: 2.5% to 6.5%
   c. Leukocytes: 15,000 to −20,000 mm^3.

Temperature Regulation

1. Heat loss of 2° to 3°C may occur at birth by evaporation, convection, conduction, and radiation.
2. Infant develops mechanisms to counterbalance heat loss.
   a. Vasoconstriction: blood directed away from skin surfaces
   b. Insulation: from subcutaneous adipose tissue
   c. Heat production: by nonshivering thermogenesis elicited by the sympathetic nervous system's response to decreased temperatures; activated by adrenalin
   d. Fetal position: by assuming a flexed position

Basal Metabolism

1. Surface area of infant is large in comparison with weight.
2. Basal metabolism per kilogram of body weight is higher than that of adult.
3. Calorie requirements are high—117 calories/kg body weight/day

Renal Function

1. Decreased ability to concentrate urine because of low tubular reabsorption rate and low levels of antidiuretic hormone
2. Limited ability to maintain water balance by excretion of excess water or retention of needed water
3. Decreased ability to maintain acid–base mechanism; slower excretion of electrolytes, especially sodium and the hydrogen ions, results in accumulation of these substances, which predisposes the infant to dehydration, acidosis, and hyperkalemia.
4. Excretion of large amount of uric acid during newborn period—appears as "brick dust" stain on diaper.

Hepatic Function

1. Decreased ability to conjugate bilirubin—causes physiologic jaundice
2. Decreased ability to regulate blood sugar concentration—causes neonatal hypoglycemia
3. Deficient production of prothrombin and other coagulation factors that depend on vitamin K for synthesis

Gastrointestinal Changes

1. Most digestive enzymes are present, with the exception of pancreatic amylase and lipase. Protein and carbohydrates are easily absorbed, but fat absorption is poor.
2. Imperfect control of the cardiac and pyloric sphincters and immaturity of neurologic control cause mild regurgitation or slight vomiting.
3. Irregularities in peristaltic motility slow stomach emptying.
4. Peristalsis increases in the lower ileum, resulting in stool frequency—one to six stools per day. Absence of stool within 48 hours after birth is indicative of intestinal obstruction.

Neurologic Changes

Reflexes are important indices of infant neural development. Absence of newborn reflexes or persistence of some reflexes beyond several months indicates neurologic immaturity or damage.

1. Rooting: when corner of mouth is touched, turns mouth toward object and opens mouth
2. Palmar grasp: pressure on palm elicits grasp (pressure on sole also elicits plantar flexion)
3. Tonic neck: when head is turned to one side with leg and arm on that side extended, the extremities on other side flex
4. Neck righting: when head turned to one side, the shoulder, trunk, and then pelvis turn to that side
5. Moro: sudden loud noise causes body to stiffen and arms to go up, out, and then inward with thumbs and index fingers in C shape
6. Babinski: scratching sole of foot causes great toe to flex and toes to fan

7. Blink: eyes close and neck flexes when sudden light is shone (eyes also close when sudden loud noise occurs)
8. Withdrawal: pricking sole of foot causes flexion at hip, knee, and ankle
9. Parachute: if held prone and quickly lowered toward a surface, arms and legs will extend

◆ Nursing Interventions for the Newborn

Performing Newborn Physical Assessment

1. Assess posture: Asymmetric posture may be caused by fractures of clavicle or humerus or by nerve injuries, commonly of the brachial plexus. Infants born in breech position may keep knees and legs straightened or in frog position, depending on the type of breech birth.
2. Assess length: ranges from 46 to 56 cm (18–22 inches).
3. Weigh newborn: average weight of male is 3,400 g ($7\frac{1}{2}$ lb); female, 3,200 g (7 lb); 80% of full-term newborns will range from 2,900 to 4,100 g (6 lbs 5 oz to 9 lbs 2 oz).
4. Assess skin for hair distribution, turgor, and color.
   a. Term infant will have some lanugo over back; most of the lanugo will have disappeared on extremities and other areas of the body.
   b. *Acrocyanosis*, bluish color in hands and feet, is common because of immature peripheral circulation.
   c. Pallor: may indicate cold, stress, anemia, or cardiac failure
   d. Plethora: reddish coloration may be caused by excessive red blood cells from intrauterine intravascular transfusion (twins), cardiac disease, or diabetes in the mother.
   e. Jaundice: physiologic jaundice caused by immaturity of liver is common beginning on day 2, peaking at 1 week, and disappearing by the 2nd week.
   f. Meconium staining: staining of skin, fingernails, and umbilical cord indicates compromise in utero unless infant was in breech position.
   g. Harlequin color change: when lying on side, dependent half of body turns red, upper half pale; caused by gravity and vasomotor instability

h. Dryness/peeling: marked scaliness and desquamation are a sign of postmaturity.

i. Vernix: in full-term infants, most vernix is found in skin folds under the arms and in the groin

5. Assess for skin lesions.

a. Ecchymoses: may appear over the presenting part in a difficult delivery; may also indicate infection or bleeding problem

b. Petechiae: pinpoint hemorrhages on skin caused by increased intravascular pressure, infection, or thrombocytopenia; regresses within 24 to 48 hours.

c. Erythema toxicum ("newborn rash"): pink to red papular rash appearing on trunk and diaper areas; regresses within 24 to 48 hours

d. Hemangiomas: vascular lesions present at birth; some may fade, but others may be permanent

e. Telangiectatic nevi (stork bites): flat red or purple lesions most often found on back of neck, lower occiput, upper eyelid, and bridge of nose; regress by 2 years of age

f. Milia: enlarged sebaceous glands found on nose, chin, cheeks, and forehead; regress in several days to a week or two.

g. Mongolian spots: blue pigmentation on lower back, sacrum, and buttocks; common in African Americans, Asians, and infants of Southern European heritage; regress by 4 years of age.

h. Cafe-au-lait spots: brown macules, usually not significant; large numbers may indicate underlying neurofibromatosis

i. Abrasions or lacerations can result from internal monitoring and instruments used at birth.

6. Examine head and face for symmetry, paralysis, shape, swelling, movement.

a. *Caput succedaneum*: swelling of soft tissues of the scalp because of pressure; swelling crosses suture lines.

b. *Cephalohematoma:* subperiosteal hemorrhage with collection of blood between periosteum and bone; swelling does not cross suture lines.

c. *Molding:* overlapping of skull bones caused by

compression during labor and delivery (disappears in a few days)

7. Measure head circumference: 33 to 35 cm. (13–14 inches), approximately 2 cm (1 inch) larger than chest. Measure just above the eyebrows and over the occiput.

8. Palpate fontanelles: enlarged or bulging may indicate increased intracranial pressure; sunken often indicates dehydration; posterior fontanelle closes in 2 to 3 months; anterior closes in 12 to 18 months.

9. Palpate sutures (junctions of adjoining skull bones): may be overriding because of molding during labor and delivery; extensive separation may be found in malnourished infants and with increased intracranial pressure.

10. Examine eyes, ears, nose, and mouth for deformity, asymmetry, or any unusual discharge.

11. Examine neck for mobility, any abnormal positioning, and tone.

12. Assess chest circumference and symmetry: average circumference is 30 to 33 cm (12–13 inches), approximately 2 cm smaller than head circumference.

13. Observe breasts for engorgement: may occur at day 3 because of withdrawal of maternal hormones, especially estrogen; no treatment required—regresses in 2 weeks

14. Assess respiratory rate, rhythm, and effort (diaphragmatic because of weak thoracic muscles), and auscultate breath sounds (mostly bronchial).

15. Assess heart rate and rhythm and auscultate heart sounds for gallop (third and fourth sounds rarely heard) and murmurs (common, and most are transitory).

16. Palpate for presence of brachial, radial, pedal, and femoral pulses; lack of femoral pulses indicative of inadequate aortic blood flow.

17. Check blood pressure: newborns weighing more than 3 kg have systolic blood pressure between 60 and 80 mm Hg; diastolic, between 35 and 55 mm Hg.

18. Assess for edema: some may be present over buttocks, back, and occiput if infant is supine; pitting edema may be due to erythroblastosis, heart failure, or electrolyte imbalance.

19. Examine abdomen for umbilical hernia or distension caused by bowel obstruction, organ enlargement, or infection. Bowel sounds are usually present an hour after delivery.
20. Examine umbilical cord: single artery associated with renal and other congenital abnormalities; redness and discharge indicate infection. By 24 hours becomes yellowish brown; dries and falls off in approximately 7 to 10 days.
21. Inspect genitalia for any abnormalities.
    a. White or pink vaginal discharge may be present because of the drop in maternal hormones; no treatment necessary.
    b. Edema may be present in scrotal sac if the infant was born in breech presentation; a frank collection of fluid in the scrotal sac is a *hydrocele*, which regresses in approximately 1 month.
22. Examine spinal column for normal curvature, closure, and presence of membranous sac, pilonidal dimple, or sinus.
23. Examine anal area for anal opening, response of anal sphincter, fissures.
24. Examine extremities for fractures, paralysis, range of motion, irregular position; count fingers and toes.
25. Examine hips for dislocation: With the infant in supine position, flex knees and abduct hips to side and down to table surface; clicking sound indicates dislocation.
26. Assess newborn reflexes (see above).

Performing Newborn Behavioral Assessment

1. Assess responses according to states of consciousness, which include quiet, deep sleep, light, active sleep, drowsy awake, quiet alert, active alert, and crying.
2. Assess sleeping patterns, which normally change with maturation of the central nervous system (CNS). Newborns usually sleep 20 hours per day.
3. Assess feeding pattern: most newborns eat six to eight times per day, with 2 to 4 hours between feedings, and establish fairly regular feeding patterns in approximately 2 weeks.
4. Assess stools
    a. Meconium (tarry, green-black stool) is usually passed in 24 hours and continues for 48 hours.

b. Transitional stools (combination of meconium and yellow stools) are passed next.

c. Milk stools (yellow) are passed by day 5.

d. Newborn has up to six stools per day in the first weeks after birth.

5. Assess voiding: voids within first 24 hours; after first few days, voids 10 to 15 times a day.

Performing Metabolic Screening Tests

Obtain blood sample as directed for the following tests:

1. *Phenylketonuria (PKU)*: inability of the infant to metabolize phenylalanine; scheduled after 48 hours of protein feeding.

2. *Galactosemia:* inborn error of carbohydrate metabolism, when galactose and lactose cannot be converted to glucose

3. *Hypothyroidism:* thyroid hormone deficiency

4. *Maple sugar urine disease* (MSUD): inability to metabolize leucine, isoleucine, and valine

5. *Homocystinuria:* inborn error of sulfur amino acid metabolism

6. *Sickle cell anemia:* abnormally shaped red blood cells with lower oxygen solubility

Bathing the Newborn

1. Ensure bathwater is 37° to 38°C (98°–100°F) and use neutral soap or plain water (if skin is dry).

2. Use cotton balls or soft disposable washcloths to wipe eyes (from inside corner outward), face, and outer ears.

3. Wash head using circular motions; tilt head back to expose skin folds to cleanse neck.

4. Bathe torso and extremities quickly to prevent unnecessary exposure and chilling.

5. Cleanse genital area of male. Retract foreskin gently to cleanse underneath, and replace quickly to prevent edema.

6. Cleanse genital area of female. Gently separate folds of the labia and remove secretions. Wipe vaginal area with cotton ball, using 1 stroke form front to back.

7. Bathe buttocks using a gentle, patting motion. Keep anal area clean and dry to prevent diaper rash. If rash does occur, apply protective ointment such as zinc oxide or A&D, or expose buttocks to air or heat lamp.

8. Teach family the bathing procedure.

Providing Umbilical Care

1. Inspect the umbilical cord stump for bleeding or foul odor, which may indicate infection.
2. Apply a drying agent such as 70% alcohol or Merthiolate to cord stump where it exits abdominal wall, using gauze or cotton swabs, three to four times a day.
3. Leave open to air; do not cover with diaper or use a dressing.
4. Teach care to family, and tell them to expect stump to dry up and fall off within 7 to 10 days.

Providing Circumcision Care

1. Place sterile petroleum gauze over area for 24 hours; change after voiding.
2. Observe hourly for bleeding for first 24 hours. If bleeds, apply gentle pressure or apply epinephrine solution as directed.
3. Position infant and diaper to prevent friction, which may cause bleeding and discomfort.
4. Teach circumcision care to family.

Feeding the Newborn

1. Give first feeding of sterile water to prevent injury to lungs if aspirated.
2. Initiate breast-feeding (see p. 938) or instruct family in bottle-feeding technique:
   a. Hold baby in semi-upright position.
   b. Position bottle so the neck of bottle is filled.
   c. Insert nipple into baby's mouth so that baby's tongue is under nipple.
   d. Bubble baby during feeding while holding upright to expel air but not feeding.
3. Test blood for glucose, using glucometer to identify hypoglycemia and need for frequent feedings.
4. Suggest feeding on demand schedule until more regular feeding schedule is established.

Ensuring Infant Safety

1. Instruct the family to contact the infant's health care provider for the following:
   a. Fever greater than 37.2°C (100°F)
   b. Loss of appetite for two consecutive feedings
   c. Inability to awaken baby to his or her usual activity state

   d. Vomiting all or part of two feedings
   e. Diarrhea: three watery stools
   f. Extreme irritability or inconsolable crying
2. Inform the family that by law infants and young children in cars are required to be in a car safety seat. Demonstrate and review the proper technique for use of the car seat.
3. Provide written instructions and educational material on infant care.
4. Provide reinforcement and reassurance to the family and ensure that they know who to call with concerns.

◆ COMPLICATIONS OF THE CHILDBEARING EXPERIENCE

Abortion, Spontaneous

Spontaneous abortion is the unintended termination of pregnancy at any time before the fetus has attained viability (20 weeks' gestation or fetal weight of 500 g [1.1 lb]). Cause is frequently unknown, but 50% are attributable to chromosomal anomalies. May also be related to exposure to or contact with teratogenic agents; poor maternal nutritional status; maternal viral or bacterial illness; chronic illness such as diabetes and systemic lupus erythematosus; smoking or drug abuse; immunologic factors; postmature or imperfect sperm or ova; and structural defect in the maternal reproductive system. Complications include hemorrhage, uterine infection, septicemia, and disseminated intravascular coagulation (with missed abortion). See Box 9 for information on therapeutic or voluntary abortion.

◆ Assessment

1. Uterine cramping, low back pain
2. Vaginal bleeding usually begins as dark spotting, then progresses to frank bleeding as the embryo separates from the uterus.

■ BOX 9   THERAPEUTIC OR VOLUNTARY ABORTION

Therapeutic abortion is the termination of pregnancy before fetal viability for the purpose of safeguarding the woman's health. Voluntary abortion is the termination of pregnancy before fetal viability as a choice of the woman. First-trimester abortions are accomplished by D&C or dilation and suction. Second-trimester abortions can be managed using prostaglandin E_2 vaginal suppositories or by IM injection of prostaglandin F_2 analogues. Late second-trimester abortions can be done using intraamniotic saline injection, hysterotomy, or hysterectomy. Complications include retained products of conception, which leads to disseminated intravascular coagulation and sepsis; hemorrhage; prostaglandin complications, including fever, diarrhea, nausea and vomiting, tachycardia, and bronchoconstriction; and surgical complications, including uterine perforation, bowel trauma, and cervical laceration.

---

3. Serum beta-human chorionic gonadotropin (hCG) levels may be elevated for as long as 2 weeks after loss of the embryo.

◆ Diagnostic Evaluation

1. Ultrasonic evaluation of the gestational sac or embryo
2. Visualization of the cervix shows dilation or tissue passing through cervical os

◆ Collaborative Management

Therapeutic Interventions

1. For threatened abortion, bed rest or limited activity may be advised and bleeding monitored.

Pharmacologic Interventions

1. For missed abortion (fetal death without passage of fetal tissue), oxytocin infusion to induce delivery
2. RhoGAM injection may be necessary for maternal and paternal Rh incompatibility.

Surgical Interventions

1. For inevitable or incomplete abortion, dilation and curettage (D&C) with evacuation is performed.
2. For history of habitual abortions (spontaneous abortions with three or more consecutive pregnancies), workup to determine cause and possible suturing of cervix if incompetent cervix is a factor

◆ Nursing Interventions

Monitoring

1. Monitor amount and color of vaginal bleeding.
2. Monitor maternal vital signs for indications of complications such as hemorrhage and infection.
3. Evaluate any blood or clot tissue for the presence of fetal membranes, placenta, or fetus.

Supportive Care

1. Report any tachycardia, hypotension, diaphoresis, or pallor, indicating hemorrhage and shock.
2. Draw blood for type and screen for possible blood administration.
3. Establish and maintain an IV with large-bore catheter for possible transfusion and large quantities of fluid replacement, if signs of shock are present.
4. Encourage the patient to discuss feelings about the loss of the baby; include effects on relationship with the father.
5. Do not minimize the loss by focusing on future child bearing; rather acknowledge the loss and allow grieving.
6. Provide time alone for the couple to discuss their feelings.
7. Discuss the prognosis of future pregnancies with the couple.
8. If the fetus is aborted intact, provide an opportunity for viewing, if parents desire.

Patient Education and Health Maintenance

1. Instruct on perineal care to prevent infection.
2. Discuss with the couple the methods of contraception to be used.
3. Explain the need to wait at least 3 to 6 months before attempting another pregnancy.
4. Teach the woman to observe for signs of infection (fever, pelvic pain, change in character and amount of vaginal discharge), and advise to report them to provider immediately.
5. Provide information regarding genetic testing of the products of conception if indicated; send the specimen according to policy.

Cesarean Delivery

Cesarean delivery is the surgical removal of the infant from the uterus through an incision made in the abdominal wall and an incision made in the uterus. Size and location of incisions vary, but abdominal and uterine incisions of choice are low and horizontal. Vertical incisions may be necessary for quicker procedures, the presence of adhesions, and other complications. Indications for cesarean delivery include cephalopelvic disproportion; uterine dysfunction, inertia, and inability of cervix to dilate; neoplasm obstructing birth canal or pelvis; malposition and malpresentation; previous uterine surgery (cesarean delivery, myomectomy, hysterotomy) or cervical surgery—evaluated on an individual basis; complete or partial placenta previa; premature separation of the placenta; prolapse of the umbilical cord; fetal distress; active herpes outbreak; breech presentation; and need for cesarean hysterectomy. Indications for cesarean hysterectomy are ruptured uterus; intrauterine infection; hemorrhage due to uterine atony that does not respond to oxytocin, prostaglandin, or massage; laceration of major uterine vessel; severe dysplasia or carcinoma in situ of the cervix; placenta accreta; and gross multiple fibromyomas.

◆ Potential Complications

1. Increase in morbidity and mortality as compared with vaginal birth

2. Hemorrhage, endometritis
3. Paralytic ileus, intestinal obstruction
4. Pulmonary embolism, thrombophlebitis
5. Increased chance of prematurity
6. Respiratory depression of the infant from anesthetic drugs
7. Possible delay in maternal–infant bonding

◆ Collaborative Management

Preoperative Care

1. Maintain NPO status (except possibly ice chips) and monitor maternal and fetal vital signs during labor.
2. Obtain blood sample for type and screen and possible crossmatch if needed; also obtain sample for baseline CBC.
3. Determine drug allergies and answer questions about anesthesia; option for regional or general, depends on the indication for surgery.
4. Establish a large-bore IV and insert a Foley catheter.
5. Administer an antacid, as directed, to reduce gastric acidity and the risk of aspiration pneumonia.
6. Administer antibiotics prophylactically, as directed.
7. Assist with abdominal skin preparation and ensure that a grounding pad for electrocautery is applied to patient.
8. Encourage presence of support person through the delivery.
9. Explain that a sensation of pressure will be felt during the delivery, but that little pain will occur. Instruct that any pain should be reported.

Postoperative Care

1. Assess maternal vital signs and fundal firmness and position every 15 minutes the first hour, every 30 minutes the second hour, and hourly until she is transferred to the postpartum unit or per facility protocol.
2. Assess type and amount of lochia and condition of the incision line or dressing.
3. Monitor urinary output and presence of bowel sounds.
4. Assess level and presence of anesthesia or pain, and medicate as indicated.
   a. Encourage use of relaxation techniques after medication has been given for pain.

b. Monitor for respiratory depression up to 24 hours after epidural narcotic administration.

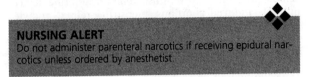

NURSING ALERT
Do not administer parenteral narcotics if receiving epidural narcotics unless ordered by anesthetist.

5. Encourage support and splinting of the abdominal incision when moving or coughing and deep breathing.
6. Encourage frequent rest periods, and plan for them after activities.
7. Encourage ambulation to reduce pain caused by gas, and decrease chance of thrombophlebitis.
8. Provide aseptic dressing changes and encourage perineal care every 4 hours or as needed.
9. Encourage infant bonding as soon as possible and, when talking of the birth, refer to it as a cesarean birth, to imply it is just another method of birth, not a surgical experience.

◆ Family Education and Health Maintenance

1. Teach the woman the "football hold" for breast-feeding so that the infant is not lying on her abdomen.
2. Teach the woman to observe for signs of infection—foul-smelling lochia, elevated temperature, increased pain, redness and edema at the incision site—and to report them immediately.
3. Assist family in planning for the assistance of friends, family, or hired help at home during the period immediately after discharge.

Ectopic Pregnancy

Ectopic pregnancy is any gestation located outside the uterine cavity. The fertilized ovum implants outside of the uterus, usually in the fallopian tube. Predisposing factors include adhesions of the tube, salpingitis, congenital and developmental anomalies of the fallopian tube, previous ectopic pregnancy, current use of an intrauterine device, multiple induced abortions, menstrual reflux, and decreased tubal motility.

◆ Clinical Manifestations

1. Abdominal or pelvic pain
2. Amenorrhea: in 75% of the cases
3. Vaginal bleeding: usually scanty and dark
4. Uterine size is usually similar to what it would be in a normally implanted pregnancy.
5. Abdominal tenderness on palpation
6. Nausea, vomiting, or faintness may be present.
7. Pelvic examination shows a pelvic mass, posterior or lateral to the uterus, and cervical pain on movement of the cervix.

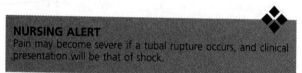

NURSING ALERT
Pain may become severe if a tubal rupture occurs, and clinical presentation will be that of shock.

◆ Diagnostic Evaluation

1. Serum beta human chorionic gonadotropin (β-hCG), when done serially, will not show characteristic increase as in intrauterine pregnancy
2. Ultrasound: may identify tubal mass, absence of gestational sac within the uterus
3. Culdocentesis: bloody aspirate from the cul-de-sac of Douglas indicates intraperitoneal bleeding from tubal rupture
4. Laparoscopy: visualization of tubal pregnancy
5. Laparotomy: may be done if there is any question about the diagnosis

◆ Collaborative Management

Therapeutic Interventions

1. Treatment of shock and hemorrhage, if necessary, with IV fluids and blood transfusions

Surgical Interventions

1. Goal is preservation of maternal life, through removal of the pregnancy and reconstruction of the tube, if possible.
2. The surgical procedure depends on the extent of tubal involvement and if rupture has occurred. Procedures include removal of ectopic pregnancy with tubal resection, salpingostomy, salpingectomy, and possibly salpingo-oophorectomy.

◆ Nursing Interventions

Monitoring

1. Monitor maternal vital signs for hypotension and tachycardia caused by rupture or hemorrhage.
2. Monitor for presence and amount of vaginal bleeding, indicating hemorrhage.
3. Monitor for increase in pain and abdominal distention and rigidity, indicating rupture and possible intraabdominal hemorrhage.
4. Monitor CBC for amount of blood loss.

Supportive Care

1. Establish an IV line with a large-bore catheter and infuse fluids and blood products as prescribed.
2. Obtain blood samples for CBC and type, and screen for whole blood, as directed.
3. Administer analgesics as needed and prescribed.
4. Remain attentive and supportive to patient preoperatively, which may be a life-threatening period.
5. Provide emotional support after surgery, and help family explore and express their grief and sense of loss over the pregnancy.
6. Refer for counseling to local bereavement group, social worker, clergy, or psychologist.

Patient Education and Health Maintenance

1. Teach signs of postoperative infection, including fever, abdominal pain, increased or malodorous vaginal discharge.
2. Reinforce that chances of another ectopic pregnancy are increased and that subsequent conception potential may be decreased, based on health care provider's explanation.

3. Discuss contraception.
4. Teach signs of recurrent ectopic pregnancy: abnormal vaginal bleeding, abdominal pain, menstrual irregularity.

Hydramnios

Hydramnios (polyhydramnios) is caused by an excessive amount of amniotic fluid. Anomalies causing impaired fetal swallowing or excessive urination may contribute to the condition. It is associated with maternal diabetes, multiple gestation, and Rh − isoimmunization. Other associated factors are anomalies of the CNS, including spina bifida and anencephaly, or anomalies of the gastrointestinal (GI) tract, including tracheoesophageal fistula. In chronic hydramnios, the fluid volume gradually increases; in the acute type, the volume increases rapidly over a few days. Complications include preterm labor, dysfunctional labor with increased risk for cesarean delivery, and postpartum hemorrhage caused by uterine atony from gross distention of the uterus.

◆ Assessment

1. Excessive weight gain, dyspnea
2. Abdomen may be tense and shiny.
3. Edema of the vulva, legs, and lower extremities
4. Increased uterine size for gestational age, usually accompanied by difficulty in palpating fetal parts and in auscultation of fetal heart

◆ Diagnostic Evaluation

1. A diagnosis is made based on the presenting symptoms and ultrasound evaluation.
2. Ultrasound evaluation will show large pockets of fluid between the fetus and uterine wall or placenta.

◆ Collaborative Management

Therapeutic Interventions

1. Depends on the severity of the condition and the cause; hospitalization is indicated for maternal distress.

2. If impairment of maternal respiratory status occurs, an amniocentesis for removal of fluid may be performed.
   a. The amniocentesis is performed under ultrasound for location of the placenta and fetal parts.
   b. The fluid is then slowly removed.
   c. Rapid removal of the fluid can result in a premature separation of the placenta.
   d. Usually 500 to 1,000 mL fluid are removed.

◆ **Nursing Interventions**

Monitoring

1. Evaluate maternal respiratory status.
2. Inspect abdomen and evaluate uterine height and compare with previous findings.
3. Monitor fetal heart rate as indicated.

Supportive Care

1. Encourage positioning with head elevated to promote chest expansion, and on left side to promote placental perfusion. If unable to position on side, use a wedge to displace the uterus to the left.
2. Provide oxygen by face mask, if indicated.
3. Limit activities, and plan for frequent rest periods.
4. Maintain adequate intake and output through fluid intake.
5. Encourage passive or active assisted range of motion to the lower extremities.
6. Provide a diet adequate in protein, iron, and fluids.
7. Assist the woman with position changes and ambulation as needed.
8. Instruct the woman to wear loose-fitting clothing and low-heeled shoes with good support.
9. Prepare patient for the type of delivery that is anticipated and for the expected finding at the time of delivery.

Patient Education and Health Maintenance

1. Instruct the woman to notify her health care provider if experiencing respiratory distress.
2. Teach the woman signs of preterm labor and the need to report them to health care provider.

Hyperemesis Gravidarum

Hyperemesis gravidarum is exaggerated nausea and vomiting during pregnancy persisting past the first trimester. Cause is unknown but may possibly result from high levels of hCG or estrogen. Psychological factors including neurosis or altered self-concept may be contributory. The persistent vomiting may result in fluid and electrolyte imbalances, dehydration, jaundice, and elevation of serum transaminase.

◆ Assessment

1. Persistent vomiting; inability to tolerate anything by mouth
2. Dehydration: fever, dry skin, decreased urine output
3. Weight loss (up to 5%–10% of body weight)

◆ Diagnostic Evaluation

1. Tests may be done to rule out other conditions causing vomiting (cholecystitis, appendicitis).
2. Liver function studies: elevated AST up to four times normal in severe cases
3. Blood urea nitrogen (BUN) and creatinine: may be slightly elevated
4. Serum electrolytes: may be hypokalemia, hyponatremia or hypernatremia
5. Urine for ketones: positive

◆ Collaborative Management

Therapeutic Interventions

1. Try withholding food and fluid for 24 hours, or until vomiting stops and appetite returns; then restart small feedings.
2. Control of dehydration through IV fluids—often 1 to 3 liters of dextrose solution.
3. Most women respond quickly to restricting oral intake and giving IV fluids, but repeated episodes may occur.
4. Rarely, total parenteral nutrition is needed.

Pharmacologic Interventions

1. Control of vomiting may require antiemetic such as prochlorperazine in injectable or rectal suppository form.
2. Potassium and vitamins may be added to IV fluids.
3. Bicarbonate may be given for acidosis.

◆ Nursing Interventions

Monitoring

1. Evaluate weight gain or loss pattern.
2. Evaluate 24- or 48-hour dietary recall.
3. Monitor intake and output.
4. Monitor vital signs for tachycardia, hypotension, and fever caused by dehydration.
5. Assess skin turgor and mucous membranes for signs of dehydration.
6. Monitor serum electrolytes and report abnormalities.
7. Monitor fetal heart tones routinely.

Supportive Care

1. Maintain NPO status except for ice chips until vomiting has stopped.
2. Advise the woman that oral intake can be restarted when emesis has stopped and appetite returns.
3. Begin small feedings. Suggest or provide bland solid foods; serve hot foods hot and cold foods cold; do not serve lukewarm.
   a. Avoid greasy, gassy, and spicy foods.
   b. Provide liquids at times other than meal times.
4. Suggest or provide an environment conducive to eating.
   a. Keep room cool and quiet before and after meals.
   b. Keep emesis pan handy, yet out of sight.
5. Encourage patient to discuss any personal stress that may have a negative effect on this pregnancy.
6. Refer to social service and counseling services as needed.

Patient Education and Health Maintenance

1. Educate the woman about proper diet and nutrition in pregnancy.
2. Educate the woman about healthy weight gain in pregnancy.

3. Ensure referral for prenatal care and social services as needed.

Induction of Labor

Induction of labor is the deliberate initiation of uterine contractions before their spontaneous onset. It is indicated when the woman's life or well-being is in danger or if the fetus may be compromised by remaining in the uterus any longer. Contraindications include genital herpes outbreak; vaginal bleeding with known placenta previa; abnormal fetal presentation; previous uterine scar (controversial); known cephalopelvic disproportion; and severe fetal distress.

◆ Collaborative Management

Therapeutic Interventions

1. Amniotomy (artificial rupture of membranes, AROM)—done to make contractions stronger
   a. Vulva is cleansed, amniohook is inserted through the cervix, and membranes are ruptured after evaluation of fetal presentation.
   b. Fetal heart tones are assessed continually for at least the next 20 minutes.
   c. Complications include umbilical cord prolapse or compression, maternal or fetal infection.
2. Stripping the membranes: separating the membranes from the lower uterine segment without rupturing the membranes
   a. Membranes and amniotic fluid then act as a wedge to dilate cervix.
   b. Maternal/fetal infection is a complication.

Pharmacologic Interventions

1. Oxytocin: given IV by infusion pump
   a. Fetal monitoring is instituted. If membranes have ruptured, an intrauterine catheter and internal scalp electrode may be used.
   b. The dose is increased every 20 to 30 minutes by 1

to 2 μU/min. The total dose should not exceed 30 μU/min.

   c. The goal is to establish a regular labor pattern—contractions occurring every 2 to 3 minutes, lasting 45 to 60 seconds, and having an intensity of 50 mm Hg (moderate).

   d. Complications include uterine hyperstimulation, fetal distress, increased rate of cesarean section, and neonatal hyperbilirubinemia, possibly from red blood cell trauma from intense contractions or decreased maturity of the neonate.

2. Prostaglandin E_2 (PGE$_2$)—used before induction of labor for cervical ripening

   a. If labor results from administration of PGE$_2$, it is similar to spontaneous labor.

   b. Prostaglandins are administered intracervically or vaginally.

   c. Uterine hyperstimulation is a complication.

◆ Nursing Interventions

Monitoring

Before Induction

1. Obtain a 30-minute strip for the fetal heart rate and uterine activity.
2. Evaluate maternal vital signs.
3. Evaluate the patency of the IV site.

After the Administration of Oxytocin

1. Continuously monitor fetal heart rate and uterine activity.
2. Assess maternal vital signs every 15 minutes until a labor pattern is established, then every 30 minutes. Temperature is taken every 4 hours unless an amniotomy has been performed and then every 2 hours.
3. Monitor intake and output records, and watch for signs of water intoxication.
4. Evaluate IV site for patency and rate control for correct rate at least hourly.

Supportive Care and Patient Education

1. Teach or review the use of relaxation and distraction techniques.

2. Before beginning any new procedure, explain the procedure to the woman and her support person.
3. Limit vaginal examinations, especially after membranes have ruptured.
4. Position mother on left side to enhance placental perfusion.
5. Have oxygen set up with a mask ready and administer as prescribed if fetal decelerations occur.
6. If hyperstimulation of the uterus or fetal distress occurs, discontinue the infusion, maintain the primary IV, and notify the health care provider immediately.

Placenta Previa

Placenta previa is the development of the placenta in the lower uterine segment, partially or completely covering the internal cervical os (Fig. 31). The cause is unknown, but a possible theory states that the embryo will implant in the lower uterine segment if the decidua in the uterine fundus is not favorable. Seen more often with history of abortion, cesarean section, and uterine scarring. Most occur in multiparas. Complications are immediate hemorrhage, shock, and maternal death; fetal mortality; and postpartum hemorrhage.

◆ Assessment

1. Characteristic sign is painless vaginal bleeding, which usually appears near the end of the second trimester or later.
2. Initial episode is rarely fatal and usually stops spontaneously, with subsequent bleeding episodes occurring spontaneously; each episode is more profuse than the previous one.
3. Bleeding from placenta previa may not occur until cervical dilation occurs and the placenta is loosened from the uterus.
4. With a total placenta previa, the bleeding will occur earlier in the pregnancy and be more profuse.

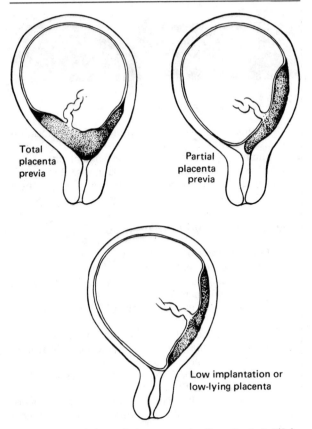

FIGURE 31 Variations of placenta previa. (From Scott, J, DiSaia, PJ, Hammond, C, & Spellacy, WN, Danforth's Obstetrics and Gynecology, 7th ed., Philadelphia, JB Lippincott, 1994).

> ### NURSING ALERT
> Never perform a vaginal examination on anyone who is bleeding. This may result in puncturing the placenta.

◆ Diagnostic Evaluation

1. Ultrasound is the method of choice, to show location of the placenta.
2. If findings are questionable, transvaginal ultrasound can improve the accuracy of diagnosis. Because of bleeding tendencies, however, this must be done by a highly skilled technician.

◆ Collaborative Management

Therapeutic Interventions

1. Bed rest and hospitalization until delivery is usual.
2. If discharged, needs availability of immediate transport to the hospital for recurrent bleeding.
3. IV access and at least two units of blood available at all times
4. Continuous maternal and fetal monitoring
5. Amniocentesis may be done to determine fetal lung maturity for possible delivery.
6. Vaginal delivery may sometimes be attempted in a marginal previa without active bleeding.
7. A pediatric specialty team may be needed at delivery because of prematurity and other neonatal complications.

Surgical Interventions

1. Cesarean section is often indicated and may be performed immediately on bleeding, depending on the degree of placenta previa.

◆ Nursing Interventions

Monitoring

1. Monitor amount and type of bleeding.
2. Monitor and record maternal and fetal vital signs.

3. Monitor for uterine contractions.
4. Monitor hemoglobin and hematocrit for amount of blood loss.
5. Monitor temperature every 4 hours unless elevated; then evaluate every 2 hours.
6. Monitor white blood cell (WBC) count for infection.

Supportive Care

1. Position mother on left side to promote placental perfusion and administer oxygen if evidence of fetal distress.
2. Establish and maintain a large-bore IV line, as prescribed, and draw blood for type and screen for blood replacement.
3. Position mother in a sitting position to allow the weight of fetus to compress the placenta and decrease blood loss during episode of bleeding.
4. Maintain strict bed rest during any bleeding episode.
5. If bleeding is profuse and delivery cannot be delayed, prepare the woman physically and emotionally for a cesarean delivery.

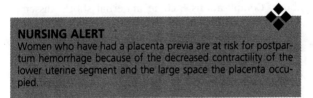

NURSING ALERT
Women who have had a placenta previa are at risk for postpartum hemorrhage because of the decreased contractility of the lower uterine segment and the large space the placenta occupied.

6. Use aseptic technique when providing care, and teach perineal care and handwashing to prevent infection.
7. Provide emotional support and discuss the effects of long-term hospitalization or prolonged bed rest.

Patient Education and Health Maintenance

1. Educate the woman and her family about the cause and treatment of placenta previa.
2. Advise the woman to inform medical personnel about her diagnosis and not to have vaginal examinations.
3. Educate the woman who is discharged from the hospital with a placenta previa about avoiding intercourse or anything per vagina, limiting physical activity; the

need for an accessible person in the event of an emergency; and to go to the hospital immediately for repeat bleeding.

◆ Abruptio Placentae

Abruptio placentae is premature separation of the normally implanted placenta in the third trimester. There are two types of abruptio placentae: concealed hemorrhage and external hemorrhage. With a concealed hemorrhage, the placenta separates centrally, and a large amount of blood is accumulated under the placenta. When an external hemorrhage is present, the separation is along the placental margin, and blood flows under the membranes and through the cervix. Women at risk for developing abruptio placentae include those with history of hypertension or previous abruptio placenta; or who have rapid decompression of the uterine cavity, short umbilical cord, or presence of a uterine anomaly or tumor. Additional risk occurs in existing pregnancies complicated by trauma, hypertension, alcohol, cigarette smoking, and cocaine abuse. Complications include maternal shock, disseminated intravascular coagulation (DIC), amniotic fluid embolism, postpartum hemorrhage, prematurity, and maternal or fetal death.

◆ Assessment

1. Concealed hemorrhage: results in a change in maternal vital signs, but no visible bleeding is present
2. External hemorrhage: Vaginal bleeding is evident along with a change in maternal vital signs.
3. Fetal heart rate may change, depending on the degree of hemorrhage.
4. Abdominal pain is often present.

◆ Diagnostic Evaluation

1. Diagnosis is usually made on clinical signs and symptoms.
2. Ultrasound is done, but it is not always sensitive enough to pick up abruptio placentae.

◆ Collaborative Management

Therapeutic Interventions

1. Hospitalization, bed rest, and continuous fetal monitoring
2. Management of hemorrhagic shock with IV fluids and blood transfusions
3. If the woman's status is stable, and there is no fetal distress, then a vaginal delivery may be considered.
4. Pediatric specialty team may be necessary at delivery because of prematurity and neonatal complications.

Surgical Interventions

1. Severe abruptions with fetal distress necessitate immediate delivery by cesarean section.

◆ Nursing Interventions

Monitoring

1. Monitor amount of bleeding and the presence or absence of pain.
2. Monitor maternal vital signs and fetal heart rate through continuous external fetal monitoring.
3. Monitor uterine contractions.
4. Measure and record fundal height, which may increase with concealed bleeding.
5. Monitor hemoglobin and hematocrit for blood loss.

Supportive Care

1. Position mother in the left lateral position, with the head elevated to enhance placental perfusion.
2. Administer oxygen through a face mask at 8 to 10 L/min.
3. Establish and maintain large-bore IV line for fluids and blood products as prescribed.
4. Encourage relaxation techniques.
5. Inform the woman and her family about the status of both herself and the fetus.
6. Encourage the presence of a support person.

Patient Education and Health Maintenance

1. Provide information to the woman and her family regarding cause of and treatment for abruptio placenta.
2. Encourage involvement from the neonatal team regarding education related to fetal/neonatal outcome.

Postpartum Hemorrhage

Postpartum hemorrhage involves a loss of 500 mL or more of blood; it occurs most frequently in the first hour after delivery. It may be caused by uterine atony (relaxation of the uterus) secondary to multiple pregnancy; hydramnios (excessive amniotic fluid); high parity; prolonged labor with maternal exhaustion; deep anesthesia; presence of fibromyoma; and retained placental fragments. Laceration of the vagina, cervix, or perineum secondary to forceps delivery, large infant, or multiple pregnancy may also cause postpartum hemorrhage.

◆ Assessment

1. With uterine atony, uterus is soft or boggy, often difficult to palpate, and will not remain contracted; excessive vaginal bleeding occurs.
2. Hemorrhage usually occurs about the tenth postpartum day with retained placental fragments.
3. Lacerations of the vagina, cervix, or perineum cause bright red, continuous bleeding even when the fundus is firm.

◆ Collaborative Management

Pharmacologic Interventions

1. For uterine atony, oxytocin is prescribed.
2. Pain medication may be needed to counter uterine contractions.

Surgical Interventions

1. If placental fragments have been retained, curettage of the uterus is indicated.
2. Lacerations may need to be repaired.

◆ Nursing Interventions

Monitoring

1. Monitor for hypotension, tachycardia, change in respiratory rate, decrease in urine output, and change in mental status—may indicate hypovolemic shock.

2. Monitor location and firmness of uterine fundus.
3. Percuss and palpate for bladder distension, which may interfere with contracting of the uterus.
4. Monitor amount and type of bleeding or lochia present and the presence of clots.
5. Inspect for intactness of any perineal repair.
6. Monitor CBC for anemia.

Supportive Care

1. Maintain a quiet and calm atmosphere.
2. Maintain or start a large-bore IV line if vaginal bleeding becomes heavy.
3. Ensure that crossmatched blood is available.
4. Infuse oxytocin, other contractile agents, IV fluids, and blood products at prescribed rate.
5. Provide information about the situation and explain everything as it is done; answer questions that the woman and her family ask.
6. Maintain aseptic technique and evaluate for infection. Report chilling, elevated temperature, changes in white blood cell count, uterine tenderness, and odor of lochia.
7. Administer antibiotics as prescribed.

Patient Education and Health Maintenance

1. Educate the woman about the cause of the hemorrhage.
2. Teach the woman the importance of eating a balanced diet and taking vitamin supplements.
3. Advise the woman that she may feel tired and fatigued, and to schedule daily rest periods.
4. Advise the woman to notify her health care provider of increased bleeding or other changes in her status.

Pregnancy-Induced Hypertension

Pregnancy-induced hypertension (PIH, preeclampsia, eclampsia) is a disorder occurring during pregnancy after the 20th week of gestation and involving edema, proteinuria, and hypertension. Eclampsia is diagnosed when convulsions occur in the absence of an underlying neurologic condi-

---

■ BOX 10 HELLP SYNDROME

HELLP syndrome is a severe complication of pregnancy-induced hypertension. It is comprised of *H*emolysis, *E*levated *L*iver enzymes, and *L*ow *P*latelets.

1. These findings are frequently associated with DIC and in fact may be diagnosed as DIC.
2. The hemolysis of erythrocytes is seen in the abnormal morphology of the cells.
3. The elevated liver enzyme measurement is associated with the decreased blood flow to the liver as a result of fibrin thrombi.
4. The low platelet count is related to vasospasm and platelet adhesions.
5. Treatment is similar to treatment for PIH with close monitoring of liver function and bleeding.
6. These women are at increased risk for postpartum hemorrhage.

---

tion in the presence of hypertension, edema, and protein-uria. Actual cause is unknown. Theories of the cause include the exposure to chorionic villi for the first time, or in large amounts, along with immunologic, genetic, and endocrine factors. Chronic hypertension, hydatidiform mole, multiple gestation, polyhydramnios, and diabetes mellitus may predispose to PIH. It is primarily seen in primigravidas and adolescents, and women older than 35 years of age are at higher risk. Complications include abruptio placentae, disseminated intravascular coagulation (DIC), HELLP syndrome (Box 10), prematurity, intrauterine growth retardation, and maternal or fetal death.

◆ Assessment

1. Hypertension, which is defined as a blood pressure of 140/90 mm Hg or greater on two occasions at least 6 hours apart

---

2. Proteinuria, oliguria
3. Nondependent edema, present after 8 to 12 hours of bed rest
4. Frequently, a sudden weight gain will occur, of 2 lb or more in 1 week, or 6 lb or more in 1 month. This often occurs before the edema is present.
5. Altered level of consciousness, visual changes, headache
6. Epigastric pain, chest pressure
7. Hyperreflexia with or without clonus

◆ Diagnostic Evaluation

1. 24-hour urine for protein greater than or equal to 300 mg.
2. Serum BUN and creatinine may be elevated.
3. Sonogram or nonstress testing to evaluate placenta and fetus.

◆ Collaborative Management

Therapeutic Interventions
1. Bed rest to help decrease blood pressure and maintain placental perfusion
2. Increased dietary protein and possibly calories to ensure adequate nutrition
3. Hospitalization for close monitoring and seizure prevention may be necessary.
4. If symptoms are uncontrollable, delivery is planned.

Pharmacologic Interventions
1. Magnesium sulfate may be given either IV or IM as loading dose, followed by maintenance dose to treat and prevent seizures.
2. Diazepam and amobarbital sodium may be used if convulsions occur that do not respond to magnesium sulfate.
3. Antihypertensive drug therapy may be used when the diastolic pressure is above 110 mm Hg or when cerebrovascular accident is impending.
   a. Hydralazine is the drug of choice; it relaxes the arterioles and stimulates cardiac output.
   b. Side effects include tachycardia, palpitations, dizziness, faintness, headache.

4. Beta-blockers may be used to rapidly control acute hypertension; however, further studies are needed on these drugs and their use in pregnancy.

◆ Nursing Interventions

Monitoring

1. Monitor blood pressure in a sitting position and in the left lateral position to detect hypertension.
2. Monitor intake and output strictly and notify health careprovider if urine <30 cc/h.
3. Monitor vital signs every hour.
4. Auscultate breath sounds every 2 hours and report signs of pulmonary edema (wheezing, crackles, shortness of breath, increased pulse rate, increased respiratory rate).
5. Monitor protein level of spot urine specimens.
6. Evaluate edema, carefully noting the presence after 12 hours or more of bed rest.
7. Monitor daily weights for gain.
8. Evaluate deep tendon reflexes and clonus.
9. Monitor fetal activity and evaluate nonstress tests to determine fetal status.

Supportive Care

1. Control IV fluid intake using a continuous-infusion pump.
2. Position woman on left side to promote placental perfusion.
3. Encourage extra protein in diet to replace protein lost through kidneys.
4. Keep the environment quiet and as calm as possible.
5. If hospitalized, side rails should be padded and remain up to prevent injury if seizure occurs.
6. If hospitalized, have oxygen and suction set up, along with a tongue blade and emergency medications immediately available for treatment of seizures.
7. Explain that PIH does not lead to chronic hypertension and usually does not occur with subsequent pregnancies.

Patient Education and Health Maintenance

1. Teach the woman the importance of bed rest in helping to control symptoms.

2. Encourage the support of family and friends while on bed rest.
3. Provide and suggest diversional activities while on bed rest.
4. Provide information on tests and procedures to evaluate maternal–fetal status, such as blood tests, sonogram, and nonstress testing.

Preterm Labor

Preterm labor is defined as uterine contractions occurring after 20 weeks of gestation and before 37 completed weeks of gestation. Risk factors include multiple gestation; history of previous preterm labor or delivery; abdominal surgery during current pregnancy; uterine anomaly; history of cone biopsy; history of more than two first-trimester abortions or more than one second-trimester abortion; fetal or placental malformation; diethylstilbestrol (DES) exposure; bleeding after the first trimester; maternal age of younger than 18 or older than 35 years; poor nutritional status; poor, irregular, or no prenatal care; emotional stress; more than 10 cigarettes smoked in a day; and recreational drug use. Complications are prematurity and associated neonatal problems, such as lung immaturity.

◆ Assessment

1. Contractions are less than 10 minutes apart.
2. Cervical changes result with cervical dilation of 2 cm or effacement of 75%.

◆ Collaborative Management

Therapeutic Interventions

1. Treatment is begun early with bed rest in a left lateral position.
2. Hydration with IV fluids and continuous monitoring of fetal status and uterine contractions

Pharmacologic Interventions

1. If conservative therapy is not successful, tocolytic therapy is instituted. These drugs should be used only when the potential benefit to the fetus outweighs the potential risk.
2. Beta-mimetic agents such as ritodrine and terbutaline
   a. These drugs stimulate the beta$_2$-adrenergic receptors, which causes uterine relaxation.
   b. Ritodrine is administered IV or orally; terbutaline may be administered IV, subcutaneously, or orally.
   c. Frequent monitoring is necessary to observe for side effects of increased pulse, shortness of breath, chest pain, decreased blood pressure, hypervolemia, decreased potassium concentration, hyperglycemia, and hyperinsulinemia.
   d. Baseline ECG and laboratory tests, including CBC with differential, electrolytes, glucose, BUN, creatinine, prothrombin time, and partial thromboplastin time, are obtained.
3. Magnesium sulfate (MgSO$_4$): interferes with smooth muscle contractility
   a. Administration is IV by infusion pump.
   b. Pulmonary edema, loss of deep tendon reflexes, decreased respirations, and hypotension are adverse reactions related to magnesium toxicity.
   c. Serum magnesium levels are monitored.
   d. Calcium gluconate is the antidote and should be at the bedside.
4. Indomethacin: prostaglandin inhibitor that inhibits contractions; given orally or rectally and usually well tolerated
5. Nifedipine: calcium channel blocker that relaxes smooth muscle; given orally, and side effects include headache, nausea, and flushing from vasodilation

◆ Nursing Interventions

Monitoring
During tocolytic therapy, monitor the following:
1. Fetal status by electronic fetal monitoring
2. Uterine contraction pattern
3. Respiratory status for pulmonary edema
4. Muscular tremors

5. Symptoms of palpations and dizziness
6. Urinary output

Supportive Care

1. Provide accurate information on the status of the fetus and labor (contraction pattern).
2. Allow the woman and her support person to verbalize their feelings regarding the episode of preterm labor and the treatment.
3. If a private room is not used, do not place the woman in a room with an occupant who is in labor or who has lost an infant.
4. Encourage diversional activities while on bed rest and encourage visits from family.

Patient Education and Health Maintenance

1. Educate the woman about the importance of continuing the pregnancy until term, or until there is evidence of fetal lung maturity.
2. Encourage the need for compliance with a decreased activity level or bed rest, as indicated.
3. Teach the woman the importance of proper nutrition and the need for adequate hydration, at least eight glasses of fluids a day.
4. Instruct the woman not to engage in sexual activity.

Preterm Rupture of Membranes

Preterm or *premature rupture of membranes* (PROM) is defined as rupture of the membranes before the onset of spontaneous labor. PROM at term may result from stretching of the membranes and fetal movements that cause the membranes to weaken. In preterm PROM, risk factors include infection; previous history of preterm PROM; hydramnios; incompetent cervix; multiple gestation; abruptio placentae. Complications include preterm labor; prematurity and associated complications; maternal infection (chorioamnionitis); and fetal/neonatal infection.

◆ Assessment

1. PROM is manifested by a large gush of amniotic fluid or leaking of fluid per vagina, which usually persists.

◆ Diagnostic Evaluation

1. Sterile speculum examination for identification of "pooling" of fluid in the vagina.
2. Nitrazine test: positive test will change pH paper strip from yellow-green to blue in the presence of amniotic fluid taken from the vaginal canal.
3. Fern test: positive test will show ferning pattern of amniotic fluid on a slide viewed under a microscope.

◆ Collaborative Management

Therapeutic Interventions

1. Once PROM is confirmed, the woman is admitted to the hospital and usually remains there until delivery.
2. The woman is evaluated to rule out labor, fetal distress, and infection, and to establish gestational age. If all factors are ruled out, the woman is managed expectantly.
3. Management of PROM at 36 weeks' gestation or greater focuses on delivery.
4. Vaginal examinations are kept to a minimum to prevent infection.

Pharmacologic Interventions

1. Tocolytics to prevent premature labor are controversial.
2. Corticosteroids to decrease the severity of respiratory distress syndrome in the premature infant are controversial.
3. Prophylactic antibiotics may be used.

◆ Nursing Interventions

Monitoring

1. Evaluate maternal blood pressure, respirations, pulse, and temperature every 4 hours. If temperature or pulse are elevated, measure them every 1 to 2 hours as indicated.
2. Monitor the amount and type of amniotic fluid that is leaking and observe for purulent, foul-smelling discharge.
3. Evaluate daily CBC with differentials, noting any shift

to the left (ie, increase of immature forms of neutrophils), indicating infection.

4. Evaluate fetal status every 4 hours or as indicated, noting fetal activity and heart rate.

5. Determine if uterine tenderness occurs on abdominal palpation, indicating infection.

Supportive Care

1. Place patient on disposable pads to collect leaking fluid and change pads every 2 hours or more frequently as needed.

2. Review the need for good handwashing technique and hygiene after urination and defecation.

3. Report immediately any change in vital signs, uterine tenderness, CBC, or fluid leakage that may indicate infection.

4. Encourage diversional activities and involvement of support person.

Patient Education and Health Maintenance

1. Explain that the goal is to await the onset of natural labor while preventing infection.

2. Explain that if signs of infection do develop, the baby will be delivered and infection will be treated.

INDEX

Page numbers followed by *f* indicate illustrations; *t* following a page number indicates tabular material; *d* following a page number indicates a display.

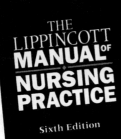
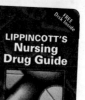
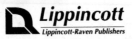